FINANCIAL MANAGEMENT *for* NURSE MANAGERS *and* EXECUTIVES

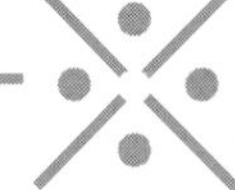

SECOND EDITION

Steven A. Finkler, PhD, CPA
Program in Health Policy and Management
Robert F. Wagner Graduate School of Public Service
New York University
New York, New York

Christine T. Kovner, PhD, RN, FAAN
Division of Nursing
School of Education
New York University
New York, New York

W.B. SAUNDERS COMPANY
A Harcourt Health Sciences Company
Philadelphia London Toronto Montreal Sydney Tokyo

W.B. SAUNDERS COMPANY
A Harcourt Health Sciences Company

The Curtis Center
Independence Square West
Philadelphia, Pennsylvania 19106

Library of Congress Cataloging-in-Publication Data

Finkler, Steven A.
Financial management for nurse managers and executives / Steven A. Finkler, Christine T. Kovner. — 2nd ed.
p. cm.
Includes bibliographical references and index.
ISBN 0-7216-7714-2
1. Nursing services—Business management. 2. Health facilities—Business management. I. Kovner, Christine Tassone. II. Title.
[DNLM: 1. Financial Management—methods—United States Nurses' Instruction. 2. Delivery of Health Care—economics—United States Nurses' Instruction. 3. Nurse Administrators—United States.
W 74 F499f 2000]
RT86.7.F46 2000
362.1'73'0681—dc21
DNLM/DLC

99-31116

FINANCIAL MANAGEMENT FOR NURSE MANAGERS AND EXECUTIVES ISBN 0-7216-7714-2

Printed in the United States of America

Last digit is the print number: 9 8 7 6 5 4 3 2 1

To Our Parents,
With love and appreciation for all you taught us.

S.A.F. and *C.T.K.*

Preface

When a publisher asks authors to write a second edition of a book, it usually means that the first edition was popular and it is time to update the content. We were extremely pleased with the success of the first edition and particularly with the comments that we received from colleagues. Contemplating writing a second edition of a book forces the authors to confront not only the success of the first edition but also what can be improved. We clearly needed more content on managed care and settings other than hospitals. Numbers and facts throughout the book had to be updated. But, as we reread the book, we were also surprised at how much did not need to be changed.

Of course, concepts such as supply and demand stay the same, but we were surprised that much of what we wrote in 1993 remains accurate today. The chapter on computers was the most outdated and required substantial revision. Also, we initially decided to eliminate the chapter on retention, because shortages were no longer an issue. But as we neared completion of our work, there was evidence of nursing shortages arising once again in some geographical areas. We revised that chapter and put it back in. We added a chapter on the nurse entrepreneur and hope that those nurses who are developing new ventures will find that chapter particularly useful. We added more material about settings other than hospitals and increased the content on financial aspects of managed care.

Our experience in the real world of health care shows us that nurse managers are expected to understand a great deal about the financial management of organizations for which they work. What they do know is often learned on the job—often without any conceptual basis. Many nurse managers do not know a great deal about financial management, but it is our experience that most of them want to know more. They have found that an understanding of financial management would be a great asset to them in their management function.

This book is for the nurses who want to know what questions to ask the finance department and what answers to give the finance department in response to its questions. Even more importantly, it is for nurses who want to manage better. All levels of nursing management benefit from an improved understanding of financial management concepts. As more nurses develop their own practices or businesses, it is essential that they understand financial management.

What about *Budgeting Concepts for Nurse Managers*,[1] written by one of this book's authors? Why write another financial management book? The budgeting book is one of great depth but limited scope. It considers only issues related to budgeting. Financial management extends beyond the realm of budgeting. When the second edition of *Budgeting Concepts for Nurse Managers* was being prepared, the idea for this book was conceived. Some reviewers argued that the first edition of the budget book was inadequate in scope. It did not discuss financial statements, economics, or busi-

[1]Steven A. Finkler, *Budgeting Concepts for Nurse Managers*, Third Edition, W.B. Saunders, Philadelphia, 2000.

ness plans. It avoided numerous other financial management issues. Other reviewers argued that its narrow focus was its strength. Ultimately a decision was made to maintain *Budgeting Concepts for Nurse Managers* as a budgeting book but also to write a broader, more inclusive text that would cover the many aspects of financial management that are of growing interest to nurses.

Why are the existing financial management texts written for business schools inadequate for this purpose? Our experience as teachers suggests to us that people learn concepts best when the examples are relevant to them. This book is not only about financial management but also about nursing and the problems and opportunities that confront nurses in providing nursing care. Business school courses often use "widget" production as the basis for their examples. Although the financial concepts of producing widgets are similar to those for the delivery of health care services, widgets are not people. Producing widgets and treating patients are inherently, fundamentally, different.

Making financial management concepts come alive to the reader requires some connection between the concept and its ultimate application. We have tried to make that connection in the nursing examples used throughout this book.

This book has been designed for use both as a textbook for graduate students and as a reference for practicing nurse managers or nurse entrepreneurs who are seeking a better understanding of financial management. Topic coverage includes all the financial management areas with which we think nurse managers should be familiar.

In preparing the book, we chose to err on the side of inclusiveness rather than on the side of omission. In our attempt to achieve completeness, more topics are included in the book than may be covered in some one-semester graduate courses on financial management for nurses. The book is particularly broad in its inclusion of topics such as economics, strategic planning, quantitative decision-making tools, and marketing. To the extent that any course skips over chapters, the students will still find those chapters to be valuable reference material for reading and study at a later date.

Some areas are discussed in greater depth than others. The level of detail for each topic reflects our belief about the depth required by a nurse manager. Each chapter has an extensive list of suggested readings if the reader wants more depth in a particular subject area. In an attempt to provide a coherent whole, chapters refer to pertinent material in other chapters. However, each chapter is virtually self-contained, so the reader can choose to read a single chapter on a particular topic or read chapters in a different order than presented.

This book is not meant to prepare the nurse manager to replace financial managers in health care organizations but rather to prepare the nurse manager for a collegial relationship with financial managers. For example, the book covers business planning. That does not mean that each nurse manager will single-handedly have to prepare a full 100-page business plan. Although entrepreneurs may need to complete a business plan, many nurse managers are more likely to need to be able to *participate* in the development of business plans. As a nurse manager you may be aided by consultants, by your own staff, or by the organization's finance department. Nurse managers need to know what a business plan is, what is in a business plan, what is important about it, how to read it, and how to make a decision based on it.

We envision this book's being used in a graduate course in financial management for nurses. It is our expectation that a faculty member can use this book in the order it is written. However, we have attempted to allow flexibility in recognition of the fact that graduate programs prepare different levels of nurse managers and have different core course requirements. Some programs have prerequisites; others may provide an entire required course on some of the topics to which we devoted a chapter such as the health care environment or economics. If students are already familiar with the content, it is not necessary to assign these chapters. We have attempted to prepare a book that can meet the needs of a variety of nursing programs, as well as those of practitioners. On the other hand, the chapters on topics such as management (Chapter 3) or marketing (Chapter 19) do not provide the depth that one would find in an entire textbook written on those topics. Given the financial management focus of this book, we are only attempting to provide an overview of those areas for students who have not yet taken a course in them and a refresher for those who have.

The topics covered are appropriate for programs that prepare chief nurse executives (CNEs) and for programs that prepare midlevel nurse managers as well. For programs preparing midlevel managers the instructor may not wish to assign all chapters. Individual instructors may choose to modify their coverage of chapters based on their students' specific needs.

An instructor's manual is available to go with this book. The manual includes questions for discussion as well as problems and their solutions. To obtain the *Instructor's Manual,* course instructors should contact the W.B. Saunders Company or their Saunders sales representative. The questions and problems can be used for homework assignments, in class, or for examinations.

Part I of the book includes chapters on the environment faced by health care organizations, how financial management fits in the health care organization, and key issues in applied economics. We believe an understanding of the material in these chapters is fundamental to the study of financial management in health care. An instructor may choose to skip some or all of the chapters in this part if the material the chapter(s) contains is a prerequisite to entry into the program or is covered elsewhere in the curriculum.

Part II discusses financial accounting, including accounting principles and analysis of financial statements. To understand costing and budgeting, we believe the midlevel nurse manager needs to be familiar with the basic accounting concepts in the first chapter in this part (Chapter 5). A thorough understanding of financial statements and financial statement analysis (Chapter 6), however, is more appropriate to the CNE level.

Part III discusses cost analysis. We believe that Chapters 7 and 8 contain content necessary for all levels of nurse managers. Chapter 9, measuring the costs of recruiting and retaining staff, may not be necessary for all midlevel nurse managers.

Part IV focuses on planning and control. The management role of making plans and then attempting to carry out those plans to the extent possible is central to the role of all managers. The chapters in this part of the book therefore contain material with which all levels of nurse managers should be familiar.

Part V deals with management of the organization's financial resources. It includes concepts such as management of cash, loans, and accounts receivable. This content will be of greater interest to managers approaching the CNE level.

Part VI discusses a variety of additional management tools and includes a chapter on the nurse entrepreneur. Although all levels of nurse managers should be at least generally familiar with these concepts, the CNE should have a more thorough understanding of them.

Part VII addresses the future of financial management with respect to nurse managers, and we believe it should be read by all levels of nurse managers.

We would like to express our thanks to the many people who helped with the preparation of this book. First we thank the many nurses whom we have taught and with whom we have worked. They have shared their knowledge and insights about the real world of financial management encountered by nurses in health organizations.

We very much appreciate the comments and suggestions made by the following individuals who commented on the previous edition and made thoughtful suggestions for the second edition:

John J. Goehle, CPA, BS Accounting
Lattimore Community Surgicenter
Rochester, New York

Lou Ann Hartley, MSN, CNAA, PAHM
Marshall University College of Nursing and Health Professions
South Charleston, West Virginia

Mary Ann Thurkettle, PhD, RN
University of San Diego
San Diego, California

We are particularly grateful to the graduate students in the Division of Nursing at New York University's School of Education. We presented earlier versions of some of the examples to them. They let us know when the examples were not clear. We also discussed concepts that are used throughout the book. Our students' comments helped us to clarify our presentation in this edition. We also thank Jonathan Rowe for his assistance with the literature search.

A special word of thanks goes to Elizabeth Kolodny for all of her help with the many logistical details in compiling the finished manuscript.

Finally, we would like to thank our readers. We thank you not only for reading this book but also for helping to improve it. We encourage you to contact us with comments, suggestions, examples, or corrections.[2] All material we receive that is used in a subsequent edition will be acknowledged in that future edition.

Steven A. Finkler
Christine T. Kovner

[2]Send all communications to Prof. Steven A. Finkler, Ph.D., C.P.A., Robert F. Wagner Graduate School of Public Service, New York University, Tisch Hall—Room 600, 40 West Fourth Street, New York, NY 10012-1118.

About the Authors

STEVEN A. FINKLER, PhD, CPA

Steven A. Finkler is Professor of Public and Health Administration, Accounting, and Financial Management in the Program in Health Policy and Management at New York University's Robert F. Wagner Graduate School of Public Service. He is a member of the National Advisory Council for Nursing Research at the National Institute of Nursing Research, National Institutes of Health.

An award-winning teacher and author, Prof. Finkler is currently engaged in a variety of research projects in the areas of health care economics and accounting.

In addition to this book, Prof. Finkler has authored more than two hundred publications including *Budgeting Concepts for Nurse Managers* (third edition, 2000); *Cost Accounting for Healthcare Organizations: Concepts and Applications* (second edition, 1999); *Finance and Accounting for Nonfinancial Managers* (CD-ROM edition, 1996); articles in *The Journal of Nursing Administration, The New England Journal of Medicine, Nursing Economic$, Journal of Neonatal Nursing, Western Journal of Nursing Research, O.R. Nurse Managers' Network, Health Services Research, Medical Care, Healthcare Financial Management, Health Care Management Review,* and other journals; and a chapter in *Managing Hospitals: Lessons from the Johnson & Johnson—Wharton Fellows Program in Management for Nurses.*

Prof. Finkler received a B.S. in Economics and M.S. in Accounting from the Wharton School. His Master's Degree in Economics and Ph.D. in Business Administration were awarded by Stanford University. Prof. Finkler, who is also a Certified Public Accountant, worked for several years as an auditor with Ernst and Young and was on the faculty of the Wharton School for six years before joining New York University in 1984. He was Editor of *Hospital Cost Management and Accounting* from 1984 through 1997.

CHRISTINE T. KOVNER, PhD, RN, FAAN

Christine Kovner is a Professor in the Division of Nursing, School of Education, New York University, where she has worked for 14 years. She was the first Agency for Health Care Policy Research (AHCPR)/American Academy of Nursing Senior Scholar. Her research interest is the cost and use of health personnel. She is the author of 50 published articles and book chapters. She is coauthor of "The Health Care Workforce" in *Health Care Delivery in the United States.*

Her study of 589 hospitals in ten states on the relationship between nurse staffing and quality in hospitals in the United States, published in *Image* in 1998, was widely discussed in the media. She is a member of the New York State Department of Health Hospital Review and Planning Council, where she serves on the Fiscal and Codes Committees.

Dr. Kovner is the editor of the newsletter *Nursing Counts* and is coeditor of *Applied Nursing Research.* She serves as a reviewer for numerous professional journals. She is a member of many professional organizations such as the American Academy of Nursing, the American Nurses Association, Sigma Theta Tau (the national honor society for nursing), the American Public Health Association, and the Association of Community Health Nurse Educators. She was awarded the Distinguished Nurse Researcher award from the Foundation of New York State Nurses Association in 1994.

Contents

PART I

A FINANCIAL MANAGEMENT FRAMEWORK 1

※ PART VII

THE FUTURE 473

PART

I

A FINANCIAL MANAGEMENT FRAMEWORK

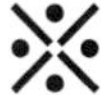

CHAPTER

1

Introduction and Overview

CHAPTER GOALS

The goals of this chapter are to:

- Provide the reader with an introduction to financial management
- Clarify the components of financial management
- Give the reader a road map for the study of financial management

※ INTRODUCTION

Few professions have seen as dramatic a change in role over the last several decades as that of the nurse manager. The nurse manager of the 1960s was predominantly a clinical manager. The role focused on ensuring the adequacy of the clinical care provided to patients. The manager was expected to accomplish those clinical activities with the resources provided.

Today the nurse manager still must accomplish that primary clinical function; it remains the essence of nursing. The responsibilities of the job, however, are much greater. Managers must be able to determine the resources they will need and then argue convincingly to get their share of resources from a limited total amount available to the organization.

The accuracy with which resource needs are projected and the efficiency with which care is provided must be much greater in the current environment. Health care services cost more than ever, and the pressures to control costs are greater than ever as well. As a result, the financial aspects of the job of the nurse manager are growing and becoming more sophisticated each year. Nurses are expected to develop and justify budgets, to use appropriate computer technology, and to minimize the cost of staff and supplies.

Many of the nonclinical managerial aspects of nursing relate to the financial management of the nursing unit, department, and the health care organization itself. This book covers a wide range of financial management topics. It is designed to meet the needs of nurse managers of all levels throughout the health care organization. Some readers may wish to selectively choose chapters that are most relevant to their needs.

※ A FINANCIAL MANAGEMENT FRAMEWORK

Part I of this book is designed to set the stage for the study of financial management. It contains four chapters. This overview chapter provides an in-depth guide to the book and should aid the reader in making an informed choice in approaching this subject matter. Chapter 2 discusses some of the essential elements of the environment of health care organizations. Chapter 3 establishes the relationships between financial and nurse managers. Chapter 4 provides a fundamental discussion of the principles and tools of microeconomics.

The Health Care Environment

Every organization must act within the confines of an existing environment. Some health care organizations are the sole providers of health care services in their geographic region; others have substantial competition. In some areas it is easier to hire new staff than in other areas.

Who are the key players in the health care industry? Who buys services? Who sells them? Who pays for them? What legal bodies make regulations that affect what health care organizations can do? The health care industry is regulated. This has created an especially difficult environment in which to operate an organization. Before one can begin to address the financial management of health care organizations, it is important to tackle the issue of government, regulation, and competition.

Organizations such as health maintenance organizations, preferred provider organizations, and other managed care companies are here to stay. These organizations are discussed in Chapter 2, which provides the foundations the nurse needs as background before addressing the more specific financial management techniques.

Financial Management and the Health Care Organization

In addition to understanding the environment within which health care organizations operate, it is useful for managers and prospective managers to understand the structure of organizations and how financial management is related to that structure.

Health care organizations are generally structured as hierarchies. Too many people work in most organizations for them all to report to one person. Therefore a pyramid structure is often established. Care givers report to a manager, who in turn reports to another manager higher in the pyramid, or hierarchial structure.

Increasingly, health care organizations are also using matrix management. Matrix management is a system in which a manager has responsibility cutting across department lines. For example, product-line management is now common. A health care product line is a specific type or group of patients. A manager is responsible for a product line, including all services needed to provide care to patients in that product line. This requires a cooperative relationship among the product-line manager and both the managers and staff of all of the organization's departments. The staff need to respond to both the product-line managers and the unit or department manager.

Although matrix management is used in some health care organizations, Chapter 3 focuses on the traditional hierarchical management structure used in the majority of health care organizations. Much of the discussion focuses on issues related to the degree of centralization created by such structure. It also considers the official and actual authority of specific individuals within the organization. Equally critical is the discussion of the distinction between the line and staff roles in an organization. Within that context the role of finance is discussed. The roles of the chief financial officer and the finance department staff are explained and compared with the roles of nurse managers at various levels in the organization.

Economics

Accounting and finance are applied areas of microeconomics. The theory of economics forms the foundations upon which all financial management is ultimately built. The essence of economics is that society has a limited amount of resources, with competing demands for them. The economic system attempts to allocate those resources in an optimal fashion.

Chapter 4 introduces the building blocks used in economics. The critical building blocks—economic goods, marginal utility, marginal cost, supply and demand, and economies of scale—are discussed. This leads into an examination of the workings of a free enterprise system.

In the free enterprise system one cannot separate human motivation from the actions of human beings. The economic system will always be the result of the interplay of resource allocation with the actions of people. As a result, it is necessary to consider the issue of incentives and their role in achieving market efficiency.

The economic system, even a free enterprise system, cannot always be relied upon to generate a perfect outcome. In fact, there may be times when the system simply fails to achieve a socially optimal result. The existence of monopolies, the absence of full information, the impact of insurance systems, and other factors may lead to less than desirable outcomes. Chapter 4 addresses these issues of market failure and of society's attempts to intervene to generate a more equitable outcome.

Economics has a bearing on nursing. It forms the framework from which resources are allocated. Chapter 4 also specifically addresses issues related to the market for nursing labor: Why do nursing shortages occur from time to time and then diminish? Is there some logic or rationale that can explain how the economic system leads to such shortages and then resolves them?

※ FINANCIAL ACCOUNTING

Accounting has often been referred to as "the language of business." One needs to be conversant with the basic principles of accounting to conduct any of the various aspects of financial management. Part II focuses on basic accounting issues.

The two principal areas of accounting are managerial accounting and financial accounting. Managerial accounting refers to the generation of any financial information that would be useful to managers in their role of managing part of an organization. Most of this book focuses on managerial accounting issues. The nurse manager also needs to understand financial accounting. Part II contains two chapters on financial accounting issues. Financial accounting provides the foundations of accounting. It focuses on generating financial information about the results of operations and the financial condition of the organization.

Financial accounting originated largely to provide information to outsiders who were lending money to an organization or investing in it, but the information generated is extremely useful for the organization's internal managers as well. Nurse managers who can assess and use this information will be at an advantage. Chapter 5 looks at the basic principles of accounting, and Chapter 6 provides a more advanced look at the analysis of financial statements.

Accounting Principles

Accounting does not represent a science. Surprisingly, accounting professors teach that accounting is closer to an art than a science. No fundamental laws of nature govern accounting. One generally agreed upon principle forms the keystone upon which all accounting is built, however: The books must balance.

This concept has become so pervasively known and accepted that the reader of this book likely takes it for granted. Everyone knows you must balance the books. But what does that really mean? Does it mean that you must break even, that you must balance the revenues against the expenses of each organization or individual? No. Clearly, some organizations make money, while others lose money. What does it mean when one says that the books must balance?

Balancing the books refers to the basic equation of accounting that describes the relationship between the valuable resources possessed by the organization and the claims on those resources by creditors and owners of the organization. That equation becomes the basis for ledgers and journals and the other technical elements of an accounting system. Chapter 5 introduces the reader to the equation of accounting and to the concepts of assets, equities, revenues, expenses, journal entries, ledgers, and generally accepted accounting principles. These concepts affect every manager in most health care organizations. A fundamental understanding of these concepts is essential to understand financial management.

Financial Statement Analysis

At higher levels of management the focus of a manager's interest in financial management must broaden. The tools of financial management become not only an integral element for being able to efficiently manage a unit or department but also the messengers of the general financial well-being of the organization.

Can the organization afford to provide nurses with a substantial raise? Can the organization reasonably be expected to replace old intensive care unit monitors with new ones? Is the organization acting in a prudent manner that will allow for its continued existence? These are just a few examples of the types of issues that become relevant as one moves up through the ranks of nursing management. The answers to these questions require information about the general financial condition of the organization.

Chapter 6 focuses on issues of analysis of financial statement information. What do the income statements and balance sheets of organizations really tell the reader? Are other elements of information also important? Are there ways to use raw financial statement information to make it more informative?

⁂ COST ANALYSIS

One of the most critical areas of financial management is the analysis and control of costs. The surplus (profit) or deficit (loss) of an organization each year depends on both its revenues and its costs. Both elements—revenues and costs—require managerial thought and attention. Cost management has been an essential role of nurse managers at all levels for a number of years. Part III examines issues related to costs.

Cost Management

The first chapter in Part III, Chapter 7, deals with basic issues of cost management. All levels of management encounter these issues in their normal activities.

The chapter introduces definitions of critical terms. The concepts of fixed, variable, marginal, and relevant costs are discussed at some length. The nature and behavior of costs are covered, with emphasis on the relationship between patient volume and costs. As volume changes over time, managers must be able to understand and predict the impact that such changes will have on costs. Techniques are provided for such prediction or estimation of future costs.

In the last decade of the 20th century the health care industry became more entrepreneurial. In an effort to find the resources to subsidize services offered at a loss, many health care organizations, even not-for-profit organizations, are constantly searching for profitable ventures. The last section of Chapter 7 provides a method to determine when a program or project or service will have sufficient volume to break even, i.e., to be financially self-sufficient. Such an approach is frequently used by organizations to determine whether to undertake a proposed new venture.

Determining the Cost of Health Care Services

Chapter 8 moves from basic cost concepts to the broader issue of cost measurement with two primary focuses. One is on how health care organizations collect cost information by unit or department and assign those costs to patients. The second is on how to determine the cost of nursing care.

The Medicare step-down cost-finding and rate-setting method is presented in Chapter 8 and compared with more recently developed costing methods. Attention is also paid to understanding product-line costing. Issues of patient classification systems and staffing are considered. Standard costing techniques are also discussed.

Determining the cost of nursing is a topic of much interest to nurse managers. As health care organizations are forced to operate in a constrained financial atmosphere, nurse managers at all levels are taking a greater role in controlling costs. To do this, nurse managers need a better understanding of the costs of providing nursing care. Such an understanding can also be useful to the advanced practice nurse who must set a price for care.

Recruiting and Retaining Staff

Chapter 9 addresses a concern that peaks during nursing shortages but requires managerial attention regardless of whether there is a current shortage of nurses. That is the issue of measuring and managing the costs of recruiting and retaining staff.

There is little question that personnel is the single greatest cost in health care. Attracting and retaining qualified staff are essential to maintaining a desired quality-of-care level. Because of the high cost of recruiting nurses, the recruitment and retention of nurses has become a financial management issue.

What can management do to keep key levels of satisfaction high? What are the tools and approaches an organization can use in attracting new nurses? What alternative sources of personnel are there? How much does nurse recruitment cost, and how does one measure that cost? These are the issues that Chapter 9 focuses on.

※ PLANNING AND CONTROL

Planning and control are elements central to the success of any organization. Planning helps the organization to know where it wants to go and to develop a plan to get there. Control helps to ensure that the plan that has been adopted is carried out.

Part IV devotes four chapters to this important topic. These chapters specifically address strategic planning, budgeting concepts, operating budget preparation, and the control of operating results.

Strategic Planning

Strategic planning is an outgrowth of the long-range planning of the 1950s. *Strategic management* is the process of integrating strategic thought throughout the management process. Organizational success largely depends on the care with which the organization acts strategically. Knowing an organization's strengths and weaknesses and being aware of its opportunities and threats are the critical elements upon which the field of strategic management has been built.

Strategic planning is discussed in Chapter 10. How are strategic plans defined? Why are they prepared? What benefits can the organization hope to achieve from strategic management? The chapter also discusses long-range plans and program budgets.

Budgeting Concepts and Budget Preparation

The budgeting aspect of planning is explored in two chapters. Chapter 11 provides an overview of the various types of organizational budgets and of the budget process. Chapter 12 goes into greater depth on the preparation of the operating budget.

The types of budgets examined include operating, long-range, capital, product-line, program, zero-base, cash, and special purpose. Each type of budget has an integral role in planning for health care organizations.

The budget process is much broader than the actual preparation of each unit's budget. The process includes preparing a timetable, doing an environmental review, and developing goals, objectives, assumptions, and priorities. It also includes budget negotiation and revision.

Capital budgeting has become more complicated in the health care industry. Health care organizations must examine the financial implications of capital acquisitions more closely. The technical appendix to Chapter 11 discusses sophisticated analytical approaches to capital budget evaluation. The methods discussed include the present cost approach, net present value, and internal rate of return.

Chapter 12 looks at specific issues related to preparation of operating budgets. The starting point for preparing the operating budget is the estimated workload. First, however, the likely number and mix of patients must be considered before a determination can be made of the resources needed to care for those patients.

The largest and most complicated element of the budgeting process relates to personnel costs. The major part of Chapter 12 is devoted to examining the issues related to staffing and to calculating labor costs. Costs of services other than personnel services and budgeting for revenues are also covered.

The last section of the chapter deals with budget implementation. A budget loses much of its value if it is largely ignored after being approved. It is vital that managers think specifically of the actions that must be taken to implement their budgets.

Controlling Operating Results

Implementation of the budget, however, does not mean that everything will come out according to the plan. Chapter 13 discusses the issue of control. That discussion includes the provision of specific tools of variance analysis, which are used to help managers to discover variations from the original plan and to keep outcomes as close to the plan as possible.

Traditional variance analysis compares the actual results to the budgeted plan. Information is provided for each line item of each budget for the most recent month and cumulatively for the year-to-date. Chapter 13 also introduces the concept of flexible budgeting, a variance analysis technique that provides better insight into the likely causes of observed variances. By subdividing variances into their underlying components, the manager is able to identify the major influences that generated the variation from the budget.

Performance Budgeting

Health care budgeting focuses to a great extent on the resources needed to provide a certain volume of services. This is a one-dimensional view of health care. Managers generally attempt to achieve many objectives. Rather than simply trying to provide care to a specific number of patients, managers try to keep patients satisfied, improve the quality of care, control costs, keep staff and other clients happy, and achieve other ends. Performance budgeting, discussed in Chapter 14, is a technique that examines the things that a department or organization is trying to achieve. With this technique the manager can develop a budgeted level of performance and cost for each of a number of objectives of the organizational unit.

※ MANAGING FINANCIAL RESOURCES

All managers of health care organizations manage resources. Determining which personnel and other resources to use and how to use them is a managerial function. Organizations have many types of resources. The people working for any health care organization are a valuable resource, as is the reputation for quality. The financial resources of the organization—specifically, its money—is another. To the same extent that clinical resources must be carefully used, financial resources must be managed efficiently.

Decisions concerning where and how to get money are one element of managing financial resources. Some resources in proprietary organizations come from investments in the organization by its owners. In not-for-profit organizations a common source of financial resources is issuance of bonds. Profits are a potential source of financial resources for all types of health care organizations. In the last 50 years it has become common for health care organizations to borrow much of the money they need.

Organizations have financial resources, which they must manage efficiently. Decisions must be made concerning how much cash to have on hand. Management techniques must ensure that cash is received as promptly as possible. In addition, managers must ensure that cash is available when needed for payrolls or interest payments. This need to have control over the inflow and outflow of cash necessitates careful management of receivables, inventories, marketable securities, payables, and leases.

Some readers may assume that the management of financial resources is the strict domain of financial managers, but that is not the case. For example, a financial manager can do little to control inventory levels. The nurse manager is in a much better position to make determinations regarding necessary inventory levels and to enforce policies established to avoid unnecessary stock-piling of inventory. Inventory usage directly affects the amount of money available to the organization. Nurse managers and financial managers must work together in the management of financial resources to arrive at an optimal outcome for the organization.

Part V of this book is divided into two chapters. Chapter 15 focuses directly on the management of the short-term financial resources of the organization. Chapter 16 is concerned with the long-term financing of health care organizations.

Short-Term Financial Resources

Short-term resources appear in the current asset and current liability sections of the balance sheet. (NOTE: The balance sheet is discussed in Chapter 5.) Such resources generally provide or require cash within a relatively short time, usually less than a year. These short-term resources and short-term sources of resources are referred to as the organization's *working capital*. Working capital is discussed in Chapter 15.

Long-Term Financing

Long-term financing relates to the alternatives the organization has for acquiring financial resources that will not have to be repaid for more than a year. To be able to acquire capital assets such as buildings and equipment, the organization must know that it can acquire money that does not have to be repaid in a short time. The choices it makes regarding such long-term financing can have dramatic effects on the ability of the organization to provide health care services and to compete in the health care marketplace. The aspects of financial management related to long-term financing are discussed in Chapter 16.

ADDITIONAL MANAGEMENT TOOLS

The health care sector has rapidly become complex. To keep up, managers must constantly expand and improve their capabilities. Part VI of this book examines some additional management tools that can help a nurse manager to cope with the complicated environment of health care.

The chapters in this part focus on information systems, forecasting and other methods for decision making, marketing, and entrepreneurialism. Each of these may be thought of as peripheral to traditional financial management, yet each represents a topic of direct current interest to nursing managers.

Management Information Systems and Computers

Computers and the information they can generate are the subject of Chapter 17. The number of uses for computers in nursing management continues to grow. Computers are used to prepare budgets, to examine variances, to write letters and papers, and to forecast patient volume and acuity, among other applications.

Chapter 17 provides basic information about computers and information systems and looks into some of the common uses of computers to generate information to aid nurse managers in their jobs.

Forecasting and Other Decision-Making Methods

An essential role of managers is to make decisions. Forecasting methods can be used to provide managers with information about the future that can be used to make a variety of decisions. Chapter 18 discusses a number of quantitative and qualitative approaches to forecasting. These include computerized techniques as well as the less high-tech but often equally effective Delphi and Nominal Group approaches.

Chapter 18 also provides an explanation of expected value, linear programming, inventory control, Gantt, Critical Path Method (CPM), and the Program Evaluation and Review Technique (PERT). Each of these is a technique for generating information for managerial decision making that has proved effective over a period of years and a range of applications.

Marketing

Health care services sell themselves. When people are sick, they seek care. Is it appropriate to try to "sell" health care services? Does marketing have a role in health care? The concept of marketing brings with it the ethical question of whether marketing can be justified in the health care industry. The authors believe that much of the ethical question stems from misunderstanding the objectives of modern marketing.

The role of marketing is to assess customer needs and respond to them. Many people perceive marketing as simply developing advertising to sell a specific product regardless of whether consumers need it. In that perception, the seller has something and wants to convince the potential customer to buy it. In a broader view of the marketing function, the role is quite different. The customers include not only potential patients but also those persons with whom nurses have contact within the organization. Marketing determines what the potential customer needs and allows the organization to produce services that fill that need. Advertising is a way to communicate that the organization is prepared to offer what the customer wants or needs.

Advertising is a very small element of marketing. Managers must understand who their customers are. They must understand what needs exist and how those needs can best be satisfied.

Certainly the organization wants the customer to buy from it rather than from another organization. To that extent the reality of competition must be considered. Marketing is discussed in Chapter 19. The main focus of the chapter is on the elements of marketing that allow the organization to use market research to be dynamic and to adaptatively respond to the changing needs of its patients. Failure to use marketing is more likely to result in selling patients services that they do not need than wise marketing management is.

How does this relate to nurses? Nurses are often the ones who most shape the product produced by health care organizations. If patients are not getting what they need, the care provided should change. If that is to happen, it is critical for nurses to be as involved as possible in determining what patients do need and how best to fulfill that need.

At the end of the 20th century, *entrepreneur* became a common word in nursing. Nurses developed their own businesses, such as a private clinical practice or a home health agency. Chapter 20 describes the characteristics of nurse entrepreneurs, identifies opportunities for business development, and discusses business plans.

⁜ NURSING AND FINANCIAL MANAGEMENT: CURRENT ISSUES AND FUTURE DIRECTIONS

The role of nurses in health care organizations has been rapidly evolving over the last several decades. Few nurse managers who left the profession in the 1980s would recognize it today. The level of responsibility for issues of financial management has increased dramatically for nurses at all levels of health care organizations.

We doubt that the rate of change is going to decrease in the near future. The share of the total economy consumed by health care services is large. The pressures to control health care spending grow stronger. Those pressures translate into more and more pressure on nurse managers to provide high-quality care in a cost-effective manner.

Nurses will respond to that need for greater efficiency by becoming more knowledgeable and by taking on an ever-increasing financial management role. To be able to control costs, nurse managers need to know what those costs are. They need timely, accurate cost information.

Chapter 21 relates to issues of the future. What will be the evolving role of financial management in nursing management? How will financial management affect the chief nurse executive? The mid-level nurse manager? The nurse policy maker? We believe that today we are seeing only the beginning of the role of nurse managers in financial management.

CHAPTER

2

The Health Care Environment

CHAPTER GOALS

The goals of this chapter are to:

- Describe the health care system
- Explain the role of each major participant group in the health care system
- Explain the financing system for health care services
- Explain how different health care providers are paid for the services they provide
- Discuss approaches developed in the last several decades to stem the growth in health care costs
- Analyze the implications of the health care environment for nurse managers

※ INTRODUCTION

Before discussing the specific tools of financial management, it is important to provide an overview of the health care system, to allow the reader to better relate the techniques of financial management to the organizations that use them.

The health care system is based on an intricate set of relationships among a number of different participants. The participants are extremely varied, including not only those who give care and those who receive health care services but also those who regulate the care that is provided and those who provide payments that supplement those made by the consumers. The actions of the participants in the health care system are affected by the economic and regulatory environment of the local, regional, and national society. The economic and regulatory environment changes continuously and is influenced by political and economic factors. These factors interplay with technological and other scientific advances in the capabilities of health care organizations to provide the highest level quality of care.

The traditional interplay among the nurse, physician, and patient is just a small part of the larger health care system. There are many different types of providers of care. Some are individually based, such as nurses and physicians; some are institutionally based, such as hospitals and nursing homes; some are organizationally based, such as health maintenance organizations (HMOs) and home care agencies; and some are societally based, such as government-sponsored care for veterans and the military.

The health care system takes into account the needs of a broad base of consumers, from the typical acute care hospital patients to those in need of drug rehabilitation, extended convalescent care, permanent nursing home care, mental health care, dental care, rehabilitative therapy, home care, and a myriad of other health care services.

The care that providers supply to consumers is subject to a complex web of regulations. For the most part such regulations stem from an intention to protect consumers. Professional nurses believe they are skilled and know what care is needed and how to provide it. The regulatory environment often seems to be an unneeded intrusion of politicians into an area in which they have little knowledge and even less expertise. The reason for the regulations is not generally to control the activities of the competent trained individual but to protect consumers from the untrained or incompetent. The well-educated nurse pays a high price for compliance with regulations. In providing care in accordance with regulations, however, one must consider what untrained, unqualified providers of care might do in an unregulated environment.

Care is paid for in a complex manner, under a set of changing rules, by a diverse group of payers. We have already reached a stage where the cost of care has become too great for most individuals to bear. One hospitalization can easily wipe out the life savings of a family. Therefore we have developed a system that uses pooled resources, many individuals each contributing some money so that the tremendous costs of a serious illness can be paid for with those pooled resources.

The nurse manager can benefit by being aware of constraints and opportunities that the environment offers. Financial decisions must take into account not only the current environment but also anticipated changes that may affect that environment in the future. Today there may be limitations on changes that nurse managers can make to run their units and departments in a more efficient manner. Over time, however, regulations change, and those constraints may fade away. Other regulations arise to pose new challenges.

This chapter begins with a description of the major participants in the health care system. Next it addresses the principal issues related to paying for health care services. Finally, several current approaches to controlling the costs of health services are addressed. Included is a discussion of the development and growth of HMOs, preferred provider organizations (PPOs), and other managed care approaches.

⁜ THE KEY PARTICIPANTS IN THE HEALTH CARE SYSTEM

Essentially, there are five key groups of participants in the health care system:

1. Providers
2. Suppliers
3. Consumers
4. Regulators
5. Payers

Providers are those persons and organizations that deliver health care services to patients. Suppliers are the manufacturers and distributors of the equipment and supplies used in the process of providing care. Consumers are those persons who receive health care services (or would, if they had adequate access to care). Regulators are those bodies that create rules with which health care suppliers and providers must comply. Finally, payers are those persons and organizations that pay for the care provided.

The remainder of this section discusses the providers, suppliers, consumers, regulators, and payers in more detail.

Providers

The providers of health care services include all persons and organizations that produce and distribute health care services. Included among providers are health professionals such as nurses and physicians and health care organizations such as hospitals, nursing homes, and home health agencies. The government is also a major provider of health care services.

In discussions of the health care environment, providers are often grouped together as if they were one entity. However, providers often have different and competing interests. The traditional providers and those about whom the most is written are nurses, physicians, hospitals, and the government.

Nurses

Most nurses work for hospitals, but many work in other settings, such as nursing homes, home care agencies, surgical centers, clinics, HMOs, physician offices, hospices, and schools.

Nurses affiliated with hospitals are almost always salaried or hourly wage employees. They work in nursing units that are part of the nursing department. The nursing department reports to the chief operating officer or chief executive officer. The organizational structure of nursing within health care organizations is addressed in Chapter 3.

The primary role of the staff nurse is to provide direct hands-on care to patients. That role has been modified over the years. In addition to hands-on care, nurses plan and coordinate the care that patients receive. They also act in a supervisory capacity, managing other individuals, such as unlicensed assistive personnel and licensed practical nurses, who provide care directly to patients. The many professional activities that fall within the domain of nursing are well known to most of the readers of this book.

Nurses are generally interested in providing the best quality of care for patients. They often believe that only educated health professionals can assess the type and quality of care that should be or is being provided to patients, and they generally believe that nursing should have autonomy over its own professional practice.

That nurses are generally employees and their income is usually related to the amount of time they work, rather than to the number of care episodes they provide, must be considered in understanding nurses' incentives. The commonly touted need to control costs in health care organizations may have a lower priority for nurses than providing excellent patient care. Many nurses see their role as providing the best possible care. They consider it the role of other managers of the organization to find the resources necessary for nurses to provide that care. On the other hand, nurse managers see the financial management of resources as a key component in their role.

Although the majority of nurses work in acute care hospitals, nurses do have a variety of options when it comes to selecting a work setting. Each opportunity has its own specific characteristics, advantages, and disadvantages. For example, the salaries paid to nurses working as employees in physicians' offices are often lower than those paid in other settings. The working hours tend to be better, however, and often the level of job-related stress is lower. Some nurses work as consultants. They tend to work long hours and to earn higher salaries, but they may lose most, if not all, patient contact. Some nurses work for managed care organizations evaluating claims. They may also lose patient contact, but they work stable, normal, nine-to-five hours, with less overtime and stress. Other nurses work as independent nurse practitioners or entrepreneurs, setting their own time schedules. Chapter 20 discusses the expanding opportunities for nurse entrepreneurs.

Physicians

Physicians provide health care both in and out of the hospital. They are generally paid for each episode of care they provide, although frequently they are paid a fee per month no matter how much care they provide. The two predominant locales for the provision of care by physicians are their offices and hospitals.

In their offices, physicians are generally owners or co-owners, although sometimes they are employees working for another physician or for a hospital that has purchased their practice. Often the structure of the physician's office is corporate.

By forming a corporation the physician limits personal liability. The corporation owning the practice is liable for paying for equipment, rent, supplies, and salaries.

Some essential health care procedures and supplies are used by physicians in their offices regardless of cost. For example, they always use sterile needles. On the other hand, physicians often add facilities to their office practice only if they believe they are financially justified. An internist's office will add an x-ray machine for taking chest x-rays only if it is seen as a profit enhancement; otherwise patients will be referred to a radiologist.

In most cases, physicians are "guests" at a hospital, rather than employees. This creates an unusual set of incentives. Most technological improvements in the quality of care offered by the hospital are paid for by the hospital. Therefore the same physician who might not replace an existing office x-ray machine with the latest model available each year is still likely to demand that the hospital purchase the latest equipment. The hospital's acquisition of such equipment does not cost the physician anything. In some cases the equipment can reduce physicians' time treating each patient or allow physicians to provide additional types of treatments, enhancing their income.

To be sure, physicians also have the motivation of desiring that their patients receive the best care possible. The fact that physicians do not personally pay for the technological and other quality-of-care enhancements at hospitals inherently must alter their incentives, however. Being a guest rather than an owner has implications for their view of financial structure of the hospital. It is in the physicians' interest for the hospital to stay in business, but there is often little perceived reason not to try to convince the hospital to acquire the latest technology to ensure that patients have the best quality of care.

Physicians can be extremely persuasive because of their role in advising patients where to go for treatment. The physician represents the primary source of patients for most hospitals. A physician affiliated with two or three hospitals, as many are, has the ability to steer patients toward any of those hospitals. In most cases, one would hope, the physician chooses some hospital characteristics that makes it most suitable for each specific patient's needs. Physicians, however, sometimes use their control over patient admissions to gain specific concessions from hospitals.

This power over admissions that physicians have is one of the most important forces in the hospital industry. Their control over admissions also affects nursing home admissions, home care agency patient referrals, and referrals to other physician specialists. In trying to understand the actions of participants in the health care system, it is essential to understand this key role that physicians play in directing patients where to go for their care.

Hospitals

Hospitals serve two primary functions. They house sophisticated technological equipment, and they are locations where patients can receive 24-hour-per-day nursing care for acute episodes. Society centralizes services, locating essential pieces of equipment and skilled personnel resources in specific locations: acute care hospitals. Patients with acute health problems go to hospitals for diagnostic tests and for treatment. A wide range of health care professionals can make use of sophisticated clinical supplies and technologies to provide patient care.

The hospital is an organizational entity with an existence apart from the individual professionals who provide care within its walls. Some hospitals are organized as for-profit companies, and many of these are publicly traded corporations whose stock can be bought and sold on national exchanges. Some hospitals are owned by governments. The majority of hospitals in the United States are established as voluntary agencies; that is, they are not-for-profit organizations, not run by corporations or government agencies. Any profits that they earn are reinvested for the benefit of the local community. Some hospitals are established as subsidiaries of larger not-for-profit organizations, such as religious organizations or universities.

The hospital's leadership consists of health care professionals and a board of directors or trustees. The board is generally made up of respected members of the community, who often are not health care professionals.

The hospital's professional leadership, together with the board, establishes overriding goals and directions for the organization and provides oversight to ensure that the organization acts to achieve those goals. Most hospitals have as part of their primary mission the provision of the highest quality of care possible. Hospitals, however, also have limited resources. In recognition of that fact, the achievement of all goals is tempered by the need to stay in business. If the hospital fails financially and stops providing service, the result will be less desirable than providing only acceptable care rather than the highest quality care.

Government

The three levels of government—local, state, and national—are large providers of health care services. The federal government operates a significant hospital system for the military and the Veterans Administration, and the federal prison system. State governments often operate a variety of health care facilities including hospitals for mental health and clinics and hospitals for prisoners. Public hospitals have existed for many decades in the United States. Local governments often become actively involved as providers of health care services. For example, many cities and counties own hospitals, nursing homes, and outpatient facilities.

The government generally provides only those services that it believes will not otherwise be provided. The government also has a role as a payer for care. That role is partly intended to ensure adequate access. Nonetheless, there are clearly situations where access is still not adequate without the direct intervention of the government as a provider of care. In some of those cases the government directly provides the care.

Other Providers

Many other types of providers of health care services are not discussed here. These include those in which nurses have a significant role, such as nursing homes and home care agencies, and those where nurses have little or no role, such as dental offices. Each type of provider has unique perspectives and problems.

Many providers share commonalities and have differences from those described above. For example, physical therapists may work for a salary at a hospital, as nurses do, or be paid on a per treatment basis, as physicians are. Some home health agencies have a goal of making profits; others are not-for-profit voluntary organizations.

Nurses who work for home health agencies may be paid a salary or be paid for each visit they provide, similar to the way physicians are paid. It is important to note the variety of providers with competing goals and interests. Even some providers working for other providers may have conflicting interests. These goals may conflict in the area of finance: physicians may make money if the hospital expends resources and loses money. For example, the addition of a lithotripter machine will probably increase the income of urologists at the hospital. The machine may be so expensive, however, that the hospital will lose money on lithotripsy procedures.

Other conflicts arise in the area of quality of care: hospitals may want to cut professional hours per patient day, while the nursing staff has a primary goal of increasing the quality of patient care. The differences in the underlying goals of each provider may carry over to the strategies that each provider uses to achieve its goals.

Suppliers

The second key participant in the health care system is the supplier. This group includes the manufacturers and distributors of all supplies and equipment used in health care organizations.

Often suppliers are not considered in discussions of the key participants in the health care system. They are virtually always for-profit corporations that are part of the general industrial complex. Are they related to health care? Suppliers make billions of dollars of sales each year. One cannot ignore their role.

Suppliers do not just provide the health care industry with the items that providers need to care for their patients. Suppliers also invent new technologies. That innovative role is a significant issue in understanding the environment in which the health care system operates.

On the one hand, there is tremendous pressure to contain the growth in health care costs. Health care before the introduction of Medicare consumed just 4% of every dollar earned. By 1996 nearly 14% of all U.S. society's earnings were spent on health care. This is not merely the result of inflation. Not only is much more money spent on health care services but also a much larger share of all money earned is spent on health care. For example, in 1965 an individual earning $15,000 spent $600 on average for health care services. In 1996, if the same individual were earning $45,000 (because of increases in wage rates), the money spent on health care would not increase proportionately to $1,800 but would have risen to $6,120! This amount includes direct payments by the individual, payments for insurance, and taxes paid to the government to support programs such as Medicare and Medicaid. Much of the growth in costs is related to innovations that allow the health care system to do more things to provide care.

Often new technologies are extremely expensive. The suppliers therefore have taken an active role that at the same time improves the quality of care that can be provided but also increases the costs of providing it.

Consumers

Consumers are the individuals who use health care services. Consumers use a variety of types of services, ranging from preventive and advisory services to diagnostic, therapeutic, and rehabilitative care, and in some cases to monitoring or custodial care.

Consumers are becoming increasingly knowledgeable about the services they want from health care providers. Access to the Internet has dramatically increased information available to consumers. Nevertheless, there is a gap in knowledge between the health care professional and the consumer of health care services. As a result, individual consumers often rely heavily on health care professionals to advise them.

Most nurses view consumers as individual clients. Nurses are educated to encourage clients to participate actively in their care. Therefore nurses work with patients to select treatment options and to choose where care will be provided.

This may not always be the case with other providers. Physicians in particular have tremendous power over consumers because of the physicians' specialized knowledge. Physicians can use this to their advantage, and perhaps their patients', by convincing hospitals to provide resources in exchange for patient admissions.

Although one usually thinks of patients as individuals, in recent years consumers have increasingly tried collective action. In the 1990s consumer groups such as the American Association of Retired Persons (AARP) actively lobbied for health care options that are in the interest of the represented group. Because many of these groups represent constituencies of voters, governments often respond to them.

Regulators

The regulatory environment in which the health care system exists is dominated by rules and regulations that affect the actions and activities of health care providers, payers, and consumers. Some regulations even regulate the activities of regulators in a technical tangle of rules that often seems to distract the health care system from the activity of providing health care services.

Regulations are generally thought of in terms of a government order that has the force of law. The government, at local, state, and federal levels, as part of its role to protect the public, has an interest in maintaining the public's health. To achieve that end a number of regulations are issued. Although regulations are generally not specifically laws, they are often promulgated by government agencies to carry out laws. Health care providers must obey the regulations or be subject to specific legal sanctions. In some instances the sanctions have strong implications for reimbursement. This would be the case, for instance, if a hospital were not eligible to receive Medicaid payments if it failed to comply with a certain state regulation.

The U.S. Constitution identifies the federal government's responsibility to protect the health and welfare of the people. In recent years this has been broadly interpreted by the federal government to develop increasing safeguards for the public's health, including regulating pharmacologic agents and monitoring communicable diseases.

In its role as a payer for health services (discussed later in this chapter) the federal government has developed regulations for providers of health care services that are paid for with federal dollars. For example, the federal government has created a number of regulations that specify who can participate in Medicare. These regulations affect providers, consumers, and even those organizations that the federal government contracts with to process Medicare claims for payment. Beginning in 1998, advanced practice nurses could be paid directly by Medicare.

The state regulatory function varies widely from state to state. In part this regulatory influence is derived from the state's function to regulate those services for which it pays, such as those provided under Medicaid. In part the regulations derive from the state's interest in protecting the public through the licensure of those professionals and organizations that provide health care. Regulations vary from rules that decree the square footage of patient rooms in hospitals, to the ratio of nurses to patients in an intensive care unit, to the information that must be provided to patients before they are discharged from hospitals.

Licensure is one of the widely applied regulations. It is not without controversy, however. Every state has laws concerning the licensing of health professionals and health care organizations that provide care. Some economists have argued that such licensing is unnecessary. Instead, they suggest disclosure. Health care organizations would have to provide consumers with information about their training or accreditation, their experience, and their outcome rates. Then consumers could decide what providers to use and how high a price they are willing to pay. Society, however, continues to insist upon licensure. The arguments in favor are that many consumers are not well informed and that licensure ensures minimum practice levels. Further, the damage that could be done by an untrained, unexamined provider is too great to warrant the risk.

Local government regulations often cover areas related to construction, fire safety, and how to handle a death. For example, in many states, regulations do not allow nurses to declare a patient dead. Often such regulations result from lobbying efforts by special interest groups such as the American Medical Association (AMA) rather than from an underlying need to protect the consumer.

Since the government, as discussed earlier, is a large provider of health care services, it is interesting to realize that the government in some instances is regulating itself. Often the federal government is exempt from local law. Therefore the building codes and licensing regulations that affect a voluntary hospital may not affect a military hospital. On the other hand, Medicare payment regulations developed at the federal level affect payments made to county-owned and operated hospitals and other health care facilities.

Only the government has the legal authority to issue regulations and to mandate adherence to them. Health providers are also subject to the regulations of voluntary accreditation and certification bodies, such as the Joint Commission on Accreditation of Healthcare Organizations (JCAHO). While adherence to the standards of these organizations is voluntary, societal and fiscal pressures are such that few hospitals elect not to be accredited by JCAHO, and few surgeons choose not to be certified by their specialty board.

Nurse managers and nursing associations can do a number of things to influence the adoption of regulations at all levels of government and by associations such as JCAHO (see Chapter 21). Change is slow, however, and not always possible.

Nurse managers must make the effort to become familiar with the various regulations that affect their organization, department, and unit. They must reflect on how those regulations affect not only day-to-day operations but also the management decisions they can make. Since regulations vary so much from state to state, it is important for nurse managers to know the regulations in the state in which they practice. There is little consensus on whether this regulation is positive or negative for the health care system. Recently, however, there has been movement toward deregulation and encouragement of free markets.

Payers

In the U.S. health care system, often the consumer of health care services does not pay for them directly. The most common payers are individuals, insurance companies, employers, and government.

In 1996 national health expenditures were $1 trillion. The rate of increase in spending for health care services stabilized in the mid 1990s but showed signs of getting out of control again near the turn of the century. Unlike other goods and services, health care costs are usually not paid for by the person using the service. The single largest payer group for health care services is the government. Among Medicare, Medicaid, and other direct government payments for health care services, the government pays for 47% of the care. Insurers and employers are the next largest payer for care, followed by individuals paying for their own care. About 32% of health care costs are paid for by private insurance and charitable funds. Only about 17% of all personal health expenditures are paid for by self-pay patients *"out of pocket."* These services and goods include over-the-counter medications, prescriptions, physician services, private duty nursing service, and institutional care.

Individual Consumers

In most aspects of our society, individuals are obligated to pay for the resources they consume. In health care, however, that is only the case for the minority of payments. Most of the money paid to health care providers does not come directly from individuals.

Given the high cost of health care services, this should not be surprising. For example, if a $300,000 house burns down, it is unlikely that it will be rebuilt with money directly from the owner. It is much more likely that the owner was paying an annual insurance premium of $1,000 to protect the house in case of a fire. Many people each pay $1,000 premiums, but only a few houses burn down. The insurance company then pays the $300,000 to rebuild the house. Similarly, those individuals who have health insurance call upon that insurance to pay for major health care services. What about the individual who has not been paying premiums and does not have insurance? If your house burns down and it is uninsured, there are two main choices. Rebuild it with your own money if you have it, or do without a new house if you do not.

Those individuals who pay providers directly for health care services are referred to as *self-pay* patients. They often are charged the highest rates. They are also the most likely to default on their payment obligations because the high cost of care is beyond their personal means.

Approximately 43 million Americans had no health insurance in 1998 and were forced to pay for all their care or seek care from public facilities that do not require payment. Other Americans, even though they have insurance for some health care costs, pay for certain kinds of care that their insurance does not cover. This sometimes includes preventive care, such as annual gynecologic examinations or mammograms; eyeglasses; medications, both prescription and nonprescription; and many home health services.

Any payers other than individual consumers who receive the care are often called *third-party payers*. The care provided to an individual is paid for not by the consumer or the provider but by a third party. The most common third-party payers are insurers, employers, and the government.

Insurers

Insurance companies take money from individuals and employers, pool the money, and then pay providers when the insured individuals consume health care services. Some insurance companies operate as for-profit corporations. Other insurers are not-for-profit organizations, existing to provide service rather than to profit from the provision of that service. Still other insurers are formed as mutual companies, returning any profits earned to their insured population in the form of dividends or reduced premiums.

Many insurers are able to demand discounted rates from many health care providers. If hospitals refuse to negotiate a discount, then the insurer can tell its insured members that they will not be paid for care received from that provider. Losing payments for all patients who are covered by an insurer can present a substantial financial blow to a health care provider.

The negotiated discount from normal charges becomes formalized through a contract drawn up between the insurer and the health care provider. The discount is referred to as a *contractual allowance* because it is a discount from standard rates, as allowed for in the contract between the payer and the provider.

Increasingly, insurance is provided by managed care organizations such as Oxford Health Plans or United Healthcare. These organizations negotiate with providers such as hospitals. In many cases these managed care organizations are requiring providers to share the risks and profits. This can result in losses for the providers if care is more costly than anticipated.

Employers

Employers, especially larger ones, have included health care benefits as a fringe benefit for many years. To a great extent that benefit used to consist of buying health insurance for the employee. For large companies, however, there are enough employees to reasonably anticipate likely claims. In such cases, employers provide health care insurance benefits to the employees without contracting with an insurance company to take the risk.

Consider if the employer had decided to offer its employees fire insurance. If the employer has 20,000 employees, it might reasonably determine from historical patterns that in any given year between five and ten houses will burn down among its 20,000 employees. Rather than buying insurance for each employee, the company may find it cheaper to simply reimburse the employees whose houses burn down. Suppose, hypothetically, that there is an average $300,000 loss when a house burns down. Ten fires would cost the company $3 million. Paying $1,000 for a policy for each of the 20,000 employees, however, would cost the company $20 million. It is cheaper to bear the risk directly.

The same thing has now taken place with health insurance. The employer still provides the benefit to the employee. As long as the health care services are paid for, the employee probably does not know if an insurance company or the employer takes the risk.

Many aspects of health care insurance claims are complicated. Was the treatment appropriate? Was it provided by a qualified individual? Is the charge appropriate? Because of these complexities, there has been a growing trend for insurance companies to work for employers as a conduit of payments from employers to health care providers.

The insurance company uses its expertise to process health insurance claims, but the employer does not buy insurance. It pays the insurance company an administrative fee for processing the claims. The employer pays all the actual costs for the claims. This gives the employer a strong incentive to limit covered benefits and to try to get employees to restrain their use of health care services.

Government

Governments, in addition to regulating care and providing care, are also the largest payer for care. The most notable area that the government is involved in is Medicare and Medicaid. Medicare services are paid for by the federal government, and Medicaid services are paid for by a combination of federal and state and sometimes local payments. There are also many other federal, state, and local programs that pay health care providers for services.

In 1996 the federal government paid for about 34% of all health care, and state and local government combined paid for about 13%.[1] The federal government pays for and provides all health care, including dental care, for members of the military. The federal government pays for and provides a more limited range of benefits for veterans. Veterans' coverage is substantial if obtained at Veterans Administration facilities. The federal government also provides health care for Native Americans and for federal prisoners. On a more limited basis the federal government provides health care in a variety of special situations, such as hospital care at the Hospital Center of the National Institutes of Health.

Most state governments provide and pay for health care in institutions for the developmentally disabled and mentally ill. Many city and county governments provide and pay for health care in locally owned hospitals and clinics that have historically provided care to the medically indigent. In addition, most local governments provide minimal services including immunizations and treatment of sexually transmitted disease. Some jurisdictions provide care for children and treatment of communicable diseases.

Other programs are usually directed at vulnerable or at-risk populations such as substance abusers, pregnant women, persons infected with human immunodeficiency virus (HIV), and children at high risk. These programs are subject to whims of local political forces and do not have the breadth of coverage and permanence of programs such as Medicare and Medicaid.

As a payer for health care services, the government takes money, usually raised from taxes, and uses it to pay for health services. In a sense this is a pooling of money, similar to an insurance system, except that often there is a redistributive element. The taxes are paid by individuals who are not likely to receive the health care services paid for by the government. Government payments to providers are only for covered groups that the government has specifically identified.

⁜ FINANCING THE HEALTH CARE SYSTEM

Many individuals and organizations provide health care services because they want to help people stay healthy or get well. However, the economic reality is that

---

[1]http//www.hcfa.gov/stats/nhe-oact/Tables/+11.htm.

most providers would not be able to provide care unless they were compensated. As is the case for other consumer goods and services, health care services represent a product that must be paid for. It is important for nurse managers to understand the major sources of revenues for health care providers.

The Medicare and Medicaid Programs

By far the most pervasive role of government in the payment for health care is as a third-party payer. This role is primarily a result of Titles 18 and 19 of the Social Security Act of 1965. These laws created Medicare and Medicaid, which commenced in 1966.

Under Title 18 the federal government administers Medicare, an insurance program for the elderly and permanently disabled. Medicare is divided into two separate elements, Parts A and B. Part A of the program, which provides payment for hospital care, is financed by taxes on earnings. Part B, the medical care portion of the program, is optional and is financed by premiums from potential patients. The amount of payments to hospitals and physicians is decided at the federal level.

The Medicare program is administered by the Health Care Financing Administration (HCFA). The actual payment system is carried out through the assignment of a number of *fiscal intermediaries*. These organizations receive an administrative fee from the government for processing bills received from providers. The intermediary receives money from HCFA and pays it to the providers based on approved claims. Often insurance companies such as Blue Cross act as intermediaries, benefiting from their own expertise in processing health care claims. HCFA is encouraging those eligible for Medicare to obtain care through a managed care organization. From the government's point of view, this is expected to decrease expenditures. From the participant's point of view, these plans often provide extra services such as pharmaceuticals in exchange for limiting options in medical and hospital care.

Under Title 19 the federal government runs the Medicaid program for the medically indigent. The program is financed by federal general tax revenues and state contributions. The percentage share paid by the federal government varies from state to state. The program is optional for states. Those states that choose to participate must pay for a minimal level of services for eligible participants. All states are currently participating. States may also cover other services in addition to the federally mandated minimum. Services paid for under this title vary widely from state to state. Reimbursement rates are decided by each state and also vary widely. Unlike Medicare, in which participation in managed care is optional, some states now mandate that patients receiving Medicaid receive care through a managed care organization.

In the quarter-century that these programs have existed, their presence has had a dramatic effect on shaping the way health care is delivered. The original intent was to improve access to care for the indigent and aged, two underserved populations. Through these programs the government, as a major payer, has gained increasing control of what care is provided to whom and how it is provided. Many believe that these programs were the most important factor in the rising health care costs over the last 30 years.

The Insurance System

Insurance has become a major source of financing for the health care system and is second only to the government in terms of the amount of money it pays to health care providers. Most Americans have private health insurance, usually provided by employers. Some individuals buy their own health insurance.

In some cases insurance companies take the risk of high claims. In other cases employers retain the risk and insurance companies just process the claims; or providers such as physicians share the risk. In any event, the consumer has the protection of insurance.

Insurance is an organized way to share the risk of the costs associated with undesirable events. An insurance *premium* is paid to buy protection against the negative event. If it occurs, the insurer provides payment to cover the loss. In this way the risk of a major financial loss is spread among all who are paying into the system, and only those who require health care services use this pooled money.

Health insurance most often covers services (benefits) rather than being an *indemnity* plan, which provides a dollar amount for a specific medical condition. The policy states that the insurer will provide payment for specified procedures and activities of specified health care providers. Historically, insurers provided a standard set of benefits. Currently employers negotiate with insurers to provide an array of benefits for a set price. This price is usually based on the previous experience of the group being insured *(group rated).*

In *community rated* plans the premium is based on the general experience of the community rather than a specific group. Some argue that community rating is the only fair way to share risks. Otherwise there will be an attempt to load high insurance costs on a small group with a high expense experience. This to some extent defeats the purpose of insurance. Others argue that community rating is inherently discriminatory, making persons at low-risk pay for the high losses experienced by distinctly different groups. Sometimes insurers handle this problem by using community rating but adding surcharges for persons at high-risk, such as smokers.

Beneficiaries often complain that "managed care doesn't cover that" or nurses complain that "the insurance company won't pay for a nurse to do that procedure." While it is accurate that the insurance company will not pay, it is important to remember that the decision about benefits is made based on the costs of coverage. If more items are included, the costs to the insurer will be higher and the premium will have to be raised, whether through a managed care organization or traditional service plan.

Moral Hazard

In theory, insurance is an ideal way to deal with the random risk of large losses. Even though some people pay a premium year after year and never collect, they benefit from the peace of mind of knowing that they are protected from a devastating loss.

In practice, however, there are a number of problems with health insurance. Most problems relate to a phenomenon known as *moral hazard.* A moral hazard reflects the fact that once insured, an individual's behavior may change.

Consider an extreme example: Why buy a home fire extinguisher when your house is insured against fire? This example is extreme because it is unlikely that fire insurance can ever adequately reimburse someone for the loss of a home. Personal items may have little dollar value but are meaningful to their owner. Therefore it is unlikely that an individual would fail to own a fire extinguisher just because the house is insured. Yet fire insurance companies often offer a discount on the premium for working fire alarms or extinguishers. Apparently, even in this extreme situation, insurers have found that moral hazard exists.

In health care the problems are significantly greater. We might argue that no one is likely to smoke simply because they know they have the safety of insurance to cover treatment for lung cancer. Yet there are other ways that health insurance policyholders can influence to some extent the number and cost of undesirable events that befall them.

Many health care services may be optional, such as some types of mental health services, some elective procedures, or even whether to go to a doctor because of a cold. Health insurance creates a problem related to buying in an economical fashion. The person who has to pay for services is likely not to consume services unless they are worth the price. If a physician charges $100 for an office visit and the patient must pay that out-of-pocket, the patient will think twice as to whether it is really necessary to see the physician. Once the patient has insurance, the price for the visit could drop to $0. At that price, all the individual is giving up is time. There is a moral hazard effect because the individual changes behavior from what it would be without insurance.

Sometimes insurers turn this to the advantage of all concerned. Many dental plans pay 100% benefits for routine preventive care but lesser percentages for other types of treatments. It is unusual for insurance to cover small losses that have a high likelihood of occurrence. The administrative costs are too high to try to pool money to cover semiannual dental checkups. However, the theory is that if full coverage is provided for dental cleanings and examinations, more people will follow a plan of routine oral examinations, reducing the likelihood of larger dental claims for more extreme treatment later.

Coinsurance, Deductibles, and Co-payments

In an effort to overcome the problems of moral hazard, insurance companies often require that beneficiaries pay *coinsurance*, a *co-payment*, or a *deductible* to make consumers bear enough of a portion of the cost of health care services that they do not use the services as if they were free.

A deductible is an amount of money the consumer must pay before the insurer will pay anything for care. Generally the insurer requires the consumer to pay the first $200 for care each year before becoming eligible for any benefits. This can forestall unneeded trips to health care providers for minor complaints. However, if a serious condition arises, the individual is likely to seek care, even if he or she must pay the first several hundred dollars of cost. In the current financial environment, it would not be surprising for the deductible to rise to as high as $500.

A co-payment is a dollar amount, usually $5 or $10, that must be paid each time a service is used. This approach is common among HMOs. Co-payments are usually so small ($5 or $10) that the consumer is unlikely to fail to seek care when really needed, but they are a reminder that care is not free. Some believe that even a small co-payment discourages unnecessary patient use of health care services.

Coinsurance is a portion of each health care payment that is the responsibility of the consumer. It is similar to a co-payment but tends to be more substantive. Generally coinsurance is stated in terms of a percentage, generally 10% to 30%, that the consumer must pay.

Insurers and the businesses that pay for insurance use these mechanisms to decrease the use of "unnecessary care." They believe that if the beneficiary must pay some of the cost, he or she will not seek care for conditions that are self-limiting or do not require medical or nursing care. Others argue that these mechanisms prevent people from seeking care early when treatment could be effective and could prevent more expensive care later.

When there is no deductible, co-payment, or coinsurance, the insurer must pay all health care claims that are valid. This is referred to as *first-dollar coverage*.

Customary and Reasonable Coverage

Whether first-dollar coverage is in effect or not, insurers often place some limitations on how much they will pay for services. This is most commonly accomplished through use of limitations at the level of *customary and reasonable charges*, and more recently, negotiated rates between the provider and the insurer.

Customary charges are based on surveys of what providers in an area are charging. Insurance companies can carry out these surveys simply by reviewing all bills that they receive over a period of time from a particular geographic region. The insurance company decides that any bills that exceed the average charge by a certain amount are excessive. The company then only reimburses up to a level that it determines is reasonable.

In some cases insurance policies contain specific limitations on payment amounts. For example, it is not uncommon to have a 50% coinsurance rate for mental health care benefits **and** a limit of $40 per visit. In a high-cost area such as New York City, psychiatrists commonly charge $150 per session. With a $40 cap and 50% coinsurance, the benefit paid would be only $20, and the patient would be responsible for the remaining $130. It is not clear to what extent this is because insurers believe there is great moral hazard in the utilization of mental health care service *vs* the extent to which mental health services are not seen as being as valuable or necessary as acute care hospital treatment or even a physician office visit because of a runny nose.

Other Sources of Financing

Government and insurance payments account for nearly three fourths of the money that goes into the health care system. Of the remaining monies going into the health care system the bulk is paid for by individuals. Even though only about 20% of all money is paid directly by consumers, this still represents nearly $200 billion each year. Some health care is paid for from philanthropic gifts.

Many payments are small and include those for over-the-counter drugs or prescriptions, an occasional physician visit, uninsured dental care, and routine eye care and eyeglasses. Such charges are paid for out-of-pocket by the large majority of persons.

Self-pay dollars for hospital and other expensive care generally come from the lower and upper classes of society; the rich tend to pay for many items that health insurance finds beyond the customary and reasonable limits. The working poor often have inadequate health insurance. They are too well off to benefit from many programs designed for the indigent but not well off enough to have a comprehensive health insurance plan. Many workers have no health insurance at all.

The last major source of funding for health care services is philanthropy. Historically, the charitable sector of society considered health care services one of its most important concerns. A lot of dollars still flow into health care organizations from philanthropic sources, although this represents a much smaller share of the total than it once did.

The reason for the decline is largely the growing role of the government and insurance. Nearly half of all health care payments come from the government. This is a much larger share than was paid by the government only 40 years ago. Further, despite the high number of uninsured Americans, there is also a growing number who do have insurance.

An additional factor has been the growth of the for-profit sector in health care. In 1997, 13% of hospital beds and 16% of hospitals were investor owned (for-profit).[2] Most of those beds are owned by large multihospital for-profit corporations.

As the industry has become more for-profit oriented and as other sources of funding have increased, the role of philanthropy as a major financer of health care services has gradually declined.

※ PAYING HEALTH CARE PROVIDERS

The preceding section addressed the issue of where the resources come from for paying health care providers. Different providers are paid in different ways. We now turn our attention to the payment systems for providers. We will focus in particular on hospitals, the largest providers of health care services.

In most industries goods and services are produced at a certain cost to the provider. Providers then add a "profit" for the cost of doing business and to cover their investment. The cost plus the profit is used to establish a charge. Consumers

[2]American Hospital Association, *Hospital Statistics 1999 Edition*, A.H.A., Chicago.

then choose to buy or not buy the product. If a company is making a large profit, other potential providers may decide to enter the industry. Competition increases, and prices are lowered (see a discussion of this process in Chapter 4). If prices become too low, some providers will no longer be able to make a profit. They will leave the industry. Eventually an equilibrium is reached at a stable set of prices, with additional competitors neither entering nor leaving the industry.

Hospital Payment

Hospital prices are not set by the process of market economics just described. The above description suggests that people are free to enter and leave the market at will. Obviously one cannot easily set up a hospital. Even if one had the money to buy or build a hospital building and equip it, a number of state permissions would be required. The need for such permissions tends to restrict entry into the industry.

These restrictions were developed at least in part because society and elected government officials believed that health care services have special characteristics. People who buy health care services do not have the knowledge to choose among providers the way consumers can choose among hotels. Once in a hospital, consumers do not have the knowledge to choose which tests they should have as they might choose which services to order in a hotel. Furthermore, the need for health care services is often sudden and unexpected and does not involve a choice. Therefore there must be a certainty that providers are competent and will provide an acceptable level of care.

Not only do we not reach a price equilibrium because of a lack of free entry into the hospital industry but prices are also controlled to a great extent by the government. Both Medicare and Medicaid impose their own pricing on hospitals.

In the last decade there has been a dramatic shift in focus on the part of Medicare payments nationwide and Medicaid payments in some states. This movement is from a cost-based system of hospital payment to a prospective payment system. We will discuss both the old cost-based system, which is still used for paying many types of providers, and the prospective payment system, which is used to pay for most Medicare inpatient care as well as some other hospital patient care.

The tremendous growth of managed care has also led to new payment approaches based on negotiated rates. This trend will be discussed. This section also addresses the issue of charity care.

Cost-based Reimbursement

Until 1983 most government payers and Blue Cross paid hospitals based on reimbursement of their costs. Hospital accountants calculated total costs to provide care and divided that amount by the quantity of care provided. Costs were calculated for most hospital services, such as the cost per diagnostic test such as a chest x-ray, and for room and board.

Even for-profit insurers and self-pay patients often paid an amount based on costs. The finance department would take costs for units of service and add a factor to develop a charge. Self-pay patients and insurers paid based on those charges.

Medicare, Medicaid, and Blue Cross each established their own definitions of allowable costs. They then paid hospitals based on the amount of those costs incurred on behalf of Medicare, Medicaid, and Blue Cross patients. The Medicare guidelines were nationwide, while the allowable costs and reimbursement levels for Medicaid varied from state to state. Blue Cross definitions varied from one Blue Cross company to another around the country. The system of payment became known as *cost reimbursement*. The difference between the full charge for a service and the cost reimbursed is referred to as a *contractual allowance*.

For the nurse there was little incentive to reduce the cost of care in this system. Supplies used were billed to patients or included in the daily room and board charge. If the unit needed more nurses to care for sicker patients, they could be hired.

Obviously the system was not this simplistic. At times there were not enough nurses to be hired. An even more significant issue was that some hospitals had large numbers of uninsured patients, from whom reimbursement of costs could not be ensured.

Charity Care

In our society, hospitals are not permitted to turn away patients in need of acute care. There have been unfortunate examples of hospitals that used extremely narrow definitions of what represents an acute episode requiring hospital care. Many hospitals have been more open in admitting all patients who truly are in need of care. Patients who either could not pay (indigent) or did not pay (bad debts) have created financial problems that were addressed in a number of ways, including government subsidies, philanthropy, and cross-subsidization.

For hospitals with high rates of poor patients, many governments developed *disproportionate share arrangements,* which provided extra payments to those hospitals. Often these arrangements were financed by taxing hospitals with fewer poor patients to provide a subsidy to those hospitals with more poor patients.

Philanthropy also covered some of the cost. However, as the government role has increased, the role of philanthropy in paying for care has declined.

Finally, charges in excess of cost for some insured and self-pay patients resulted in enough revenues to offset the losses on bad debts and charity care. This is often referred to as *cross-subsidization.* Payments from one group of patients cover costs for another group of patients. Many would argue that the costs of poor patients should be borne by society through a general tax. In the cross-subsidization approach only those individuals who are hospitalized are taxed for care of the poor.

The role of charity care by hospitals is unclear. In some states, such as New York, all inpatients who pay for their care either directly or through a third party (except for Medicare) bear at least part of the cost of all indigent patients through a surcharge on their hospital charges. One could therefore argue that not-for-profit hospitals in New York do not provide charity care. In that case, why would hospitals have not-for-profit status and be exempt from taxes? That question has led to nationwide controversy in the last decade.

In recent years changes in financial reporting requirements have been passed that focus on charity care. Each year hospitals must indicate on audited financial statements the amount of charity care they have provided. This should reveal the extent to which hospitals provide care to the needy and also some information on how that care is financed.

While there are skeptics who do not believe that hospitals provide much charity care, in some cases the burden of charity care has overwhelmed hospitals, and a number of hospitals have had to merge or close. Such mergers accelerated after the introduction of prospective payment systems.

Prospective Payment Systems

Following the implementation of Medicare and Medicaid in 1966 the cost of hospital care began to escalate dramatically. Since government was paying a large share of these costs, it was in the government's (and taxpayers') interest to slow this escalation of costs. In 1983, Congress authorized HCFA to pay hospitals for care of Medicare inpatients on the basis of a prospective payment system (PPS) called *Diagnosis Related Groups* (DRGs). A similar system is being developed for care of hospital outpatients and for home care. With *prospective payment* a hospital has predetermined prices for services rather than simply being reimbursed for whatever costs are incurred.

Developed at Yale University, DRGs are a classification system that groups similar patients into categories that reflect the amount of care required. These groups were constructed to reflect similar medical diagnoses requiring about the same amount of hospital time. Medicare DRGs are based on factors including patient age, medical diagnosis, whether an operating room procedure was performed, complications, and co-morbidity.

It should be noted that a DRG is not assigned to a patient until the patient is discharged. The DRG assigned is based on the illness that required the admission. In most cases a good estimation of what the DRG will be can be made at admission.

Under the DRG payment system hospitals are no longer paid on the basis of the cost of care but on a predetermined amount based on the DRG. If the hospital stay costs the hospital more than the DRG rate, the hospital loses the difference. If the stay costs less than the rate, the hospital keeps the surplus. The rates paid are based on the national costs of each DRG, adjusted for annual inflation and expected productivity gains.

For certain specialty hospitals (such as pediatric, psychiatric, and oncology) DRGs are not used. But, for the most part, DRGS are a dominant force in hospital payment, particularly if the hospital cares for many Medicare patients.

Negotiated Rates

Generally negotiations are for a percentage discount from the hospital's normal rates. Sometimes a flat charge per patient day is agreed to, regardless of services provided. In some cases managed care organizations negotiate capitated rates, which are a flat monthly payment per member regardless of his or her consumption of medical services.

For nurses the rules have changed. The total revenue to the hospital for many patients is fixed regardless of the costs incurred in treating these patients. It *does* matter how many catheter kits are used, and it *does* matter if the patient has one less x-ray, because those items cost the hospital money. Most important, it matters how long the patient stays in the hospital. The most important predictor of hospital cost is the patient's length of stay. If on average it costs $1,000 per day to stay in a hospital, the patient who stays two extra days will cost the hospital as much as $2,000 more than the patient who stays fewer days. Consequently, there is increasing pressure on nurse managers to decrease patient length of stay. In those organizations where the nurse manager is fiscally accountable for the unit, it is vital for the manager to understand the importance of the reimbursement system. For those patients whose care is paid according to a negotiated rate, using fewer resources means more profit for the hospital.

Nurse Payment

Almost 60% of nurses work in hospitals, and most nurses in hospitals are paid an hourly wage by their employer. Overtime is paid for hours worked in addition to base. Nurse managers are likely to be paid a salary. In general they are not paid overtime but are given compensatory time off. In fact, most nurse managers work more than their scheduled hours without additional compensation.

Several hospitals are now experimenting with alternate payment systems for staff nurses. These include paying nurses a salary with no additional compensation for overtime; paying nurses a salary plus bonus, based on the productivity of the nursing unit; and paying a group of nurses a set amount of money to provide care for a specified period of time. As hospital management attempts to increase productivity, it is anticipated that alternate methods of payment will expand.

Many nurses work in organizations other than hospitals. In most cases they are employees working for an annual salary or an hourly wage. In some cases there are profit-sharing arrangements or bonuses. Nurses in some home health care settings are paid on a per visit basis. Nurses are rarely paid directly by insurers or consumers of care. Most often these payments are made to an organization, which pays the nurse.

Some nurses are self-employed and receive payment directly from patients or insurers. Private duty nurses often are paid directly, as are nurse psychotherapists. Nurse practitioners, nurse psychotherapists, and nurse midwives are sometimes paid directly by insurers. Professional nurses have been lobbying for "third-party reimbursement for nurses." Nurses argue that they should be reimbursed in the same way physicians are. They provide the nursing care. They argue that they should be able to authorize care and should be directly reimbursed for it.

There is substantial evidence that when nurses provide care that would otherwise be provided by physicians, money is saved. Examples are prenatal care or well-child care. (No empirical studies could be located that discuss the impact of reimbursing nursing care that was not substitutive.) However, the concept of direct payment to nurses has met with resistance from payers. Payers apparently believe this care will be additive and will increase total health care costs rather than lowering them.

It should be noted that the benefit structure of employees' health insurance is determined by the employer, not the government. Therefore, if employers wanted this benefit and were willing to pay for it, their insurers would provide it. It would appear that the nursing profession could make substantial progress in the area of payments for nurses if it lobbied effectively. Effective lobbying led to Medicare's directly paying advanced practice nurses.

Physician Payment

Physicians have traditionally been paid by patients, either directly or through the patient's insurance company. Their income is usually directly related to the number of care episodes they provide. In recent years, however, a number of changes in physician payment have been occurring.

First, the percentage of physicians who are salaried employees has been growing dramatically. Physicians have long been salaried employees in some hospitals, such as some academic medical centers. However, as the costs of opening a practice continue to increase, fewer physicians have opened their own practices. Within a few years it is likely that the majority of physicians will be salaried employees.

Another major change in physician payment was introduced by Medicare early in the 1990s. This change reoriented the payment scale for different types of physicians. The intent was to reemphasize the importance of cognitive skills and to deemphasize the importance of procedures. Medicare hoped to provide higher payments to physicians for making diagnoses and lower payments to physicians for performing surgery and other high-tech procedures. Recently it has become common for physicians to be paid either a rate per patient per month, without regard for the amount of care provided, or a fee per episode of care. For example, a specialist such as a psychiatrist is paid $2,000 to treat an episode of depression rather than a fee for each patient visit.

Home Health Agency Payment

Home health agencies are paid by government, insurers, and directly by patients. Most agencies bill on a per visit basis for professional nursing services and on an hourly basis for unskilled aide care. Certified home care agencies provide skilled nursing care and other services. They are authorized to receive direct payment from Medicare for the services they provide; in addition, they receive payment from Medicaid, insurers, and directly from patients.

Home care agencies that are not certified to receive payment from Medicare may receive payments from Medicaid, other third-party payers, and directly from patients. Both certified and noncertified agencies usually are reimbursed by third-party payers on a cost basis. In essence, the agency calculates its allowable costs, divides by the number of visits, and calculates a per visit charge. Assuming that this reimbursement per visit covers their costs, it is in the agency's interest to provide more rather than fewer visits. Agencies may not be able to cover their costs. Some costs are not allowable by the third-party payers. Some agencies provide care to people who have no insurance and cannot pay.

Home health care costs have been escalating, and it is anticipated that in a few years some form of episode-of-care reimbursement will be instituted. Congress has mandated that HCFA develop such a system for Medicare patients. It is now common for managed care organizations to negotiate payments for episodes of care for home health agencies. In such cases the agency is paid a set fee to care for the patient without regard for the number of visits provided.

Nursing Home Payment

Although nursing homes provide short-term care for patients recovering from injuries such as a hip fracture, most nursing home residents are institutionalized for approximately two years. Paying for long-term care is a major national policy issue for the 21st century. Most nursing home care is paid for by Medicaid. However, in most cases people are not eligible for Medicaid until they have used up all their savings and become impoverished.

⁜ METHODS USED TO CONTROL PAYMENTS FOR CARE

With the rapid rise of health care costs over the quarter-century following the introduction of Medicare and Medicaid, there has been a growing push to control spending. This has given rise to a number of approaches. Most prominent among them is the development of HMOs, PPOs, and other managed care efforts.

Health Maintenance Organizations

HMOs provide health care services to individuals or groups in exchange for a monthly payment. The payment is the same whether the individual uses services or not. This contrasts with the fee-for-service approach, in which an individual pays specifically for those health care services consumed. HMOs were first popularized in the 1960s as a way to contain health care costs and to improve health. However, the basic type of organization had existed for many decades prior to the 1960s. Two noteworthy examples are the Kaiser-Permanente Health Plan, which is a dominant force in the west, and the large Health Insurance Plan (HIP) in New York. In 1996, about 21% of the population was enrolled in HMOs, and by 1997, 81% of employee's were enrolled in some type of managed care plan.[3] The developers believed that the insurance system was designed to pay for "sickness care." Most insurance pays only for care for people who are sick. Why not develop an insurance system that would pay to keep people well?

In HMOs, preventive care is paid for and there is an emphasis on keeping people well and out of the hospital. Not only should HMOs improve care, but they also have the potential to lower costs by eliminating unnecessary care and by detecting health problems early.

For the HMO system to work there needs to be an incentive for physicians (the *gatekeepers*) to use less expensive outpatient care and to hospitalize patients only when necessary. The incentive is money. In most HMOs physician groups are paid on a *capitation* basis; that is, they are paid a flat fee per patient, regardless of the amount of care that the patient consumes.

Patients pay a flat premium, or capitation charge, called the PMPM (per member per month charge). If the population stays well and does not use a lot of health

---

[3]KMPG Peat Marwick, *Health Benefits in 1997*, June 1997.

services, the physician group shares in the money that is not spent. However, the physicians are at risk. If the patient population consumes a lot of health care resources, physician payments are lower.

From the patients' point of view, there is usually little or no charge for most health care visits. Preventive care is encouraged. The patient does not have to pay the doctor and then be reimbursed.

There are two principal types of HMOs: the group model and the individual practitioner association (IPA). In the group model, all the HMO's physicians are employees of the HMO. They provide care only to patients of the HMO in HMO-owned facilities and affiliated hospitals. All HMO members get their care from a physician who is part of the group. This substantially limits choice in selecting a physician.

In the IPA model, physicians have their own private practice and treat many of their patients on a traditional *fee-for-service* basis; that is, they charge patients for each episode of care and each service provided. However, for members of the IPA HMO that chose the physician as their primary provider, the physician provides the care in exchange for a portion of the HMO's PMPM charge. The IPA model keeps the physicians at risk. They earn less if the covered HMO members consume a lot of health care services. They earn a higher amount if HMO members consume relatively few services.

IPAs tend to have far more affiliated physicians than group model plans. In the group approach, the HMO must have enough members to keep its physicians busy. The IPA model allows the physicians to have their own non-HMO patients. Therefore an HMO with the same number of members can offer a much larger number of physicians. This provides more choice to members of the HMO. Further, it uses the physicians' offices. Therefore the HMO doesn't have to make nearly as large an investment in clinical offices and equipment.

However, some observers think that IPA doctors are not as committed to the ideals of the HMO approach as are members of a group model HMO. There is a large rift in the industry between those dedicated HMO physicians who believe that HMOs not only can be less expensive but also can provide more appropriate care and those physicians who view HMO IPA affiliation as just another way to get more patients into their offices.

For HMOs to work, patients must get all their care from physicians affiliated with the HMO. If patients could go to other providers, those providers might order expensive tests or hospitalization when outpatient care and less expensive tests would do. Therefore most HMOs view the primary care physician as a gatekeeper. This primary physician prevents patients from consuming unnecessary treatments by specialists and from gaining unneeded admissions to the hospital.

In addition, most HMOs have arrangements with specific hospitals to provide care. Often the HMO negotiates a discounted rate for hospital care. In such cases patients' choice of hospitals is limited. Many consumers do not like HMO restrictions on choice of physician and hospital.

Preferred Provider Organizations

PPOs are arrangements between providers (e.g., physicians, hospitals) and third-party payers. The providers agree to provide care for set prices, usually less than the current prevailing rate. The payers agree to steer large numbers of patients to that provider. Incentives are given to insured individuals that encourage them to receive their health care services from these preferred providers.

Arrangements for discounts from preferred providers are most often made by insurers or employers. In some cases state governments negotiate PPO arrangements for Medicaid care.

If clients choose to receive care from a preferred provider, they often have lower out-of-pocket expenses. For example, the coinsurance for each episode of care may be 0% or 10% if the preferred provider is used, but 30% if the preferred provider is not used. Sometimes deductibles are waived if care is from the preferred provider. Although the systems restrict the provider options for patients, many employers prefer this method because it lowers expenses. Insurers (and the employers who pay their premiums) believe that PPOs decrease costs.

There is a saying in the PPO industry that "if you've seen one PPO, you've seen one PPO." Each arrangement tends to be unique. It is difficult to make generalizations about PPOs.

Point of Service

In the latter half of the 1990s, one of the most rapidly growing forms of managed care was point of service (POS) plans. Typically these plans offer a choice of in-network or out-of-network care. In-network care often operates as an HMO, with HMO-type coverage. Out-of-network benefits allow choice of provider but reimburse the patient as if they were in a PPO and chose not to use the preferred provider.

Managed Care

Managed care is a term often used to refer to HMOs or to any system in which an attempt is made to control consumption of health care resources. More formally, managed care is a system in which someone acts as an intermediary between the patient and the provider of services. The role of physician as gatekeeper was discussed above. In a managed care system a designated person (often called the case manager) rather than the physician authorizes the provision of the services. While a major goal of managed care is to decrease costs by decreasing unnecessary services, case management can also ensure that patients get appropriate and timely care.

Most insurance companies now have managed care. They may require prior approval for all but emergency care and refuse to pay for care that was not authorized. Managed care programs often require a second opinion for surgical procedures and may require that only certain facilities and providers be used. Among the current criticisms of HMOs, PPOs and other managed care insurers is the criticism that patients are being unduly restricted to care that may jeopardize their health.

※ IMPLICATIONS FOR NURSE MANAGERS

Managers cannot operate effectively in a vacuum. The purpose of this chapter was to discuss the various elements of the health care system to provide an explanation of the environment in which nurse managers work.

There are a number of key players or participants in the health care system. These include not only the providers of care and the patients but also the health care suppliers, regulators, and payers. In health care much of what an organization and professional can or cannot do is influenced by forces external to the organization. These forces may be government regulatory bodies, insurance companies, or consumer groups. Changes in payment systems to health care organizations have implications for how care is provided. Changes in the regulation of health professionals have implications for what ancillary workers can and cannot do. Without considering the role of each participant and the relationships among all the participants, one risks making decisions that do not take all relevant factors into account.

Many things are done by health care providers that may not make obvious sense. Some of these things can be understood if the manager considers the system of financing the health care system. Health care providers have become dependent on revenues from Medicare, Medicaid, insurance, and self-pay patients. However, the payments being made have placed a great stress on the economy.

In reaction to that financial stress, the government has focused on prospective payment and managed care. Insurers have placed hurdles such as coinsurance, deductibles, co-payments, and limits on customary and reasonable charges, as well as restrictions on the specific care that will be reimbursed. With decreasing funding from philanthropic sources, providers must be ever more diligent to carefully remain financially solvent. The main payers are attempting to restrict payments, while at the same time a growing number of patients are not covered, even by government programs for the indigent, and cannot afford to pay for their care.

In further response to the need to control health care costs, more programs have been created to manage these costs. The most prominent among these are HMOs, PPOs, POS, and managed care. Potentially, in most health care provider organizations the nurse manager will have to deal directly with each of these cost containment alternatives. Nurse managers will have to become more conscious than ever of the costs of running units and departments. There is likely to be a growing need for information that can be used in negotiations and decisions that relate to HMOs, PPOs, POS plans, and other managed care efforts.

KEY CONCEPTS

Key participants Major groups involved in the organization and delivery of health care are the providers, suppliers, consumers, regulators, and payers.

Providers Health workers such as nurses or physicians and health care organizations such as nursing homes or hospitals that dispense health care services to people. The most important providers of care are hospitals, nurses, physicians, and the government. However, many other types of providers are essential to providing the total range of health care services. Different providers have different goals and incentives, and different methods.

Suppliers Manufacturers and distributors of supplies and equipment used by health care providers. Suppliers have a dramatic impact on the health care industry as a result of their development on new technologies.

Consumers Individuals who receive health care services. Generally consumers of health care are less knowledgeable about health care purchases than they are about the purchase of other goods and services.

Regulators Federal, state, and local governments have the legal authority to regulate the health care industry as part of their function of protecting the public. Health providers are also subject to the regulations of voluntary accreditation and certification bodies such as the Joint Commission on Accreditation of Healthcare Organizations.

Payers Individuals or organizations that pay for health care services provided to consumers. The most common groups of payers are individuals, insurers, employers, and the government.

Third-party payer Organization or government ("third parties") that pays for health care services consumed by individuals.

Contractual allowances Discounts from normal charges that are given to large payers of health care services.

Health care financing Government is the largest payer for health care services, providing about 47% of the funding. Insurers and employers are the next largest group, followed by individuals.

Medicare and Medicaid Government programs that pay for health care services for the aged, permanently disabled, and some indigent individuals. The Medicare program is administered by the Health Care Financing Administration, and payments to providers are made through fiscal intermediaries.

Insurance system Most people in the United States have private health insurance. In exchange for a premium, often paid for by an employer, individuals receive health insurance coverage. The premium rates are set based either on the experience of a specific group (group rated) or the community as a whole (community rated). To discourage unnecessary use of health care services, insurance usually has deductibles, co-payments, and coinsurance.

> **Deductible** Amount the individual must pay each year before insurance begins to pay for care. This payment is usually several hundred dollars.
>
> **Co-payment** Dollar amount that must be paid by the individual each time a health service is used. For example, some pharmaceutical plans require that a $5 or $6 fee be paid for each generic prescription, and $10 or $12 for a brand-name drug.
>
> **Coinsurance** Percentage of charges that must be paid by the beneficiary, usually 20%.

Out-of-pocket expense Money the individual must expend directly for health care services not covered by insurance or other third-party sources.

Customary and reasonable charges Limits set by insurers on the amount that they will consider for payment, based on surveys of typical charges in the community.

Cost-based reimbursement Payments made to providers based on reimbursement to the provider for the cost incurred in providing care.

Prospective payment Payments made to providers based on a fixed price for each specific type of patient. Payments are not made in advance of treatment.

Diagnosis Related Groups (DRGs) Medicare prospective payment system. Patients are placed in specific groups (DRGs) based on their principal diagnosis, surgical procedure, age, and other factors. Payment for each patient within a specific group is the same. The payment is a predetermined fixed amount and is not dependent on the costs incurred in treating the patient.

Health maintenance organization (HMO) Health care organization that agrees to provide health care on a capitation basis. The HMO is paid a set fee per member per month to provide all specified health care services to enrolled patients.

Preferred provider organization Organization that agrees to provide care for a group of individuals, such as an employee group, based on a negotiated set of fees. These fees are often lower than the prevailing fees in the community. In contrast to HMOs, the providers are paid on a fee-for-service basis.

Point of service organization Organization that offers members either in-network, HMO-type coverage with low coinsurance and deductible rates but limited choice or out-of-network care with greater choice but higher deductible and coinsurance rates.

Managed care System for organizing the delivery of care in which someone other than the provider of care controls the services the patient uses. These systems are usually used to control and limit the use of services. However, they are also used so that people do not receive unnecessary care, which subjects the patient to unnecessary risk.

SUGGESTED READINGS

Bean, Kent H., "Under New Management," *Health Systems Review,* Vol. 30, No. 4, July/August 1997, pp. 33–34.

Bryce, C. L., and K. E. Cline, "The Supply and Use of Selected Medical Technologies," *Health Affairs,* Vol. 17, No. 1, January/February 1998, pp. 213–224.

Burns, Lawton R., Gerri S. Lamb, and Douglas R. Wholey, "Impact of Integrated Community Nursing Services on Hospital Utilization and Costs in a Medicare Risk Plan," *Inquiry,* Vol. 33, No. 1, Spring 1996, pp. 30–41.

Campbell, Claudia, Homer Schmitz, and Linda C. Waller, *Financial Management in a Managed Care Environment,* Delmar's Health Information Management Series, Delmar Publishers, Albany, N.Y., January 1998.

Campbell, Sandy, "The Newest Gatekeepers: Nurses Take on the Duties of Primary Care Physicians," *Health Care Strategic Management,* Vol. 15, No. 3, March 1997, pp. 14–15.

Donaldson, M. S., K. D. Yordy, K. N. Lohr, and N. A. Vanselow, eds., *Primary Care America's Health in a New Era,* National Academy Press, Washington, DC, 1998.

Fuchs, Victor, *Who Shall Live?* Basic Books, New York, 1974.

Gabel, J., "Ten Ways HMOs Have Changed During the 1990s," *Health Affairs,* Vol. 16, No. 3, 1997, pp. 134–145.

Ginzberg, Eli, *Tomorrow's Hospital: A Look to the Twenty-First Century,* Yale University Press, New Haven, Conn., 1996.

Gold, M. R., R. Hurley, T. Lake, T. Ensor, and R. Berenson, "A National Survey of the Arrangements Managed-Care Plans Make with Physicians," *New England Journal of Medicine,* Vol. 333, 1995, pp. 1678–1683.

Grimaldi, Paul L., "Managed Care Glossary Update," *Nursing Management,* Vol. 28, No. 8, August 1997, pp. 22–25.

Handy, Joanne, "Alternative Organizational Models in Home Care," *Journal of Gerontological Social Work,* Vol. 24, No. 3–4, 1995, pp. 49–65.

Holman E. J., and E. Branstetter, "An Academic Nursing Clinic's Financial Survival," *Nursing Economic$,* Vol. 5, No. 15, September-October 1997, pp. 248–252.

Hu, Teh-Wei, Sean D. Sullivan, and Richard Scheffler, "HMO and PPO Growth and Hospital Utilization and Payment: A Recursive Model," *Advances in Health Economics and Health Services Research,* Vol. 13, 1992, pp. 225–241.

Kennedy, G., S. Rajan, and S. Soscia, "State Spending for Medicare and Medicaid Home Care Programs," *Health Affairs,* Vol. 17, No. 1, January-February 1998, pp. 201–212.

Kovner, T. K. "Health Maintenance Organizations and Managed Care," In T. Kovner and S. Jonas, eds., *Health Care Delivery in the United States,* 6th edition, Springer, New York, N.Y., 1999, pp. 279–306.

Levit, K. R., H. C. Lazenby, and B. R. Braden, "National Health Spending Trends in 1996: National Health Accounts Team," *Health Affairs,* Vol. 17, No. 1, January-February 1998, pp. 35–51.

Mechanic, David, "Managed Care: Rhetoric and Realities," *Inquiry,* Vol. 31, No. 2, Summer 1994, pp. 124–128.

Morrisey, M. A., J. Alexander, L. R. Burns, and V. Johnson, "Managed Care and Physician/Hospital Integration," *Health Affairs,* Vol. 15, No. 4, Winter 1996, pp. 62–73.

Robinson, James C., "Administered Pricing and Vertical Integration in the Hospital Industry," *Journal of Law and Economics,* Vol. 39, No. 1, April 1996, pp. 357–378.

Rosenberg, Charles E., *The Care of Strangers,* Basic Books, New York, N.Y., 1987.

Safiiet, Barbara J., "Health Care Dollars and Regulatory Sense: The Role of Advanced Practice Nursing," *Yale Journal on Regulation,* Vol. 9, No. 2, Summer 1992, pp. 417–488.

Snow, Charlotte, "Mergers, Affiliations Spell Survival for VNAs," *Modern Healthcare,* Vol. 26, No. 48, November 25, 1996, p. 38.

Stahl, Dulcelina A., "The Phases of Managed Care: Where Does Subacute Care Fit?," *Nursing Management,* October 1996, pp. 8–9.

Starr, Paul, *The Social Transformation of American Medicine,* Basic Books, New York, N.Y., 1982.

Thorpe, K. E., "The Health System in Transition: Care, Cost and Coverage," *Journal of Health Politics, Policy and Law,* Vol. 22, No. 355, April 1997.

Wunderlich, G. S., F. A. Sloan, and C. K. Davis, *Nursing Staff in Hospitals and Nursing Homes: Is It Adequate?,* National Academy Press, Washington, DC, 1996.

CHAPTER

3

The Role of Financial Management Within the Health Care Organization

CHAPTER GOALS

The goals of this chapter are to:

- Explain the role of management in organizations
- Explain the structural hierarchy of organizations in theory and practice
- Distinguish between formal and informal lines of authority and between the line and staff roles of managers
- Assess the advantages and disadvantages of centralized *vs* decentralized management approaches
- Describe the role of financial managers in health care organizations
- Describe the financial responsibilities of the chief nurse executive and other nurse managers
- Discuss the interactions between nurse managers and financial managers in health care organizations
- Introduce and explain the concept of responsibility accounting, including cost and revenue centers
- Discuss issues of politics in budget determinations
- Describe the role of networking

INTRODUCTION

The primary role of nurses is the delivery of patient care. Nurses are educated for that set of activities, and for most nurses it is the reason they chose nursing. Historically, anything to do with money or financial resources was seen by most nurses as the purview of administration. Most nurses did not know about budgets or organizational resources and did not want to know about them. They wanted to keep people healthy and provide nursing care to those who were not healthy. Some nurses had to be involved with money; they became nursing administrators. According to some nursing leaders, a number of these nurses even abandoned nursing and became hospital administrators.

Over the last quarter of the 20th century, however, there was increasing pressure for health care organizations to control costs and to provide care efficiently. Health care organizations tried to accomplish this with as little nursing intervention in the area of management of resources as possible. In most cases, financial managers tried to simply provide nursing departments with a budget and to tell nurse managers to hold to the budgeted level of spending. That approach proved unworkable.

Managers who spend the money know the most about the resources that are needed. They must be involved in the planning process if the budget is to be realistic. To control costs, nursing departments, home health agencies, and ambulatory care organizations must be directly involved in a wide array of financial activities. In some organizations this means that nurses are taking on an increasing burden of financial calculations. In other organizations nurses are hiring nonclinical persons with MBA degrees to work for them as staff members. Those individuals do the actual financial calculations. In either case, ultimately nurses are responsible for the content of those calculations. Nurse managers must have sufficient financial skills either to develop or to supervise the development of financial information needed to run their organizations. This is necessary not only to provide acceptable quality of care but also to provide that care on a cost-effective basis.

In today's health care environment it is acceptable for nurses to know and to be concerned about the organization's money. A growing number of undergraduate and graduate programs in schools of nursing include financial management in their programs.

This chapter is intended to explain the role of financial management in the structure of organizations and how nursing and nurse managers fit into that organizational structure from a financial management perspective. To accomplish that, we include issues such as lines of authority, formal and informal linkages, interrelationships among managers, and the role of politics and power in health care organizations.

⁜ THE ROLE OF MANAGEMENT

Health care organizations include a wide variety of providers of health care services, such as hospitals, nursing homes, home health agencies, and others such as nursing centers. Regardless of the type of organization, certain management functions must be carried out. Three of the most important of these are planning, control, and decision making.

Planning is essential for the efficient management of the organization. Through planning, managers consider possible options available to the organization and steer its path. Without planning the organization drifts like a rudderless ship. With planning the organization is able to set a direction and make progress in moving toward it. Strategic planning and budgeting, two topics covered in this book, are essential elements of the planning process.

Control is a critical management task. Once the plan has been established, it must be implemented. Control refers to the managerial tasks related to ensuring that the plans of the organization are carried out as closely as possible. Control is necessary for carrying out the plans, assessing progress, and determining what can be done when progress is not satisfactory.

Decision making is perhaps the overriding role of management. Plans will not carry any weight unless someone makes decisions that are necessary to carry them out. Control will lack authority if no one makes decisions to correct problems that arise when the plan is not met. Organizations do not progress without change. Change cannot occur without someone's having the authority to make decisions and exercising that authority.

These basic elements of the role of management apply to all managers within the organization. Only when managers apply these principles can organizations most efficiently achieve their goals.

⁜ THE HIERARCHY OF HEALTH CARE ORGANIZATIONS

To make plans, control the organization, and make and carry out decisions, each organization has a managerial *hierarchy.* The hierarchy establishes the authority and responsibility that different individuals have within the organization.

Each organization has a governing board, generally referred to as the board of trustees or board of directors. The board has the ultimate responsibility for the decisions made by the organization. The board is generally made up of respected individuals from the community and business world. Most of the board members are *not* full-time employees of the organization.

Ultimately the financial condition of the organization is the responsibility of the board. The board has the final approval over adoption of the annual budget and provides the direction for setting that budget. The board adopts a mission statement that sets the overall direction of the organization. It also adopts goals and objectives that tell the organization's managers what they should be trying to do to accomplish the mission. An administrator, often called the chief executive officer (CEO) or president, reports to the board and is responsible for managing the organization. As is typical in bureaucratic organizations, a variety of managers report to the CEO.

The Top Management Team

It is unusual to find any moderate to large organization that can be run by one manager; too many different functions must be carried out. As a result, there are many managers, each with a specialized set of activities and scope of authority. For the single top manager to know what each manager is doing, there is a hierarchy of managers. Instructions may be passed down through the hierarchy, along with the authority to carry out the instructions. To facilitate this process, many organizations form a top management team, which acts together on making major organizational decisions. In addition, information is passed up through the hierarchy. For example, various nurse managers often directly observe events about which the higher levels of management should be informed.

Many large organizations have an associate administrator as part of this team, often called the chief operating officer (COO) or executive vice president for operations, who is responsible for the day-to-day operations of the organization. The team also includes a chief financial officer (CFO), who is responsible for the financial aspects of running the organization. The CEO, COO, and CFO attend board meetings. The CEO is often a member of the board.

Until the recent past the chief nurse executive was called the director of nursing. In recent years the titles vice president for nursing and vice president for patient services have gained widespread use. The titles chief nurse executive (CNE) and chief nursing officer (CNO) are also used. There is still a wide gap, however, between organizations that consider the CNE a key member of the top management team consisting of the CEO, COO, CFO, and CNE and those that consider the CNE on a par with a number of other department heads who report to a member of the top management team. The trend is recognition of the special role played by the CNE, who controls approximately half of most health care organizations' budgets and an even greater share of the organizations' salaries. In home care agencies the CNE controls most of the entire budget. In more and more health care organizations the CNE is included in the top management team and is taking on functions such as attending board meetings and participating in the organization's most important decisions.

There is some controversy in nursing over the appropriateness of this trend. As the CNE becomes part of the top management team, the responsibility of that position shifts from responsibility for and management of the nursing department to responsibility for and management of the organization. Instead of looking downward at the nursing department, CNEs are starting to look outward at the overall actions of the organization and how they affect the organization as a whole. The result is that nursing is gaining in prestige as a member of the inner circle of management. The CNE is privy to more information and is a key player in the most important decisions of the organization. However, some would argue that the role that CNEs serve in such situations lessens their ability to be an advocate for the needs of nursing in the organization. The role removes the CNE even further from the patient and from an awareness of the needs of staff nurses.

We believe that the trend is appropriate. Nursing controls too great a part of the resources of health care organizations to be excluded from the key decisions that affect those organizations. However, we also believe that CNEs must be cognizant of the difficult position in which this trend places them and must make a special effort to ensure that the needs of the organization are balanced with the needs of the nursing department and its managers and staff.

Line *vs* Staff Authority

To carry out its mission and its specific goals and objectives, the organization has a hierarchy of managers who are supervised by the CEO or by the top management team. The types of managers that exist in an organization can be divided into two major classes based on their *line function* or *staff function.* The line function is the element of running an organization that is related directly to the production of its goods and services. In the case of health care organizations, the line function is carried out by the managers and departments that provide patient care. Most nurse managers are considered *line managers.* Their managerial efforts go to the direct care of patients.

In contrast, the staff function concerns providing auxiliary assistance or service to the line managers and their departments. Finance officers are *staff managers.* The role of finance as a staff department is to carry out necessary functions for running the organization that are indirect to the provision of care. Finance makes sure that there is money to buy the things that the organization needs and to pay for them. It also provides necessary information about the finances of the organization.

Line managers do not report to staff managers. Therefore the finance department does not have authority over any line operations of the organization. Nevertheless, the information provided by finance is often used by line managers to help them make more effective managerial decisions. Nursing managers must understand the staff role played by finance and make use of them as a resource.

To better understand the distinction between staff and line authority, one must understand the framework of both formal and informal lines of authority and responsibility within an organization.

Formal Lines of Authority

Organizations have formal chains of command that define lines of authority and responsibility. Of interest in this book is how the nursing department fits within the overall organizational structure and its relationship to the organization's financial management. Also of interest is the nursing organization, whether a small nurse-run clinic or a large temporary nurse agency. As managed care becomes more common, nursing organizations are developing new ways of relating, often through contracting.

The formal lines of authority for most organizations are specified in the form of an organization chart. An organization chart provides a diagrammatic perspective of the interrelationships. Each position on the chart has supervision over the position below it connected by solid lines. Each position reports to those above. Other positions on the same level on the chart are on a similar level of the organizational hierarchy. There is often communication between individuals on the same level, but there is not a direct reporting relationship.

It is also common to have formal relationships that do not represent the same degree of authority or control. For instance, a manager at one level in the organization may report to a line manager directly above. The director of the dietary department may report to the chief operating officer but may also report information on a regular basis to the chief of the medical board, who is concerned about the impact of nutrition on the quality of care. However, the chief of the medical board is not the supervisor of the dietary manager and has only limited ability to make decisions and give instructions in that area. Such formal but limited relationships are indicated on organization charts by dashed lines.

Informal lines of authority may also exist. However, they are completely outside the official policy of the organization and do not appear on the organization chart.

The most complex health care organizational structures are found in integrated delivery systems. Within these systems, hospitals usually have the most complex organizational structure. Figure 3–1 shows an organizational chart for a hospital of moderate size. Solid lines indicate direct paths of formal authority and responsibility. As can be seen in the figure, the vice president for nursing reports to the executive vice president, who reports to the president, who reports to the board of trustees. The vice president for nursing is on the same level as the five other senior management staff.

It is worthy of note that while the CFO is highly placed in the organization, only financial departments report to that individual. None of the direct providers of care report to the CFO.

Figure 3–2 shows the organizational chart for the nursing department in a major medical center (not shown on the chart). In this organization, the CNE reports to the CEO of the medical center. Within the nursing department are associate directors of the various clinical services. Both organizations follow traditional organizational models, with nursing as a separate department and most nurses who work in the organization reporting through nursing. Note, however, that the operating room director reports to the executive director of nursing in the medical center (see Fig. 3–2).

The medical staff at most hospitals are not employees of the hospital but are voluntary staff. Therefore they also are not part of the direct-line hierarchy in the hospital. Nevertheless, a hospital cannot function without medical staff any more than it can function without nursing staff. There are established relationships between the medical staff and the employees of the organization.

The dotted line in Figure 3–1 indicates the relationship of the medical staff to the hospital. Most hospitals have a medical board, which has responsibility for the quality of medical care in the organization. Both Joint Commission on Accreditation of Healthcare Organizations and state regulations require that this be a formal relationship, but the relationship is not the same as that of employee and employer.

Figure 3–3 shows the organizational chart of a large government-owned hospital. Note that physicians are employees of the hospital and therefore directly accountable to the chief executive officer.

Figure 3–4 shows the organizational chart for a home health agency. Although the chart shows a solid line from staff to patient care manager, this does not

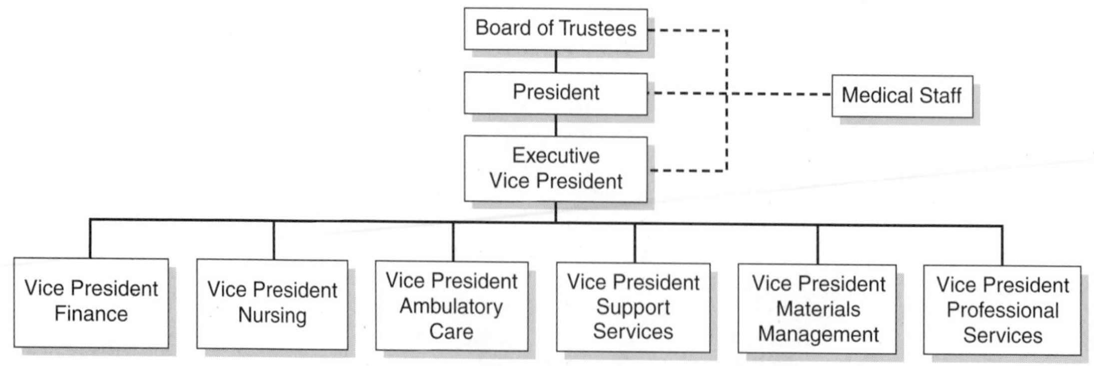

FIGURE 3–1. Organization chart for voluntary hospital.

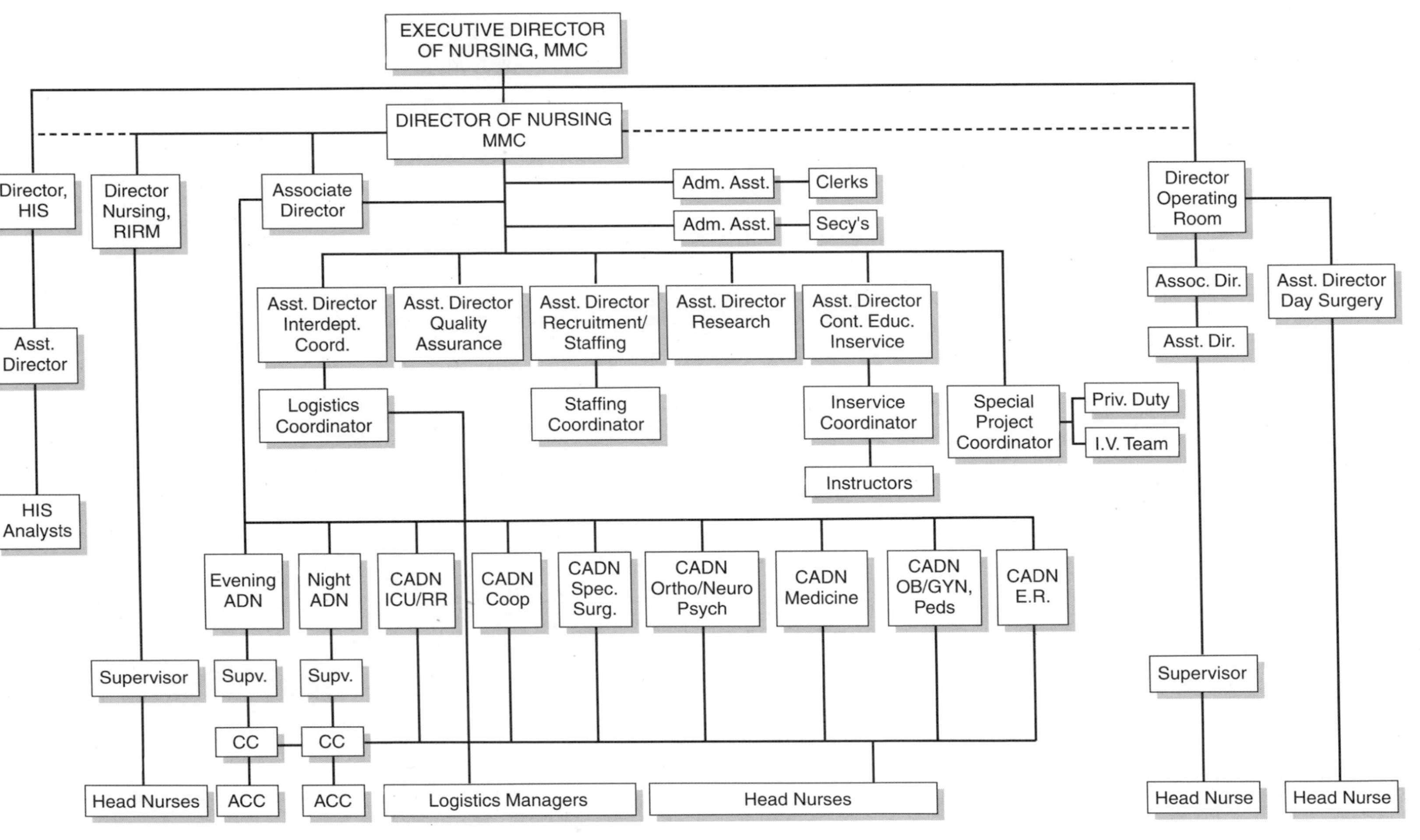

FIGURE 3–2. Organization chart for major medical center *(MMC)* nursing and related departments.

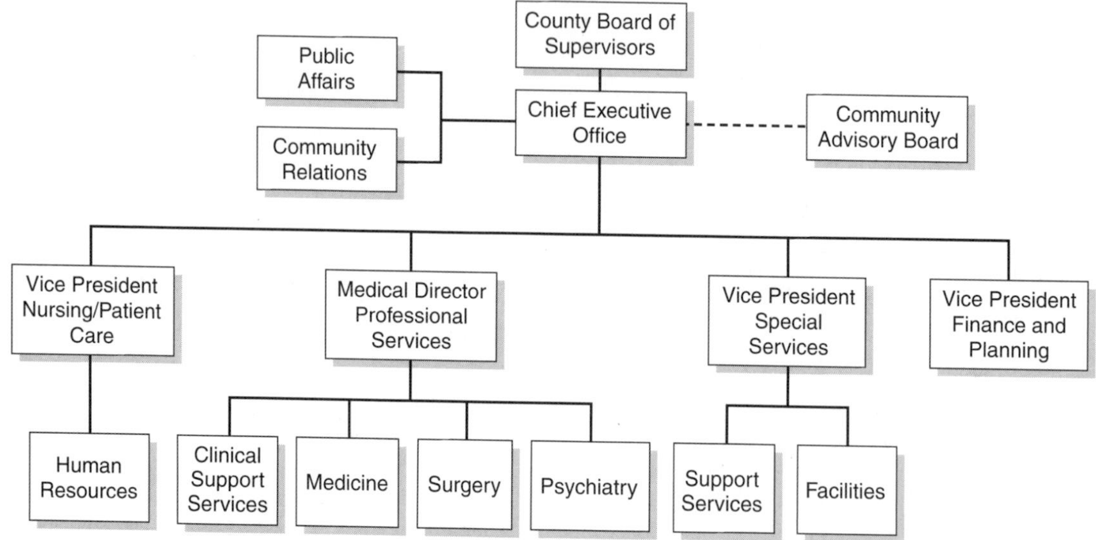

FIGURE 3–3. Organization chart for government hospital.

necessarily reflect how staff are paid. They may be paid on a fee-for-service or per visit basis, but still report directly to a patient care manager.

Integrated delivery systems often include a variety of health care organizations with varying levels of formal relationships. Figure 3–5 shows a simple integrated health system that owns health organizations, including a physician–nurse practitioner ambulatory care center. Some managed care organizations own facilities (e.g., hospitals), professional practices (e.g., multispecialty group practices), and other services (e.g., laboratories). Other managed care organizations own only the insurance and management components and contract for all health provider services.

Informal Lines of Authority

The organization charts shown above include only the formal relationships. Informal relationships are not part of the official authority structure of the organization. As such, they come and go, often with the individual in a specific position. Informal relationships develop gradually over time. Although they have no

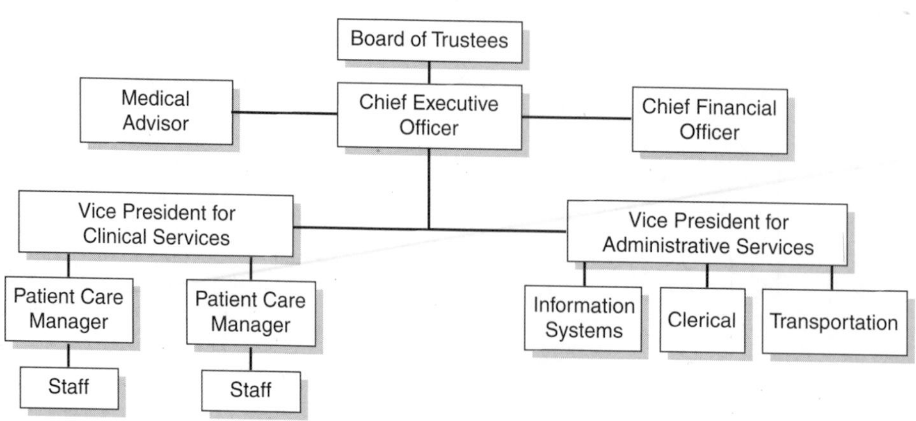

FIGURE 3–4. Organization chart for home health agency (not-for-profit).

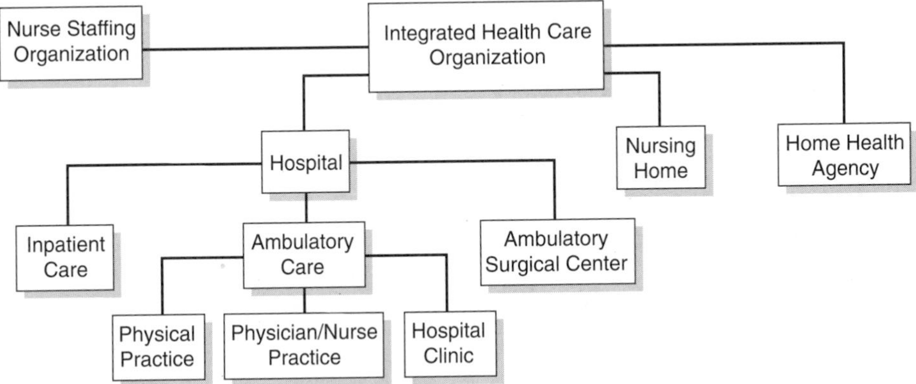

FIGURE 3–5. Organization chart for integrated health system (not-for-profit).

official standing, often they become an accepted part of the way an organization operates.

Most texts of organizational theory point out that informal lines of authority are often as important, if not more important, as the formal lines of authority. Informal lines of authority are based on the history of the organization, the key players in the organization, and resources controlled by the various players. Depending on the specific history in any particular health care organization, in some organizations the CNE may have more or less authority and responsibility than the organizational chart indicates. This could develop over time from the presence of a CNE with a particularly strong personality. The gains of one occupant of a position may even carry over to the successor. So may the losses.

Not long ago in many health care organizations the director of nursing was an individual who believed that nursing was a strictly clinical function. This director relied heavily on the finance department to handle all issues related to money and resources. Even if the formal structure of the organization gave the director of nursing certain authority, it was often not taken. Informal structures then took over, filling the void. As such directors are replaced over time with CNEs who believe that they should have greater control over nursing resources, it often requires a battle to regain the authority that officially resides in the nursing department. Informal structures can be as hard to overcome as formal ones.

In some organizations, individual key players may have special relationships. The CNE may be married to the chief of surgery. This personal relationship allows each access to information that he or she might not normally have. These two players may then form a coalition for certain decisions.

In other cases key employees have a special relationship with people important to the hospital. The director of volunteers may be the brother of the major employer in town. The employer pays for care of employees who use the hospital. In some organizations, key players share a common history: they went to school together; they both worked together at another hospital; they may socialize at a place of worship. Each of these special relationships has implications for the sharing of information and support that occurs in the process of running a hospital.

A third source of informal authority is control of resources. A common maxim is, "He who controls information controls the organization." Financial information is an example of information frequently not shared in organizations. Another resource includes employees. The nursing department usually is the largest hospital department in terms of employees.

But number of employees may not be as influential as bottom-line results. Nursing is generally seen as a cost center rather than a profit center. Nursing must work to keep its expenses within budgeted expectations. Certain other departments are profit centers. The results of activities in those departments may be reflected in a departmental profit. Historically the profit generated is used as a bargaining chip when resource allocation decisions are made. This means that some managers may be able to exercise greater influence than others. In some cases, managers may bypass the formal lines of authority and jump over one or more levels in the organization, using their power to gain resources to achieve their goals.

Other elements also serve to reinforce informal lines of authority. Physicians admit patients to the hospital. Patients represent revenue. Therefore physicians have power. The implicit (and sometimes explicit) threat to refer their patients elsewhere allows the medical board to have significant impact in decisions.

Often informal relationships are worked out in hospitals to exchange services. For example, the head nurse on 3 North makes sure that when the mother of the supervisor of housekeeping is a patient in the hospital, she receives special attention. When 3 North needs extra housekeeping help, the housekeeping department may be more responsive.

Centralized *vs* Decentralized Organizations

Health care organizations tend to be centralized and bureaucratic. As they became more complex and employed more specialized workers, authority for decision making became centralized. There is, however, a growing trend toward decentralization in many of these organizations. For example, a 600-bed hospital may be divided into four 150-bed "minihospitals." The unit-based council developed in many shared-governance models in nursing is an example of decentralization. As Finkler states, "To a great extent the degree of decentralization rests upon the confidence top management has in the management team throughout the hospital, and on the quality of the performance measurement system in place."[1]

One author suggests that management should be limited to no more than five layers and prefers no more than three.[2] He argues for increased authority and responsibility for unit managers, including higher spending authority.

Decentralization enhances the development of unit-based managers, puts authority for making decisions with the people who have the current information, allows management by exception rather than by rule, and allows a quick response to both client need and environmental change.

For an organization to grow and thrive it must continually develop its management staff. Decentralization permits the organization to foster management skills and identify those successful managers who can be promoted within the organization. A second advantage of decentralization is that the best information on which to make decisions is often at the unit level. Unit managers are in constant contact with clients and staff. They know and understand the needs of these groups better than a nurse manager sitting in a central office.

A third advantage of decentralization is the ability to decentralize exceptions to rules. Although large bureaucratic organizations need policies and rules, exceptions are inevitably necessary. Decentralization allows exceptions to be made at the unit level when appropriate.

Finally, timeliness is enhanced in a decentralized organization. Centralized organizations take a great amount of time to make decisions as information moves up and then back down through the organizational hierarchy. In a decentralized organization, decisions can be made in a more timely and efficient manner.

Although there is a trend toward decentralization, it does have disadvantages. Health care organizations function in a regulated environment. This environment

---

[1]Steven A. Finkler, "Responsibility Centers," *Hospital Cost Management and Accounting*, Vol. 3, No. 9, December 1991, p. 1.

[2]Tom Peters, *Thriving on Chaos*, New York, Alfred A. Knopf, 1987, p. 359.

requires accountability for a myriad of details. External regulators have requirements on everything from how supplies should be stored to what to tell a patient before discharge. In decentralized hospitals a system for ensuring regulatory compliance may be the greatest challenge.

Other problems exist as well. Decentralization requires that top management provide the necessary education to train managers. Inevitably, managers will make errors. Communication is a critical factor in decentralization.

Because more decentralized decisions are made, there must be a working communication system so that top management is informed of decisions in a timely fashion. It is likely that unit-based managers and top managers will have conflicting goals. The unit-based nurse manager will have as a goal providing high-quality care with the least stress to the staff. Although those goals are consistent with top management, the cost of providing this care will be of less concern to the nurse manager than to top administration. Systems have to be put in place to motivate the unit manager to achieve the organization's goals and/or a framework for unit managers to participate in setting organizational goals.

Nurse managers at the unit level will likely make some mistakes; they are human. The organization must tolerate some mistakes and have in place a system to assist managers to learn from, rather than be punished for, exercising judgments.

To successfully achieve decentralization requires a commitment from the organization for education. Most unit managers in health care organizations have a baccalaureate degree at most and few years of experience. Yet the expectations for management skills are those of someone with graduate education. This is particularly apparent with regard to financial decision making. To our knowledge, budgeting concepts are not taught in undergraduate nursing programs, yet it is often these undergraduates who in three to five years become the nurse manager of a unit.

For decentralization to work there must be a commitment from the organization to have unit-based managers with the appropriate management skills, including financial management.

※ THE ROLE OF THE CFO AND OTHER FINANCIAL MANAGERS

The CFO is in charge of all the financial functions of the organization. The financial resources of cash and investments and their sources—loans, contributions, and retained profits—are the domain of the finance function. The generation of accounting information for external reports is the function of financial accounting. The generation of accounting information for use by the organization's own managers is the function of managerial accounting. Financial managers also must consider the organization's internal control system. The CFO is responsible for all these functions.

The Finance Function

All organizations, whether in the health care industry or not, must manage their financial resources. These resources include *cash, marketable investments,* and *accounts receivable.* Finance is also responsible for managing the sources of these resources, such as notes and accounts payable, loans, and payroll. The finance function includes making and maintaining relationships with banks and other sources of funds for the organization.

Cash must be managed. This includes safeguarding it against misappropriation, ensuring that cash resources are handled efficiently, and ensuring that the organization has sufficient cash for its needs. In the finance function, financial managers consider the timing of cash inflows and outflows from the organization. If it becomes apparent that there will be insufficient cash at times to meet the organization's needs, arrangements must be made to get additional cash. This may require arranging for loans, pushing harder on fund-raising efforts, or increasing capitalization in a for-profit organization.

Finance also actively works to maximize the benefit of accounts receivable. Accounts receivable are amounts owed to the organization for the care it has provided. Those amounts might be owned by individuals, insurance companies, or the government. Careful management is required to ensure that the organization collects all possible receivables in a timely manner. Eventually some receivables will prove uncollectible. All large organizations have bad debts. Active management, however, can minimize bad debts. Active management can also result in receivables being collected as quickly as possible. The sooner receivables are collected, the sooner the money is in the organization's bank accounts earning interest for it.

When money is collected for the patient care provided, it is either immediately spent or invested. Part of the finance function is to make decisions regarding appropriate investments. It requires care to determine how to invest the money so as to earn a high return for the organization while safeguarding the money so that the risk from any investment is minimal. Health care organizations do not want to miss the chance to earn high returns on available cash, nor can they afford to lose their investment by taking excessive risks.

Finance officers also manage cash indirectly by managing the payment of the organization's obligations. In some cases, to keep cash invested (earning a return for the organization) the finance managers will defer payment of obligations for a period of time. A choice may be made to pay the telephone bill a month late. This choice must be balanced against the possible negative consequences of the action. The phone bill must not be paid so late that telephone service is discontinued; supplies bills must not be paid so late that suppliers stop providing needed clinical supplies to the organization.

If it becomes apparent that there will be insufficient cash to meet obligations, even with borrowing, fund raising, and management of receivables and payables, finance officers will raise the possibility of cost cutting throughout the organization. Such cost cutting cannot be authorized without the approval of the CEO. The CFO is not directly above the department managers in the chart of organization.

Therefore, decisions such as requiring cost cutting must be made by the CEO and COO. Ultimately, the CEO is responsible to the board. If the organization becomes bankrupt because of insufficient cash to pay obligations as due, the CEO is responsible. If quality of patient care declines because of cost cutting aimed at saving cash, the CEO is responsible. As a result, the CEO will at times approve requests by the CFO to take actions that affect the departments providing care.

More often, the CEO will push to find other financing alternatives that do not affect care. While most nurse managers become aware of efforts to cut costs to reduce cash expenses, they are not aware of other efforts. Negotiations with banks to increase the amount they will lend, or with suppliers requesting that they allow deferred payments, are kept within the finance area. In most organizations a wide variety of approaches will be assessed and attempted before cost cutting that might affect patient care is implemented.

In the final analysis, however, the finance department can only ensure the long-run existence of the organization if total spending is kept to a level that can be met by total receipts. Since even borrowing money requires cash payments (at least interest), the finance department's efforts to control the organization's sources and uses of money will ultimately have an effect on the operations of the clinical and administrative departments.

The Financial Accounting Function

The financial accounting function of the organization's finance department is different from the finance function. Financial accounting has nothing to do with the decisions of whether to borrow money and, if so, how much and from where. Nor does it concern the efficient management of cash resources, accounts receivable, investments, or obligations of the organization. It is concerned with collecting information about the finances of the organization and translating that information into a form that can be reported to interested individuals outside the organization.

A wide range of individuals is interested in the finances of health care organizations. These include government regulators and payers; stockholders, in the case of for-profit organizations; and possible donors, suppliers, and lenders. A great deal of effort by the finance department is consumed by the various reporting requirements of different outside users.

The Managerial Accounting Function

Of particular interest to nurse managers is the managerial accounting function of the financial managers of the organization. This function relates to providing financial information that can be used to better manage the organization. This is a give-and-take process. Financial managers often request financial information from nurse managers. However, managerial accounting should be a two-way street. Nurse managers need to learn how to get useful managerial accounting information from financial managers. Understanding the role of managerial accounting should help in that regard.

The first key element of managerial accounting is to aid in the general management role of planning. Planning is an essential role of management. The organization carries out much of its planning via the budgeting process. The financial managers are responsible for putting together an overall financial plan for the organization that achieves certain goals. Those goals may include growth, expansion of services, or just financial stability. From the perspective of the financial manager, the plans of all the departments must be aggregated to generate a plan for the organization that is workable.

Managerial accounting is also concerned with the role of management in the area of control. To implement a plan there must be a variety of control reports that managers use. These reports can ensure that suppliers get paid only for items actually delivered and that employees get paid only for an appropriate number of hours or days. The reports may focus on the spending of each department and each area of each department. From the perspective of the finance department, enough information is generated for control to allow the top management team to have the information it desires.

Other managers in the organization, however, have the right to request information in a form that is useful for their control needs. Nurse managers should place demands on accounting to provide information that is both timely and useful. Realize that information does not make decisions; managers do. But managers cannot take actions to control spending if they do not have information about what is happening. Therefore there should be a demand for all the information that is needed and for that information to be in a usable format.

Note that there is stress on the usability of data. It is not simply an issue of there being too little information. Certainly, receiving too little information leaves managers without the ability to make informed decisions; however, too much information may obscure the relevant data needed to make an appropriate decision. Line managers must work with the finance department to specify what information is needed and what presentation would be most useful.

One of the most critical problems of management in health care organizations is that too often finance tells line managers what information they need and the format it will be provided in. There is a terrible lack of communication in most organizations. Line managers do not get the information they need, and staff feels abused because the information they provide is not used. There should be a major effort to have periodic meetings between staff and line managers to discuss whether the information generated by staff meets the needs of the line managers and, if not, why not.

Internal Control Function

Internal control refers to the process and systems that ensure that decisions made in the organization are appropriate and receive appropriate authorization. This requires a system of accounting and administrative controls. According to noted accounting authorities,

> *Accounting control* comprises the methods and procedures that are mainly concerned with the authorization of transactions, the safeguarding of assets, and the accuracy of accounting records. Good accounting controls help *increase* efficiency; they help *decrease* waste, unintentional errors, and fraud.
>
> *Administrative control* comprises the plan of organization (for example, the formal organization chart concerning who reports to whom) and all methods and procedures that help management planning and control of operations. Examples are departmental budgeting procedures and performance reports.[3]

It is extremely important that health care organizations not waste any of their resources. Accounting controls must be in place to minimize the chances of theft or of errors that will detract from the organization's resources. Fraud and embezzlement must be prevented to the extent possible. Therefore there must be a system of checks and balances that prevents the possibility of one person's withdrawing significant sums of money and misappropriating them. Generally, two signatures are needed for the disbursement of cash, so that there is less chance of theft.

Organizations can help minimize risks by following a few general rules:

- Hire qualified, reliable people.
- Create a separation of functions that prevents the disbursement of cash based on authorization by one individual.
- Require authorization before disbursement of resources.
- Require documentation of all financial transactions.
- Establish formal procedures.
- Create physical protection, such as safes and locks.
- Enforce vacation and rotation-of-duties policies that ensure that more than one person carries out each task related to money each year.
- Bond employees (i.e., purchase insurance policies to protect the organization against theft by employees).
- Provide for an independent check of financial transactions.

No organization can ever guarantee that it will not lose financial resources. However, it is the role of the financial managers of the organization to establish controls that minimize the possibility of such losses.

※ THE ROLE OF THE CNE IN FINANCIAL MANAGEMENT

In identifying the knowledge and skills required for nurse managers, Mark, Turner, and Englebardt differentiate two levels.[4] They describe the nurse *executive* as the senior nurse responsible for managing nursing in the entire organization and the nurse *manager* as responsible for an area or program within the organization. We

---

[3]Charles T. Horngren and George Foster, *Cost Accounting—A Managerial Emphasis,* 6th edition, Prentice-Hall, Englewood Cliffs, NJ, 1987, p. 910.

[4]Barbara A. Mark, Jean T. Turner, and Sheila Englebardt, "Knowledge and Skills for Nurse Administrators," *Nursing and Health Care,* Vol. 11, No. 1, April 1990, pp. 185–189.

prefer the generic term nurse manager to refer to both and use the term CNE when referring to the nurse executive, while using mid-level or first-line manager when referring to nurses who manage parts of the organization.

This section discusses the role of the CNE in the financial management of the organization and of the nursing division. Financial management includes management of the financial resources of the organization. This includes not only cash and obligations but ultimately the expenses incurred by the organization and the revenue it generates. In almost all health care organizations the CNE has the authority and responsibility for the expenses incurred by the nursing department. In some health care organizations the CNE also has responsibility for generation of revenues.

Responsibility for expenses means that the CNE is the person who is ultimately answerable for all expenses incurred by the department. The CNE is directly involved in the negotiation process that establishes the level of resources that will be available for the department, and is accountable for any spending above or below the planned level.

Responsibility is starting to extend to revenues as well. Few hospitals hold the CNE accountable for revenues. However, many other types of organizations, such as home health agencies, assign the CNE the authority and responsibility for both expenses incurred and revenues generated. For example, home health agencies are reimbursed on a per visit basis. The manager sets appropriate standards for visits per nurse and charges per visit and authorizes other expenses. In such cases the CNE becomes accountable not only for the amount spent but also for the revenues.

In addition to their responsibility for nursing, many hospital CNEs, often those with the title vice president for patient services, are responsible for nonnursing departments. These often include the emergency room and the operating room and sometimes departments such as social work or other professional services. In many home health agencies the CNE is responsible for all services provided by the agency. In many organizations the CNE is responsible for new product development, such as an outreach program to the elderly or development of ambulatory surgery.

As a member of the senior management team the CNE must have the financial skills of equivalent senior managers. The CNE should have a thorough grounding in applied economics, be familiar with basic accounting principles, and have the skills to analyze financial statements. In addition to these basic skills, the CNE must be highly competent in cost management. To do this the manager must understand how to determine the cost of nursing services. To effectively manage costs it is necessary for the CNE to be effective at strategic planning and controlling operating results.

As a member of the senior management team the CNE must understand the management of the financial resources of the organization. This includes working-capital management and sources of financial resources. All but the smallest health care organizations have financial officers. CNEs need not be financial officers; however, they must understand financial management enough to ask the right questions, comprehend the answers, and participate in senior management decisions about financial management.

※ THE ROLE OF MID-LEVEL NURSE MANAGERS IN FINANCIAL MANAGEMENT

The authority and responsibility of mid-level nurse managers (e.g., clinical assistant director of nursing, patient care managers) varies widely from one health care organization to another. In small nursing agencies the mid-level nurse manager is responsible for costs and revenue. The manager of eight nurses in a home health agency may be responsible not only for personnel and related expenses but also for the amount of revenue generated by the staff. In most hospitals, however, mid-level nurse managers are responsible only for direct expenses in their area.

The level of decentralization will determine the knowledge and skills needed by mid-level and first-line nurse managers. It is clear that first-line nurse managers require budgeting skills. While these managers do not require all the knowledge and skills of the CNE, they should be familiar with most of the concepts.

In preparation for writing this book, the authors interviewed a number of CNEs, and mid-level and first-line managers. Those we spoke with differentiated the depth of knowledge required among levels of nurse managers more than they differentiated among content areas. Most of those we spoke with agreed that in addition to budgeting, the mid-level managers must have basic knowledge about applied economics and the financing of health care. In addition, they should understand cost management, including the basic principles of determining the cost of nursing care. Mid-level managers should have skills in both strategic planning and forecasting. Most of those we interviewed believed that mid-level and first-line managers needed skills in inventory control at the level for which they were responsible but did not need skills in managing other short- or long-term financial resources. They did not think this group needed to be able to read a financial statement. All agreed that the level of skills required depends on the type of organization and level of decentralization of the organization.

For example, many mid-level managers should have skills in securing grants for demonstration projects, research, or ongoing financial needs, while most mid-level managers would not need to understand corporate stock issuance or bond ratings.

To competently manage the unit or program, nurse managers need financial skills for planning, control, and decision making. Using forecasting skills they can estimate services to be delivered in the future and likely labor and supplies needed to provide the services (or evaluate the forecasts provided by other parts of the organization). With this information and solid budgeting skills they can prepare a budget and, more important, interpret the variance reports either created by themselves or supplied centrally.

※ INTERACTIONS BETWEEN FISCAL AND NURSE MANAGERS

Nurse managers have lateral relationships with fiscal managers. As the CNEs in many organizations become part of the top management team, they become peers of the fiscal officers. At all levels of the organization, however, nurse managers have no formal authority to require information or services. Although the CEO may require that fiscal managers provide information to nurse managers, often the format is not presented in a way that is useful to nurse managers. Therefore a collegial relationship between nursing and finance is essential.

Relationships between fiscal departments and nursing are strained in some organizations. Many fiscal officers continue to believe that nurse managers do not need a substantial amount of financial management information. People in the fiscal department may feel threatened when nurse managers ask questions. One CNE told us that when she pointed out systematic inaccuracies in the data she was receiving from the fiscal department, the CFO became hostile. She eventually was fired, in part because she was raising questions that were discomforting.

A substantial amount of team building, informal communication, and networking is necessary for nurse managers and fiscal departments to generate and use financial information that is useful for the organization. It is up to both nursing and finance to work in a cooperative manner. In some cases nursing may have to invest in the nursing-finance relationship for a while before dividends start to be received. Nevertheless, establishing a good working relationship with the people who work in finance can be worth the investment.

※ RESPONSIBILITY ACCOUNTING

The previous sections have focused on the role of financial managers, the role of nurse managers, and their interactions. There has been a presumption that all managers attempt to the best of their abilities to carry out their activities in the best interests of the organization. The organization, however, needs a way to assess the performance of its managers. That is the role of responsibility accounting. *Responsibility accounting* is an attempt to measure financial outcomes and to assign those outcomes to the individual or department responsible for them so that performance can be assessed.

It is important to note that the performance of a manager is not necessarily the same as the performance of a unit or department. The distinction is primarily concerned with the issue of ability to control outcomes. The philosophy of responsibility accounting is that managers should be held accountable for things that they can control and should not be held accountable for things that are beyond their control. Therefore there should always be an attempt to evaluate a unit's or department's performance separately from its manager.

For instance, top management may be concerned that the cost of providing care exceeded expectations because an unexpected shortage of nurses resulted in the use of additional overtime and high-cost per diem agency nurses. In that case, the performance of the nursing units will likely be below expectations. On the other hand, the unit managers should be evaluated on how well they managed the situation. In light of the shortage of nurses, did they make economical choices about when to use overtime, when to hire per diem agency nurses, and when to leave a position unfilled for a shift?

Nurses should always bear this principle in mind, both in their interactions within the nursing department and between the nursing department and the remainder of the organization. Managers should be held accountable only for the things they can control. Without implementation of such a philosophy managers develop a pervasive negative attitude. When they are considered to have failed because of causes beyond their control, they lose all incentive to attempt to be efficient in the use of resources that are within their control. Why work hard when you will fail no matter what you do?

Managers must also believe that they will be evaluated in a fair manner. In essence, they must trust that the system will generate a fair evaluation of their performance. The performance evaluation of managers in most health care organizations centers on the use of responsibility centers.

Responsibility Centers

A *responsibility center* is a part of the organization, such as a department or a unit, for which a manager is assigned responsibility. There are three general categories of responsibility centers: cost, revenue, and profit.

A cost center has responsibility only for the control of expenses. Most nursing units in hospitals are cost centers. This makes sense given the basic concept of responsibility equal to control. The typical first-line nurse manager cannot exercise any control over revenues. This manager does not generate patients, nor is that position responsible for the prices charged to patients. Therefore it is logical to hold that individual accountable only for expenses.

Units that are solely revenue centers are rare. That would imply that they can control revenues but have no control over expenses. Usually marketing departments are considered revenue centers because the organization wants to see specifically how much revenue the marketing effort is generating.

The most common alternative to a unit that is a cost center is a profit center. A profit center is responsible for both revenues and costs. Therefore it is both a cost center and a revenue center. It is responsible for the expenses it incurs as well as the revenues it generates. Most hospital operating rooms are profit centers. In some hospitals patient care units are now considered profit centers. Many nurses working in ambulatory settings are responsible for managing profit centers. However, health care terminology differs from that used in most industries. The health care industry, traditionally not-for-profit, prefers to avoid use of the term profit and therefore to avoid use of the term profit center. It has become the practice in health care organizations to use the term *revenue center* to refer to all responsibility units that are both revenue centers and cost centers.

One weakness of hospital management has been its perception of the results of cost centers and revenue centers. Resources have often been more tightly constrained for cost centers than for revenue centers. The reason for this is that cost centers at the end of a year show a large balance of expense without any counterbalancing revenue. Revenue centers, on the other hand, show revenue and expense. Many revenue centers show profits. Those profits have been used as a justification for more liberal allocation of resources to those departments. Similarly, managers of revenue centers have at times been perceived as being better managers. This has worked unfairly against nursing departments, which have been considered cost centers.

That approach tends to be somewhat irrational. Expenses are not inherently bad and do not indicate poor management. Patient care cannot be provided without incurring expenses, and there would be no revenue at all without incurring the expenses of departments such as nursing. On the other hand, the existence of profits does not necessarily indicate good management. Evaluations of managers should be based on a standard of comparison. That standard is generally the budget. Both cost and revenue centers should be evaluated against the budgeted amount to assess the performance of the manager.

Even this approach is somewhat simplistic. The budget is based on an expectation of what will happen. If patient volume increases, then expectations need to be adjusted. More patients result in more revenues, but more expenses as well. Managers must be evaluated in comparison with the budget after it has been adjusted for patient volume and, if possible, patient acuity. The ultimate goal is to evaluate the contribution of the manager apart from factors that are outside the manager's control. That is the only way that managers will perceive that the organizational structure is fair. Fairness is a necessary perception to get the maximum effort from managers.

INCENTIVES AND MOTIVATION

The issue of fairness in the evaluation of managers raises the question of goals and attitudes. Organizations are made up of people as much as they are made up of buildings and equipment, if not more so. Individuals, however, have their own interests as persons as well as employees. It is possible that their own interests will conflict with those of the organization that employs them. In that case it is vital to attempt to achieve goal congruence. *Goal congruence* simply means that the wants and desires of the organization and its employees are consistent. Organizations develop a set of incentives for their employees. The goal of those incentives is to encourage employees to work toward achieving the organization's goals.

Large organizations tend to have many layers of management. Each manager in each layer must work constantly to achieve the goals of the organization to have the most effective results. However, there is reason to believe that in most organizations, managers may have reason not to work in the best interests of the organization. This is because what is in the best interests of the organization may not be in the best interests of the individual manager.

Most nurses entered the profession because of a desire to help people and to serve. They did not expect to get rich. Nevertheless, an individual manager may want a big salary, a large office with fancy furniture, and a large staff. The organization would prefer that the manager work for a low salary in a small office with old furniture and minimal staff. Individuals are not bad because they would prefer more money and more perquisites. The organization is not bad because it wants to conserve its resources so it can use them to provide more patient care. Yet there must be some meeting of the minds or there will be a constant tension between the wishes of the individuals and the wishes of the organization.

Goal congruence is the meeting of the minds. It is achieved in most cases through a system of incentives. The organization must put forth a system of incentives that makes it worthwhile for the individual to do what is in the interests of the organization. First-line nurse managers must find a way to provide incentives to the nursing staff. Mid-level nurse managers must find incentives for first-line nurse managers. Associate directors of nursing must find incentives for mid-level managers. CNEs must find incentives for the associate and assistant directors of nursing.

Incentives can be provided in a variety of ways. Some organizations use bonuses; others use merit pay increases. Another approach is to provide managers with a letter from their supervisor discussing budget performance. Often simple, explicit recognition of a manager's hard work to achieve the organization's goals is a sufficient motivating tool to gain the benefits of goal congruence. The question of incentives and motivation is discussed further in Chapter 13.

POWER AND POLITICS

Power, authority, and influence have no standard definitions. Hampton, Summer, and Webber have noted that "influence is the process by which one person follows another's advice, suggestion, or order; power is a personal or positional attribute that enables one to influence; and authority is only one of several bases of power—one granted to an influencer-manager by higher organizational officials."[6] These authors suggest that power can take many forms, and suggest six:

- Coercive power is based on fear of punishment.
- Reward power is based on hope for reward.
- Legitimate power is based on the belief that the influence has formal authority.
- Referent power is based on charismatic leader traits.
- Expert power is based on the leader's special expertise.
- Finally, representative power is based on the democratic delegation of power to a leader.

It is postulated that referent and expert power are most important for managers of professionals. That is, the managers of professionals will be most effective in influencing if they are charismatic leaders and are seen as experts by others.[7]

Access to information and resources in health care organizations can serve as a base for power development. Because health care organizations are often large and complex, it is difficult to have all the information required to make many decisions. Thus those who control the information are in a position to be powerful and to influence decision making.

Control of financial information by "administration" and the power associated with it has been seen by many as a reason for the level of nurses' influence in the organization. While the cynic might argue this control has been intentional, others would argue that many nurses have not sought this information. As nurses understand financial management and gain access to and develop financial information, their ability to influence decision making may improve.

NETWORKING

Because managers are often dependent on others over whom they have no authority, the use of power is critical to the effective manager. Effective managers

---

[6]David R. Hampton, Charles E. Summer, and Ross A. Webber, *Organizational Behavior and the Practice of Management*, Scott, Foresman, & Company, Glenview, Ill., 1987, p. 150.

[7]Ibid.

develop relationships with people in the organization whom they depend on for information and with whom they build coalitions to influence the goals and resource allocation of the organization.

Networking was the buzz word of the 1990s. "I'm going to a networking event," and "I'm networking at lunch today" were heard in health organizations. Networks have been described as horizontal as well as vertical. For most managers lateral relationships are often more important than vertical relationships in achieving goals. For example, for the unit manager in a hospital, resources required from dietary and housekeeping are critical to running the unit. Typically the nurse manager has no direct authority over the housekeepers and dietary aides who perform activities on the unit. Nurse managers must therefore rely on their lateral supervisors, peers, and subordinates to effectively achieve the unit's goals.

Numerous articles have appeared in the nursing literature about networking—what it is, how to do it—and blessing it as a strategy. It is also argued that trade is the basis of networking. Managers trade information and services. They trade the ability to get things done. Effective managers work on building relationships with others so that when they need something (information, services) they can get it. This occurs both within and outside the organization.

※ IMPLICATIONS FOR NURSE MANAGERS

Control of information about both revenues and expenses is the key to financial control. In organizations where this information is not shared, control is not possible. A second factor is responsibility and authority for revenues in addition to the responsibility for expenses. Efforts on the part of both fiscal managers and nurse managers to share information and cooperate are necessary for successfully managing an organization.

KEY CONCEPTS

Management's role Most essential elements are planning, control, and decision making.

Board of trustees or board of directors Governing body that has the ultimate responsibility for the decisions made by the organization. The board sets the overall direction and adopts goals and objectives for the organization. The CEO reports to the board and is responsible for managing the organization.

Managerial hierarchy Structure that establishes the authority and responsibility of different individuals within the organization. The board is at the top, with the CEO reporting to the board. The COO reports to the CEO. The CFO and CNE may report to either the CEO or COO, depending on the specific organization. The COO, CFO, and CNE each have a number of managers who report directly to them.

Line and staff functions Line function is the element of running a health care organization that is related directly to the provision of patient care. Nurse managers are considered line managers. In contrast, the staff function concerns providing auxiliary assistance or service to the line managers and their departments. Finance officers are staff managers.

Lines of authority Formal lines of authority may be either direct (full authority), such as the associate director of nursing reporting to the CNE, or indirect (limited authority), such as the director of dietary reporting to the chief of the medical staff. Informal lines of authority carry no official authority but may have a substantial de facto impact.

Chief financial officer (CFO) In charge of all the financial functions of the organization. These include those related to the sources and investment of the organization's financial resources, the generation of accounting information for making external reports, and the generation of accounting information for use by line managers. It also includes the function of internal control.

Chief nurse executive (CNE) In charge of all nursing functions in the organization. This primarily includes all nursing care provided to clients. Other responsibilities include managing the human and financial resources of the nursing department to achieve the health care mission of the department.

Mid-level nurse manager Responsible for nursing functions on more than one nursing unit or area. This includes all nursing care provided to clients. Other responsibilities include managing the human resources for the manager's area of responsibility. Responsibilities usually include financial management.

First-line manager Responsible for one patient care unit, area, or group of nursing staff. This includes all nursing care provided to clients. Other responsibilities may include some financial management.

Responsibility accounting Attempt to measure financial outcomes and assign those outcomes to the individual or department responsible for them. The performance of a manager is not necessarily the same as the performance of a unit or department. Managers should be held accountable only for things they can control.

Responsibility center Part of the organization, such as a department or a unit, for which a manager is assigned responsibility. Health care organization responsibility centers are generally divided into cost centers and revenue centers.

Power "A personal or positional attribute that enables one to influence."[8] Access to information and resources in health care organizations can serve as a base for power development. Thus those who control the information are in a position to be powerful and influence decision making. Control of financial information is sometimes used to influence decisions.

Networking Effective managers develop relationships with people in the organization on whom they depend for information and with whom they build coalitions to influence the goals and resource allocation of the organization. The relationships are often made informally through a shared history (e.g., attending school together) or through a shared professional experience (e.g., participation in professional association activities). Trade is often the basis of networking. A person with information or services, such as financial information, may trade that information for something such as a prompt reply when a request is made.

[8]David R. Hampton, Charles E. Summer, and Ross A. Webber, *Organizational Behavior and the Practice of Management*, Scott, Foresman, and Company, Glenview, Ill., 1987, p. 150.

SUGGESTED READINGS

Adams, D., "Teaching the Process of Delegation," *Seminars for Nurse Managers*, Vol. 2, No. 4, December 1995, pp. 171–174.

Campbell, Claudia, Homer Schmitz, and Linda C. Waller, *Financial Management in a Managed Care Environment*, Delmar's Health Information Management Series, Delmar Publishers, Albany, N.Y., January 1998.

Evan, K., K. Aubry, M. Hawkins, T. A. Curley, and T. Porter-O'Grady, "Whole Systems Shared Governance: A Model for the Integrated Health System," *Journal of Nursing Administration*, Vol. 25, No. 5, May 1995, pp. 18–27.

Havens, D., "An Update on Nursing Involvement in Hospital Governance: 1990–1996," *Nursing Economic$*, Vol. 16, No. 1, January-February 1998, pp. 6–11.

Havens, D., "Is Governance Being Shared?" *Journal of Nursing Administration*, Vol. 24, No. 6, 1994, pp. 59–64.

Jones, K., "The Ins and Outs of Financial Management: An Introduction," *Seminars for Nurse Managers*, Vol. 1, No. 1, 1993, p. 4.

MacDonald, G., "Shared Governance—A Unit Based Concept," *Axone,* Vol. 17, No. 1, September 1995, pp. 3–5.

Prince, S. B., "Shared Governance, Sharing Power and Opportunity," *Journal of Nursing Administration,* Vol. 27, No. 3, March 1997, pp. 28–35.

Storfjell, J. L., and S. Jessup, "Bridging the Gap Between Finance and Clinical Operations with Activity-Based Cost Management," *Journal of Nursing Administration,* Vol. 36, No. 13, December 1996, pp. 12–17.

Zachry, B. R., R. L. Gilbert, and M. Gragg, "Director of Nursing Finance: Controlling Health Care Costs," *Nurse Management,* Vol. 26, No. 11, November 1995, pp. 49–53.

CHAPTER

4

Key Issues in Applied Economics

CHAPTER GOALS

The goals of this chapter are to:

- Introduce applied economics and discuss the notion of scarce resources
- Define economic goods and services and the role of utility in determining the demand for goods and services
- Explain the law of supply and demand and the functioning of free markets
- Define the concept of elasticity of demand
- Define and explain economies of scale
- Consider the role of incentives in economic behavior
- Discuss market efficiency and market failure
- Distinguish between redistribution of resources to improve economic efficiency *vs* redistribution for improved equity
- Explain the economic view of the market for nurses and periodic nursing shortages
- Discuss the implications of economics for nurse managers

※ INTRODUCTION

Economics is the study of how scarce resources are allocated among their possible uses. The rapid growth of managed care in the 1990s reduced payments to health care providers and forced managers to make difficult choices in the spending of their limited resources.

Costly new drugs, treatments, and technologies strain the capacity of society to pay the costs of health care. Wage increases further increase the cost of health care services. Americans have been consuming both more care and more expensive care. Maintaining and improving the quality of health services costs an ever-increasing amount, even if the care is provided in a totally efficient manner.

How are the pressures to increase spending reconciled with the constraints imposed by government and managed care organizations to control spending? Fundamentally, that is a question of applied economics, the topic of this chapter. As a management or policy tool, economics is used to help individuals, organizations, and society make optimal use of their limited resources.

The tools of economics are developed from a structure built upon analysis of the behavior of individuals and organizations. This chapter discusses how the law of supply and demand governs how a free market operates. The specific prices charged for products are based on the cost of producing the product. Another important pricing factor is how strongly consumers react to changes in prices. These concepts are discussed in this chapter. Next the chapter focuses on the role of incentives.

Individual behavior is often reactive. Therefore, it is possible for an organization or the government to generate desired behavior by creating appropriate incentives.

After the discussion of incentives, the chapter concentrates on issues of market efficiency in the provision of health care services. The basic notions of market efficiency and of redistribution of society's scarce resources are discussed, and a variety of issues related to the failure of the free market are explored.

The chapter concludes with a discussion of how economists might view the reasons for periodic nursing shortages and of the implications of applied economics for nurse managers.

※ FUNDAMENTAL CONCEPTS OF ECONOMICS

Economics is the study of the allocation of scarce resources among alternative possible uses. Included in such study are the actions and behaviors of patients, health maintenance organizations (HMOs), other insurance companies, providers of health care services, and the government. Given the limited nature of resources, efficient use of resources is desired. By studying behavior, economists are able to attempt to ensure that resources are used in an optimal manner.

Economic Goods

Consumers purchase *goods* or *services* provided by suppliers. These goods or services are referred to as economic goods. Goods and services are any items that consumers wish to acquire or to use. Such goods and services provide a benefit to the consumer. Consumers generally acquire goods and services through exchange. While it is possible to *barter* or exchange some goods or services for other goods or services, most exchanges are facilitated by the use of money. Each good or service has a monetary price.

Consumers have a combination of wealth and income available to make purchases. *Wealth* is the value of all of the resources the consumer currently owns. *Income* is the increase in wealth, or the amount of additional resources the consumer gains over a period of time. Additional dollars of income may come either from working or from profits on investments. The wealth and income of all consumers is limited. No one can afford to buy everything. Therefore consumers make choices in the things they purchase.

Utility

When consumers purchase goods and services, they gain a benefit from them. The benefit may be physical. For example, without food and water one would die. There is a clear physical benefit from acquiring enough food and water to survive. Other benefits are psychic. Chocolate may be perceived by some to be a pleasurable food. It is not required for subsistence, but it may well be desired. Economists refer to the physical and psychic benefit one receives from goods or services as the *utility* of those items. The more benefit received, the greater the utility.

Utility helps determine how much an individual would be willing to pay to acquire a good or service. Suppose that the price of water is 10¢ a glass. Water is needed for survival, so its utility to the consumer may well exceed 10¢ by a substantial amount. If the utility exceeds the price, the consumer will buy the water at the 10-cent price.

Suppose that the price of chocolate is $1 per bar. One person may not be wild about chocolate. Given the limitation of that person's total wealth and income, a chocolate bar may have utility that makes the chocolate's value only 50¢. That person would not buy the bar for $1. Other people may get such high psychic benefit from chocolate that they would be willing to pay up to $5 a bar. Some people would buy chocolate for $1. Not everyone receives the same utility from a specific good or service. In other words, the value of different goods and services is different to different people.

The more income an individual has, the more he or she can buy. However, income can also take a nondollar form. Each year individuals receive a dollar salary from their job, and they also gain some leisure time. That leisure time is itself a form of income. Leisure represents an economic good. It can be consumed. Or, like other economic goods, leisure time can be exchanged. A nurse may choose (in some cases) to work more overtime to make more money. In that case the nurse has decided that there is something that can be purchased with the extra money earned that is worth more than the extra eight hours is worth as leisure time. The additional utility of the extra dollars exceeds the utility of the leisure time.

It is assumed that rational individuals will act so as to maximize their total utility. To maximize total utility, a mix of goods must be consumed so that the last unit of each type of item consumed yields the same marginal utility per dollar spent. This accomplishes the purchase of a set of goods and services that, in aggregate, provides the most benefit.

Marginal Utility

As an individual makes purchases, actions are taken as if the *marginal utility* (or *marginal benefit*) of each additional purchase is evaluated. The marginal benefit represents the additional benefit or utility gained from a purchase of one more unit of a particular item. A person may have a high marginal utility for one glass of water. However, a second glass of water is not worth quite so much. The twentieth glass of water on a given day may not have much additional utility at all.

How much water is the individual likely to consume? The consumer will select a set of goods and services so that the last unit of each yields the same marginal benefit per dollar spent. By doing this, total utility will be maximized. Any other combination of goods and services would mean that some money was spent on items that provided less utility per dollar than could have been obtained from another item.

Not all individuals have the same marginal utility values. If we were evaluating chocolate, some individuals would value the first piece more highly than others would. The same is true for the second, tenth, and hundredth piece. This is true for any good. However, by aggregating information about the marginal benefit or utility for all individuals, we can develop information about the overall demand for the good or service.

Marginal Cost

Economists call the price paid for the good or service the *marginal cost.* It tells what it costs the consumer to purchase one more unit of that item. As a result of the argument just presented about utility, economists conclude that any consumer can maximize utility by setting the marginal benefit of purchases equal to the marginal cost. That is, one purchases units of each good or service until the marginal benefit of another unit is just equal to the marginal cost.

This is also a useful concept for suppliers. They will make a profit when the price they charge exceeds the cost of making the good or providing the service. Therefore we would not expect to see a service sold at less than the marginal cost of the resources needed to produce it. Pricing based on marginal costs is discussed further in Chapter 7.

Savings

What if the consumer has made a series of purchases but feels that the benefit from an additional purchase of any item is not worth the price charged, even though there is still some money left over? In that case, the individual receives more benefit from saving money than from spending it. Many individuals reach a point where the utility of saving money exceeds the utility of additional expenditures. What benefits can be realized from saving money? Several examples of the benefits individuals have from saving as opposed to direct consumption are protection against future unemployment, creation of a pool of money for a future vacation or retirement, and accumulation of money for a child's college education.

⁜ SUPPLY AND DEMAND

Free Enterprise

Economics is governed by the law of supply and demand. *Supply* is the amount of good or service that all suppliers in aggregate would like to provide for any given price. *Demand* is the amount of the good or service that consumers would be willing to acquire at any given price. The United States economy is based on a system of free enterprise, or capitalism. In such a system any individual can choose whether to invest wealth or capital in a business venture. That venture provides goods and services to the public. Workers can choose whether to work for that venture at the wages offered. Consumers can choose whether to buy the products of the venture at the seller's price. The central theme of the system is freedom of choice.

In theory such a system would also result in optimal use of society's scarce resources. Supply and demand are automatically equated by a process known as the *market mechanism*. Suppose that there are consumers who would like to purchase a product, and suppliers who would like to sell that product. That represents the basis for there to be a *market* for that product. A *free market* (the basis for the capitalistic system) is simply a situation in which sellers are free to charge whatever price they like for their product, and buyers are free to purchase or not purchase at the price sellers are charging. Exchange may take place if the buyers and the sellers reach a mutually agreeable price.

In a free market system, suppliers compete with each other for the inputs—labor, materials, and capital—and to sell their outputs. Competition may take a number of forms. One hospital might compete for nurses by offering them better working conditions. Another might offer more holidays and vacations. One hospital might compete for patients by emphasizing quality of care. Another might stress the convenience of using its facilities. Throughout the economy, the most widely used basis of competition is price. Higher wages are paid to attract employees, and lower prices are charged to attract customers.

In practice, free markets do not always exist, and unregulated competition does not always result in optimal use of society's scarce resources. If prices are not set by the results of active competition, but by an individual seller or buyer or by a regulator such as the government, the market is not a free market. Buyers may still have the option of buying at the stated price. But sellers are not free to set whatever price they choose. This chapter discusses market failure and regulatory intervention at greater length later.

An Example of Supply and Demand

For simplicity, consider a health care product for which there is clearly a free market: toothpaste. This preventive health care item fits all the various requirements for a free market. It is widely available, there are a number of competitors, and consumers have a fair degree of choice in whether to make a purchase. Suppose that the suppliers of toothpaste were to charge $5 per tube. At a price that high, many companies would be willing to supply toothpaste because there would be substantial profits. However, few people would want toothpaste so badly that they would be willing to pay the price. Some people might, but not many. Suppliers would be trying to sell more toothpaste than people are willing to buy.

Suppose that there is a total demand of 100 tubes of toothpaste at the $5 price, but there are 10 suppliers who would each like to sell 100 tubes. Obviously, they cannot each sell 100 tubes. They could each sell 10 tubes, but at that low volume the costs of setting up for production would be so high that it would not be worthwhile. *Equilibrium* is a situation in which the quantity of a good or service offered at the stated price is the same as the quantity that buyers want to purchase at that price. Equilibrium is a stable situation. Buyers and sellers are in agreement, and prices fluctuate little, if at all. If supply and demand are not equal at a given price, then the market is in *disequilibrium.* When there is disequilibrium, as there is in this toothpaste example, there is pressure to either raise or lower the price until equilibrium is achieved.

One supplier will no doubt cut its price in an effort to corner the market. Other suppliers will follow suit or else choose not to produce that product.[1] Eventually a point is reached where the quantity buyers demand at a given price is the same as the supply at that price, in a fully functioning free market.

The amount of any item that a consumer wants depends on the price of that item. However, it depends on other factors as well. The utility of water is much higher if water is the only liquid available than it would be if the consumer also had a choice of milk, wine, and soft drinks. Such other items are referred to as *substitutes.* The demand of an individual for a specific good or service is also determined in light of the amount of wealth and income a consumer has, and the specific preferences of the individual. The aggregate demand for a good or service depends on how these factors affect all consumers.

Suppose the price offered by toothpaste suppliers drops to $3. At that lower price, more people are willing to buy toothpaste. Assume the quantity demanded at that price is 420 tubes. The suppliers lowered the price in an effort to compete for the original demand for 100 tubes. At the lower price the number of tubes demanded has increased. On the other hand, at a price of $3, the profits per tube are not as great. Some suppliers will leave the industry. At that lower price, suppliers want to sell only 600 tubes, not 1,000. But 600 tubes offered at that price is still greater than the 420 tubes demanded at that price. The market is not yet in equilibrium.

Price will fall further. At a price of $2.50, buyers want to buy 500 tubes and sellers want to offer 500 tubes. The demand and supply are now the same, and they are in equilibrium. It is possible to draw a graph that estimates how many tubes of toothpaste would be demanded by consumers for any given price. The *demand curve,* D, indicates the quantity of toothpaste (horizontal axis) that would be desired by consumers for any given price (vertical axis). Similarly, the *supply curve,* S, indicates the quantity that would be offered by suppliers at any given price. Figure 4–1 presents both the demand and supply curves on one graph. Equilibrium is achieved when the demand and supply curves intersect. Only at that point is there a price that generates exactly the same amount of demand and supply. What is the total dollar size of the toothpaste industry? In equilibrium, a total of 500 tubes are sold at $2.50 per tube. Therefore, multiplying the quantity times the price, we find that the industry generates $1,250 of charges or revenue.

Note that there is some unfilled demand, even at equilibrium. The demand curve continues to a volume of 900 tubes. That means that consumers could use 900 tubes.

---

[1]Note that if a supplier does not match the lower price other suppliers offer, no one will buy from that supplier in a fully functioning free market. Why pay more for exactly the same item? Examples of multiple prices do exist, however. For instance, convenience stores charge higher prices but do not go out of business. This is because the products offered are not identical; in addition to toothpaste, the convenience store is offering convenience.

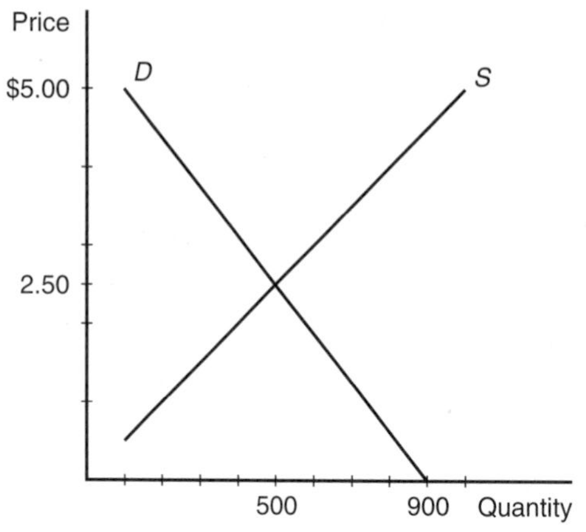

FIGURE 4–1. Supply and demand for toothpaste.

But what is the price at 900 tubes? It is zero. The demand would be that high only if the product were offered for free.

ELASTICITY OF DEMAND

In the above toothpaste example, the quantity demanded rose steadily as the price fell. It is a general assumption of economics that demand and price are *inversely* related. That is, as price goes down, the quantity demanded rises, or as price rises, the quantity demanded declines. However, an open question is how much more will be demanded as the price declines. Suppliers find this question very interesting. Are profits likely to rise more if prices are raised or lowered? How responsive is a change in demand to a change in price?

The obvious solution is to look at the supply and demand curves and determine how much would be demanded at any given price. However, the specific demand curve for each product, such as that seen in Figure 4–1, is not generally known. Economists draw such diagrams as an analytical tool, to study what would happen if a certain pattern of demand existed. Measurement of demand is much more difficult to accomplish. Generally, demand curves are estimated based on a combination of available evidence and suppositions or assumptions.

On the basis of such estimates, economists attempt to determine whether demand is elastic or inelastic. *Elastic* demand is a situation in which an increase or decrease in price results in a proportionately greater change in demand. *Inelastic* demand is a situation in which a decrease in price results in a proportionately smaller decrease in demand.

Suppose that a product's price is cut by 10%. If the increase in demand is more than 10%, the demand is said to be elastic. The more the quantity demanded increases, the more elastic the demand is. Similarly, if the price of the product is increased by 10% and the quantity demanded falls by more than 10%, the demand is considered elastic.

If the quantity demanded were to rise by very little in response to a decline in price, it would hardly be worthwhile for the supplier to cut the price. All customers would get the lower price, but the supplier would get very few new customers. On the other hand, if demand were very elastic, a small price cut would result in a large number of additional customers. In that case the price cut might be worthwhile.

Certain types of health care services have generally been considered inelastic. When consumers are sick, they want medical care. They tend to be not very sensitive to the price. For example, if a consumer needs a visiting nurse to come to the house, the difference in charge between $80 and $88 may not affect demand substantially.

Suppose that a for-profit home health agency wishes to increase its profits. Currently the average cost to the agency to provide each visit is $78, and the average price charged per visit is $80. The agency provides 1,000 visits per month and makes a profit of $2,000 per month ($80 price less $78 cost equals a profit of $2 per visit, times 1,000 visits equals a profit of $2,000).

What would happen if the price were raised by 10%, to $88? If the demand is inelastic, the number of visits might fall by only 5%. In that case the agency would only have 950 visits (a 5% decrease in volume), but the price for each one would be $88 (a 10% rise in price). The profit of $10 per visit ($88 price less $78 cost) for 950 visits would be far greater than the profit of $2 per visit for 1,000 visits.

On the other hand, suppose a competing visiting nurse association charges only $80 for a similar service. In that case, the demand for the for-profit agency's services might be highly elastic. The 10% price increase could result in a 90% decrease in the quantity demanded. The profit of $10 per visit on 100 visits would not be as good as the profit of $2 per visit on 1,000 visits. Elasticity of demand depends not only on how essential the good or service is but also on the existence of competition in the marketplace.

ECONOMIES OF SCALE

A critical concept in health economics is *economies of scale.* Many decisions nurse managers make require a knowledge of the cost per patient. However, that cost is not constant. The cost per patient varies due to economies of scale. Economies of scale refer to changes in the cost per patient as the number of patients changes. Having more patients is referred to as a larger scale of operations.

All organizations tend to have some costs that are *fixed* and some that are *variable.* Fixed costs stay the same as the volume of patients increases. For example, rent on a nursing home building remains the same regardless of whether the nursing home is half, three quarters, or 100% full. Variable costs increase as the number of patients increases. When one considers all the costs of providing care, the cost per patient decreases as the number of patients increases, because there are more patients to share the fixed costs.

Increasing Returns to Scale

Suppose that the fixed costs for a nursing home include rent, heat, and the salary of the administrator, for a total of $100,000 per month. Variable costs include nursing staff, medications, and dietary, for a total of $70 per patient day. If there are 2,000 patient days a month, the cost per patient day is $120, as follows:

Total Fixed Cost	$100,000
Total Variable Cost: $70/day × 2,000 patient days	140,000
Total Cost	$240,000
Divided by Total Patient Days	÷ 2,000
Total Cost per Patient Day	$120

However, what if there were 4,000 patient days a month? The fixed cost would still be $100,000. The total variable cost would be $280,000 ($70 per patient day × 4,000 patient days). The total cost would be $380,000. The cost per patient day would now be only $95 ($380,000 ÷ 4,000 patient days). The cost per patient day has declined as a result of economies of scale, sometimes referred to as *increasing returns to scale.* Large volumes make it less costly to treat each patient because of the sharing of fixed costs by the larger number of patients.

Decreasing Returns to Scale

At extremely large volumes, however, *decreasing returns to scale* are encountered. Decreasing returns refers to the fact that at very large volumes the cost per patient tends to increase. There are several reasons for this. For one thing, when full capacity is reached (e.g., all beds are full), fixed costs rise. It may be necessary to add a new facility. Another problem is that at very large size it becomes more expensive to acquire resources. There may not be any nurses available to staff the extra volume, and this may drive up the costs of labor.

The implications of this is that there is a least cost volume for any organization. At that volume all economies of scale have been realized, but decreasing returns to scale have not yet set in (Fig. 4–2). Cost C represents the least cost per patient. That cost occurs at a volume of Q patients.

⁜ ECONOMICS AND INCENTIVES

In the earlier hypothetical toothpaste example, each consumer or supplier acted in his or her own best interest. Suppliers decided whether they wanted to provide a product at different prices, and consumers decided whether they wanted to buy the product at various prices. The decision of each consumer or supplier individually was aggregated to derive a total demand curve and a total supply curve. The lesson that individuals act in their own best interests is central to economics, and in turn it leads to an important lesson about incentives.

Whenever an action is taken, whether by government, an organization, or an individual, that action may affect other individuals or organizations. Much as in physics, for every action there is a corresponding reaction. Managers and policymakers must be aware that the actions they take may give individuals and organizations incentives to behave in a certain way.

For instance, many health care insurance companies use deductibles, coinsurance, and copayments. A deductible is a portion of health care cost that the individual must pay before insurance covers any of that individual's costs. Coinsurance is a percentage of each health care bill that the individual must pay out-of-pocket. A copayment is a specific amount, such as $10 per physician visit. Why are these used? The rationale is that if insurance fully covers all costs, the consumer will use health care services for many little problems that do not need medical attention. By making individuals bear some of the cost, they have a personal financial incentive to be more judicious in the use of health services. The lower the cost to the consumer, the greater the demand, as evidenced by demand curves.

The issue of incentives is a concept of economics that has wide applications. Should your employer offer bonuses? One reason to do so is to give the individual an incentive to work harder in the interests of the organization. The bonus provides the individual with more resources. Those resources can be used for consumption or for savings, to result in greater total utility.

Consider another example. Should hospitals be paid on a cost reimbursement

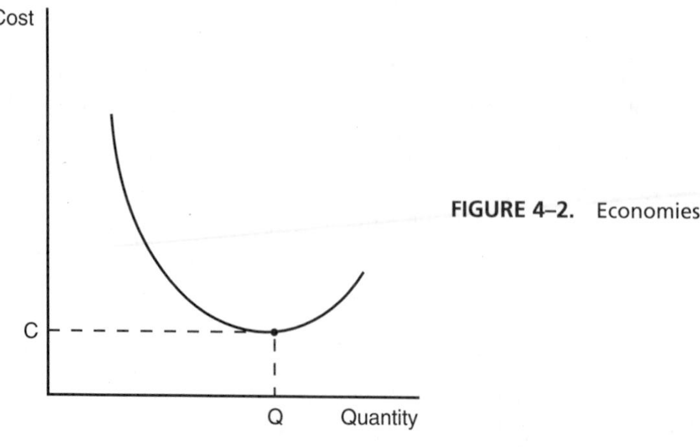

FIGURE 4–2. Economies of scale.

basis? For many years that is how Medicare paid hospitals. It was determined, however, that this gave hospitals an incentive to have high costs. Therefore the cost reimbursement system was replaced with the Diagnosis Related Groups (DRG) system. The DRG system does not reimburse the hospital for its costs; it pays a fixed amount, based on the type of patient, regardless of length of stay or cost.[2] The hope was that DRGs would give hospitals an incentive to shorten length of stay and decrease costs.

⨳ MARKET EFFICIENCY

One can view the health services field as having three key economic questions:

1. How much?
2. How?
3. For whom?

How much health services are to be provided? How are they to be produced? And who will receive them? The first two questions relate to efficiency of production; the third relates to distribution of society's scarce resources. The efficiency of the market is judged by how well it responds to these three questions.

In the case of a fully functioning free market, the three questions would solve themselves. How much production would depend on the supply and demand curves. Finding the equilibrium price and quantity would determine how much.

The how would also be solved at equilibrium. The supplier who is most efficient at the task would be able to offer the service at the lowest cost. As price declines until supply and demand intersect, the less efficient producers will drop out of the competition. When equilibrium is achieved, it means that the existing suppliers must be using efficient techniques or they would have been forced out of business. This means that *technical efficiency* has been achieved. Technical efficiency means that the services are produced using the minimum possible amount of resources for the quantity and quality of output achieved.

For whom is also solved by equilibrium. Any potential buyers who are able and willing to pay the equilibrium price or more will receive the goods or services. Anyone who can or will only pay less than that price will not receive the goods or services. This represents *distributional efficiency.* The market efficiently distributes goods based on the utility of the various consumers.

However, market efficiency does not address the issue of equity or fairness. Is the free market outcome fair for those who are poor? The question of fairness raises the issue of redistribution of resources.

⨳ REDISTRIBUTION OF RESOURCES

Government and management tend to have very different objectives. The management of an organization may desire to determine how to best provide patient treatment. It uses economics to find the least costly ways to provide a particular level or type of care. This is technical efficiency. The government is interested in distributional efficiency and equity. Could society be made better off by redistribution of resources?

Collective Action

Resource redistribution is more than simply taking resources from the rich to help the poor. It is based on a much wider notion of welfare than the use of welfare

---

[2]For patients who have an unusually long length of stay there is supplemental payment. However, that payment is kept low so that hospitals do not have an incentive to extend patient stays.

payments to the poor. The government taxes everyone so that it can have public sewer systems, police, and fire protection. It would be too expensive for any one individual to buy his or her own police department or fire department. The government acts as a central collection organization, taking contributions (taxes) from each individual and putting them all together to be able to do what any one person cannot, such as having fire and police protection. There is little disagreement that such protection is needed and worthwhile.

This is an example of distributional efficiency through government collective action. The government optimizes the result through its redistribution of resources, making everyone better off than they would be without the intervention.

Equity Improvement

A more controversial aspect of resource redistribution concerns taxing one group of individuals to provide a benefit to another group. For example, taxes paid by the working class tend to support Medicare payments made for the elderly. This makes some individuals better off, but some worse off.

Should such redistribution from current workers to the aged take place? That is a value judgment, not an economic calculation. In the fire or police example, collective action makes everyone better off. Attempts to improve societal equity often improve the utility of some people at the expense of others. How much redistribution should take place? Again, that is a value judgment. Society must make those value decisions. Then economics can focus on whether the money is being used efficiently to achieve society's goals.

※ MARKET FAILURE

Except for issues of collective action or equity improvement requiring resource redistribution, the free market is generally assumed to be an efficient mechanism. Left to its own devices, it should always find equilibrium between supply and demand. However, it is often contended that the marketplace for health care services is not perfectly efficient. There is a condition referred to as a *market failure.* Market failure means that the market does not function fully and freely. This results in an inability to reach supply and demand equilibrium without intervention. The government often steps in to try to correct market failure.

Market failure can result from a number of different factors. Sometimes government intervention itself is responsible for the failure. Another factor is lack of full information on the part of the consumer. Yet another is failure of consumer actions to fully account for the market price because consumers are not directly responsible for full payment for their health care service consumption. Market failure can be caused by lack of full competition, as occurs if either sellers or buyers have monopoly power. Finally, failure can occur when the actions of individuals do not result in optimal output because their actions do not consider externalities that they generate. All these factors are discussed here.

Government Intervention

Free market economics does not generally result in satisfying all demand. It only results in providing products to consumers who are able and willing to pay a price high enough to make it worth the while of producers to supply the product. In the health care marketplace, society has generally agreed that at least some elements of health care should be provided to individuals who cannot afford to pay for their care. This represents an equity redistribution of resources based on a value judgment by society.

In redistributing resources, an attempt should be made to avoid creating market distortions. The consequences of redistribution should be carefully analyzed.

Consider, for example, that society does ensure that an individual in terrible pain from an abscessed tooth who appears at an emergency room receives care for that tooth, for free if necessary. This is accomplished either through government payment for the services or through legislation mandating that the care be offered whether the patient can afford to pay the charge or not.

Suppose that a member of Congress argues that the nation is spending $2,000 for emergency care for poor individuals with tooth abscesses that could be saved had those individuals had toothpaste. In our earlier example we noted that at equilibrium, 500 tubes of toothpaste are purchased at $2.50 a tube. However, if toothpaste were free, 900 tubes would have been consumed. There is an unmet demand of 400 tubes because of the $2.50 price. The member of Congress might note that this unmet need is the result of people being too poor to spend their meager resources on toothpaste. At $2.50 a tube, it would cost the government only $1,000 to buy 400 tubes of toothpaste. This is half as much as is being spent on avoidable emergency care. Therefore it would be both cheaper and more socially responsible and morally correct to distribute toothpaste and prevent those abscesses. Is that a correct economic analysis?

What happens if the government acts as a buyer for the health care service, be it toothpaste or emergency abscess care? Will the supply curve change? No. The suppliers have calculated their costs, and the curve indicates how much supply they will offer at any given price. What about the demand curve? If the government says it will buy care for poor people, the amount of care demanded at any specific price has changed. To ensure that everyone has toothpaste, 900 tubes must be purchased. The supply curve in Figure 4–3 indicates that the price at which that volume will be available is $4.50 per tube.

What are the implications of this government decision? First, society must raise taxes by enough to cover the cost of toothpaste provided to those who did not buy it at the market price of $2.50. Since the free market equilibrium was 500 tubes, the government must buy 400 tubes. At what price? Assuming the government pays the market price, it would have to pay $4.50 per tube.

However, the government has also introduced another change. At the higher price of $4.50 per tube, the original demand is less than 500 tubes. It is only 180 tubes (see Fig. 4–3). There are a number of people who were able to buy the toothpaste at a price of $2.50 but who are unwilling or unable to pay $4.50 for it. The government policy, however, will ensure that they get the toothpaste by buying it for them. Thus, in the new equilibrium 180 tubes of toothpaste are bought by consumers at a price of $4.50 per tube, and 720 tubes are bought by the government at a price of $4.50 per tube.

Prices have nearly doubled as a result of government intervention. The number of people providing their own care has fallen from 500 to 180. The 180 are each

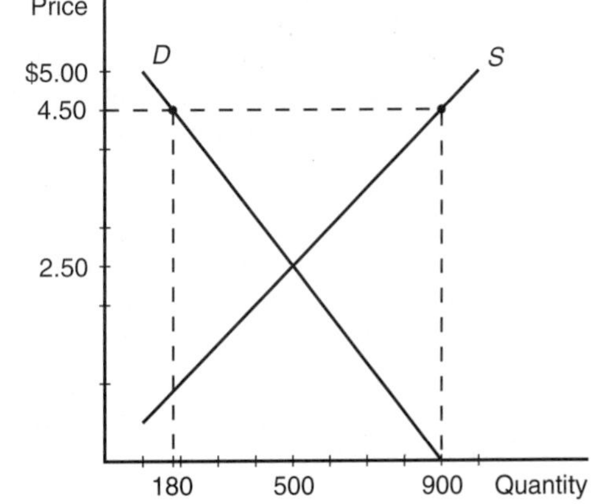

FIGURE 4–3. Supply and demand for toothpaste with government intervention.

paying nearly twice as much. In addition, there will be a tax of $3,240 to pay for the 720 tubes at $4.50 per tube. This compares with the $2,000 tax that was paid to take care of abscesses. It turns out that the new policy of toothpaste instead of abscesses is substantially more expensive, not less expensive as had been proposed.

What is the total size of the toothpaste industry? There are 900 tubes sold at $4.50 per tube, for a total charge of $4,050. Earlier there had been 500 tubes sold for $2.50 each for a total of $1,250. The good intentions of the government to provide direct care to avoid tooth abscesses has caused the number of tubes sold to nearly double and the revenues of the industry to increase nearly fourfold. Is it any surprise that health care costs rose dramatically in the decades following the introduction of Medicare and Medicaid?

Therefore, is it obvious that Medicare and Medicaid were mistakes? No, it is not. Perhaps society should be willing to spend substantial additional amounts of money to avoid tooth abscesses, diseases, morbidity, and mortality. Economics is a science, not a political party. Economics is essential because it allows us to analyze the impact of a policy.

Economists would argue that it is inappropriate to adopt a new policy, such as government payment for toothpaste, without considering the likely economic implications of that policy action. Once the costs of the action are known, economics does *not* make recommendations for or against the policy.

Lack of Full Information

A critical factor causing widespread market failure in health care is that the consumer typically has far less information than the seller. This lack of information makes it difficult for the buyer to make a rational, informed decision.

Consider an extreme hypothetical example. A consumer has a cough, and the doctor examines him. The doctor concludes that there is a 99.9% chance that the patient simply has a cold. If the patient has a cold, the cough will probably go away in a week or so. After 2 weeks perhaps 5% of patients will still have a cough.

If the cough does not go away, the doctor could then order an x-ray to determine if the patient has some more serious condition, such as tuberculosis or lung cancer. Assume that in one in a thousand cases there is a more serious condition.

What if the doctor, who happens to own an x-ray machine in his office, prescribes a chest x-ray for each person with a cough. The doctor has a personal incentive to do this, since a profit can be earned on each of 1,000 x-rays. Waiting two weeks and then prescribing an x-ray for the 5% who are still coughing will result in only 50 x-rays. In either case the doctor diagnoses the serious condition. However, in one way he can earn far more money.

Assume that no patient will incur a significant detriment by waiting the two weeks for the x-ray. When the physician recommends an x-ray, the patient is usually not an informed buyer. The physician recommends that the x-ray be taken to rule out any serious problem. The unknowing patients agree to the x-ray.

Had the patients been fully informed that they could save their money, wait two weeks, and then come back with no risk, many might opt to do so. The lack of complete information takes away an important element of choice from the patient.

This type of market failure can be corrected by a system of regulations. For example, the government could dictate when it is appropriate to prescribe a chest x-ray. The government has provided such restrictive regulations only reluctantly. The health services community has argued, successfully to a great extent, that the potential risk to the health of patients from extremely high regulation outweighs the economic benefits of reductions in inappropriate utilization.

Lack of Direct Patient Payment

The failure of the market to be efficient because of a lack of information is exacerbated by the fact that many patients have Medicare, Medicaid, Blue Cross, or some other insurance plan that will pay part or all of the cost of the x-ray. The high cost of health care services has induced many individuals to acquire health insurance. Health insurance represents a pooling of resources.

On the surface, insurance is clearly a good thing. Rather than some people being lucky and healthy and having little if any cost, while some are unlucky and ill and have costs that wipe out their life savings, everyone pays a set insurance premium, such as $2,000 per year. However, there are problems with insurance. Once the individuals have purchased the insurance, there is little incentive for them not to consume great amounts of health care services.

The impact of insurance is similar to the example in which the government purchased toothpaste. Once individuals are fully insured (assuming neither deductible nor co-payment), the price to them for health care services drops to zero. In that case, their demand is based on a price of zero. Market failure results in suboptimal use of resources. Health resources are consumed until their marginal utility is nearly zero, because of the zero cost. This drives up the total costs of providing health care services.

Monopoly Power

Market failure is often associated with lack of full competition. The basic foundations of free markets assume that there are a large number of buyers and a large number of suppliers for any good or service. If there is only one seller, that seller is referred to as a monopoly. Sometimes there are natural monopolies, where it only makes sense to have one supplier. Many public utilities fall into that category. Duplication of power plants and power lines would be technically wasteful. In such cases, government regulates prices to prevent the supplier from charging an excessive amount.

In small communities, hospitals may effectively be natural monopolies. It is too costly to build more than one hospital for the community. In that case, the hospital has the potential to charge substantially more than a hospital in a city with 100 hospitals. In the latter case, an individual wanting elective surgery could shop around for a hospital offering a reasonable price.

Another element of market failure in health care is that consumers often use the health care facilities and organizations used by their physician. Rather than having to compete directly for patients, hospitals, nursing homes, and home care agencies need only compete for physician referrals. Once the physician makes a recommendation, the patient is often locked in, even if there are other suppliers available. When it comes to the patient's health, especially if there is any chance of death or permanent disability, each health care provider is viewed as unique. For example, if the patient hears that a surgeon is good, the patient will be reluctant to shop around for another surgeon who is cheaper or who operates at a less expensive hospital. Thus monopoly power sometimes exists for health care providers even in the absence of single supplier monopolies.

If there is monopoly power, the price may not be driven down to a normal equilibrium level. The monopoly might find that more profits can be made at a higher price. Figure 4–4 considers this situation. Equilibrium is at the intersection of the supply and demand curves, with price P1 and quantity Q1. However, what if the monopoly charges price P2? Consumers will only purchase quantity Q2 at that higher price. However, the price is so high that the monopoly may make more profit selling less volume at a high price than by selling a higher volume at the equilibrium price. This is a result of the relatively inelastic demand for health care services.

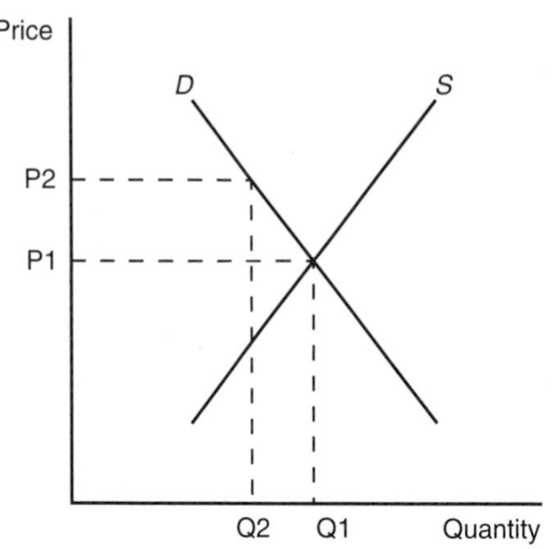

FIGURE 4–4. Example of monopoly power.

Increases in price may not lower the quantity demanded substantially. With competition, prices would fall to the equilibrium level; without competition, it pays for the provider to keep the price above equilibrium.

The government has traditionally tried to regulate public utility monopoly prices by fixing them at level P1. At that level consumers purchase Q1 quantity of services, and a free market outcome is achieved through intervention.

To the extent that the government pays health care providers directly for Medicare and Medicaid, the government is involved directly in setting the prices it is willing to pay. However, full regulation of health care pricing has not yet taken place, as it has in the case of public utilities. That means that many health care providers may have the ability to set artificially high prices to generate excessive profits.

Monopsony Power

At the same time, however, HMOs, other insurance companies, and employers are starting to exercise the power of large buyers. Blue Cross has exercised such power for many years. Just as it is possible to have a monopoly where there is only one seller, it is possible for there to be just one buyer. If there is only one buyer, it is called *monopsony.*

In recent years, there has been a great proliferation of HMOs and *preferred provider organizations* (PPOs; see Chapter 2). Insurance companies or employers direct their members or employees to use certain providers of health care in exchange for lower prices. In effect, the insurance companies are behaving as monopsonists. They control the buying of health care services for their populations. That provides them with market power to help them gain a better purchase price for the services.

Just as a supplier with monopoly power can dictate the price at which it sells a good or service, a monopsonist can dictate the price it pays to buy a good or service. For instance, suppose that the only employer for nurses in a geographic area is the local hospital. That hospital would be a monopsony.

The monopsony buyer pays low wages, which reduces the amount of supply. Fewer nurses are willing to work at such low wages. However, the savings from the lower wage offsets the financial losses from the inability to hire more staff. This may result in less care being provided. It is conceivable that part of the reason nursing shortages are frequently observed is that health care providers maintain an artificially low wage level for nurses because of their exercise of monopsony power.

Government-induced Inefficiency

Another problem creating market failure is the potential lack of incentive on the part of health care organizations to minimize costs of production. The government is often the cause of this technical inefficiency, because many government programs pay health care organizations their costs for providing care to specific groups of patients.

Without economic analysis, it might seem prudent for the government to reimburse an organization for its costs. It should save money, because the government will not have to pay for any profit. However, it provides a perverse incentive. It encourages organizations to keep costs high. Why work hard to control costs if you will be paid whatever you spend? There is no reward for low cost. History has shown that schemes that reimburse costs are not good tools for restraining the growth of health care costs.

Externalities

A last principal cause of market failure is the existence of *externalities.* Externalities exist when an action by an individual or organization has secondary effects on others that are not taken into account. For example, if a factory pollutes the skies, it may have found the cheapest way to produce its product, but as a side effect its pollution hurts people. Externalities may present additional costs or benefits to those affected. If a person goes to a hospital and is cured of a contagious disease, it benefits all those who might have caught the disease from that person.

If external costs and benefits are not taken into account, a nonoptimal amount of output may be produced. There could be too much pollution or too little health care. This represents a market failure. A mechanism is needed to correct the output level. In the case of pollution, the factory can be fined for polluting to make it realize the full costs of the pollution, including its negative external effect on others. This can cause it to reduce its output of pollution. In the case of health care, the government can tax all individuals for the positive external benefits they receive, and use the money collected to pay subsidies for health care.

In fact, the government does take that approach frequently. The government role is essential because of its ability to take collective action. As in the case of police and fire protection, the government can use collective action to benefit society.

※ THE MARKET FOR NURSES

A problem that has plagued the health care industry periodically for decades is a shortage of nurses, often followed by a surplus. These shortages have come and gone, with at least some shortages being noted in every decade since World War II. A critical issue is determination of whether nursing shortages occur because of market failure or whether the market is in fact functioning normally. The answer has serious ramifications for what the government should do to alleviate nursing shortages when they occur.

It is often argued that the primary cause of most nursing shortages is not a decreasing supply but an increasing demand. The number of nurses needed increases more rapidly than the supply. The result of an increase in demand with supply unchanged is a shift of the demand curve from D to D′ in Figure 4–5A. The new equilibrium, B, has a substantially higher wage than the original equilibrium, A. This higher wage entices more individuals to become educated as nurses. With higher wages, the profession is relatively more attractive than it was at the lower wage. This results, after a number of years, in an increased supply of nurses. Figure 4–5B shows the eventual shift in the supply curve as newly trained nurses enter the work force. The new supply, S′, removes the pressure for salaries to increase (faster than the general level of wages in society). And a new equilibrium exists at point C.

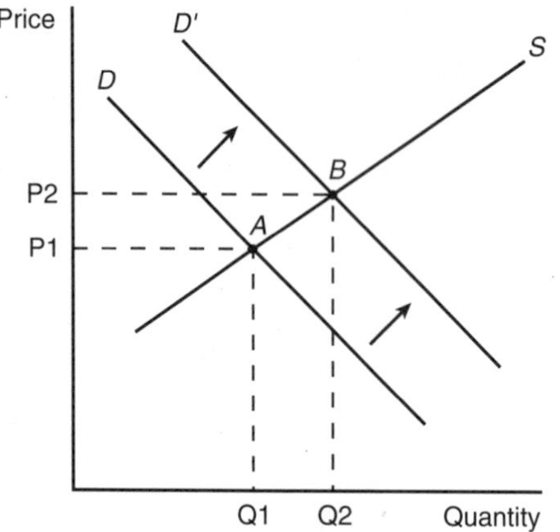

FIGURE 4–5A. Increase in demand for nurses.

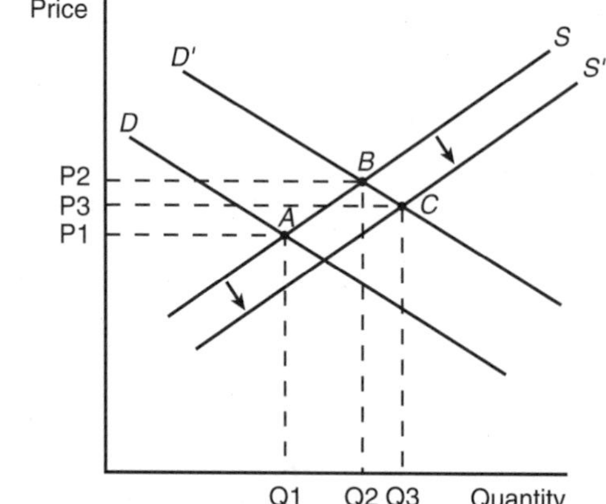

FIGURE 4–5B. Increase in supply of nurses.

Note that the equilibrium at C has a lower wage than that at point B. Wages, however, often do not adjust downward. Instead, a period of time may occur during which wages rise extremely slowly, if at all. The higher supply removes the pressure on employers to raise wages.

In fact, more nurses, Q3 as compared with Q2, are available. If the price stays at P2, an even greater number of nurses will be available. Consider where the P2 price would intersect with the S′ curve. It is at a quantity substantially higher than Q2 or Q3.

This analysis assumes that everyone has reasonably complete information. It is not likely, however, that employers know how much salaries must rise to reach an equilibrium. Therefore they raise salaries, but not enough, and then wait for the long-run education of more nurses. After several years, if the number of nurses being educated has not risen sufficiently, wages will again rise, gradually seeking the level at which enough nurses will be educated to meet the demand. If demand is continuing to rise during this period, it is difficult for supply to catch up.

The problem is made more complicated by the fact that other industries are also trying to attract qualified labor. The economic analysis of one industry is incomplete because it fails to consider possible increases in demand and wages in other industries.

Therefore the observed shortages of nurses could be the result of lack of information about the price at which sufficient individuals will be enticed into the industry. Or it could be the result of a moving target. Increasing demand plus wage increases in other industries could create a situation where prices are rising to attract more nurses, but simply not fast enough to eliminate the shortage. Both of these arguments revolve around the lag in perceptions until people realize that higher wages are available for nurses, followed by the time it takes to educate new nurses after they decide to enroll in nursing schools.

On the other hand, if this were the case, there should be increases in the numbers of students in nursing schools. It would be easy enough for the health care industry to consider whether wages are high enough by examining whether more students are applying to nursing schools and continuing to raise wages until applications start to rise.

If that is not the case, one might argue that the larger employers of nurses are :ting in a monopsonist fashion, artificially keeping wages low and enduring a ıortage of nurses in exchange for avoiding a higher total payroll cost.

IMPLICATIONS FOR NURSE MANAGERS

Accounting and finance are often viewed as elements of applied economics. We live in a society whose entire financial structure is built around a system of economics. That economic system permeates all institutions and organizations. It dictates the allocation of society's scarce resources.

The health care system, however, is largely an example of the failure of the economic system. Lack of information, monopoly power, and a variety of other factors cause the laws of supply and demand to fail to achieve normal free market equilibrium level. These failures lead to a need for a government role to help achieve efficient economic resource allocation.

Externalities and the power of collective behavior hold a special role in health care because of the value to everyone of living in a society that is basically healthy. This means that there is a further need for government intervention.

Compounding the need for a government role even further is the fact that most members of society believe that some degree of resource redistribution is essential for equity as well as for efficiency. This can allow the poorest members of society to be guaranteed at least a minimal level of health care services.

Within this complicated economic environment are nurses—nurses who want to know why their organizations do not provide more resources to their departments; nurses who want to know why salaries cannot be raised to levels that compensate more adequately for their skills and the sacrifices they make; nurses who want to know why everyone is not guaranteed the highest level of care.

The answers to these questions are complex. However, an understanding of the basic law of supply and demand and the inherent limited nature of all resources is a starting point in obtaining answers to these questions. The complications of market failure further explain why health care is one of the most highly regulated industries and why health care is sometimes viewed as best provided by a not-for-profit organization with a mission of providing care rather than a mission of maximizing profits.

As the reader goes through the remaining chapters of this book, the laws of supply and demand and the scarcity of resources should be kept in mind. The importance of incentives in understanding the likely behavior of individuals should be considered. The efficiency generated by economies of scale should be thought of. The elements of economics are fundamental to the realm of financial management issues faced by nurse managers.

KEY CONCEPTS

Economics Study of how scarce resources are allocated among their possible uses. As a management or policy tool, economics is used to ensure that individuals, organizations, and society make optimal use of their limited resources.

Economic goods Goods or services acquired by consumers that provide physical or psychic benefit. Goods or services are generally acquired through an exchange process.

Utility Benefit gained by consumers from either consuming or saving resources. Marginal utility is the additional utility gained from consuming one more unit of a particular good or service. Total utility is maximized by purchasing a set of goods and services such that the marginal utility or marginal benefit is the same for each item.

Supply and demand Supply is the amount of a good or service that all suppliers in aggregate provide at any given price. Demand is the amount of the good or service that consumers are willing to acquire at any given price. At an equilibrium price, the quantity offered and the quantity demanded are identical.

Free enterprise, capitalism, or market economy System where each individual can choose whether to invest wealth or capital in a business venture; workers can choose whether to work for that venture at the wages offered, and consumers can choose whether to buy the products of the venture at the requested price.

Elasticity of demand Degree to which demand increases in response to a price decrease, or decreases in response to a price increase. In general, the demand for health services is considered highly inelastic.

Economies of scale Cost of providing a good or service falls as quantity increases because fixed costs are shared by the larger volume. However, eventually large volume may lead to decreasing returns to scale, due to capacity constraints or shortages of labor or supplies.

Incentives Economics assumes that individuals and organizations act in their own best interests. Incentives such as health insurance deductibles are used to make it be in the individual's interest to act in a desired manner. They are often used by management to result in an improved use of an organization's scarce resources, or by government to improve the use of society's scarce resources.

Market efficiency In a fully functioning free market economy, resources are optimally allocated and used as a result of the supply-and-demand mechanism.

Redistribution of resources Even in a relatively efficient market, some government redistribution of resources can provide collective action that makes everyone better off, such as the provision of police and fire protection. Economic analysis can determine which redistributions can make everyone better off and no one worse off. Other redistributions of resources are done to improve equity. They may make some individuals better off and some worse off. Such redistribution requires an equity value judgment. Economics cannot determine a "correct" level of redistribution.

Market failure Situation in which the free market does not operate efficiently. Market failure may be the result of:

> **Government intervention** The role of the government in guaranteeing basic medical care to all individuals creates a distortion in the normal equilibrium, the effects of which should be minimized to the extent possible.
>
> **Lack of full information** There is a tremendous gap between the knowledge of the patient and the health care provider concerning what services are needed and how important they are. This lack of information prevents the consumer from making a rational, informed decision.
>
> **Lack of direct patient payment** The existence of health insurance allows individuals to consume more services than they would if they had to directly pay the full cost of the services.
>
> **Monopoly or monopsony power** Organizations with monopoly or monopsony power can sometimes make excess profits by maintaining prices of final products at a level higher than equilibrium, and the prices of inputs below equilibrium.

Government-induced inefficiency Decreases in technical efficiency may occur as a result of government reimbursement to health providers based on the cost of care provided.

Externalities An action by an individual or organization may have secondary effects on others that are not taken into account. These side effects may present additional costs or benefits to those affected.

SUGGESTED READINGS

Blair, Roger D., and Jeffrey L. Harrison, *Monopsony: Antitrust Law and Economics,* Princeton University Press, Princeton, NJ, 1993.

Cleverley, William O., *Essentials of Health Care Finance,* Aspen Publishers, Gaithersburg, MD, 1997.

Folland, Sherman, Allen C. Goodman, and Miron Stano, *The Economics of Health and Health Care,* Prentice Hall, Upper Saddle River, NJ, 1996.

Frech H. E. III, *Competition and Monopoly in Medical Care,* AEI Press, Washington, DC, 1996.

Getzen, Thomas, *Health Economics: Fundamentals and Flow of Funds,* John Wiley & Sons, New York, NY, October 1996.

Herzlinger, Regina E., *Market-Driven Health Care,* Addison-Wesley Publishing Company, Reading, MA, 1997.

Perkins, David, and Ann D. E. Clewer, *An Introduction to Health Economics: Theory and Cases,* Prentice Hall, Upper Saddle River, NJ, 1998.

Phelps, Charles E., *Health Economics,* 2nd edition, Addison-Wesley Publishing Company, Reading, MA, 1997.

Philip, Jacobs, *The Economics of Health and Medical Care,* Aspen Publishers, Gaithersburg, MD, December 1996.

PART

II

FINANCIAL ACCOUNTING

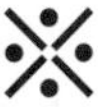

Financial accounting is the area of financial management that focuses on collecting and reporting information about the financial position of an organization and the results of its activities. Chapter 5 discusses the basic principles and terms of accounting and addresses the compilation of accounting information into financial reports that can be used by the organization's managers and other interested individuals. Chapter 6 explains the techniques commonly used to analyze and interpret the financial position of an organization and the financial results of its activities. ※

CHAPTER

5

Accounting Principles

CHAPTER GOALS

The goals of this chapter are to:

- Explain why accounting is important to health care organizations
- Describe the basic framework of accounting, including the fundamental equation of accounting
- Introduce the balance sheet and income statement
- Define a wide range of common accounting terminology
- Explain the process of recording accounting information and then summarizing and reporting that information
- Introduce and define the most common and important generally accepted accounting principles
- Describe the use of fund accounting in not-for-profit health care organizations
- Discuss the implications of financial accounting for nurse managers

※ INTRODUCTION

Accounting is a system that lets us keep "account" of things. Health care organizations have formalized accounting systems to track the financial well-being and financial success of the organization. The financial well-being and profitability of an organization may not be the most important elements of the organization's *mission* (see Chapter 10 for a discussion of organizational mission). The primary goals of the organization may relate to the types of care provided and the population served. The provider of health care services may not be hoping to financially profit from the provision of care. Nevertheless, the financial well-being and financial success of the organization are critical, because the organization must be financially viable to be able to meet the central elements of its mission.

Unless satisfactory financial results are achieved, the organization will be unable at best to acquire the latest technologies or expand services and, at worst, to pay its bills. The organization will then have to cease providing any care at all.

Therefore, a critical job of financial managers is to compile a set of financial reports, called *financial statements,* that convey to the reader information about the organization's financial position and the results of its activities. This information can be used by banks to decide whether to lend money to the organization, by philanthropists to determine whether to give it money, and by suppliers to decide whether to extend it credit. They can also be used by the organization's managers to decide whether the organization's financial results are satisfactory and how they could be improved.

The information contained in these reports can help nurse managers to know whether the organization has sufficient resources to provide larger raises, more staff, or capital expenditure requests, or whether the organization will need to substantially cut expenses just to avoid going out of business. Power is often said to reside with those who possess information. Certainly, an ability to understand and interpret the financial results of the organization is critical to ensuring that nursing receives an appropriate share of available organizational resources. Thus the study of financial accounting and the financial statements generated is not just an "academic" exercise but provides nurse managers with tools necessary for critical analysis of the financial status of the organization.

All organizations have a great number of financial transactions. Even a small nursing practice has hundreds or thousands of events each year that have a financial impact. A small home health care agency has thousands of such events during the year, and a large medical center may have tens of millions of such events. The job of accounting is to develop a system that can record each of the many events that have financial implications, summarize them, and report them in a manner that is useful to managers and other interested individuals.

This task is accomplished via the techniques of *financial accounting*. Financial accounting is a system that records historical financial information, summarizes it, and provides reports of what financial events have occurred and of the financial impact of those events. Accounting is not a science. It is based on a generally accepted set of conventions, rules, and terminology.

This chapter begins with an explanation of the basic framework upon which modern accounting rests. Next it introduces the central financial statements, which are called:

- Statement of financial position (or balance sheet)
- Statement of operations (or income statement)
- Statement of changes in net assets (or changes in equity)
- Statement of cash flows.

Understanding these financial statements is difficult, if for no other reason than that the accounting terminology they use is new to some readers. A section on terminology is provided in this chapter.

The chapter then discusses how financial information is recorded and reported by health care organizations. Such reporting often follows a set of rules referred to as generally accepted accounting principles (GAAP). There are specific reporting requirements or GAAP that health care providers must follow. Several of the most important of these principles are discussed. The chapter concludes with a brief discussion of accounting's implications for nurse managers.

※ THE BASIC FRAMEWORK OF ACCOUNTING

Accounting systems are established based upon one widely accepted *axiom*. This axiom is the basic equation of accounting:

Assets = Liabilities + Owner's equity

Assets are valuable resources that are owned by the organization. They may be either physical, having substance and form, such as a table or building, or intangible, such as the reputation the organization has gained for providing high-quality health care services. *Liabilities* are legal financial obligations the organization has to outsiders. Essentially they represent money that the organization owes to someone. These liabilities represent claims against the organization's assets. *Owner's equity* represents the amount of an organization's assets that the organization itself or its owners own.

The left-hand side of the equation represents all the valuable resources of the organization and is simply referred to as the asset side of the equation. The right-hand side of the equation represents all the claims against those valuable resources. These claims, both from outsiders and from owners, are referred to as *equities*. Therefore the right-hand side of the equation is referred to as the equity side. The equation is often referred to as the organization's assets and equities.

The owner's equity is a *residual* amount. When one subtracts the claims of outsiders from the total value of the organization's assets, whatever is left belongs to the organization or its owners. Imagine if you were to buy a house for $200,000 by placing $40,000 as a down payment and borrowing $160,000 from a bank. The $200,000 would represent the value of the house, which is an asset. The $160,000 would represent the mortgage obligation, which is a liability, and the $40,000 would be considered your *equity* in the house, which is an owner's equity. Note that if the house value were to rise or fall, the liability would remain unchanged. If the house suddenly became worth $250,000, the liability would still be $160,000, and your equity in the house would have risen to $90,000.

Since the owner's equity is a residual value, which rises and falls in response to changes in the assets and liabilities, the equation will always remain in balance. The owner's equity balance will be whatever it must be for the equation to be in balance. That forms the basis for all bookkeeping or accounting.

For proprietary or for-profit organizations, the owners may be sole proprietors, partners, or stockholders, depending on whether the organization is legally established as a *proprietorship, partnership*, or *corporation*. The owner's equity belongs to the owners of the organization. In the case of a not-for-profit organization, there is no owner per se. The organization exists for the good of the community at large. No individuals are entitled to benefit from any profits that might be generated by the organization. For not-for-profit organizations, the owner's equity is referred to as the *net assets* because it is equal to the organization's assets less its liabilities. This represents the balance of the funds after liabilities have been subtracted from assets.

※ THE CENTRAL FINANCIAL STATEMENTS

Financial information is conveyed to its ultimate users in the form of reports referred to as financial statements. The four key statements are the statement of financial position (the balance sheet), the statement of revenues and expenses (the operating or income statement), the statement of changes in net assets, and the statement of cash flows. The first two are discussed here, and the remaining two in Chapter 6.

The Balance Sheet

The most essential of the organization's financial reports is a document officially called the statement of financial position. This document is informally referred to as the balance sheet. The role of the balance sheet is to indicate the financial position of the organization at a specific point.

The balance sheet summarizes the fundamental equation of accounting. The assets are shown on the left side (or top) of the statement. The equities (liabilities plus owner's equity or net assets) are shown on the right side (or bottom) of the statement. A balance sheet for the hypothetical ABC Health Care not-for-profit organization appears in Table 5–1. The basic structure of financial statements is similar for different types of organizations.[1] Note that the total of the assets and the

---

[1]There are some differences in the specific detail of financial statements, depending on the type of organization. These differences reflect the diverse nature of health care organizations. The accounting industry official guide for accounting for health care organizations (*AICPA Audit and Accounting Guide: Health Care Organizations*, American Institute of Certified Public Accountants, New York, N.Y., 1996) includes illustrative financial statements for hospitals, nursing homes, continuing care retirement communities, home health agencies, health maintenance organizations, and ambulatory care organizations.

※ TABLE 5–1

ABC Health Care
Statement of Financial Position
as of June 30, 2000
(000s omitted)

Assets			Equities	
Current Assets			**Current Liabilities**	
Cash		$ 150	Wages payable	$ 1,123
Marketable securities		220	Accounts payable	2,430
Accounts receivable, *net* of $436 allowance for bad debts		2,319	Notes payable	500
Inventory		832	Deferred revenue	300
Prepaid assets		46	Taxes payable	145
Total current assets		$ 3,567	Total current liabilities	$ 4,498
Fixed Assets			**Long-Term Liabilities**	
Property, plant, and equipment	$43,470		Mortgage payable	$ 3,560
Less accumulated depreciation	17,356		Bonds payable	20,000
Net property, plant, and equipment		$26,114	Total long-term liabilities	$23,560
Sinking fund		1,737	**Net Assets**	
Investments		341	Unrestricted	$ 5,412
Goodwill		3,231	Temporarily restricted	520
Total fixed assets		$31,423	Permanently restricted	1,000
			Total net assets	$ 6,932
Total Assets		$34,990	**Total Equities**	$34,990

equities must always be equal. This is a result of the fundamental equation of accounting, which is required to always be in balance. If ABC Health Care were a for-profit organization, the net assets section of the balance sheet would be replaced. This is discussed later in this chapter.

The Operating Statement

When services are provided to patients, a charge is generally made. The monies received or expected to be received in exchange for services are called *revenues*. The costs of providing services are *expenses*. The revenues less the expenses represent the profit or loss of the organization.

Most organizations in industries other than health care refer to a statement that compares revenues to expenses as an income statement. This is logical because revenue less expense is defined as *net income* or *profit*. However, the not-for-profit firms in the health care industry have historically preferred not to use the words profit or income because they imply that the organization is profiting from the provision of health care. Instead, the income statement is referred to as the operating statement or statement of operations. Income is referred to as operating income or the increase in unrestricted net assets.

In practice, most not-for-profit organizations do earn a profit. This book uses the term "not-for-profit" rather than the common term "nonprofit." The term nonprofit implies that the organization does not make a profit. That is not a correct inference. A key goal of for-profit companies is to earn a profit. In not-for-profit organizations, a profit may be earned, but that profit is not the primary goal. Not-for-profit

※ TABLE 5–2

ABC Health Care
Statement of Operations
for the Fiscal Year Ending June 30, 2000
(000s omitted)

Revenues	
Patient revenues	$18,230
Other operating revenues	1,919
Total	$20,149
Expenses	
Wages for clinical services	$10,325
Patient care supplies and food	934
Housekeeping services	654
Operation and maintenance of plant	1,221
Administrative services	2,343
Depreciation and amortization	1,433
Bad debt expense	436
Interest	2,333
Total	$19,679
Operating Income	$ 470

organizations are exempt from a variety of taxes and are sometimes referred to as tax-exempt organizations.

However, profits *are* a necessary element for all health care organizations, even so-called not-for-profit organizations, for several reasons. First, to fulfill their mission many health care organizations must adopt new, expensive technologies as they become available. Profits earned on current patients help to pay for the adoption of new technology tomorrow. Second, many health care organizations want to expand both the range of services they offer and the number of people served. Such expansion requires the reinvestment of profits. Finally, the effect of inflation is to constantly increase the cost of replacing buildings and equipment as they wear out. Some profits must be earned to allow for replacement at higher prices.

Therefore, not-for-profit health care organizations do not exist for the purpose of making a profit, but making a profit does not represent improper behavior. Rather, it is indicative of an organization that will remain healthy enough to continue to provide services to its community.

An example of an operating statement for the hypothetical ABC Health Care appears in Table 5–2. If ABC Health Care were a for-profit organization, this statement would appear exactly the same as it does in Table 5–2.

※ ACCOUNTING TERMINOLOGY

Accounting is often referred to as the language of business. Numerous accounting terms become part of the everyday vocabulary of running an organization. Given the background you now have in the basic framework of accounting and the balance sheet and statement of operations, we can turn our attention to introducing the most common terms.

Assets

Some of the most common terms related to assets include:

- Liquid or liquidity

- Current assets
- Cash equivalents
- Marketable securities
- Fixed or long-term assets
- Liquidate
- Accounts receivable
- Allowance for uncollectible accounts or allowance for bad debts
- Prepaid assets
- Depreciate
- Depreciation
- Accumulated depreciation
- Sinking fund
- Goodwill
- Intangible
- Amortization

All these terms are discussed in this section. Consider Table 5–1. One of the first things to note about the balance sheet is the remark "000s omitted" (in the heading of the statement). This means that all numbers have been rounded off to the nearest thousand dollars. For example, cash of $150 is really cash of $150,000. There are several reasons for this optional rounding. One reason is that the financial statement is less cumbersome to read if some rounding is done. More important, financial statements are not as accurate as most people assume. Most accounting systems have many clerical errors. To eliminate all the errors would be extremely costly. Therefore, financial statements should be thought of as being reasonably, not precisely, accurate. Rounding off the numbers for presentation purposes helps to convey that the numbers are not exact measures.

The balance sheet presents the organization's assets in order of liquidity, from the most liquid to the least liquid. *Liquid assets* are cash or other assets that can quickly be converted to cash to pay the liabilities of the organization. Buildings and equipment, rent paid in advance, and investments set aside for future building expansions are examples of illiquid assets (having little liquidity). Organizations that have a great amount of cash and other liquid assets are relatively safer than those that are "illiquid." The most liquid assets are placed near the top of the balance sheet to give them prominence. This is done because one primary purpose of financial statements is to convey the financial stability of the organization—its ability to continue in business.

The first section on the asset side of the balance sheet is *current assets*. These are the resources that are cash, can be converted to cash within one year, or will be used up within one year. Current assets are often referred to as short-term or near-term assets. Current assets are more liquid than assets that are not current.

Within the current assets category, assets are grouped by liquidity. The first asset listed is cash. Cash includes not only money on hand but also *cash equivalents*, such as savings and checking accounts and short-term certificates of deposit. The next item is *marketable securities*. This includes investments in stocks and bonds. Similar investments are also included on the balance sheet under the heading of fixed asset or long-term asset investments. *Fixed or long-term assets* are assets that will not be used up or converted to cash within one year. The primary difference between marketable securities and fixed asset investments is intent. If management intends to sell, or *liquidate*, the stocks or bonds within one year of the balance sheet date, they are marketable securities. If the intent is to hold those securities for more than a year, they are fixed asset investments.

The next current asset listed after marketable securities is *accounts receivable*. These are amounts owed to the organization by purchasers of the organization's goods or services. Often a transaction occurs "on account." This means that payment is not made immediately. Instead, an account is opened that tracks the transaction until payment is made. For the provider of the service there is an account receivable. For the consumer of the service there is a mirror image, referred to as an account payable.

Accounts receivable are shown on the balance sheet "net." This refers to the fact that health care organizations often have bad debts; that is, there are some patients for whom payment is never received, even though the patients were expected to be able to pay for the care. Although the health care provider may not know who will not pay, an estimate must be made, and the amount of receivables shown on the balance sheet should be only the net amount that the organization estimates it will receive. If the gross amount of receivables outstanding were shown on the balance sheet, there would be an overestimate of the value of that asset. Therefore there is established an *allowance for uncollectible accounts,* sometimes called an *allowance for bad debts.* In Table 5–1 the total accounts receivable are $2,755,000, but when we subtract an estimated uncollectible portion of receivables equal to $436,000, the net accounts receivable are shown as $2,319,000.

Inventory is the next item listed in current assets. This represents the various supplies that will be used to provide goods or services. If a home health agency sells walkers and wheelchairs to its clients, it may keep a stock of them on hand. Also a wide variety of medical supplies such as sutures is needed for the patients to be treated. Those items purchased and then used in providing services are not considered expenses as soon as they are purchased; rather, they become a valuable resource, inventory, which becomes an expense only as it is used up.

The last item shown in current assets in Table 5–1 is *prepaid assets.* This represents assets that have been paid for and have not yet been used but will be used within one year. This includes items such as fire insurance premiums or rent paid in advance. These items are not expected to be converted back into cash, but they will be used up within one year, so they are considered current assets.

Fixed assets are listed on the balance sheet after current assets. Fixed assets consist primarily of property, plant, and equipment. This refers to the land, buildings, and pieces of equipment owned by the organization. Land is expected to last forever. However, buildings and equipment physically wear out with the passage of time. From an accounting perspective, they are said to *depreciate,* or decline in value or productive capability.

Suppose that a building costs $40 million when it is new, and it is expected to last forty years. Rather than show the entire cost of the building as an expense in the year it is purchased, accountants require that the cost be spread out over the expected useful lifetime of the building. The allocation of the $40 million cost over forty years is referred to as *depreciation.* The amount of the original cost allocated as an expense each year is the depreciation expense for that year. The total amount of depreciation that has been taken over the years the organization has owned the asset is referred to as the *accumulated depreciation.*

For instance, if the organization is taking depreciation expense of $1 million per year on the $40 million building and they have owned the building for ten years, the accumulated depreciation is $10 million and the net value is $30 million. The financial statement will show the original cost, the accumulated depreciation, and the net value. Note, however, that financial statements do not list each building and each piece of equipment. Instead, all similar items are combined and shown as one summary amount. In Table 5–1 the property, plant, and equipment represent the buildings owned by the organization, the land, and all pieces of equipment.

During the years that buildings and equipment get old, the organization tries to charge enough for its services to be able to collect an adequate amount of money to replace these assets when they have exhausted their useful life. However, sometimes the organization spends that money for current activities rather than saving it to replace long-term assets. To ensure adequate accumulation of resources for future major investments in buildings and equipment, the organization will sometimes establish a *sinking fund.* This is simply a segregated group of investments that can be used only for a specified purpose, generally replacement of plant and equipment or repayment of a loan taken to purchase that building and equipment.

The only asset on the example balance sheet that has not yet been discussed is *goodwill*. This is an *intangible* asset. It represents a measure of the value of the organization that goes beyond its specific physical assets. This includes good relationships with suppliers, a favorable reputation for high-quality care, and other similar values that are not easily quantified. Although most organizations have goodwill, they do not show it or any other intangible assets on their financial statements. This is because accountants have trouble measuring the true value of an organization's goodwill.

The only time that intangible assets appear on a financial statement is when the organization has purchased the intangible asset from someone else. Generally this occurs when one organization acquires another organization and has paid more than the value of that organization's specific tangible assets. In that case, accountants assume that the excess paid must have been a payment for the general goodwill of the organization. Otherwise, rather than buy the organization, one would have simply purchased similar tangible assets. Therefore, the excess paid is shown as goodwill, and the cost of the goodwill is depreciated over time.

The term depreciation, however, is only used for identifiable physical assets. Depreciation of intangible items is referred to as *amortization*. Amortize means to spread out or allocate. The cost of the intangible asset is spread out or allocated over the expected useful lifetime of the asset.

Equities

Equities consist of liabilities and owner's equity. The terms to be discussed in this section include:

- Current liabilities
- Long-term liabilities
- Wages payable
- Accounts payable
- Notes payable
- Taxes payable
- FICA
- Deferred revenues
- Mortgage payable
- Bonds payable
- Unrestricted net assets
- Temporarily restricted net assets
- Permanently restricted net assets

Liabilities are divided on the balance sheet into current liabilities and long-term liabilities. Current liabilities are obligations that are expected to be paid within one year. Long-term liabilities are obligations that are not expected to be paid within the coming year.

Current liabilities in Table 5–1 include wages payable, accounts payable, notes payable, deferred revenue, and taxes payable. Wages payable simply represent amounts that are owed to employees. Accounts payable generally represent amounts owed to suppliers (such as pharmaceutical or medical supply companies). Notes payable represent obligations to repay a loan. Depending on when the loan must be repaid, some notes payable are long-term liabilities. Taxes payable represent taxes owed to a local, state, or federal government. For-profit organizations must pay real estate, sales, and income taxes. Not-for-profit organizations are generally tax exempt. However, even if an organization is not-for-profit, it will likely have tax obligations. These usually relate to payroll deductions for employee income taxes and Social Security taxes (FICA) as well as unemployment and workmen's compensation taxes.

Deferred revenues are somewhat more complex. These represent payments that the organization has received in advance of providing its services. For example, suppose that under an arrangement with an employer in the area, your organization will provide primary care to that employer's employees. The employer makes quarterly payments in advance. The payment at the end of this year covers care to be provided in the first three months of next year. The money has been received, but the organization has not yet delivered any care. This money received will represent revenue in the future, but that recognition is deferred until the quarter of a year has passed and the services have been provided. Until then this deferred revenue is treated as a liability. This is because the organization is liable to repay the money it received if it does not keep its part of the bargain and provide the agreed-upon care.

Table 5–1 indicates two types of long-term liability: *mortgage payable* and *bonds payable.* A mortgage payable represents a loan secured by a specific asset. Mortgage payments, including interest and a portion of the liability balance, are generally made monthly. If the organization defaults on its required payments, the lender can take the asset and sell it to recover the balance of the loan.

A bond payable represents a formal borrowing arrangement where a certificate represents the debt. The certificate is legally transferable. For instance, one person lends money to a hospital and receives the bond certificate. The individual can sell that certificate to another person. The hospital is then obligated to repay the money borrowed to the new owner of the bond. Often, interest on bonds is paid only twice a year (semiannually), and the principal amount borrowed is not repaid at all until the maturity or termination date of the bond. Bondholders often are general creditors. Their loan to the organization is secured in general by all the assets of the organization rather than by a specific asset. When insufficient cash is available to make bondholder payments, the organization is often forced into bankruptcy. Therefore bonds may be a riskier way for organizations to borrow money than mortgages. However, the interest rate paid on bonds is often lower than would be obtainable with a mortgage.

The last equity section on the balance sheet is net assets or owners' equity. Note that no part of this section represent an available source of cash. This balance represents a claim of ownership of assets. All the valuable resources of the organization are on the asset side of the balance sheet.

There are three parts to the net assets section of the balance sheet of not-for-profit organizations, as seen in Table 5–1. These are *permanently restricted net assets, temporarily restricted net assets,* and *unrestricted net assets.* Permanently restricted net assets are generally the result of endowment gifts. Assets that have been given as a permanent endowment gift can never be spent by the organization. The donation is invested, and the income from the investment can be used for operating expenses. Temporarily restricted net assets are the result of gifts that have conditions. The conditions relate to a specific use for the donated assets, or a specific action the organization must undertake before using the assets, or a specific time period before the assets can be used. For example, the assets may not be able to be used until a research center is organized, or until five years have passed. All net assets that are neither permanently nor temporarily restricted are unrestricted.

As a reader of the balance sheet tries to evaluate the financial position of the organization, the segregation within net assets is helpful. In viewing the assets on the left side of the balance sheet, we know that a portion of them will be required to pay all of the liabilities of the organization. The net asset section of the balance sheet further informs the reader of the additional portion of the assets that cannot ever be spent because they are part of permanent endowment, as well as the portion of the assets that cannot be spent until some condition has been met. One should be careful to note that even unrestricted net assets do not necessarily represent liquid resources that can be used for any purpose the organization desires. It is likely that the unrestricted net assets of the organization have already been invested in the organization's land, building and equipment.

If ABC Health Care were a for-profit (or proprietary) organization, the balance sheet's assets and liabilities would appear the same as they do in Table 5–1. However, the owner's equity section of the right side of the balance sheet would be different. For-profit organizations would typically have Stockholders' Equity as the main owners' equity heading, instead of Net Assets.[2] A typical owners' equity section for a for-profit organization might appear as:

Stockholders' Equity	
Common Stock at Par Value	$ 100
Additional Paid-in Capital	900
Retained Earnings	5,932
Total Stockholders' Equity	$6,932

For-profit corporations sell shares of ownership in the organization. The corporation receives money it needs to operate a business, and the individuals receive shares of stock that represent ownership of the company. In many cases, corporations have issued stock that has a stated, or *par,* value. Par value is a technical legal concept that protects the stockholders from being sued for the debts of the corporation. Generally, one must pay more than the par value to buy stock from a corporation.

For example, a new nurse practitioner company might issue 1,000 shares of $1 par value stock, at $10 per share. The corporation would receive $10,000 in cash (i.e., 1,000 shares × $10 issue price per share = $10,000). The stock would show up in the Stockholders' Equity section of the balance sheet as Common Stock at Par Value $1,000 (i.e., 1,000 × $1 par value = $1,000) and Additional Paid-In Capital $9,000. The additional paid-in capital is simply the difference between the par value of the stock issued and the actual amount that the organization received for the stock it issued.

The retained earnings line in the Stockholders' Equity section represents the amount of profits that have been earned by the organization over the years, which have not been distributed to the owners in the form of a dividend. Often organizations retain profits and use them for expansion of services offered. However, retained earnings are not cash but a claim on ownership of a portion of the assets on the left side of the balance sheet.

Revenues and Expenses

Table 5–2 presents an operating statement for discussion. The terms to be discussed based on this statement include:

- Revenues
- Gross revenues *vs* net revenues
- Operating revenues
- Contractual allowances
- Gifts, donations, and contributions
- Wage, patient care supply, depreciation, administrative, and other operating expenses
- Bad debts
- Charity care

The decade of the 1990s produced a number of important changes in health care financial statements. Before 1990, health care organizations started their operating statement with gross patient revenues. Gross revenues are the charges for all service

[2]For-profit organizations can be organized as sole proprietorships or partnerships, rather than corporations. However, the corporate form is popular because it limits the liability of owners to the amount they have invested in the organization. In contrast, sole proprietors and partners are liable for all of the debts of an organization that they own.

care provided. However, in many cases, health care organizations received less than 100% of their charges from some payers. Some were too poor to pay anything (charity care); some patients just never paid their bill (bad debts); and some payers received discounted prices (contractual allowances). Therefore statements of revenues and expenses would subtract from patient revenues an amount for contractual allowances, bad debts, and charity care. This approach is no longer permitted.

Consider a car dealership that negotiates the price at which each car is sold. Would the auto dealer report revenue as the total of the actual amounts that all the cars were sold for, or the total of the sticker (list) prices? Clearly, the sales are the sum of the negotiated prices, not the artificially high list prices shown on the car stickers. The old health care approach was comparable to showing the total of the sticker prices of the cars rather than the total of the agreed-upon prices.

Under the current generally accepted accounting principles (GAAP), the operating statement starts with net patient service revenues and other operating revenues (such as gift shop or cafeteria sales).[3] Patients who pay for their own care, as opposed to those having Medicare, Medicaid, or HMO insurance, may well pay a different price than these large "third-party payers" do. In many cases governments and large customers (e.g., HMOs) pay a rate lower than the hospital charges. These discounts are referred to as *contractual allowances.* Sometimes they are mandated by law rather than resulting from a contractual agreement. Current accounting rules require that patient revenues be shown after discounts have been deducted. The amount of contractual allowances does not have to be shown on financial statements.

Expenses are subtracted from revenues on the operating statement. Expenses are the costs related to generating the revenues of the organization. These include wages, patient care supplies, depreciation, administrative costs, and a wide variety of other types of costs.

Bad debts are shown on the financial statement as an operating expense. Thus the care provided to patients who ultimately do not pay the hospital, although they were expected to pay, are included as revenues. They are then subtracted as a bad debt expense. This contrasts with the accounting treatment for charity care. Most health care organizations provide at least some care to patients who they do not expect will be able to pay for that care. Under GAAP, charity care is excluded from revenues.

A major controversy surrounds the appropriateness of tax-free, not-for-profit status of health care organizations. The amount of charity care provided is one piece of information that is critical for those interested in this controversy. Under GAAP, the amount of charity care provided must be disclosed, either on the financial statement in parentheses or in the notes that accompany the financial statements (see Chapter 6 for a discussion of such notes). It is incumbent on each health care organization to carefully define the difference between bad debts and charity care.

※ THE RECORDING AND REPORTING PROCESS

How does one develop financial statements? The statements are based on recording each individual event that has a financial impact on the organization, aggregating that information, and finally developing a summarized form to convey it.

---

[3]American Institute of Certified Public Accountants, AICPA, *Audits of Providers of Health Care Services,* New York, N.Y., 1990.

Journal Entries

When a financial event occurs, it is recorded in a *general journal*. The general journal is called the book of original entry because it is the first place that the accounting system makes recognition of the event. When the event is recorded, it is called a *journal entry*. The general journal provides a complete chronological financial history of the organization.

The entries are recorded in the journal using *double-entry accounting*. This term would seem to imply that the entry is recorded twice. That is not the case. Journal entries are made based on the fundamental equation of accounting. That equation begins the year in balance. Every financial event must leave the equation in balance. For instance, suppose that a patient pays the organization $100 in cash. How does that affect the financial records of the organization? Clearly, the organization's cash has risen by $100. But if we simply record a cash increase of $100, can the equation remain in balance?

We must examine the impact on assets, on the left side of the equation, and equities (liabilities and net assets), on the right side

Assets	=	Liabilities	+	Net Assets
Cash +$100				

Cash has increased the left side of the equation by $100, but the right side is unchanged. The equation does not balance. In double-entry accounting, whenever one change is made to the accounting equation, at least one other change must be made as well. In this case, suppose that the patient had just received the care. The $100 is revenue for the organization. Revenues represent an increase in net assets. Therefore the change to the equation should have been the following double entry:

Assets	=	Liabilities	+	Net Assets
Cash +$100				Revenues +$100

Suppose that the patient had received care two months ago and was just now paying for that care. At the time the care was provided the organization would have recorded the revenue because it was legally entitled to be paid for the care provided. At that time it would also have recorded an account receivable, an asset representing the legal right to receive payment. What would be recorded when the payment was received?

Assets		=	Liabilities	+	Net Assets
Cash	+$100				
Accounts receivable	−$100				

The left side of the equation has increased due to the receipt of cash and decreased due to the reduction in the account receivable from the patient. The equation remains in balance. Double-entry bookkeeping does not require both sides of the equation to change; it only requires the equation to still balance after the transaction. In this manner, any financial event can be recorded, leaving the fundamental equation in balance.

As a technical way to minimize arithmetic errors, accountants use *debits* and *credits* (abbreviated *Dr.* and *Cr.* based on the Latin roots of the words). A debit is simply an increase in an item on the left side of the equation. A credit is simply an increase in an item on the right side of the equation. Decreases are the opposite; for example, a decrease in an asset is a credit. The bookkeeping rule, debits must equal credits, is a way to help ensure that the equation is in balance.

For example, an increase on the left side of the equation and an increase on the right side will cause both debits and credits to increase by a like amount. An increase on the left side and a matching decrease on the left side will also cause debits and credits to increase by a like amount, since assets increase with a debit and decrease with a credit.

The use of debits and credits is a technical device and does not have any real substance. Nevertheless, because assets can either be debited or credited, depending on whether they rise or fall, as can equities, the technique is complicated. It is further complicated by the fact that the organization looks at the world from its viewpoint, while we generally look at the world from our own viewpoint. For instance, when we receive a debit memo from the bank, it reduces our cash balance. Therefore cash would seem to decrease with a debit.

However, cash is an asset, and assets increase with a debit. A decrease should be a credit! The seeming paradox is caused by the fact that we view the world from our perspective, not the bank's. When you have money in a bank, you have essentially loaned that money to the bank. The bank has a liability (right side of the equation) to pay you back. The bank issues a debit memo, meaning that it owes you less money. Its liability to you has decreased. When a liability decreases, the result is a debit. This views the world from the perspective of the bank. From *your* perspective, however, your asset has decreased, resulting in a credit on your records.

The bookkeeping use of debits and credits is further complicated by the fact that the same term can mean something good or bad. If your organization provided care and received payment, that is financially good. Revenue (an equity) goes up with a credit; therefore a credit is a good event. Cash (an asset) goes up with a debit; therefore a debit is a good event. However, when you pay cash, the asset amount decreases. That is a credit, and is not necessarily good. The lay usage that a credit is good ("He's a credit to the organization") is ambiguous. (Is he a credit like revenue or a credit like money leaving our account?)

When journal entries are made, they are sometimes specified in detail in a *subsidiary journal,* with only a summary entered in the general journal. For example, if the organization treats 100 patients on a given day, the many entries related to the revenue and accounts receivable from each patient may be recorded in the subsidiary revenue journal, with only a total summary amount shown in the general journal.

Ledgers

Although the journal provides a complete permanent financial chronological history, it is somewhat cumbersome to use. If one wanted to know how much cash the organization had, one would have to go back to each journal entry, see whether it changed the cash balance, and sum all the journal entries that had an impact on cash. To simplify this process, accounting uses a set of *ledgers.*

A ledger is referred to as a book of accounts. Each page in the book represents a different item that we would like to keep track of or keep "account" of. When the journal entry is recorded, each item in the journal entry is *posted* to a ledger account. Posting means to copy over or transfer the item. Thus, when a patient pays $100 that had been owed for two months, in addition to the journal entry shown above, the accountant would also add $100 to the cash ledger account and deduct $100 from the accounts receivable ledger account. At some point, if we would like to know how much cash we have, we do not have to go through all the individual journal entries; instead we can simply go to the ledger and look at the balance in the cash account.

As with the journal, there are also *subsidiary ledgers.* Thus the general ledger does not have a page for each patient who owes the organization money but one master account for accounts receivable. However, a subsidiary accounts receivable ledger keeps track of the balance owed to the organization by each and every patient.

In today's computerized environment, only smaller organizations (e.g., small home care agencies) keep manual journals and ledgers. Instead, these records are generally maintained in computer files. Whether the accounting system is manual or computerized, journals and ledgers are essential tools for recording financial events.

Reporting Information

When journals and ledgers are maintained, it is a straightforward process to report the financial results of the organization. At the end of an accounting period the accumulated balance in each ledger account is reported on the appropriate financial statement. Asset and liability accounts are used to prepare a balance sheet. Revenue and expense accounts are used to prepare an operating statement. The excess of revenues over expenses (i.e., the net income) represents a profit that is retained in the organization. It causes the net assets at the beginning of the year to increase to its level at the end of the year.

The organization can generally choose a year-end date that is convenient. *Fiscal years* do not have to coincide with the calendar year. In some states there is a regulation that mandates a particular year end. Unless that is the case, most organizations choose to end their year when they are at a relatively slow time, so that the extra bookkeeping needed at year end does not pose an unnecessarily great burden.

The use of ledger account balances to create financial statements allows a tremendous number of financial events to be summarized. The financial statements in turn convey to the user information about the organization's financial condition and the financial results of its activities.

※ GENERALLY ACCEPTED ACCOUNTING PRINCIPLES

Accounting is a set of rules, not a clear-cut science. These rules are generally followed by both *internal* and *external accountants.* Each organization has its own accountants who keep track of financial information throughout the year as it occurs. Those accountants are referred to as internal accountants. There are also accountants who work for separate certified public accounting companies. Those accountants are referred to as external accountants or external *auditors.* Many organizations hire certified public accountants (CPAs) to *audit* or examine their financial records once a year.

A CPA is someone who has been licensed by the state. Licensing as a CPA indicates a level of expertise in accounting and auditing. *Auditing* is a function that examines the accuracy and completeness of financial records. In an audit by a CPA the financial records of the organization are examined to discover significant errors, to evaluate the organization's accounting system, and to determine whether financial statements have been prepared in accordance with generally accepted accounting principles.

Generally accepted accounting principles (GAAP) are rules established by the Financial Accounting Standards Board (FASB). CPAs are required to indicate whether an audited set of financial statements is in compliance with GAAP. Many health care organizations are required to have financial statements that have been audited by a CPA. Therefore, the majority of health care organizations follow GAAP. A few of the most common and important GAAP include:

- Entity concept
- Going-concern concept
- Matching principle and cash *vs* accrual accounting
- Cost principle
- Objective evidence
- Materiality
- Consistency
- Full disclosure

The Entity Concept

The *entity* is the person or organization that is the focus of attention. A large medical center that includes a hospital, nursing school, medical school, and long-term care facility is an entity. Accounting records may be kept for that entity as a whole. However, the hospital, nursing school, medical school, and long-term care facility are also entities. Financial records could be maintained separately for each of these subentities. When financial statements are prepared, it is important to identify the specific identity of the entity to which the statements relate.

All accounting transactions must take the perspective of the entity for which the financial statements report. For example, suppose that we are interested in learning about the finances of the nursing school. Suppose further that the nursing school purchased some supplies from the hospital but has not paid for them. On the financial records of the entity we are looking at, there would be an account payable to indicate the obligation to pay for the supplies. On the records of the hospital entity there would be an account receivable because it has not yet been paid for the supplies it provided.

Going Concern

The second critical GAAP is that of the *going concern*. There is a presumption when accounting records are prepared that the entity is going to continue in business into the future. If there is a strong possibility that the entity is going to go out of business, a special indication of that fact is required. The reason for this stems from the fact that assets may be valuable to an ongoing organization but have much less value if the organization goes out of business.

The Matching Principle and Cash *vs* Accrual Accounting

The simplest way to record revenues and expenses is on a *cash basis*. When cash is received, revenue is recorded. When cash is paid, expense is recorded. This easy approach does not necessarily give a fair picture of what has happened to the organization in any given fiscal year. Suppose that we provide care to a patient who immediately pays the organization. However, our staff will not be paid their biweekly salary until the second day of the next year. The profit for the year will be overstated because it does not reflect all the costs of providing the care.

Consider further what happens when a building is purchased on the cash basis of accounting. The entire cost of the building would be an expense in the year we pay for the building. In that year the organization would show a huge loss.

To avoid such results that do not truly reflect how well the organization did in a given year, accountants rely on the matching principle, which gives rise to *accrual accounting*. The matching principle requires that organizations record expenses in the same year as the revenues they help to generate. Thus revenue and related expense are matched. Revenues are recorded in the accounting period that the organization becomes legally entitled to them. Even if the cash is not yet received, the organization accrues (i.e., accumulates or adds) the revenue to other current year revenue to find the total revenue for the year.

Accrual accounting helps the organization provide a full picture of current year activities. For example, vacation days that are earned this year but not yet taken by year end must be accrued. The vacation expense is recorded as part of the current year expenses because the vacation expense is a part of the cost of the labor that treated patients and generated revenue this year. Accrual accounting also gives rise to depreciation, ensuring that part of the cost of a fixed asset is recorded as an expense in each year that the fixed asset is used to generate revenues, rather than all in the year the asset is purchased.

Accrual accounting is more complicated than cash accounting. However, because it provides a fairer picture of what has occurred in each year, it is required for most organizations.

The Cost Principle

The cost of any resource is the amount that the organization pays to acquire that resource. Assets are generally recorded on the balance sheet at a value equal to their cost.

There are some exceptions to this straightforward concept. For example, depreciation charges off the original cost of some assets over a period of years. Therefore the net plant and equipment value will appear on the balance sheet at a level lower than the original purchase cost.

The cost principle, seemingly innocuous, creates serious problems in the interpretation of balance sheet information because over time the value of many assets may vary from their original cost. For example, land may rise substantially in value. Nevertheless, it remains on the balance sheet at its cost. This is largely the result of the principle of *objective evidence.*

Objective Evidence

The principle of objective evidence holds that information reported on financial statements should be based on objective, verifiable evidence. This is evidence that a wide group of different individuals could all be expected to agree upon.

For example, there could be considerable discussion concerning what a patient monitor is currently worth. Some might argue that it is worth what we paid for it. Others might contend that it is worth what we could sell it for. Another choice is that it is worth the amount we would have to spend if we were to replace it today. Yet another view would be that its value is based on the revenues it allows the organization to generate. Each of these perspectives has some merit; however, most of them are subjective measures.

How much revenue will a hospital generate because it has a particular patient monitor? That is clearly subject to speculation. We cannot know what future revenues will be. How much could we sell the monitor for? Again, a speculative question, unless we actually sell the monitor, which we have no intention of doing. Accountants wish to avoid speculation because it makes it hard to interpret financial statement information. Was the estimate of value made by an optimist or pessimist? It is much simpler to use objective, verifiable evidence.

As a result, accountants record the value of assets at their cost, since we can generally get agreement on the exact amount that was paid to acquire an asset. On the up side, the user of the financial statement does not have to worry about the introduction of bias in valuing the asset. On the down side, balance sheet information often is not a good measure of what assets are really worth. In many cases the assets that appear on financial statements substantially underestimate the value of the assets owned by the organization.

In contrast, however, recent changes to GAAP require marketable securities to be shown at their fair market value. Prior to recent rule changes, such assets were shown on the balance sheet at their cost. The market value was shown only if it was lower than the cost. This rule was changed because stock and bond market quotations are considered objective evidence.

Materiality

The accounting process requires the recording of thousands, millions, and even billions of individual financial transactions. Practice has shown that it is generally impossible to undertake such a task and expect it to be error free. In general, errors occur with any accounting system, and to try to eliminate all errors would be extremely costly. Therefore, accounting systems are designed to try to minimize the number and size of errors.

How many errors of what size are acceptable? To answer that question, accountants rely on the concept of *materiality*. Individual error, or all errors in aggregate, if not material in amount can be tolerated. What amount represents a material error? Is it $5, or $500, or $50,000? The answer to that question depends on a number of factors, such as the size of the organization. Accountants do not have a standard dollar cutoff that can be arbitrarily applied to all organizations; rather, they focus on the likely users of the financial information. An error in a financial report that would cause a user of the financial statement to change a decision is material.

Suppose we expect the organization's financial statements to be used by a bank when it decides whether to lend money. Assets overstated by a small amount would probably have no effect on the bank's loan decision. If assets are mistakenly overstated by a substantial amount, the bank might lend money that it would not have loaned if it had known the correct amount of assets. That would be a material misstatement of financial position. Therefore, accountants must decide what amount of money in a given situation is so large that it would likely affect the decisions of users of the financial statement. Then the accountant must attempt to ensure that if any errors of that magnitude occur, they are discovered and corrected before the financial statements are disseminated.

Note that the final financial statements are therefore not expected to be error free. They are only expected to be free of any material errors.

Consistency

In some instances, organizations have choices among alternative allowable accounting methods. The choice may have an impact on the balance sheet and statement of revenues and expenses of the organization. In such cases, the organization should be consistent in its choice from year to year. To vacillate would confuse users of the financial statement who might be attempting to compare the organization's financial performance from year to year.

Full Disclosure

Financial statements should be a fair representation of the financial position and results of operations of an organization, in accordance with GAAP. The principle of full disclosure is simply a catchall. This principle requires disclosure of any information that would be needed for the financial statements and accompanying notes, taken as a whole, to present a fair representation of the finances of the organization.

In the case of health care organizations the principle of full disclosure requires that an audited set of financial statements include a balance sheet and an operating statement. However, such disclosure would also generally require a cash flow statement, a statement of changes in net assets, and a set of explanatory notes. These items are discussed in Chapter 6.

FUND ACCOUNTING

Historically, not-for-profit organizations developed specialized accounting methods to deal with the unusual *fiduciary* nature of the organizations. A fiduciary is someone in a position of trust. The fiduciary of a not-for-profit organization controls assets that belong to the community. For-profit corporations can be expected to be closely monitored by the stockholders of the organization. Not-for-profit organizations have no owners, and therefore there are fewer "watchdogs" making sure that managers work to carry out the mission of the organization. The response to this problem was to divide authority, preventing any one manager of a not-for-profit organization from having excessive control over the organization and its assets. This divided authority was accomplished by using *fund accounting.*

Fund accounting is a system of separate financial records and controls. Distinct funds are established. Each fund has control over certain portions of the assets of the organization, and each fund has its own separate set of financial records. One could prepare a balance sheet for each fund. Typical health care organization funds include the *general operating fund,* which is considered *unrestricted* and can be used for any valid organization purpose. Other funds are typically *restricted,* and their assets can be used only for their stated purpose. These funds include the *endowment fund,* the *building fund,* and a variety of *special purpose funds.* Donor restrictions can be removed only by the donor.

Historically, a different manager has control over each fund. This, for example, prevents the chief operating officer, who is in charge of day-to-day operations, from embezzling the endowment fund. It also prevents the comingling of funds (i.e., mixing together in one pot). That way donors are assured that endowment funds will not be used to pay for current activities.

The name *fund accounting* is logical because the organization divides the resources or funds available to it into separate categories, called funds. The term *fund balance* then results from the idea that when the liabilities of each fund are subtracted from its assets, the remaining amount is the balance owned by the organization, or simply the fund balance. The fund balance represents the net assets for one specific fund.

Over the last half-century the use of separate fiduciaries for each fund has mostly been discontinued. For example, the chief executive officer of most organizations has substantial control over all of the organization's funds. Nevertheless, many not-for-profit health care organizations continue to use fund accounting because it helps provide assurance that restricted assets are used for their intended purpose.

Although many not-for-profit health care organizations use fund accounting for internal purposes, all funds must be combined when audited financial statements are prepared. It is believed that viewing the results of operations and the financial condition of the organization as a whole gives the reader a better understanding of the organization.

⁜ IMPLICATIONS FOR NURSE MANAGERS

Basic accounting concepts are critical tools for nurse managers on two levels. First, nurse managers must be able to communicate with financial managers of the organization. Second, accounting provides information that is of critical value to nurse managers as they help to steer the overall direction of the organization.

The need to garner resources for nursing and to work with the organization to control the use of resources requires that nurse managers be able to communicate with financial managers, to be able, at least to some extent, to talk their language. Many aspects of basic accounting become part of the lives of most managers. For example, journal entries are a common bookkeeping element that most managers become familiar with, at least on a mechanical level.

Going beyond that mechanical level and learning about things such as GAAP allows the nurse manager to comprehend why certain things are done, such as depreciating capital equipment. It should also serve to put many of the bookkeeping tasks nurse managers perform into their broader context.

Further, however, nurse managers must look beyond their departments to focus on what the organization as a whole must do to survive and thrive in a difficult economic environment. An understanding of accounting and financial statements is critical to being able to assess the financial position of the organization. That information in turn is needed to be able to participate in an informed manner concerning the critical strategic decisions faced by health care organizations.

Chapter 6 takes the nurse manager a step further in developing a capability to understand the organization's financial situation with a discussion of interpretation and analysis of information contained in financial statements.

KEY CONCEPTS

Accounting System to track financial events and provide information essential to undertaking the financial well-being and financial success of the organization.

Fundamental equation of accounting Assets = Liabilities + Net Assets. Assets are the valuable resources owned by the organization; liabilities are amounts the organization owes to outsiders; net assets, or owner's equity, is the portion of the organization's assets owned by the organization or its owners.

Balance sheet Financial statement that presents the financial position of the organization at a specific point in time.

Operating or income statement or statement of revenues and expenses Financial statement that presents the financial results of the organization's activities for a specific period.

Depreciation Allocation of a portion of the cost of an asset with a multiyear life into each of the years the asset is expected to be used to help generate revenues.

Journal Book (or computer file) in which the financial events of the organization are recorded in chronological order, following the rules of double-entry accounting, which require every transaction to affect at least two different financial accounts, to keep the fundamental equation of accounting in balance.

Ledgers Set of individual accounts. Information from the journal is transferred (posted) to the ledger accounts so that the balance in any account can be easily determined and reported on financial statements.

Generally Accepted Accounting Principles (GAAP) Set of rules adopted by the accounting profession that facilitates interpretation of financial statements by users outside the organization.

Fund accounting Optional accounting system used by not-for-profit health care organizations that establishes a complete distinct set of accounting records for separate groupings of the organization's assets. These groupings consist of a general unrestricted operating fund and a series of restricted funds set aside for specified purposes such as endowment or new buildings.

SUGGESTED READINGS

American Institute of Certified Public Accountants, *AICPA Audit and Accounting Guide for Health Care Organizations*, AICPA, New York, N.Y., 1996.

Emery, Douglas R., John D. Finnerty, and John D. Stowe, *Principles of Financial Management*, Prentice Hall, Upper Saddle River, N.J., 1998.

Finkler, Steven A., *Finance and Accounting for Nonfinancial Managers*, revised and expanded edition, Prentice Hall, Upper Saddle River, N.J., 1996.

Gapenski, Louis C., *Financial Analysis and Decision Making for Healthcare Organizations: A Guide for the Healthcare Professional*, Irwin Professional Publishers, Burr Ridge, Ill., January 1997.

Granof, Michael H., *Government and Not-for-Profit Accounting: Concepts and Practices*, John Wiley & Sons, New York, N.Y., 1998.

Guy, Dan M., C. Wayne Alderman, and Alan J. Winters, *Auditing*, 2nd edition, Harcourt, Brace, Jovanovich, San Diego, Calif., 1990.

Harrison, Walter T., and Charles T. Horngren, *Financial Accounting* (Charles T. Horngren Series in Accounting), Prentice Hall, Upper Saddle River, N.J., January 1998.

Horngren, Charles T., and Gary L. Sundem, *Introduction to Financial Accounting,* 7th edition, Prentice Hall, Upper Saddle River, N.J., 1998.

Keown, Arthur J., J. William Petty, David F. Scott, Jr., and John D. Martin, *Foundations of Finance,* 2nd edition, Prentice Hall, Upper Saddle River, N.J., 1998.

Larkin, Richard E., *Wiley Not-for-Profit GAAP 98,* John Wiley & Sons, New York, 1998.

Levy, V. M., *Financial Management of Hospitals,* Wm Gaunt & Sons, Holmes Beach, Fla., January 1998.

McKeon, Tad, *Home Health Financial Management,* Aspen Publishers, Gaithersburg, Md., January 1996.

McLean, Robert A., *Financial Management in Health Care Organizations,* Delmar, Albany, N.Y., 1996.

Neumann, Bruce R., Jan P. Clement, and Jean C. Cooper, *Financial Management: Concepts and Applications for Health Care Organizations,* Kendall/Hunt Publishing, Dubuque, Iowa, May 1997.

Samuels, David I., *The Healthcare Financial Management/Budgeting Toolkit,* Richard D. Irwin, Burr Ridge, Ill., December 1997.

Stickney, Clyde P., and Roman L. Weil, *Financial Accounting: An Introduction to Concepts, Methods, and Use,* 8th edition, Dryden Press, Fort Worth, Tex., 1997.

Ward, William J., Jr., *Health Care Budgeting and Financial Management for NonFinancial Managers: A New England Healthcare Assembly Book,* Auburn House Publishers, Westport, Conn., January 1994.

Zelman, William N., Michael J. McCue, and Alan R. Milikan, *Financial Management of Health Care Organizations: An Introduction to Fundamental Tools, Concepts, and Applications,* Blackwell Publishers, Cambridge, Mass., January 1998.

CHAPTER

6

Analysis of Financial Statement Information

CHAPTER GOALS

The goals of this chapter are to:

- Introduce the techniques for interpretation and analysis of financial statements
- Explain the role and nature of an independent audit and the information available in an audited report
- Introduce and describe the statement of cash flows
- Introduce and describe the statement of changes in net assets
- Discuss the types of information contained in notes that accompany financial statements
- Discuss how to assess the financial performance of an organization, including the use of the statements, notes, and ratio analysis
- Provide definitions of common ratios and examples of ratio analysis
- Distinguish between financial statements and other management reports
- Consider the implications of financial statement analysis for nurse managers

⁜ INTRODUCTION

Much of accounting is useful for any manager carrying out the day-in and day-out activities of an organization. Understanding the general financial status of the organization can help managers to better focus their department's efforts to help the overall organization. In addition, as nurse managers work to gain a more central role in management of the organization as a whole, it becomes important to be able to understand as much as possible about the overall financial well-being of the organization. Nurses want to become part of major decisions, such as whether to add or replace equipment and buildings, and the choice of how to finance such expansions. To get involved in broader issues than the management of a unit or department, it is absolutely necessary to be able to interpret and analyze information about the financial status of the organization.

Chapter 5 discussed the fundamental concepts of financial accounting. The framework of accounting, terminology of accounting, the balance sheet (statement of financial position), the operating statement, recording and reporting accounting information, generally accepted accounting principles (GAAP), and fund accounting were all covered. That provides a foundation for understanding the accounting elements of the organization. However, it does not provide the reader with the tools necessary to interpret and analyze the information that the accounting process can make available. Those tools are the subject of this chapter.

One of the most useful financial documents is the annual *audit* report. This report includes key financial statements, notes to the financial statements, and an opinion letter from an independent auditor. The information contained in an audit report provides a solid foundation for gaining an understanding of the historical results and current financial condition of the organization. This chapter begins with a discussion of the independent audit.

An audit report includes the balance sheet and operating statement (see Chapter 5). It also generally includes a statement of cash flows and statement of changes in net assets. All of these statements are essential for gaining a full understanding of the finances of the organization, and a discussion of them is included in this chapter.

GAAP require that an audit report contain full disclosure of relevant items. To comply with that principle, audited financial statements include a set of notes that provide vital information in addition to that contained in the financial statements themselves. An explanation of the nature and typical contents of the notes follows the discussion of the statement of cash flows and statement of changes in net assets.

All managers should first carefully read the auditor's opinion letter, the financial statements themselves, and the notes that accompany them, to gain a thorough understanding of the organization's finances. In addition, the technique of ratio analysis is widely used to provide additional insights. This chapter focuses on several critical types of ratios.

Not all information that a manager might desire is in the audit report. Additional financial documents, called management reports, can be generated to provide managers with a wealth of additional data. The chapter concludes with a discussion of management reports and how they differ from traditional financial statements and with a discussion of the implications of this chapter's contents for nurse managers.

※ THE INDEPENDENT AUDIT

An audit is an examination of the organization's financial statements and supporting documents. Many individuals and businesses need financial information about the organization. This includes the organization's own managers, as well as philanthropists, banks, bondholders, vendors (i.e., suppliers), and regulatory agencies. Users from outside the organization want to feel certain they can rely upon the information contained in the financial statements. For this reason many, if not most, health care organizations engage a certified public accountant (CPA) to perform an independent audit of their financial statements.

There are a number of purposes for an independent audit. The first is to examine the internal controls that the organization has built into its accounting system to minimize arithmetic and other clerical errors and to reduce the chances of embezzlement or fraud. The second is to examine through sampling some accounting records to determine whether it is reasonable to conclude that material errors have not occurred, or to find them and allow them to be corrected if they have occurred. The next purpose is to determine whether the financial statements are a fair representation of the financial results of the organization in accordance with GAAP. The credibility of a health care organization's accounting information is often supported by the results of an independent audit.

When a CPA firm completes an audit, it issues two letters: the *management letter* and an *opinion letter.* These letters are essentially the end product of what may represent months of detailed investigation.

The management letter is a letter from the CPA to the board of trustees or directors of the organization; its contents are generally not disclosed to the public. This letter discusses the strengths and weaknesses of the *internal control* system of the organization. Accountants test records on a very limited basis. It cannot be expected

※ **EXHIBIT 6–1.** *Opinion Letter*

Report of the Independent Auditors

To the Directors of ABC Health Care:

We have audited the accompanying statements of financial position of ABC Health Care as of June 30, 2000 and 1999, and the related statements of operations, changes in net assets, and cash flow for the years then ended. These financial statements are the responsibility of the ABC Health Care's management. Our responsibility is to express an opinion on these financial satements based on our audits.

We conducted our audits in accordance with generally accepted auditing standards. Those standards require that we plan and perform the audit to obtain reasonable assurance about whether the financial statements are free of material misstatement. An audit includes examining, on a test basis, evidence supporting the amounts and disclosures in the financial statements. An audit also includes assessing the accounting principles used and significant estimates made by management, as well as evaluating the overall financial statement presentation. We believe that our audits provide a reasonable basis for our opinion.

In our opinion, the financial statements referred to above present fairly, in all material respects, the financial position of ABC Health Care as of June 30, 2000 and 1999, and the results of its operations, changes in net assets, and cash flow for the years then ended in conformity with generally accepted accounting principles.

Steven A. Finkler, CPA
March 20, 2001

that accountants will uncover all errors, frauds, or embezzlements in their limited examination. Therefore it is important for the organization to have a system that limits the opportunity not only for errors but also for theft or fraud. In the management letter the auditor provides advice on how to strengthen the system. Also noted are apparent weaknesses that would cause the organization's activities to be inefficient, although that is not the main focus of a financial audit.[1]

The opinion letter is also addressed to the board of trustees or directors, but this letter is more often presented to interested parties, such as potential creditors. All internal managers have a stake in understanding how well their organization is doing. Therefore all internal managers should make a point of obtaining a copy of the opinion letter and audit report each year. An example of the opinion letter is presented in Exhibit 6–1. The opinion letter in the exhibit notes that financial statements from the years 2000 and 1999 have been audited. The tables in Chapter 5, for simplicity, showed information for only one year. However, it is general practice to provide at least two years' worth of audited information at a time so that the user can compare the previous year's results with the current year's.

The standard opinion letter has three paragraphs: an opening or introductory paragraph, a scope paragraph, and an opinion paragraph (see Exhibit 6–1). Additional paragraphs are included if unusual circumstances require further explanation.

The opening paragraph describes what the auditor was hired to do. Many CPA firms provide a range of consulting services to health care organizations. This paragraph explains to the user that an audit was undertaken and explicitly points out that the health care organization's management bears the ultimate responsibility

---

[1]It is also possible to engage the CPA or other consultant to conduct an operations audit. Such an audit focuses not on the financial records of the organization but on the efficiency with which the organization carries out all the various tasks related to providing its products or services. While such an operations audit is beyond the scope of routine annual financial audits, it may provide the organization with a number of suggestions to improve the way services are provided.

for the contents of the financial statements. Auditors merely examine the statements that are management's representation and ultimate responsibility.

The scope paragraph describes in brief what is done as part of an audit of financial statements. This paragraph explains the type of procedures auditors follow in carrying out an audit, including complying with a set of generally accepted auditing standards.

The opinion paragraph describes whether the financial statements provide a fair representation of the financial position, results of operations, changes in net assets, and cash flows of the company in the opinion of the auditor. An opinion, such as this one which says the financial statements "present fairly," indicates that in the opinion of the auditor, exercising due professional care, there is sufficient evidence of conformity to GAAP. This is referred to as a *clean* opinion.

In some cases the audit opinion letter also contains additional paragraphs containing explanations. This is generally the case if there is significant uncertainty or a material change in the application of GAAP. When extra paragraphs are included, the user should be alerted to the need to exhibit caution, and the contents of that paragraph or paragraphs should be closely examined.

※ BALANCE SHEETS AND OPERATING STATEMENTS

Reviewing the auditor's opinion letter is the first step in the analysis of financial statements. Any unusual elements of the letter should be noted for later investigation. The next step is a careful review of the statement of financial position (balance sheet) and the operating statement. These statements were introduced in Chapter 5.

It is important to read through each statement carefully. Are there any numbers that seem out of line, too high or too low? Are there indications of strength or weakness? Do things seem to be improving or getting worse? These two statements alone are inadequate to gain a full understanding of the organization's finances. However, they provide critical information for starting to gain an overall picture of the organization's financial status.

※ THE STATEMENT OF CASH FLOWS

An audited report also includes a statement of cash flows. Recall that GAAP includes a principle of matching revenues and related expenses in the same accounting period, the one in which the revenues are legally earned. However, the result of that principle is that the statement of revenues and expenses is prepared on an accrual basis. It reports the amount of revenue the organization is entitled to, not how much it has received in cash.

However, the flow of cash in and out of an organization is also critical. It is important to know how much revenue the organization is entitled to. But bills must be paid with cash. Knowing when the revenue is received in cash is critical. One must be able to know if there will be enough cash to undertake desired projects or purchase capital equipment and whether the organization has sufficient cash to be financially stable. Therefore, a statement of cash flows is generally required.

The balance sheet tells how much cash the organization has at the end of each accounting period. By comparing this balance from year to year, one can see how much the cash balance has changed. However, that does not explain where the organization gets its cash or how it uses its cash.

It is possible for even a profitable organization to become bankrupt. Financial viability depends not only on whether revenues exceed expenses but also on whether there is enough money in the bank to pay bills as they become due. A major investment in equipment may appear to be financially sensible because over the life of the equipment a profit will be made on the treatment of patients with that equipment. However, in the year the equipment is purchased, cash may be needed to pay for the entire cost of the equipment, even though only one year's depreciation will appear as an expense on the operating statement. The organization may not have the necessary cash.

The statement of cash flows provides information on where the organization's cash comes from and where the cash goes. This provides a substantially improved sense of what things the organization will have sufficient cash to undertake. Table 6–1 is a simplified example of a statement of cash flows. (Note that parentheses on a financial statement indicate a subtraction or negative number.) This cash flow statement is similar for both proprietary and not-for-profit health care providers.

For the most recent year, which ended on June 30, 2000, what does this statement tell the manager? The organization's receipts came from patient care and, to a lesser extent, from other operating activities. Cash used for operations went primarily into wages, supplies, and interest. However, note from the statement that cash also comes from and is used for investing and financing activities. For example, $350,000 of cash was generated from earnings on investments.

It is also interesting to note that for hypothetical ABC Health Care, even though there was a positive cash flow of $1,061,000 from operating activities, the cash for the year decreased by $389,000 from a starting balance of $539,000 to an ending balance of $150,000. If cash falls again next year by $389,000, the organization will run out of cash.

In fact, it would appear that the organization did run out of cash during the current year! Note that there was a $500,000 loan from a bank that was taken out during the year (Cash Flows from Financing Activities, in Table 6–1). Why did this happen? In trying to interpret financial statements, the first question to ask is whether operating activities are self-sufficient. Is enough cash being generated from those activities to sustain their cost? In this case, the answer is yes. Even though overall cash is falling, and in fact a loan had to be taken out, there was a positive $1,061,000 cash flow from operations in 2000.

※ TABLE 6–1

ABC Health Care
Statement of Cash Flows
for the Fiscal Years Ending June 30, 2000 and 1999
(000s omitted)

	2000	1999
Cash Flows from Operating Activities		
Collections from patients and third-party payers	$ 17,825	$ 16,232
Collections from other operating activities	1,919	1,432
Payments to suppliers	(2,122)	(1,876)
Interest payments	(2,333)	(2,290)
Payments to employees	(14,228)	(12,055)
Net cash from operating activities	$ 1,061	$ 1,443
Cash Flows from Investing Activities		
Earnings from restricted investments	$ 350	$ 350
Increase in sinking fund	(300)	(280)
Net cash from investing activities	$ 50	$ 70
Cash Flows from Financing Activities		
Payments of mortgage principal	$ (2,000)	$ (1,800)
Borrowing from bank	500	0
Net cash used for financing activities	$ (1,500)	$ (1,800)
Net Increase/(Decrease) in Cash	$ (389)	$ (287)
Cash, Beginning of Year	539	826
Cash, End of Year	$ 150	$ 539

The problem appears to be caused by a $2 million payment of mortgage principal. The cash excess from operations was not enough to offset the large mortgage payment, and additional borrowing was necessary. From the point of view of an internal manager, the next important question is whether a similar payment will be required in the coming years and, if so, whether there will be sufficient cash to cover it.

The balance sheet for ABC Health Care appears in Table 6–2. Looking at the long-term liabilities, you will see that at the current rate of payment it will take nearly two more years to fully pay off the mortgage (i.e., $2 million of principal was paid in 2000, and there is still an outstanding balance of $3,560,000).[2] This is disturbing. It means that if 2001 is about the same as 2000, it will be necessary to borrow another $500,000 from the bank. What if 2001 is worse than 2000?

Trends are extremely important in examining financial information. Is 2001 likely to be better, the same, or worse than 2000? Table 6–3 presents comparative operating statements for ABC Health Care. Note from those statements that the increase in unrestricted net assets fell dramatically from 1999 to 2000. The cash flows statement (see Table 6–1) shows that net cash flow from operating activities fell nearly $400,000 from 1999 to 2000 (i.e., from $1,443,000 to $1,061,000).

Does ABC have a cash crisis now? No. It has cash in the bank. Is it facing a cash flow crisis? That may well be the case. Even though the organization has had profits in the past and even though it generates a positive cash flow from its activities, it is rapidly draining its cash resources.

What response should be taken? That is a difficult question. ABC has a number of options. It could actively work to cut costs to allow the positive cash flow from activities to better cover its needs to repay the mortgage. Or it could refinance the mortgaged item, spreading smaller payments farther into the future. The ability to do that would largely depend on the likely remaining useful life of the mortgaged property.

Or it could increase the *unsecured* $500,000 loan that had already been taken out. The organization could use its cash flow statement to show a bank, well in advance of a cash crisis, that there is a current need for additional cash. However, that need will only persist for several years, until the mortgage is paid off. At that point, the positive cash flow from operating activities can be used to repay the bank.

If the organization and its managers face the coming cash crunch in advance, a variety of options are available. However, without a document such as the statement of cash flows to examine and analyze, the organization might think everything is okay. Then one day when the cash runs out and the managers have no understanding of why, the consequences may be far more severe, often leading to employee layoffs (and reduced patient quality of care) or worse. The process of financial analysis allows actions at an early stage, when there is time to find the most palatable solution.

⁜ STATEMENT OF CHANGES IN NET ASSETS OR EQUITY

There is a fourth financial statement for health care organizations: the statement of changes in net assets or equity (Table 6–4). This statement reconciles the net assets, or owners' equity from the end of the previous year to the end of the current year.

This statement is valuable because it shows the changes within each class of net assets: unrestricted, temporarily restricted, and permanently restricted. This provides the financial statement user with information on both temporary and

[2] In actual practice, the mortgage liability would be split into (1) the portion to be paid within the next year, which would be shown as a current liability under the title of Current Portion of Long-Term Debt, and (2) the portion to be paid more than one year into the future. Therefore the exact amount of mortgage principal to be paid in the coming year would be known by the manager.

※ TABLE 6–2

ABC Health Care
Statement of Financial Position
as of June 30, 2000 and 1999
(000s omitted)

Assets	2000	1999	Equities	2000	1999
Current Assets			**Current Liabilities**		
Cash	$ 150	$ 539	Wages payable	$ 1,123	$ 1,018
Marketable securities	220	230	Accounts payable	2,430	2,575
Accounts receivable, *net* of $436 and $328 allowance for bad debts	2,319	1,722	Notes payable	500	0
			Deferred revenue	300	0
			Taxes payable	145	176
Inventory	832	342	Total current liabilities	$ 4,498	$ 3,769
Prepaid assets	46	52			
Total current assets	$ 3,567	$ 2,885	**Long-term Liabilities**		
Fixed Assets			Mortgage payable	$ 3,560	$ 5,560
			Bonds payable	20,000	20,000
Property, plant, and equipment	$43,470	$43,470	Total long-term liabilities	$23,560	$25,560
Less accumulated depreciation	17,356	16,085	**Net Assets**		
			Unrestricted	$ 5,412	$ 4,942
Net property, plant, and equipment	$26,114	$27,385	Temporarily restricted	520	170
Sinking fund	1,737	1,437			
Investments	341	341	Permanently restricted	1,000	1,000
Goodwill	3,231	3,393	Total net assets	$ 6,932	$ 6,112
Total fixed assets	$31,423	$32,556			
Total Assets	$34,990	$35,441	**Total Equities**	$34,990	$35,441

※ TABLE 6–3

ABC Health Care
Statement of Operations
for the Fiscal Years Ending June 30, 2000 and 1999
(000s omitted)

	2000	1999
Revenues		
Patient revenues	$18,230	$17,578
Other operating revenues	1,919	1,432
Total	$20,149	$19,010
Expenses		
Wages for clinical services	$10,325	$ 9,525
Patient care supplies and food	934	802
Housekeeping services	654	589
Operation and maintenance of plant	1,221	1,003
Administrative services	2,343	2,050
Depreciation and amortization	1,433	1,433
Bad debt expense	436	328
Interest	2,333	2,083
Total	$19,679	$17,813
Increase in Unrestricted Net Assets	$ 470	$ 1,197

※ **TABLE 6–4**

ABC Health Care
Statement of Changes in Net Assets
for the Fiscal Year Ending June 30, 2000
(000s omitted)

	Net Assets		
	Unrestricted	**Temporarily Restricted**	**Permanently Restricted**
Net assets July 1, 1999	$4,942	$170	$1,000
Increase in unrestricted net assets	470		
Restricted contributions and grants		0	0
Investment income		350	
Net assets released from restrictions		0	
Change in net assets	$ 470	$350	$ 0
Net assets June 30, 2000	$5,412	$520	$1,000

permanent restrictions, investment income restricted for specific purposes, and net assets released from restrictions.

Alternatively, the statement for a for-profit organization shows how the issuance of stock increases owners' equity and how the payment of dividends reduces it.

※ NOTES TO FINANCIAL STATEMENTS

The purpose of financial statements is to convey information to individuals interested in the financial situation of the organization. However, in most instances the statements themselves are inadequate to provide complete information. Additional information is conveyed by appending notes to the financial statements. The purpose of these notes is to ensure full disclosure of all relevant information needed for the financial statements to constitute a fair representation of the financial position, results of operations, and cash flows of the organization in accordance with GAAP.

Financial statements without notes may be inadequate for several reasons. In some cases, organizations are allowed a number of choices of how to record and report financial results, for instance, how to report inventory. Two identical hospitals with exactly the same inventory might report a different asset value on the balance sheet and a different operating income, depending on the accounting choice made for reporting inventory. A note must disclose the choice that was made, so that the reader can compare financial statements of different organizations on an informed basis.

Sometimes notes are required to disclose particular types of information that do not otherwise appear on the financial statements. For example, financial statements of health care organizations must disclose the amount of charity care provided by the organization. This specific information may be of interest to users of the financial statements and in most instances would not be available without the notes that accompany the statements.

On occasion there is some important fact that the statements simply do not capture. For instance, a pending malpractice suit would have no impact on the financial statements. No payment or loss occurs until the case has been decided. However, a large potential loss may be of significant importance to users of the financial statement. Until the case is concluded, the lawsuit represents a *contingent* liability. There may be liability or there may not; it is contingent on the uncertain outcome of the suit. Disclosure of such a possible loss is made in the notes that accompany the statements.

A typical set of notes begins with a summary of significant accounting policies. This is a general statement covering a wide variety of issues. The entity for which the statements were prepared is described. Other information might include organizational policy with respect to charity care. Exemption from income taxes might be noted. Accounting treatment of donor pledges that have not yet been received in cash may be explained. Many other items of general background information may be contained as well.

Following the summary of accounting policies are a number of notes on specific topics. Many organizations include at this point a note calculating the amount of charity care provided. The relationship between the organization and third-party payers is often intricate, involving the rights of the third parties to conduct their own audits and revise the amounts due. Such relationships often merit a specific note. The property, plant, and equipment information shown on the balance sheet is often presented in a highly summarized form; more detailed information is provided in a note. Malpractice issues, pension plans, and commitments such as future lease payments represent the most common types of notes. Other notes explain unusual circumstances.

While the notes are sometimes quite involved and may seem peripheral to some readers, accountants believe that the information they contain is essential. To help convey that fact, each financial statement has a footnote on the same page as the statement, referring the readers to the notes that accompany the financial statements.

※ RATIO ANALYSIS

In addition to a review of the financial statements themselves and the notes that accompany them, a third major component of interpretation of financial statement information is ratio analysis. A *ratio* is a comparison of the relationship between two numbers. This is accomplished by dividing one number by another. Sometimes the result is multiplied by 100% to convert it into a percentage. A number of examples are given below. The comparison often yields insights that would otherwise not be gained.

In hospitals and other inpatient facilities, one of the most common ratios is not developed from financial statement information. It is the occupancy rate, which is the number of occupied beds divided by the total number of beds, multiplied by 100%. Suppose that a hospital has 150 occupied beds on average. Is that good or bad? Generally, the more beds occupied, the better from a financial perspective, for reasons related to costs, which will be discussed in Chapter 7. However, that still does not make clear whether 150 is good or bad. If the hospital has only 160 beds, then the occupancy rate is 94% (150 ÷ 160 × 100%), which is very good. If the hospital has 300 beds, the occupancy rate is only 50% (150 ÷ 300 × 100%), which is not very good. The fact that there are 150 filled beds does not convey valuable information; the ratio of 94% occupancy or 50% occupancy is more informative.

The issue of comparisons is at the root of ratio analysis. Not only is one number compared to another, but often ratios are compared to each other. A ratio by itself may not clearly be good or bad. Therefore, in ratio analysis one generally asks the question, "Good or bad relative to what?" The easiest comparison is of a ratio with itself for the same organization over time. Suppose that the current occupancy rate is 70%. Knowing that the occupancy rate for the last three years has fallen from 90% to 80% to 70% tells us something very different about the organization than knowing that the ratio has risen from 50% to 60% to 70%. In both cases the occupancy ratio is 70%, but one would draw very different conclusions about the status of the organization after considering the trends over time.

A second type of comparison is of the ratio for the organization with information for the entire industry. For example, the Center for Healthcare Industry Performance Studies[3] annually calculates a large number of different financial ratios, such as those shown below, for hospitals all over the country. A hospital can compare its own ratios with those of other hospitals throughout the country or region. Further, with that service hospitals can compare themselves with others of like size. Other health care industries, such as nursing homes, home care agencies, and nursing schools, have their own associations that sometimes generate ratios on an industry-wide basis.

A third focus for comparison should be with a specific similar competitor. Comparing the ratios for your organization with those of another organization just like yours can provide a number of important insights about differences. Investigation of those areas can yield important information for improving the functioning of your organization.

Before the specific classes of ratios are discussed, several notes of caution are appropriate. First, one cannot rely on the information from just one or a few ratios. Second, keep in mind that ratios draw information from financial statements that may be misleading.

Any one ratio is much like one mosaic tile. One can tell very little about a mosaic from just one tile. A large number of tiles are needed to develop a pattern. It is quite possible for one ratio to cause a user to draw wrong conclusions. What if a health care organization is in desperate financial condition? As a result of severe financial losses, the organization sells one of its buildings. Immediately after the building is sold, the organization will have a large amount of cash. Ratios that look at liquid assets will imply that the organization is in an extremely strong financial position. With the building gone, however, losses may become even greater. Only a thorough review can provide information on which to base inferences.

Ratios generally use numbers from the financial statements. GAAP require land and some other assets to be valued at their cost. However, often assets are worth far more than their cost. Therefore, ratios that concern assets that have risen in value may be misleading to the user. Another problem is that GAAP allow choices of accounting method in some cases. When one prepares a ratio, the information concerning choice (which is generally specified in the notes) is lost, to some extent. When comparisons are made of ratios from different organizations, it is difficult to take into account the differing accounting choices made by those organizations.

Except for the occupancy ratio, the ratios discussed here are from financial statement information. However, as you become familiar with the concept, bear in mind that a ratio is simply a comparison of one number with another. The ratios discussed below are not an exhaustive list; many additional ratios can be conceived of and calculated. They may be financial, using information from the financial statements; they may be financial, but use information not available on financial statements (perhaps departmental budget information); or they may be nonfinancial, such as the occupancy ratio. Managers should attempt to consider relationships that can generate new informative ratios.

The five major classes of financial statement ratios are common size, liquidity, solvency, efficiency, and profitability. Each is discussed below.

Common Size Ratios

The first type of ratio is the common size ratio. Several typical common size ratios are defined in Exhibit 6–2. The goal of common sizing is to make an organization comparable to other organizations of different sizes. For example, the hypothetical ABC Health Care has $150,000 in cash at the end of June 30, 2000 (see Table 6–2). Is that the right amount of cash? Organizations want to have neither too little cash

[3]Center for Healthcare Industry Performance Studies, Columbus, Ohio; 800-859-2447.

※ EXHIBIT 6–2. *Some Key Common Size Ratios*

$$\text{Cash to total assets} = \frac{\text{Cash}}{\text{Total assets}}$$

$$\text{Accounts receivable to total assets} = \frac{\text{Accounts receivable}}{\text{Total assets}}$$

$$\text{Current assets to total assets} = \frac{\text{Current assets}}{\text{Total assets}}$$

$$\text{Current liabilities to total equities} = \frac{\text{Current liabilities}}{\text{Total equities}}$$

$$\text{Total expenses to total revenues} = \frac{\text{Total expenses}}{\text{Total revenues}}$$

$$\text{Operating income to total revenues} = \frac{\text{Operating income}}{\text{Total revenues}}$$

(potential for inability to pay bills and bankruptcy) nor too much cash (wasted investment opportunities). But how much is appropriate?

Suppose that XYZ Health Care has $300,000 in cash. Does that mean that ABC has too little or that XYZ has too much? Before that question can be answered, the cash balance must be viewed in light of the relative size of each organization. A larger organization would be expected to need more cash for its activities. We are really interested in which organization has relatively more cash.

The common size ratio helps by putting everything into perspective based on organizational size. Each asset is divided by total assets to find its ratio as a percentage of total assets. Each liability and fund balance is divided by total equities. Each item on the operating statement is divided by total revenues. Thus cash for ABC is $150,000, compared with total assets of $34,990,000 (cash and total asset values from Table 6–2).

$$\text{Cash to total assets} = \frac{\text{Cash}}{\text{Total assets}}$$

$$\text{Cash to total assets 2000} = \frac{\$150{,}000}{\$34{,}990{,}000} \times 100\%$$

$$= .4\%$$

Dividing the cash by total assets and multiplying by 100% to convert to a percentage, we find that ABC's cash is four tenths of 1% of its assets. Assume that XYZ has total assets of $15 million. Its $300,000 of cash would then be 2% of total assets. Assume that XYZ's 2% cash to total assets ratio has been fairly stable over the last few years; that is, it was about 2% in the previous several years and the most recent year.

We still do not know if XYZ has too much cash or ABC has too little. However, now the relative portions of assets held in cash are known. This one ratio alerts management to the possibility that cash levels may be too low. This would tend to confirm some of the conclusions drawn from an examination of the cash flows statement. At the end of 1999, ABC's cash of $539,000 was 1.5% of total assets. From 1999 to 2000 the cash to total assets ratio fell from 1.5% to .4%. This downward trend over time further confirms the possibility that ABC is dangerously low on cash.

Similarly, a common size ratio can be developed for each class of asset, liability, fund balance, revenue, and expense. For example, interest of $2,333,000 is 12% of total revenues (see Table 6–3; $2,333,000 ÷ $20,149,000 × 100%) for 2000. For the previous year, interest was 11%. This increase is slight but might reflect the increasing dependence ABC has on borrowed resources. Again, a comparison with

XYZ or with the industry, also showing trend information over time, would be useful.

Liquidity Ratios

One key point of any ratio analysis is an attempt to determine whether the organization has sufficient assets that are cash or will become cash soon to pay current liabilities as they come due. The common size cash ratio is one attempt to look at liquidity. In addition, a class of ratios focuses specifically on the question of liquidity. Several common liquidity ratios are defined in Exhibit 6–3.

The most widely used liquidity ratio is the current ratio. This compares current assets with current liabilities. Rules of thumb are often dangerous, because each industry and each organization within an industry has special circumstances. Nevertheless, a rule of thumb of a current ratio of 2.0 has become widely accepted. This implies $2 of current assets for every dollar of current liabilities. The reasoning is that current liabilities generally must be paid within several months. However, current assets may take longer to be converted into cash. For example, inventories must first be consumed in providing patient care to be converted into accounts receivable; then accounts receivable may take several or more months to be collected.

For ABC Health Care, using information from Table 6–2, the current ratios for 1999 and 2000 were:

$$\text{Current ratio} = \frac{\text{Current assets}}{\text{Current liabilities}}$$

$$\text{Current ratio 1999} = \frac{\$2{,}885{,}000}{\$3{,}769{,}000}$$

$$= .77$$

$$\text{Current ratio 2000} = \frac{\$3{,}567{,}000}{\$4{,}498{,}000}$$

$$= .79$$

Over this short period, the ratio was fairly constant. Often it is desirable to view ratios over a longer time frame, perhaps three to five years, to fully observe trends or patterns. Plotting ratios on graphs each year can be particularly helpful. For example, Figure 6–1 shows three possible five-year comparisons for the current ratio for ABC Health Care. Each one tells a story at a glance.

Assume that Figure 6–1B shows the actual five-year history of ABC. While there is no clear trend here, the relatively low current ratio (as compared with a rule of thumb of 2.0) is cause for some concern. One would probably want to see some comparative industry data to determine if this is typical of the industry (e.g., hospital, nursing home, home care agency) in which ABC operates.

Another widely used liquidity ratio is the quick ratio. This ratio, recognizing the time that may be needed before inventory is used up in the normal process of activities, looks at only those current assets that are likely to be quickly available as cash. These are cash itself, marketable securities (which can be sold immediately),

※ EXHIBIT 6–3. *Some Key Liquidity Ratios*

$$\text{Current ratio} = \frac{\text{Current assets}}{\text{Current liabilities}}$$

$$\text{Quick ratio} = \frac{\text{Cash} + \text{Marketable securities} + \text{Accounts receivable}}{\text{Current liabilities}}$$

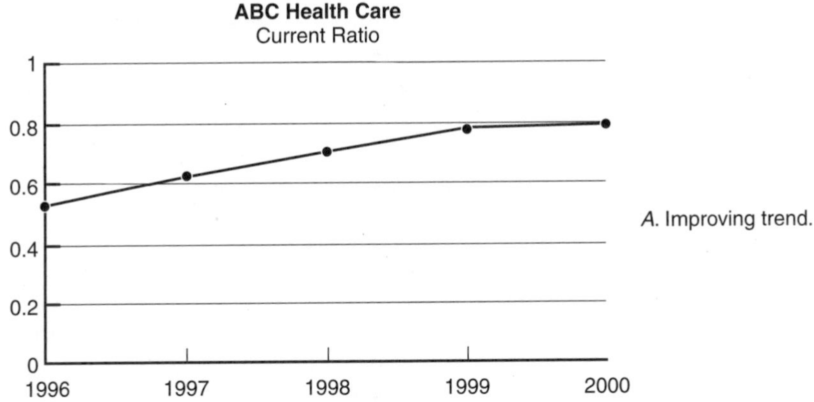

A. Improving trend.

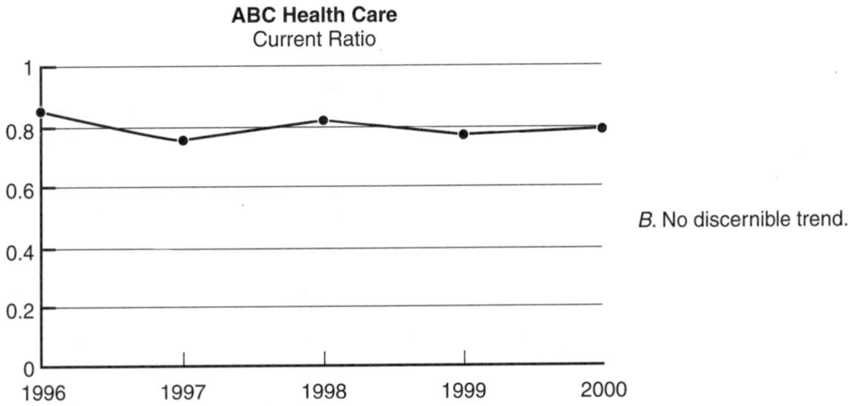

B. No discernible trend.

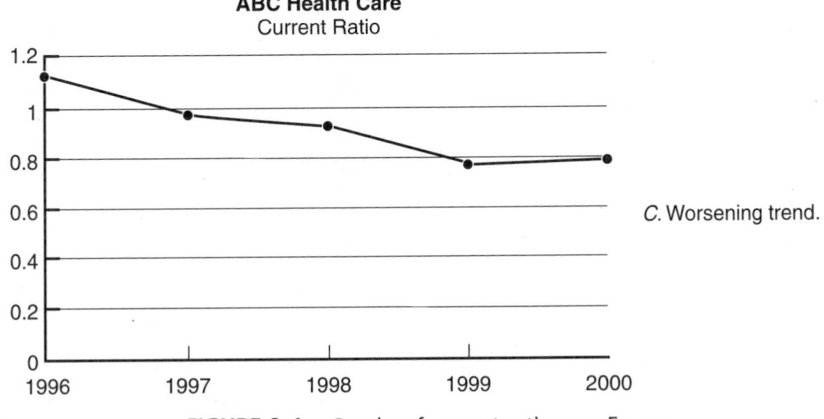

C. Worsening trend.

FIGURE 6–1. Graphs of current ratio over 5 years.

and accounts receivable (which can be used as collateral for a loan if necessary). For ABC, the quick ratio over the last two years, using data from Table 6–2, is:

$$\text{Quick ratio} = \frac{\text{Cash} + \text{Marketable securities} + \text{Accounts receivable}}{\text{Current liabilities}}$$

$$\text{Quick ratio 1999} = \frac{\$539{,}000 + \$230{,}000 + \$1{,}722{,}000}{\$3{,}769{,}000}$$

$$= .66$$

$$\text{Quick ratio 2000} = \frac{\$150{,}000 + \$220{,}000 + \$2{,}319{,}000}{\$4{,}498{,}000}$$

$$= .60$$

These results are not dramatically different from those of the current ratio. However, there is a falloff in the ratio from 1999 to 2000 that might warrant further attention, especially in light of the other things that have turned up concerning the organization's cash flow. Keep in mind that the major focus of the liquidity ratios is on the ability of the organization to meet its obligations over the coming year.

Solvency Ratios

In contrast, solvency ratios are an attempt to interpret the organization's ability to meet its payment obligations over a longer period of time, such as the next five years. Several common solvency ratios are defined in Exhibit 6–4. These ratios emphasize cash payments that must be made every year to avoid default. Such payments include interest and principal payments on loans.

The total debt to equity ratio is a generic ratio looking at long-term solvency. If this ratio is high, creditors are supplying a substantial portion of all resources used by the organization. This in turn makes it more difficult for the organization to borrow further, if it were to become necessary.

For instance, suppose that a for-profit home care agency had $2 million in assets, $1 million in debt, and $1 million in stockholders' equity. The assets might consist of accounts receivable, inventory, buildings, and equipment. Creditors would perceive that there were $2 of assets available to protect every dollar loaned to the organization. Even if the organization fell on hard times, it could sell off assets to pay creditors. In bankruptcy sales, however, buyers know that the seller must sell; therefore they often pay less than the assets might otherwise be worth.

In this example, even if each asset were sold for only half its balance sheet value, there would be enough money to pay creditors 100% of the amount owed them. But what if there were $1,500,000 of debt and only $500,000 of stockholders' equity? Then each asset would have to be sold for three quarters of its balance sheet stated value,

※ EXHIBIT 6–4. *Some Key Solvency Ratios*

$$\text{Total debt to equity} = \frac{\text{Current liabilities} + \text{Long-term debt}}{\text{Net assets}}$$

$$\text{Interest coverage} = \frac{\text{Cash flow from operating activities} + \text{Interest expense}}{\text{Interest expense}}$$

$$\text{Debt service coverage} = \frac{\text{Cash flow from operating activities} + \text{Interest expense}}{\text{Principal payments} + \text{Interest expense}}$$

$$\text{Plant age} = \frac{\text{Accumulated depreciation}}{\text{Annual depreciation expense}}$$

not just for half, for creditors to recover their money. This means that creditors are less content if the debt to equity ratio rises.

Discontent on the part of creditors may block the ability to borrow, which in turn may generate a cash crisis. Therefore it is important to monitor and control the debt to equity ratio. Total debt is equivalent to total liabilities. For ABC Health Care:

$$\text{Total debt to equity} = \frac{\text{Current liabilities} + \text{Long-term debt}}{\text{Net assets}}$$

$$\text{Total debt to equity 1999} = \frac{\$3{,}769{,}000 + \$25{,}560{,}000}{\$6{,}112{,}000}$$

$$= 4.8$$

$$\text{Total debt to equity 2000} = \frac{\$4{,}498{,}000 + \$23{,}560{,}000}{\$6{,}932{,}000}$$

$$= 4.0$$

The rule of thumb commonly used for a debt to equity ratio is 1. That implies liabilities of \$1 for every \$1 of net assets. In the health care industry, this ratio is often higher, typically going as high as 3. In both 1999 and 2000 the total debt to equity ratio is high for ABC, as computed above. In 1999 there was almost \$5 of debt for each dollar of fund balance. However, the trend is good. Although the ratio remains high, it has fallen dramatically. This is a positive sign. It tends to indicate that the problems ABC faces are related to short-term liquidity but not necessarily to long-term solvency. On the other hand, because of the high debt to equity ratio, it may not be possible for ABC to borrow in the short term to solve its short-term cash liquidity problems.

Examination of the interest coverage ratio provides information about the ability of the organization to meet its current interest payments. Often failure to meet interest payments creates the crisis that results in bankruptcy. The top half, or numerator, of this ratio consists of two parts. First, the cash flow from operations is taken from the cash flow statement (see Table 6–1). Next, interest paid (also from Table 6–1) is added to this amount. This is because the amount paid for interest was available for that purpose, in addition to the cash that was left over after all expenses, including interest, were paid.

$$\text{Interest coverage} = \frac{\text{Cash flow from operating activities} + \text{Interest expense}}{\text{Interest expense}}$$

$$\text{Interest coverage 1999} = \frac{\$1{,}443{,}000 + \$2{,}290{,}000}{\$2{,}290{,}000}$$

$$= 1.6$$

$$\text{Interest coverage 2000} = \frac{\$1{,}061{,}000 + 2{,}333{,}000}{\$2{,}333{,}000}$$

$$= 1.5$$

The interest coverage is not particularly encouraging. The cash flow into the organization that is available to pay interest is only enough to pay the interest due about one and a half times over. This means that if for any reason the cash coming into the organization were to fall by an amount equal to half the amount of interest itself, there might be a default.

This indicates a need to closely examine not only interest but also the required principal payments. The numbers for cash flow from operating activities, cash payments for interest, and principal payments can all be found on the statement of cash flows (see Table 6–1). The debt service coverage ratio provides that information:

$$\text{Debt service coverage} = \frac{\text{Cash flow from operating activities} + \text{Interest expense}}{\text{Principal payments} + \text{Interest expense}}$$

$$\text{Debt service coverage 1999} = \frac{\$1{,}443{,}000 + \$2{,}290{,}000}{\$1{,}800{,}000 + \$2{,}290{,}000}$$

$$= .91$$

$$\text{Debt service coverage 2000} = \frac{\$1{,}061{,}000 + \$2{,}333{,}000}{\$2{,}000{,}000 + \$2{,}333{,}000}$$

$$= .78$$

The debt service coverage ratio paints a bleak picture for ABC. Apparently, to cover both interest and debt principal payments, the organization spends more money than it brings in. In fact, that has been the case. In 1999 the organization's cash fell by nearly $300,000. In 2000, the cash balance fell by nearly $400,000, and in addition the organization borrowed $500,000 from the bank.

This would not appear to be a financially stable position. On the other hand, the large mortgage payments that were made in 1999 and 2000 would appear to continue only for about two more years before the mortgage is fully repaid, as noted in the earlier discussion of the cash flow statement. The organization's managers, however, should be specifically taking actions to provide for the cash that will be needed to make those payments. Also, the $20 million bond payable must be examined. When is it due? What plans are being made to repay that principal? Even if the payment is not due for ten years, there should be a plan now for actions that must be taken to ensure that cash will be available to pay the bond liability when it comes due.

Care should be taken in interpreting these ratios, however. Any one ratio gives only a part of the overall picture. For instance, ABC owns investments and marketable securities worth more than $600,000, and these can be used to offset much of the cash shortfall during the coming year, if necessary.

Another focus of solvency ratios is on whether the organization is keeping its plant up to date. Failure to reinvest in physical facilities is often a symptom of an organization that is going to be in financial trouble in the future. Failure to keep facilities up to date often reduces the competitiveness of an organization, worsening the financial problems that caused it to be unable to keep its facilities up to date in the first place.

In the case of ABC Health Care,

$$\text{Plant age} = \frac{\text{Accumulated depreciation}}{\text{Annual depreciation expense}}$$

$$\text{Plant age 1999} = \frac{\$16{,}085{,}000}{\$1{,}433{,}000}$$

$$= 11.2$$

$$\text{Plant age 2000} = \frac{\$17{,}356{,}000}{\$1{,}433{,}000}$$

$$= 12.1$$

The accumulated depreciation (from Table 6–2) represents all the depreciation charged over the years on the organization's existing buildings and equipment. By dividing that total by one year's depreciation (from Table 6–3) one can find approximately how many years the assets have been depreciated. It appears that the

※ **EXHIBIT 6–5.** *Some Key Efficiency Ratios*

$$\text{Patient revenue per day} = \frac{\text{Patient revenue}}{365}$$

$$\text{Day's receivables} = \frac{\text{Accounts receivable}}{\text{Patient revenue per day}}$$

$$\text{Revenue to assets} = \frac{\text{Total revenue}}{\text{Total assets}}$$

buildings and equipment for this organization have aged from about eleven years old on average to about twelve years old on average.

In other words, the plant has aged approximately one full year in the last year. That is cause for concern. It means there has been no significant updating of facilities or addition of equipment in the last year. If additional buildings or equipment had been purchased, the current depreciation would be higher because there would be depreciation on those new facilities. That in turn would make the ratio lower. The average age of plant would decline or at least rise less rapidly. In light of what is known about the organization's cash situation, this is not surprising. Nor is it a serious problem, unless it is allowed to continue for more than just a few years.

The average age of plant, which uses accumulated depreciation from the balance sheet and depreciation expense from the operating statement, is another ratio that would benefit greatly from some comparison with specific competitors and the industry in general. Are ABC's facilities comparatively old or new?

Efficiency Ratios

Ratios can be used as an indicator of whether the organization is being run efficiently. This is done on an organization-wide basis. Organizations may have many inefficiencies. The ratio technique will not specifically identify particular inefficiencies; rather, it can provide some overall measures to assess total relative efficiency of the organization. Several common efficiency ratios are defined in Exhibit 6–5. These are often referred to as asset turnover ratios.

The efficiency measure that tends to receive the most attention is days receivables. This is a measure of how long it takes, on average, to collect receivables. Once money has been collected, it can be invested and earn interest or can be used in some other beneficial way to aid the organization. While money is tied up in uncollected receivables, it provides no direct benefit to the organization. Therefore, generally one wants to keep the average collection period short. The day's receivable ratio is often called the average collection period ratio.

To calculate day's receivables, one first measures the patient revenue per day. This simply requires dividing the total patient revenue by the number of days in the year. If the total accounts receivable is then divided by the patient revenue per day, the result is the number of days worth of patient billings that are tied up in accounts receivable. For ABC,

$$\text{Patient revenue per day} = \frac{\text{Patient revenue}}{365}$$

$$\text{Day's receivables} = \frac{\text{Accounts receivable}}{\text{Patient revenue per day}}$$

$$\text{Patient revenue per day 1999} = \frac{\$17{,}578{,}000}{365} = \$48{,}159$$

$$\text{Day's receivables 1999} = \frac{\$1{,}722{,}000}{\$48{,}159} = 35.8$$

$$\text{Patient revenue per day 2000} = \frac{\$18{,}230{,}000}{365} = \$49{,}945$$

$$\text{Day's receivables 2000} = \frac{\$2{,}319{,}000}{\$49{,}945} = 46.4$$

In the health care industry it is not uncommon for it to take substantial periods of time before receiving payment for some patients. Therefore the 35.8 average days until collection in 1999 would be considered a fairly good result. And without knowing the 1999 ratio, the 46.4 day result for 2000 would not necessarily be considered bad. However, the trend from 1999 to 2000 is not good. It represents a substantial deterioration.

It might be that this was caused by slowing of payments by insurance companies or Medicaid and Medicare. Such slowing may be beyond the control of the organization. Or it might be caused by lack of attention to prompt mailing of bills, accurate documentation of bills, or vigorous collection efforts. Such events should be within the organization's control. Ratios are limited. They cannot explain underlying events or causes. However, they are effective for alerting managers to situations that need attention.

Another popular efficiency ratio is revenue to assets. This ratio tells how many dollars of revenues have been generated by each dollar invested in assets. It is foolish to waste resources. It does not make sense to use far more assets to provide care than are necessary. If your organization generates $1 of revenue for each dollar of assets invested, while other organizations in your field generate $3 of revenue for each dollar of assets, it would seem to imply that your organization is not efficient in the use of its assets. For ABC,

$$\text{Revenue to assets} = \frac{\text{Total revenue}}{\text{Total assets}}$$

$$\text{Revenue to assets 1999} = \frac{\$19{,}010{,}000}{\$35{,}441{,}000} = .54$$

$$\text{Revenue to assets 2000} = \frac{\$20{,}149{,}000}{\$34{,}990{,}000} = .58$$

Without industry comparisons, these numbers tell relatively little. The increase from .54 to .58 would seem to be an improvement. However, bear in mind that relatively little, if any, fixed assets were acquired this year. Thus revenues rose without the addition of assets. However, while that makes this ratio look better in the short run, it has other potentially negative long-run consequences. Once again we see that individual ratios cannot be considered by themselves.

Profitability Ratios

The last major class of ratios is profitability ratios. As noted earlier, it is appropriate for not-for-profit organizations to earn a profit. Even if profits are not part of the organizational mission, they are essential to accomplishing that mission. Therefore it is sensible to focus at least some attention on the success of the organization in earning profits. Several common profitability ratios are defined in Exhibit 6–6.

※ **EXHIBIT 6–6.** *Some Key Profitability Ratios*

$$\text{Operating margin} = \frac{\text{Operating income}}{\text{Total revenue}} \times 100\%$$

$$\text{Profit margin} = \frac{\text{Change in net assets}}{\text{Total revenue}} \times 100\%$$

$$\text{Return on net assets} = \frac{\text{Change in net assets}}{\text{Net assets}} \times 100\%$$

The first two ratios considered in Exhibit 6–6 are simply common size ratios. However, they focus attention directly on profits. The operating margin considers revenues and expenses before unusual gains or losses. That focus keeps attention on the normal day-in and day-out activities of the organization.

The operating margin considers what percentage of each dollar of revenues is left as profit before considering unusual items. The profit margin looks at *all* revenues, expenses, gains, and losses, and measures what percentage of revenues is left as an excess of revenues over expenses (i.e., net income or change in net assets). Because of the problems with consistent definition of gifts as revenue or gains, it is important to place more weight on the profit margin than on the operating margin when interorganizational comparisons are made. For ABC, there were no unusual gains or losses, so the operating and profit margins are identical. Using data from Table 6–3, they are:

$$\text{Profit margin} = \frac{\text{Change in net assets}}{\text{Total revenue}} \times 100\%$$

$$\text{Profit margin 1999} = \frac{\$1{,}197{,}000}{\$19{,}010{,}000} \times 100\% = 6.3\%$$

$$\text{Profit margin 2000} = \frac{\$470{,}000}{\$20{,}149{,}000} \times 100\% = 2.3\%$$

The profit margin has fallen off considerably. If this is simply a one-year aberration, it may not be important. If it represents a trend of declining profitability, it is important. A ratio such as this represents a warning sign that cannot be ignored.

Another important profit measure is the return on net assets. Essentially, either the owners (of a for-profit organization) or the community (in the case of a not-for-profit organization) has invested valuable resources in the organization. One can compare the change in net assets with the total net assets to get a measure of the financial return the community is earning from its investment. In the case of ABC the ratios are:

$$\text{Return on net assets} = \frac{\text{Change in net assets}}{\text{Net assets}} \times 100\%$$

$$\text{Return on net assets 1999} = \frac{\$1{,}197{,}000}{\$6{,}112{,}000} \times 100\% = 19.6\%$$

$$\text{Return on net assets 2000} = \frac{\$470{,}000}{\$6{,}932{,}000} \times 100\% = 6.8\%$$

However, this ratio is only a part of the return to the community. The community also receives the benefits related to the health care services provided. One should exercise extreme care in using the return on net assets (also called return on equity) ratio. It does not serve as a full measure of the benefits generated by the use of the assets invested in the organization because it ignores the health benefits to the community.

It is entirely possible to use a wide variety of additional ratios in each of the areas discussed above or to create other ratios. The essence of ratio analysis is to find two numbers that, when compared, yield some beneficial insight.

※ MANAGEMENT REPORTS

The financial statements generated by the accounting process are potentially of great value to managers of a health care organization. However, it should be noted that they are designed primarily with outside users in mind. They focus on reporting the financial history of the organization. By contrast, management reports focus on the future.

The role of management reports is to provide any information that can aid the manager to improve the organization's future results. Unlike financial accounting reports, which are limited by the specific rules of GAAP, management reports need only be useful. GAAP serve a purpose in providing a sound basis of comparability for outsiders to use. An outsider familiar with GAAP can learn much about the organization from financial statements prepared following GAAP. Internal users of information need not be limited by that desire for comparability or by an ability to understand an organization from the outside.

Another problem with GAAP financial statements is that they tend to be highly summarized. There is no detailed information by department. To operate efficiently, organizations assign responsibility to a large number of unit and department managers. These managers cannot control results without having information specific to their departments. Managers can use department-level information to calculate ratios. Those ratios can then be tracked over time to assess whether there is improvement or deterioration in financial results at the department level.

Therefore it is not only allowable but also desirable for internal managers to request a wide variety of additional financial information. It is possible to structure any set of reports that contain information that management believes will help in managing the organization better. Such reports need not follow GAAP. Throughout the remainder of this book, a number of different financial reports are discussed that will aid the manager in the process of managing efficiently and effectively.

IMPLICATIONS FOR NURSE MANAGERS

Nurse managers should endeavor to obtain a copy of their organization's financial statements, preferably audited financial statements. There will often be resistance to providing such statements. Information represents power, and some individuals do not want to share power. "Why do you need those statements?" they may well ask. "Your concern should be with the management of your department." Yet how can one manage a department in isolation from what is happening to the organization as a whole?

Management of a department takes place within the organization. Often restrictions are placed on salary increases or capital acquisitions. Are those restrictions justified? If they are, then the financial managers should be pleased to share the financial statements with you to prove how bad things really are. Doing so is an excellent way to help rally all members of the organization in support of the organization in its financial crisis. On the other hand, if the hard times are really not so hard, then managers have the right to know that too.

It is critical that the chief nursing executive be a part of the organization's top management team. That job should not be focused on running the nursing department but on helping the organization make the correct organization-wide decisions. Understanding the finances of the organization is critical to such decisions.

Even at lower levels of nursing management, it makes little sense to try to manage in a vacuum. All members of the management team can be more effective the better they understand their organization and its finances.

KEY CONCEPTS

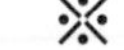

Independent audit Examination of an organization's financial statements and supporting documents by an outside independent auditor. The audit examines the organization's internal controls, searches for material errors, and determines whether the statements have been prepared in accordance with GAAP.

Opinion letter Letter from a CPA indicating whether the audited financial statements conform to GAAP.

Analysis of financial statements Review of the opinion letter, the balance sheet, operating statement, cash flows statement, statement of changes in net assets, notes to the financial statements, and ratios related to the financial statements.

Statement of cash flows Financial statement that shows where the organization's cash came from and how it was used over a specific period.

Statement of changes in net assets Financial statement that summarizes items that affect the organization's unrestricted, temporarily restricted, and permanently restricted net assets.

Notes to the financial statements Supplementary and explanatory information; a critical element of an overall presentation of the organization's financial information. These notes are required to ensure that adequate and full disclosure of all relevant information, in accordance with GAAP, is made.

Ratios Comparisons of one number with another, to provide some insight or understanding of the finances of the organization that would not be realized from looking at each number individually. Ratios should be compared over time and also with the industry norms and with specific competitors.

Common size ratios Comparison of financial statement numbers with a key number on the financial statement to take into account the relative size of the organization.

Liquidity ratios Comparisons aimed at determining the organization's ability to meet its obligations over the coming year.

Solvency ratios Comparisons aimed at determining the organization's ability to meet its obligations over the long term.

Efficiency ratios Comparisons aimed at determining the relative efficiency of the organization's use of its resources.

Profitability ratios Comparisons aimed at determining the relative profitability of the organization.

Management reports Any report other than the four central financial statements, prepared to provide managers with information to aid in management of the organization.

SUGGESTED READINGS

American Institute of Certified Public Accountants, *AICPA Audit and Accounting Guide for Health Care Organizations*, AICPA, New York, N.Y., 1996.

Cleverley, William O., *Essentials of Health Care Finance*, Aspen Publishers, Gaithersburg, Md., February 1997.

Davidson, Sydney, C. Stickney, and R. Weil, *Accounting: The Language of Business*, 8th edition, Thomas Horton and Daughters, Glen Ridge, N.J., 1990.

Defliese, Philip L., Henry R. Jaenicke, Vincent O'Reilly, and Murry B. Hirsch, *Montgomery's Auditing*, John Wiley & Sons, New York, N.Y., 1990.

Emery, Douglas R., John D. Finnerty, and John D. Stowe, *Principles of Financial Management*, Prentice Hall, Upper Saddle River, N.J., 1998.

Ferraro, McDuffie, A.M. Jerome, and J.S. Chan, "Communicating the Financial Worth of the CNS through the use of Fiscal Reports," *Clinical Nurse Specialist*, Vol. 7, No. 2, March 1993, pp. 91–97.

Finkler, Steven A., *Finance and Accounting for Nonfinancial Managers*, revised and expanded edition, Prentice Hall, Upper Saddle River, N.J., 1996.

Gapenski, Louis C., *Financial Analysis and Decision Making for Healthcare Organizations: A Guide for the Healthcare Professional*, Irwin Professional Publishers, Burr Ridge Ill., January 1997.

Granof, Michael H., *Government and Not-for-Profit Accounting: Concepts and Practices*, John Wiley & Sons, New York, N.Y., 1998.

Guy, Dan M., C. Wayne Alderman, and Alan J. Winters, *Auditing*, 2nd edition, Harcourt, Brace, Jovanovich, San Diego, Calif., 1990.

Horngren, Charles T., and Gary L. Sundem, *Introduction to Financial Accounting,* 7th edition, Prentice Hall, Upper Saddle River, N.J., 1998.

Keown, Arthur J., J. William Petty, David F. Scott, Jr., and John D. Martin, *Foundations of Finance,* 2nd edition, Prentice Hall, Upper Saddle River, N.J., 1998.

Larkin, Richard E., *Wiley Not-for-Profit GAAP 98,* John Wiley & Sons, New York, N.Y., 1998.

Levy, V.M., *Financial Management of Hospitals,* Wm Gaunt & Sons, Holmes Beach, Fla., January 1998.

McKeon, Tad, *Home Health Financial Management,* Aspen Publishers, Gaithersburg, Md., January 1996.

McLean, Robert A., *Financial Management in Health Care Organizations,* Delmar, Albany, N.Y., 1996.

Neumann, Bruce R., Jan P. Clement, and Jean C. Cooper, *Financial Management: Concepts and Applications for Health Care Organizations,* Kendall/Hunt Publishing, Dubuque, Iowa, May 1997.

Pelfrey S., "Managing Financial Data," *Seminars for Nurse Managers,* Vol. 5, Vol. 1, March 1997, pp. 25–30.

Samuels, David I., *The Healthcare Financial Management and Budgeting Toolkit,* Richard D. Irwin, Burr Ridge, Ill., December 1997.

Stickney, Clyde P., and Roman L. Weil, *Financial Accounting: An Introduction to Concepts, Methods, and Use,* 8th edition, Dryden Press, Fort Worth, Tex., 1997.

Suver, James D., Bruce R. Neumann, and Keith E. Boles, *Management Accounting for Healthcare Organizations,* 3rd edition, Pluribus Press, Westchester, Ill., 1992.

United Hospital Fund, *Hospital Watch,* 55 Fifth Ave., New York, N.Y., quarterly.

Ward, William J., Jr., *Health Care Budgeting and Financial Management for Non-Financial Managers: A New England Healthcare Assembly Book,* Auburn House Publishers, Westport, Conn., January 1994.

Zelman, William N., Michael J. McCue, and Alan R. Milikan, *Financial Management of Health Care Organizations: An Introduction to Fundamental Tools, Concepts, and Applications,* Blackwell Publishers, Cambridge, Mass., January 1998.

PART

III

COST ANALYSIS

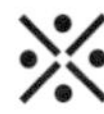

One of the most critical areas of financial management is analysis and control of costs. Costs represent half of the financial equation. The surplus (profit) or deficit (loss) of an organization each year depends on its revenues and its expenses or costs. Both elements, revenues and costs, require managerial thought and attention. Cost management has been an essential role of nurse managers at all levels for a number of years. Revenue management is an area of growing interest for nurse managers.

The first chapter in this part of the book, Chapter 7, deals with basic issues of cost management. The chapter introduces definitions of critical terms. The nature and behavior of costs is discussed. The relationship between patient volume and costs is stressed. Techniques are also provided for the prediction or estimation of future costs. Finally, the chapter provides a method to determine when a program or project or service will have sufficient volume to break even, that is, be financially self-sufficient.

Chapter 8 moves from basic cost concepts to the broader issue of cost measurement. There are two primary focuses: One is on how health care organizations collect cost information by cost center and assign that information first to revenue centers and ultimately to patients. The second is on how to cost out nursing services.

The Medicare step-down cost-finding and rate-setting methods are presented and contrasted with more recently developed methods. Attention is also placed on understanding product-line costing. Issues of patient classification systems and staffing are considered. Standard costing techniques are discussed.

Costing out nursing is a topic of much interest to nurse managers. As health care organizations are forced to operate in a constrained financial atmosphere, chief executive officers look to nurse managers at all levels to take a greater role in controlling costs. Financial reimbursement for nursing services is also discussed.

Chapter 9 addresses a concern that peaks during periods of nursing shortages but that requires managerial attention regardless of whether there is a current shortage of nurses. That is the issue of measuring the costs of recruiting and retaining staff. Ways to measure those costs and to include them in the budget are discussed.

Nurse managers must have a solid background in costing out nursing to understand the costs of their units and services. This will aid them in managing staff and other resources effectively. ※

CHAPTER

7

Cost Management

CHAPTER GOALS

The goals of this chapter are to:

- Define basic cost terms
- Explain the underlying behavior of costs and the importance of that behavior for decision making
- Provide tools for cost estimation
- Explain how costs can be adjusted for the impact of inflation
- Provide the tool of break-even analysis

※ INTRODUCTION

Cost control is a major element of the job of all nurse managers. Understanding costs and their behavior provides the manager with the ability to understand the expenses incurred in the cost centers under their authority. The skillful management of costs is an essential element of the financial success of any health care organization. However, cost management is complicated.

Many cost terms commonly used are not well understood. Direct costs, indirect costs, average costs, fixed costs, variable costs, and marginal costs are concepts that managers use and must clearly understand. This chapter stresses the definitions of these and other key terms.

The relationship of fixed and variable costs is the most fundamental cost concept. The total costs incurred by health care organizations depend directly on the interplay between fixed and variable costs. Building upon those concepts is the issue of volume. Volume ultimately becomes a critical aspect of almost every successful health care organization and of every failing one.

Health care organizations are not static; they are constantly in a state of flux and change. Services are added; other services are deleted. Some areas of the organization expand; others contract. To a great extent these changes are dictated by clinical factors. However, every change has an impact on organizational cost. In each case managers should determine whether the financial impact of a proposed change will be favorable or unfavorable for the organization. While an unfavorable financial impact may not mean that a service must be deleted, a good manager makes decisions based on as much information as possible. One approach, called marginal cost analysis, is critical to generating information for such decisions.

Another important area of cost management is cost estimation. What will costs likely be in the coming year? That question requires careful management attention. This chapter provides several techniques to help in exploring that topic.

The last major topic covered in this chapter is break-even analysis. It addresses the issue of the volume of patients required for a program or service to become financially self-sufficient.

⁜ BASIC COST CONCEPTS

The most critical of cost concepts is referred to as *cost behavior.* Cost behavior is the way that costs change in reaction to events within the organization. If patient volume rises by 5%, what do costs do? What if patient volume falls 5%? How can one predict whether total costs will exceed revenues or remain less than revenues? Which factors are related to stable costs and which to rising costs?

Cost behavior depends on the specific elements of cost in any cost center or organization. A *cost center* is any unit or department in an organization for which a manager is assigned responsibility for costs. Some types of costs are stable, changing little, if at all, even in response to significant changes in patient work load. Other costs are highly changeable, reacting directly to other changes in the organization.

The goal of this section is to lay out a framework upon which to develop an understanding of how costs behave in health care organizations.

Definitions

Cost measurement is more complex than one might expect. When someone asks what something costs, accountants have trouble responding with a direct answer. The reason is that the appropriate measure of cost depends substantially on the intended use for the cost information. Finding out what it cost to treat each patient last year is very different from calculating what it might cost to treat one more patient next year. The cost per patient when 100 patients are treated may be very different from the cost per patient when 500 patients are treated.

To make sense in this complicated area, all managers (nurse managers and accountants) must rely heavily upon a consistent set of definitions. These definitions provide the basis of a common language so that when a cost per patient is cited, all managers can interpret that information in the same way and effectively communicate with each other.

Service unit A basic measure of the product or service being produced by the organization, such as discharged patients, patient days, home care visits, emergency room treatments, or hours of operations.

Cost information is often collected on a service unit basis. Managers need to know the cost per service unit. Within one health care organization a number of different types of service units may exist. For example, the operating room may use hours of operations, while a medical/surgical unit uses patient days.

Direct costs

a. Costs that are incurred within the organizational unit for which the manager has responsibility are referred to as direct costs of the unit.

b. Costs of resources for direct care of patients are referred to as the direct costs of patient care.

Indirect costs

c. Costs that are assigned to an organizational unit from elsewhere in the organization are indirect costs for the unit.

d. Costs within a unit that are not incurred for direct patient care are indirect costs of patient care.

Direct costs are a particularly difficult concept because their definition relates to the object of the analysis. If one were interested in the direct cost of patient care (definition b above) in a specific medical/surgical unit, that cost would not include the cost of the unit manager's time spent on administrative duties or the cost of clerical personnel in the unit. It likewise would not include the cost of a nurse restocking a supply cart. It would, however, include the cost of clinical supplies used, as well as the cost of nursing time spent with a patient.

From a different perspective, however, all of these costs are direct costs. That perspective applies when one is contrasting all the costs assigned to a unit or department. For the unit as a whole (definition a above), all nursing salaries and clerical salaries incurred within the unit are direct costs. Costs assigned to the unit from outside, such as laundry or housekeeping, are indirect costs to the unit. Similarly, a portion of the salary of the chief nurse executive (CNE) and of nursing administration are indirect costs to a specific unit. However, from the perspective of the nursing department as a whole, rather than that of one unit, the salary of the CNE is a direct cost.

Laundry costs are considered indirect by both the unit manager and the CNE. The labor and other costs of the laundry department are clearly incurred neither directly within individual nursing units nor within the nursing department as a whole, even though nursing may control the amount of laundry it uses (definition c above). But that does not mean that laundry costs are considered indirect costs by everyone. The manager of the laundry department would consider all costs incurred in that department direct costs. Perspective is critical in the classification of a cost as direct or indirect. From a focus on patient care, indirect costs would include all costs that are not direct patient care costs (definition d above).

Full cost Total of all costs associated with or in an organizational unit or activity. This includes direct and indirect costs.

For example, all the costs of a hospital would represent its full or total costs. Moving to the department or unit level, it is important to include not only direct costs but also all indirect costs. Full costs include an appropriate share of laundry, administration, billing, engineering, medical records, housekeeping, and so forth. The question of what is an appropriate share of costs to assign to each cost center is difficult and is addressed in Chapter 8.

Average cost Full cost divided by the volume of service units.

Many questions faced by managers require information on the cost per patient, per treatment, or per patient day. This represents the average cost. Each cost center may use its own service units and calculate its own average cost.

Fixed costs Those costs that do not change in total as the volume of service units changes.
Variable costs Those costs that vary directly with changes in the volume of service units.

The salary of the CNE does not change day by day as the census changes. Therefore the costs of the CNE are fixed costs. Supplies that are used for every patient are variable. The more patients, the more supplies used.

The definition of the service unit measure is crucial in defining fixed and variable costs. For example, while most clinical supplies used in a hospital vary with the number of patient days, surgical supplies are more likely to vary with the number of surgical procedures, and clinic supplies will likely vary with the number of clinic visits.

Relevant range Normal range of expected activity for the cost center or organization.

Fixed costs are fixed over the relevant range. Suppose that a thirty-bed nursing unit anticipated an average occupancy rate of 75%. It would not be unreasonable to expect the unit to have an 80% or even 85% occupancy rate. However, a rate of 160% would clearly be beyond the reasonable anticipated rate for that unit. To accommodate that many patients the hospital would have to add another nursing unit.

Within the normal relevant range, the costs for the salary of the nurse manager would be fixed. However, if occupancy reached 160%, there might well be expansion to two units, with a manager for each. The fixed costs would rise. They are only fixed within the relevant range.

Marginal costs Extra costs incurred as a result of providing one more service unit, such as one extra patient day.

Marginal cost information is critical in the decision-making process. Managers are often interested in how costs change when the number of patients cared for changes. This differs to some extent from variable costs. Suppose that a hospital does not currently provide liver transplantation. What would be the marginal costs of adding liver transplantation to the hospital's range of services?

Since no transplants are done currently, it is probable that the hospital would need equipment, supplies, and personnel to provide that service. The supplies represent a variable cost. For each transplant done, the hospital will need additional clinical supplies. However, the equipment represents a fixed cost. Once the equipment is purchased, it can be used for many transplants. Since both the supplies and the equipment are needed for the first transplant, both the supplies and equipment costs are marginal costs of adding that service.

If one considers the total costs incurred by an organization before it makes a change and the total costs after it makes the change, the difference in costs represents the marginal costs of that change.

Mixed costs Costs that contain both fixed and variable cost elements.

An example of a mixed cost is electricity. The operating room uses some electricity every day to light hallways and for other purposes not related to the number of patients. That portion of electric usage is a fixed cost. Much of the electricity used by the department is used in the operating suites. The more surgeries, the more electricity used. Therefore it has a variable component as well. Similarly, a home health agency would have mixed costs for transportation if it used agency-owned cars. Some costs would be fixed, such as annual maintenance, and some costs would vary with the number of home visits.

Mixed costs create some problems for managers. If the number of service units for a cost center rose by 10%, one would expect fixed costs to stay unchanged. One would expect variable costs to rise by 10%. Mixed costs would be expected to rise but by some amount greater than zero and less than 10. Later in this chapter methods will be provided for estimating the change in mixed costs resulting from a change in patient volume.

Step-fixed or step-variable cost Costs that are fixed over small ranges of activity that are less than the relevant range.

Often nursing units require a fixed number of nurses on duty for a range of patients. Within that range of patients, the nursing personnel cost remains fixed. However, if the number of patients increases by a large enough number, additional personnel will be needed. That personnel level is then fixed over a new, higher range of activity.

The key to step costs is that they are fixed over volume intervals but vary *within* the relevant range.

Fixed *vs* Variable Costs

The total costs of running a department are generally divided into those costs that are fixed and those costs that are variable. The concepts of fixed and variable costs are often conceptualized with the use of graphs. In the following example the service unit measure is assumed to be patient days. Figure 7–1 provides an example of fixed costs. Specifically, the graph shows the annual salary for a unit nurse manager for the coming year. The salary is $60,000.[1]

That salary is a fixed cost for the organization. The salary paid to a nurse manager is not dependent on any patient-volume statistic. In Figure 7–1 the vertical axis shows the cost to the institution. As one moves up this axis, costs increase. The

---

[1]This is a hypothetical number. First-level nurse manager salaries vary with geographic region, institution size, and institution type.

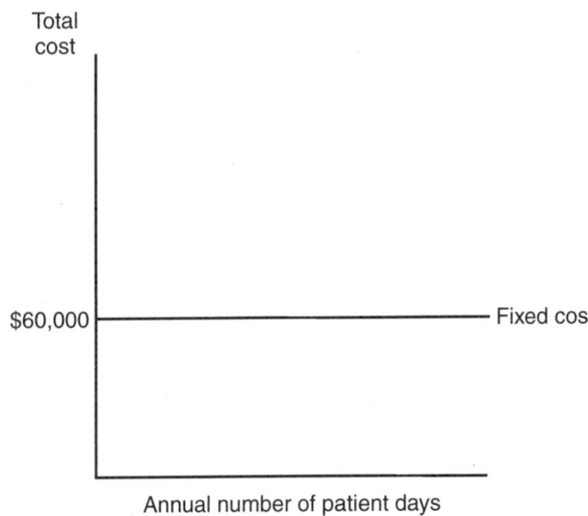

FIGURE 7–1. Fixed costs: cost for a nurse manager.

horizontal axis shows the number of patient days. The farther to the right one moves, the more patient days the institution has.

Note that the fixed costs appear as a horizontal line. This is because regardless of the volume, the salary for the nurse manager will remain the same. Thus the cost is the same for 8,000, 10,000, or 12,000 patient days.

Variable costs vary with the volume of service units. Suppose that each patient's temperature is taken twice a day. If the hospital's thermometers use disposable thermometer covers, then one would expect use of disposable covers to vary directly with patient volume. Assuming that each thermometer cover costs $.50 and that two a day are used for each patient, then the cost of those items is $1 for each patient each day. The more patient days, the more the cost for that disposable item in the total nursing unit budget.

Consider Figure 7–2. This graph plots the cost for disposable thermometer covers as they vary with patient volume. As in Figure 7–1, the vertical axis represents cost, and the horizontal axis represents patient volume. Unlike Figure 7–1, which showed

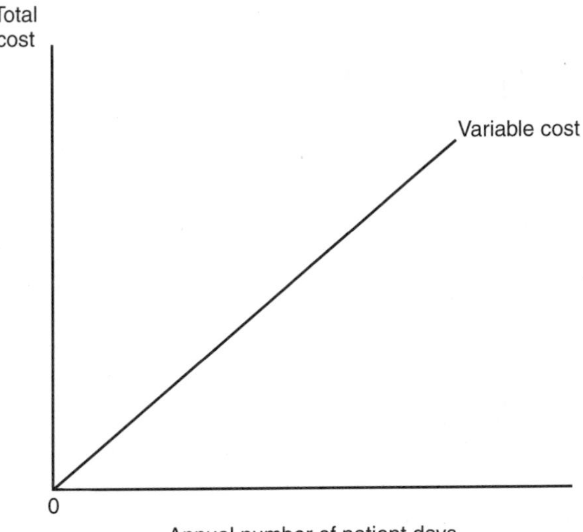

FIGURE 7–2. Variable costs: costs of a disposable supply item.

some amount of cost even at a volume of zero, this graph shows zero cost at a volume of zero, since zero patient days implies that none of this particular supply is used. The total variable cost increases by $1 for each extra patient day.

For instance, in Figure 7–3, dotted lines have been inserted to show the cost when there are 10,000 patient days, and the cost when there are 50,000 patient days. As you can see, $10,000 is spent on the disposable item if there are 10,000 patient days, and $50,000 if there are 50,000 patient days.

The total of the fixed and variable costs is shown in Figure 7–4. This figure combines the fixed costs from Figure 7–1 with the variable costs from Figure 7–3. Note that in the graph the total costs start at $60,000, even if volume is zero, because of the fixed costs of the nurse manager.

Cost Graphs and the Relevant Range

One potential problem exists with this type of graphic analysis of fixed and variable costs. That concerns the *relevant range*. The relevant range represents the likely range of activity covered by a budget.

Variable costs increase proportionately over the relevant range. However, it is unlikely that the hospital will pay $.50 for each disposable thermometer cover at *any* volume level. If purchases increase substantially, the hospital will probably get a price reduction per unit. On the other hand, if purchases decreased substantially, the hospital would possibly have to pay more per unit. However, the variable costs may reasonably be considered to increase proportionately over the relevant range.

It was noted earlier that fixed costs are not fixed over any range of activity. If a nursing unit has zero patient days, the hospital will close the unit and not have any fixed cost for a nurse manager. If patient volume rises substantially and exceeds the capacity of the unit, the hospital might need to open a second unit and incur the additional cost of a second nurse manager. The costs, however, are fixed over the relevant range.

Essentially, variable costs do not increase by exactly the same amount per unit

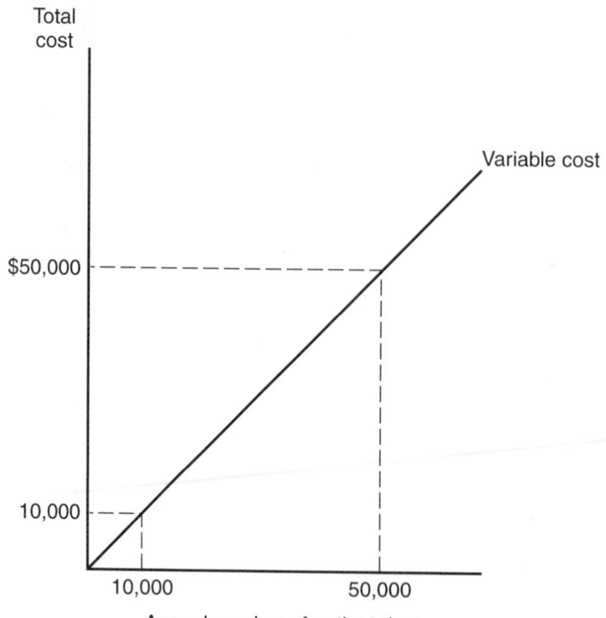

FIGURE 7–3. Variable costs: costs of a disposable supply item at volumes of 10,000 and 50,000 patient days.

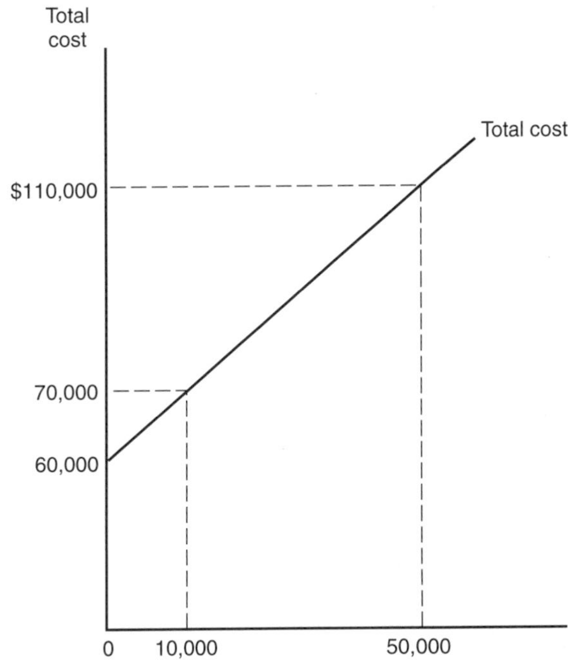

FIGURE 7–4. Total costs for unit.

over *any* range of volume, and fixed costs do not remain fixed over *any* range of volume. However, for most budgets, volume expectations for the coming year do not assume drastic changes.

When fixed and variable costs are graphed, the relevant range issue is often ignored; costs appear fixed over all ranges of activity in the graph. However, the user of the graph should bear in mind that the graph's information is only accurate within the relevant range.

Many costs are *step fixed* and vary within the relevant range but not smoothly. They are fixed over intervals shorter than the relevant range. See Figure 7–5 for a graphic representation of step-fixed costs.

For example, staffing patterns may be such that a nursing unit will use five nurses over a range of work load. If that range is exceeded, the unit will have to use six nurses. Clearly, more patient days or greater average acuity requires more nursing care hours. However, if the staffing pattern is about 4.2 hours of nursing time per patient day, the unit would not expect to hire a nurse for an additional 4.2 hours every time the patient-day census increased by one.

As long as there is a staffing chart that tells how many nurses are needed for any volume of patient days, the presence of step costs does not present a major budgeting problem.[2] Generally, because of the use of overtime and agency nurses, a step-fixed pattern of cost is estimated by treating the staffing costs as if they were variable. While this will not give a precise result, it is usually a reasonable approximation.

The Impact of Volume on Cost per Patient

If a nurse manager were to ask what it costs to treat patients in the unit, accountants would probably answer, "It depends." Costs are not unique numbers

[2]Note that such staffing charts often give the volume of patient days, adjusted for acuity level. See Chapter 12 for a discussion of using acuity for staffing calculations.

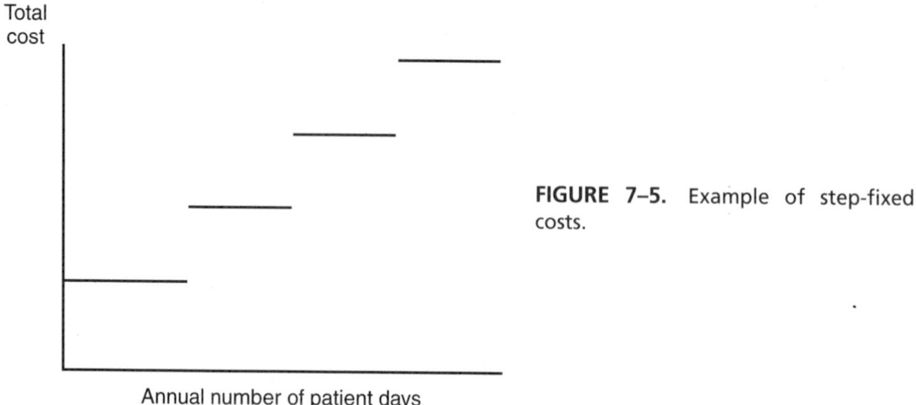

FIGURE 7–5. Example of step-fixed costs.

that are always the same. The cost to treat a patient depends on several critical factors. One of these is the volume of patients for whom care is being provided.

Suppose that a unit has fixed costs of $200,000 and variable costs per patient day of $200. Using this hypothetical data, what is the average cost per patient day? If there are 3,000 patient days for the year, the total costs are the fixed cost of $200,000 plus $200 per patient day for each of the 3,000 patient days. The variable costs are $600,000 (i.e., $200 per patient day × 3,000 patient days). The total cost is $800,000 (i.e., $200,000 fixed cost + $600,000 variable cost). The cost per patient is $267 (i.e., $800,000 total cost ÷ 3,000 patient days) per patient day.

However, what if there are only 2,500 patient days? Then the variable costs, at $200 per patient day, are $500,000, and the total cost is $700,000. In that case the cost per patient day is $280. The cost is higher because there are fewer patients sharing the fixed costs. Each patient day causes the hospital to spend another $200 of variable costs. The $200,000 fixed cost remains the same regardless of the number of patient days. If there are more patient days, each one shares less of the $200,000 fixed cost. If there are fewer patient days, the fixed cost assigned to each rises.

Table 7–1 calculates the fixed, variable, total, and average cost per patient at a variety of patient volumes.

Figure 7–6 shows the average cost at different patient volumes. The cost declines as the volume of patient days increases, because more patients are sharing the fixed costs. In Chapter 4 this result was referred to as economies of scale.

Suppose there are only 500 patient days. The total variable costs of $200 per patient day are $100,000, and the total cost is $300,000. The cost per patient day is $600, more than double the previous cost per patient results at 2,500 and 3,000 patient days.

In trying to understand costs, it is critical to grasp the concept that because fixed

※ **TABLE 7–1.** *Fixed, Variable, Total, and Average Costs at Various Patient Volumes*

Volume (A)	Fixed Cost (B)	Variable Cost (C = $200 × A)	Total Cost (D = B + C)	Average Cost (E = D/A)
1	$200,000	$ 200	$200,200	$200,200
50	200,000	10,000	210,000	4,200
100	200,000	20,000	220,000	2,200
500	200,000	100,000	300,000	600
1,500	200,000	300,000	500,000	333
2,500	200,000	500,000	700,000	280
3,000	200,000	600,000	800,000	267

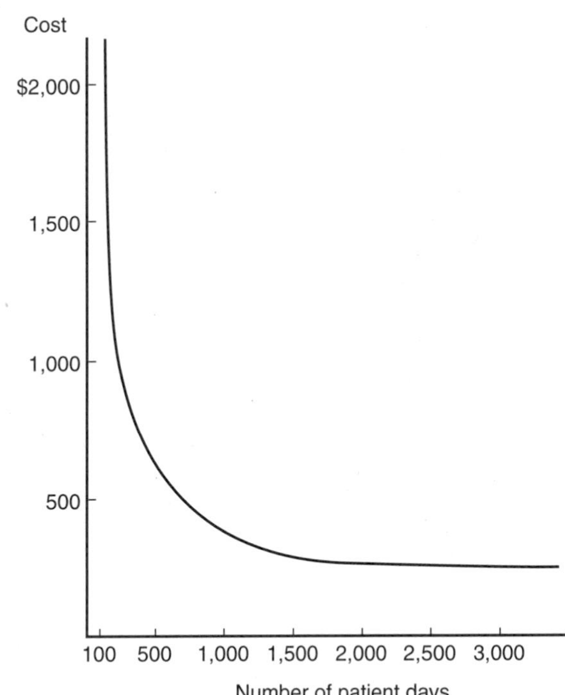

FIGURE 7–6. Average cost per patient day.

costs do not change in total, the cost per patient or per patient day does change as volume changes. The greater the volume, the greater the number of patients available to share the fixed costs. There is no unique answer to the question, What is the cost per patient day? That question can only be answered by giving the cost per patient day assuming a specific volume of patients. The volume of patients is critical.

One implication of this result is that health care organizations almost always find higher volume preferable to lower volume. As volume increases, the average cost per patient declines. If prices can be maintained at the original level, the declining cost will result in lower losses or higher profits.

Marginal Cost Analysis

Another costing concern is the issue accountants and economists refer to as *marginal cost analysis*. Decisions to change the volume of a service or to change the specific types of services offered should be based on marginal rather than average costs.

If someone were to ask the nurse manager the cost of treating a particular type of patient, the answer should be, "It depends." The previous section pointed out that it depends on the number of patients. It also depends on what the answer will be used for. If the question is just one of historical curiosity, the average cost is an adequate response. However, if the information will be used for decision making, that response may well be incorrect.

Suppose the hospital was trying to decide whether to negotiate with a health maintenance organization (HMO) to accept additional patients of the same average acuity and mix as the 2,500 patient days the hospital currently has. The HMO has offered $250 per patient day for 500 patient days. From the earlier calculations, the cost per patient for 500 patient days is $600! However, the hospital would not be providing only 500 patient days of care. It already has 2,500 patient days. From the earlier chart, the average cost is $280 per patient day at 2,500 patient days. At 3,000 patient days the average cost would be $267. Given that information, would it pay to accept the additional patients at a price of only $250?

It definitely would. Why should the hospital accept $250, if the additional patient days will cost at least $267? Actually the additional patient days will not cost at least $267. All the patients, on average, will cost that amount. The $267 includes a share of both fixed and variable costs. If the unit is going to have at least 2,500 patient days regardless of the HMO negotiation outcome, then the fixed costs of $200,000 will be incurred no matter what. The fixed costs will not change if the hospital has the extra 500 patient days.

Decisions such as this one require *marginal analysis*. The "margin" refers to a change from current conditions. "A patient on the margin" refers to adding one more patient or reducing volume by one patient. Marginal costs are the costs for treating one more patient.

On the *margin* in this case, if the hospital were to take the additional HMO patients, it would have more variable costs but would not have any additional fixed costs (assuming that 3,000 patient days is within the relevant range). Each extra patient causes the hospital to additionally spend only the variable costs of $200 per patient day. That is less than the $250 the HMO has offered to pay. The hospital will be better off by $50 for each additional patient day.

The additional costs incurred for additional patients are often referred to as the *marginal, out-of-pocket, or incremental costs*. If fixed costs were to rise because the relevant range was exceeded, those costs would appropriately be included in the incremental costs along with the variable costs. The key element in marginal costing is that the only costs relevant to a decision are those that change as a result of the decision.

The decision may be to add a new service or to close down an existing one. It may be to expand volume (as shown in the above HMO example) or to contract volume. In any case where a decision is being made that contemplates changing patient load, the essential information to be considered is the revenues and costs that change. Effective managerial decisions require that the manager know the amount by which total costs will increase and the amount by which the total revenues will increase or, alternatively, the amount by which both will decrease. Costs that do not change in total for the organization are not relevant to the decision. Fixed costs generally do not increase when additional patients are added (within the relevant range), and therefore they do not affect marginal costs.

Marginal cost analysis is sometimes referred to as *relevant costing*. The concept of so-called relevant costing is that all decisions should be made based only on those costs that are relevant to the decision. The simplest way to think about this concept is to consider costs before and after a change. The only relevant costs are those that change as a result of the decision. The approach applies equally to revenues.

In the hospital-HMO example, suppose that prior to the HMO negotiation the hospital was receiving $275 for each of its 2,500 patient days. Total revenue ($275 × 2,500) was $687,500. Total costs were $700,000 (calculated earlier). The hospital was losing $12,500, the amount that the $700,000 total costs exceeded the $687,500 of revenues. If the HMO business is accepted, the additional revenue would be $250 times 500 patient days, or $125,000. The total costs for 3,000 patient days (calculated earlier) are $800,000. The cost increase of going from 2,500 patient days to 3,000 patient days is only $100,000 (i.e., $800,000 total cost for 3,000 patient days *vs* $700,000 total cost for 2,500 patient days).

The total costs with the HMO patients are $800,000, and the total revenues are $812,500 (i.e., the original $687,500 + $125,000 revenue from the HMO). The unit has gone from a loss of $12,500 to a profit of $12,500. The costs have increased by $100,000, and the revenues have increased by $125,000. The amount by which the extra revenues exceed the extra costs for the 500 HMO patients accounts for the turnaround from a loss to a profit. This should not be surprising. The extra revenue per patient day is $250. The additional cost per patient day is $200. The difference

※ **TABLE 7–2.** *ABC Hospital Liver Transplant Program Financial Projections*

Operating Expenses	
Nurse program supervisor	$ 70,000
OR nurses (RN: circulating, scrub)*	100,000
Technician*	35,000
Orderlies*	14,000
OR receptionist/secretary*	24,000
Benefits*	55,000
Medical supplies*	150,000
Allocation of building depreciation	10,000
Allocation of OR equipment depreciation	20,000
Telephone allocation*	5,000
Office supplies*	3,000
Allocation of malpractice insurance and overhead not included above*	130,000
Total	$616,000

*Expense items assumed to vary directly with the number of operations.

NOTE: These numbers are hypothetical and do not reflect the true costs related to liver transplantation.

between incremental revenue of $250 per patient day and incremental cost of $200 per patient day is a profit of $50 per patient day. This extra profit of $50 for each of the 500 HMO patient days accounts for exactly the $25,000 profit from the HMO patients.

Had the hospital used average cost information for its decision, it would have turned away the extra business and lost the chance to gain a $25,000 profit. The $250 revenue is less than the $267 average cost. However, the average cost is not relevant for such decisions because it incorrectly assumes that each extra patient will cause the hospital to have additional variable and fixed costs. The incremental cost is relevant because it considers only the additional revenues and additional costs that the hospital will have as a result of the proposed change.

Relevant Cost Case Study

Assume that a hospital is trying to decide whether to perform liver transplant surgery.[3] The finance department has prepared a financial projection of the expenses for the service, which appears in Table 7–2. Which elements of the table are not relevant costs for the decision?

The first questionable item in the financial projection is the cost of the program supervisor. It is quite possible that one individual will be given the responsibility for the liver transplant program. However, one must question whether a new manager will be hired just for that position or whether the responsibility will be assigned to a manager who would be working on various other things in any case. Does the hospital actually spend more for supervisors if it has this program than it would if it did not? If the answer is that no more money is spent on supervision if the program exists than if it does not, then the cost is not relevant.

The costs of the staff in the operating room during the transplantation are probably relevant. By adding more patients, more nursing staff will be needed. The same is true of the technician. On the other hand, it is not clear that the secretary and orderly are relevant costs. The manager must assess whether the addition of the program will necessitate having an additional full- or part-time secretary or orderly. If existing staff carry a heavier burden with no staff additions, the costs are not

[3]This discussion is not intended to be a comprehensive analysis of all the relevant and nonrelevant costs related to liver transplantation. Its purpose is merely to provide the reader with some examples of costs that are not relevant to a particular decision.

relevant unless additional overtime is incurred. In that case, it would be the overtime cost that was relevant.

Allocation of building overhead is clearly a nonrelevant cost. The building will depreciate in any case. Unless remodeling is done to accommodate the program or unless the organization must acquire additional space, building depreciation should not be considered in making a decision regarding whether to offer the program. The same is true for equipment depreciation. Assuming that no additional equipment is acquired for the program, depreciation is not a relevant cost. On the other hand, some new equipment will likely be required, and depreciation of any equipment specifically purchased for the program is a relevant cost.

Malpractice insurance is a peculiar item. In some hospitals it is based on past experience. In other hospitals it is based on the sum of the riskiness of the patients and services of the hospital. Liver transplantation can be a risky operation. However, patients are aware of that. An assessment must be made concerning whether this program increases the risk of lawsuits and malpractice findings against the hospital. If so, the malpractice insurance costs will probably increase as a result of the program, and the cost is considered relevant.

Accountants may still argue that a portion of the nonrelevant cost items must be assigned to the program so that the full costs of the liver transplantation program will be known. "All costs must be allocated to all activities to be fair, or else why should any costs be allocated to any activities?" Managers would argue that it is preferable not to allocate any costs rather than to allocate costs in such a way as to result in poor managerial decisions. If it is decided not to add the liver program because of costs allocated to it that are not relevant, then the accounting system is a hindrance to the organization's success. The analysis of the new program must allow the manager to know how much *more* cost the organization will have with the program than without the program.

Whether preexisting costs are allocated to the program or not, the important thing to keep in mind is that when decisions are made, relevant costs are the only costs that should be considered.

※ COST ESTIMATION TECHNIQUES

One of the most difficult parts of financial management is the prediction of costs. This is an essential component of financial management. Budgets contain cost estimates. Trying to predict how much will be spent on each type of expenditure in the coming year presents great problems for both inexperienced and experienced managers. Managers must have ways to estimate such costs.

One approach is to simply look at what happened this year and predict that it will occur again next year, with an increment for inflation. At the other extreme is an approach that says it is desirable to do better next year than this year, so it is appropriate to budget a certain percentage less than was spent this year. In each case, the approach is far too simplistic. A priori, there is no reason to believe that next year will be just like this year, and simply wishing to spend less than this year will not make it so.

Some sort of clear method is needed that will allow prediction of what will happen next year based on the past. Some way to formally consider why that prediction may not come true is also needed. Finally, if costs are to be reduced below the predicted outcome, there must be a specific plan that the nurse manager believes can accomplish the cost cutback.

This section considers several methods of cost estimation. Not all elements of the budget are simply costs. Items such as the number of patient days must be predicted as well. A discussion of general forecasting is presented in Chapter 18. Here the focus is solely on prediction of costs.

Often historical information about costs incurred can be a great aid in predicting what costs will be in the future. This is especially true in the case of mixed costs, which have both fixed and variable cost elements. Cost estimation techniques look at historical information and compare the change in cost over time with the change in volume over time to isolate fixed and variable costs.

If costs rise as volume rises, what could account for the increase in costs? Fixed costs, by definition, do not change as volume changes. Therefore any change in cost as volume changes must be attributable to the variable cost. By seeing how much costs change for a change in volume, it is possible to calculate the variable cost per unit. Once the variable cost per unit is known, the total variable cost for any volume can be determined by multiplying the variable cost per unit by the volume. Then fixed cost can be determined as well. The difference between the total cost for any volume and the total variable cost for that volume is the fixed cost. The fixed and variable cost information can then be used to estimate costs for the coming year, based on a forecast of the volume in the coming year.

There is one critical problem in the flow of logic that allows cost estimation. Changes in cost over time are assumed to be the result only of changes in volume. However, to some extent changes in cost over time are the result of other changes. One possible type of change is evolving clinical practice. For example, a new technology may require more IV solutions than were needed before its patients had access to that technology. Managers should always adjust any estimates they make for the impact of any changes that they anticipate.

Another problem is inflation. If inflation were a constant percent that was the same each year, one could argue that past inflation could be ignored and inflation would automatically be built into predictions for the future. However, inflation rates tend to fluctuate from year to year. Over a period of years the fluctuations can be substantial. Therefore, to be able to predict fixed and variable costs, the data should be adjusted for the effect of inflation.

Adjusting Costs for Inflation

Suppose that a nurse manager is interested in determining how much the total RN staff costs of the unit will be for fiscal year 2001.[4] This hypothetical unit is staffed with a minimum of ten full-time equivalent (FTE) RNs for any volume up to 9,000 patient days at a certain acuity level. The cost of those ten FTEs is fixed because the unit will always have at least that cost. As volume increases above 9,000 patient days, additional nursing time will be needed. In 1999 patient days numbered 9,800, and the cost including fringe benefits was $500,000. In 2000 the patient days totaled 11,000 and the cost was $580,000. The cost increase of $80,000 was attributable to both the increased volume and inflation.

Most readers are probably familiar with the consumer price index (CPI), the most widely used measure of inflation. The CPI and many other indexes of inflation, such as the hospital market basket index, were developed by or for the federal government. The CPI measures the relative cost of a typical basket of consumer goods. Whatever the basket of goods cost in the base year is considered to be 100% of the cost in that year, or simply 100. The index is revised, and a new base year is established from time to time. If it costs twice as much to buy the same goods in a year subsequent to the base year, the index would be 200% of the base year costs, or simply 200.

The U.S. Department of Commerce, Bureau of the Census, annually publishes the *Statistical Abstract of the United States.* Included in that book are "Indexes of Medical Care Prices." There are several quite useful indexes under that heading, including the index of medical care services and the hospital daily room rate index.

In this example the nurse manager wants to find the variable cost per patient day

---

[4]A fiscal year may start at any convenient date, not necessarily January 1. For example, a fiscal year could begin on July 1 and end on June 30. In that case, fiscal year 2001 would refer to the year from July 1, 2000, through June 30, 2001.

of nursing labor for 2001 using current dollars as of the end of fiscal year 2000. If information from 1996 through 2000 is used, the nurse manager will have to find the value of an appropriate index in each of those years. The financial managers in most health care institutions can provide nurse managers with appropriate indexes adjusted for labor costs in the specific geographic area. Failing that, most library reference sections can be of assistance with current index information. Assume that an appropriate index has values as follows:

1996	258
1997	287
1998	318
1999	357
2000	395

Suppose also that the following cost and volume information is available:

Year	Patient Days	Cost
1996	8,000	$328,000
1997	8,700	364,000
1998	8,850	404,000
1999	9,800	500,000
2000	11,000	580,000

It appears that costs have risen from 1996 to 2000, even though volume is below 9,000 patient days in each of those years. Because the staffing is fixed at ten FTEs for any volume below 9,000 patient days, the cost is expected to be about the same in each of those three years and to increase only as volume increases above 9,000 patient days, thus requiring more nursing staff. The cost information, however, is not comparable because of the impact of inflation. To make the numbers reasonable for comparison purposes, they must be restated in *constant dollars,* that is, in amounts that have been adjusted for the impact of inflation.

That adjustment can be done by multiplying the cost in any given year by a fraction that represents the current value of the index divided by the value of the index in the year the cost was incurred. This is not a complicated procedure. For example, in 1996 the cost was $328,000. The hypothetical index value is 395 for fiscal year 2000. In 1996 it was 258. Multiply $328,000 by the fraction 395⁄258. The result is $502,171, which is the 1996 cost adjusted to year 2000 dollars. Now the $580,000 spent when there were 11,000 patient days in 2000 can be compared with $502,171, the constant-dollar cost of 8,000 patient days in 1996. In a similar fashion all the data can be restated in year 2000 dollars, as in Table 7–3.

Inflation accounts for changes in prices. One example of a change in prices is a change in wages. Wage rates are the price an organization pays for labor. Note that adjusted for inflation, there was very little change in costs from 1996 to 1998, the period during which the staffing was fixed because patient days were less than 9,000. However, the actual dollars spent in those years, before adjusting for inflation, rose from $328,000 to $404,000. Such an increase might at least partly reflect the impact of rising salaries.

TABLE 7–3. *Adjusting Costs for Inflation*

Year	Patient Days	Original Cost		Index Fraction		Adjusted Cost
1996	8,000	$328,000	×	395/258	=	$502,171
1997	8,700	364,000	×	395/287	=	500,976
1998	8,850	404,000	×	395/318	=	501,824
1999	9,800	500,000	×	395/357	=	553,221
2000	11,000	580,000	×	395/395	=	580,000

These index values are hypothetical. Managers should consult their organization's financial managers for an appropriate inflation index and its actual values for their specific geographic region.

High-Low Cost Estimation

The high-low approach is a relatively simple, quick-and-dirty approach to cost estimation. It is unsophisticated and therefore not terribly accurate, but in many cases it may be good enough. It certainly is better than simply taking a guess.

The key to the high-low method is the fact that fixed costs do not change at all in response to changes in volume. The way the method works is to look at the organization's cost for a specific item over a period of approximately five years. Costs adjusted for inflation should be used, as described above.

The use of five years is arbitrary. It might be more appropriate to use a longer period, but one would not want to use data from much less than five years. Less than five years should be used only if there have been substantial changes in the unit that make earlier data no longer relevant. For the period chosen, find the highest volume and the lowest volume and compare the costs at these two volumes.

The amount by which the costs changed from the lowest to highest volume should be compared with the amount by which the volume changed. In the example from the previous section, the highest volume in the last five years was 11,000 patient days, and the cost for nursing labor that year for the department was $580,000. The lowest volume in the last five years was 8,000 patient days, and the constant dollar inflation adjusted cost in that year was $502,171. In this case, inflation-adjusted costs increased by $77,829, while volume increased by 3,000 patient days. If $77,829 is divided by 3,000 patient days, the result is $25.94 per patient day. Although it is certainly likely that nursing labor is a step-fixed cost and therefore will not go up by $25.94 for *each* additional patient day, that volume provides a reasonable measure of the amount of additional nursing services needed per patient day when there are significant changes in volume.

If the variable cost per patient day is $25.94, what is the fixed cost? The yearly total variable cost is first found by multiplying the variable cost per patient day by the number of patient days ($25.94 × 8,000 = $207,544). The total nursing labor cost for 8,000 patient days was $502,171 in 1996; if $207,544 is the variable cost, then the remainder, $294,627, represents the fixed cost. Similarly, for 11,000 patient days at $25.94 per patient day, the variable cost is $285,373; given a total cost of $580,000 in 2000, the fixed cost would be $294,627. The fixed cost is expected to be the same at either volume level, because by definition it is fixed.

This fixed and variable cost information can be used in preparing next year's budget. If 12,000 patient days are expected, then costs will be expected to rise by $25.94 times 1,000 patient days, or $25,943. The fixed cost portion will not change. Since this information was calculated using 2000 constant dollars, both the fixed and variable costs will have to be adjusted upward for the expected 2001 salary increases or, more generally, for the expected impact of inflation during the next year.

The high-low method is not accurate because it considers only the experience of 2 years. One or both of the 2 years chosen may have had some unusual circumstance that would skew the costs in that year. A superior prediction is possible if some method is used that takes more experience into account. *Regression analysis* can provide such a prediction.

Regression Analysis

The volume of patient days and the total cost for those days for a number of years can be plotted on a graph. The horizontal axis represents volume, and the vertical axis represents cost. The result is a scatter diagram. The points on the graph each represent a volume and the cost at that volume. If a line is drawn approximating the points, it can be used for future predictions. By selecting any expected volume on the horizontal axis, it is possible to go vertically up to the line and then from the line move horizontally across to a point on a vertical cost axis. That point represents the

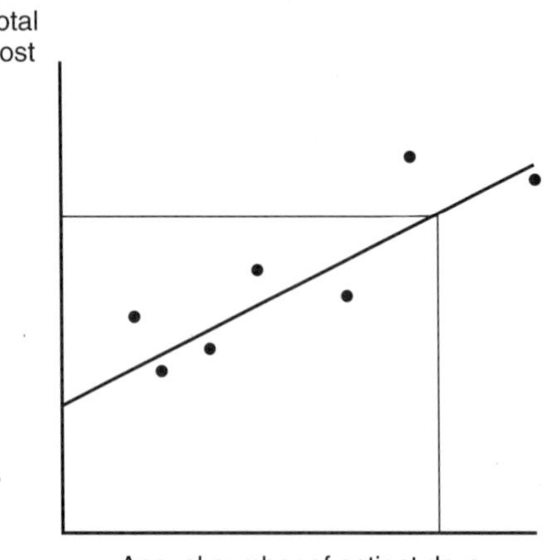

FIGURE 7–7. Predicting costs from scatter diagram.

prediction of cost. For example, Figure 7–7 shows a scatter diagram with a line drawn approximating the points.

The difficulty in drawing the diagonal line connecting those points is properly placing it so that it will give accurate predictions. Regression analysis is a technique that applies mathematical precision to a scatter diagram. Regression technique can select the one line that is effectively closest to all the individual points on the scatter diagram and that will therefore best predict cost for the future. This can fairly accurately break costs down into their fixed and variable components.

Simple linear regression analysis can take all available past information into account in estimating that portion of any cost which is fixed and that portion which is variable. The phrase simple linear regression refers to several issues. First, it is simple in the sense that there is only one *dependent* variable and one *independent* variable. Cost is the dependent variable that is being estimated. Cost depends on the value of the independent variable.

An independent variable is a *causal* factor. For example, the most significant causal factor for nursing costs might be patient days. The more patient days, the greater the costs for nursing. Patient days *cause* costs to be incurred. For the admissions department of the hospital, it is not patient days but rather the number of patients that is important, since admission time is the same for each patient regardless of the ultimate length of stay.

The second part of the phrase simple linear regression refers to the presumption that cost behavior can be shown in a linear fashion, that is, using a straight line. What if a slightly lower price per disposable supply unit is paid for every increase in volume (e.g., $.75 for one unit, $.7499 per unit for two units, $.7498 per unit for three units, and so on)? In that case, Figure 7–2 is not an accurate reflection of how variable costs change. It is necessary to draw a curved line on the graph, but the mathematics involved with curved lines instead of straight lines are far more complicated. Variable costs are generally treated as if they are linear even if that is only an approximation of their true behavior.

Finally, the term regression refers to trying to regress, or bring all the points from the scatter diagram as close as possible to the estimated line.

For example, suppose that the CNE desires to make a rough starting prediction for the total cost of all nursing units in a hospital for the coming year. If last year there were 50,000 patient days and this coming year patient days are expected to be 52,000, then there is a 4% expected increase in the number of patient days. However, it cannot be assumed that all nursing costs will go up by 4%, because some costs, like the salary of the CNE, are fixed and will not rise in proportion to the number of patient days.

The high-low method is one way to make the prediction, but the high-low method relies on only two data points. Far greater accuracy in breaking out fixed and variable costs is possible if the past years' costs on a very detailed basis are examined, cost item by cost item, to determine which were fixed and which were variable. That is a very time-consuming procedure. Gathering information costs money, and even if the information is gathered, there are always some costs that cannot be separated into fixed and variable components without some estimating method, because they are mixed costs. For example, nonmedical supplies, such as paper, pens, and forms, are needed to some extent regardless of patient volume. On the other hand, the more patients, the more nonmedical supplies used.

How can costs be divided into their fixed and variable components and less money be spent on gathering information than if each line item from past years is examined? Regression analysis can help to separate these mixed costs.

Mixed Costs and Regression Analysis

Suppose it is known that last year the combined cost of the salary of the nurse manager and the disposable supplies was $110,000 and that the number of patient days was 50,000. This uses the information represented in the graphs presented in Figures 7–1 through 7–3. The volume of patient days is expected to rise to 52,000 next year. Should the $110,000 cost be increased by 4% because volume is increasing by 4%? No, it should not. Some costs are fixed. Only variable costs increase as volume increases.

One would expect costs to increase by $2,000, or $1 for each extra patient day, because it is known in this simple example that variable costs for the disposable thermometer covers were $1 per patient day. However, in dealing with a more realistic example with many different fixed, variable, and mixed costs, the variable costs per patient day are not necessarily known. Suppose that the historical information in Table 7–4 were available (already adjusted for inflation using the indexing techniques). If the high-low technique were used to evaluate the fixed and variable costs, there would be a very strange result. The highest cost is $110,000, and the lowest cost is $101,000; thus costs have risen by $9,000. At the same time volume has increased from 40,000 patient days to 50,000 patient days, or an increase of 10,000. When $9,000 is divided by 10,000 patient days, a variable cost of $.90 per patient day results. Is that an accurate estimate? No, because it is known that the variable cost is $1 per patient day. What might be the cause of the discrepancy?

It is possible that 1991 was the first year that the disposable thermometer covers were used. Perhaps many of them were defective and were thrown away, or perhaps some were wasted because of lack of familiarity with using them. In any case, if more than $1 per patient day was spent on disposable thermometer covers in the low-volume year, then the costs were unduly high in that year. Therefore, the change

※ **TABLE 7–4.** *Historical Data for Thermometer Cover Costs*

Year	Patient Days	Cost
1991	40,000	$101,000
1992	42,000	102,000
1993	43,000	103,000
1994	44,000	104,000
1995	45,000	105,000
1996	46,000	106,000
1997	47,000	107,000
1998	48,000	108,000
1999	49,000	109,000
2000	50,000	110,000

in cost from 1991 to 2000 looks unrealistically low, and the variable cost measure is unrealistically low.

At the other extreme, had there been unusual waste (perhaps the fault of the nurses, but possibly due to quality problems with a large batch of the disposable item) in the most recent, high-cost year, the change in cost would look especially high, and the variable cost per unit would have come out to more than $1. As has been stated before, if one relies on just two data points, as the high-low method does, results are subject to the whims of unusual events in either of those years.

In reality, one would not expect to use exactly $1 per patient day on disposable supplies in any year. For one reason or another, some patients will have their temperature taken only once on a given day. This might be caused by admission to the hospital late in the day, for instance. On the other hand, patients with fever will no doubt have their temperature taken more often. A more likely pattern of costs is shown in Table 7–5.

Simply looking at this list does not provide a lot of insight about fixed and variable costs. Figure 7–8 shows a scatter diagram for these points. One can roughly see how costs increase as volume increases. A straight line cannot be drawn through all the points on this scatter diagram. However, the regression technique uses all the available information to select a line that will provide the best estimate in the absence of any other information.

Regression analysis uses information about the dependent and independent variables in the past to develop an equation for a straight line. As part of that process it calculates a constant value and a coefficient for the independent variable. If the dependent variable is the cost, then the constant represents the fixed cost and the coefficient of the independent variable represents the variable cost.

Regression analysis is a statistical technique. A detailed discussion of statistics is beyond the scope of this book. However, many mechanical approaches to regression have made it a workable tool in health care institutions. Regression can be performed on many hand-held calculators. A wide variety of statistical programs and spreadsheet programs for personal computers also have regression capability.

Turning back to the scatter diagram in Figure 7–8, it is possible to use regression analysis to predict what the costs will be for the nursing unit next year if there are 52,000 patient days. Regression analysis will determine a specific line to plot through this scatter diagram that will give the best possible estimate of fixed and variable costs and therefore allow prediction of the cost next year.

Basically, the process requires several simple steps. First determine the cost associated with each volume of patient days. For instance, when there were 40,000 patient days, the cost was $101,000. The independent variable, patient days, is often referred to as the X variable because it is plotted on the horizontal axis. The dependent variable, cost, is often referred to as the Y variable because it is plotted on the vertical axis.

TABLE 7–5. *More Likely Historical Cost Pattern*

Year	Patient Days	Cost
1991	40,000	$101,000
1992	42,000	101,800
1993	43,000	103,600
1994	44,000	103,800
1995	45,000	105,300
1996	46,000	106,700
1997	47,000	106,900
1998	48,000	108,800
1999	49,000	108,900
2000	50,000	110,000

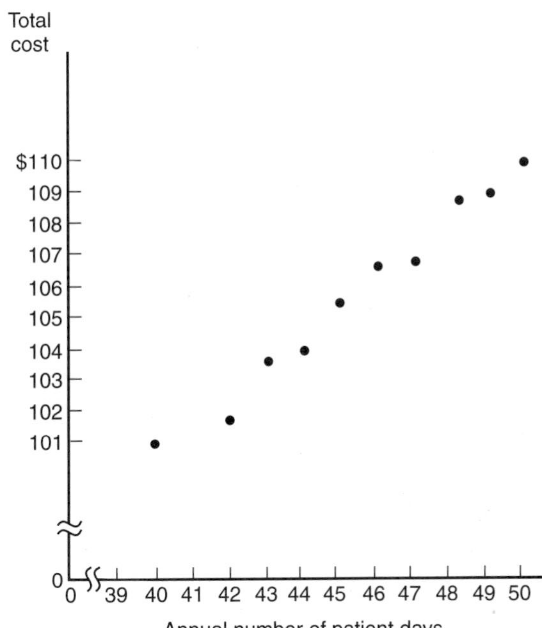

FIGURE 7–8. Scatter diagram of total costs for nursing (costs and patient days in thousands).

Any computer program will require that you provide the X values and the Y values for each year. Having provided that information, it is generally only necessary to give a command to compute the regression to complete the process. It is important not to let the extremely quantitative nature of regression theory learned in a statistics course discourage you from attempting to use this tool. In practice, very little mathematics are required of the user. Regression is a tool to help you manage better. The major difficulty in using regression is simply fear of the process.

In the example, regression analysis using the data in Table 7–5 predicts that the fixed cost is $62,255 and the variable cost is $.96 per unit. Figure 7–9 shows the resulting line. If extended, it would have its intercept at $62,255, increasing with a slope of .96. These figures are not exactly the expected variable cost of $1 per patient day and fixed cost of $60,000 for the salary of the nurse manager. They are, however, better estimates than the estimates the high-low method would give. The high-low approach predicts a fixed cost of $50,000 and variable cost of $.90 per patient day. Regression analysis is an inexpensive, potentially very useful, and relatively simple way of estimating fixed and variable costs and helping to predict future costs.

For any number of patient days predicted, it is now possible to multiply by .96 and then add $62,255 to get a forecast of future costs. With many computer regression packages, the process is made even simpler by requiring only that the forecast volume be entered into the computer along with the historical data. The computer will then generate the estimated cost for the coming year automatically based on the forecast volume. Remember, however, that it is necessary to adjust upward the resulting cost for expected increases due to inflation for the coming year.

While you will soon find this approach quite simple, it is useful only as a tool to aid you in managing. It should not be allowed to take over the role of your judgment. The mathematical model is quite accurate in predicting the future if nothing has changed. It is your role as a manager to know if there are reasons that costs are likely to change from their past patterns.

For instance, if you know that 1991 was the first year disposable thermometer covers were used and that there was an awful lot of waste that year, you might want to eliminate that year from the analysis. If you do, your regression results will show

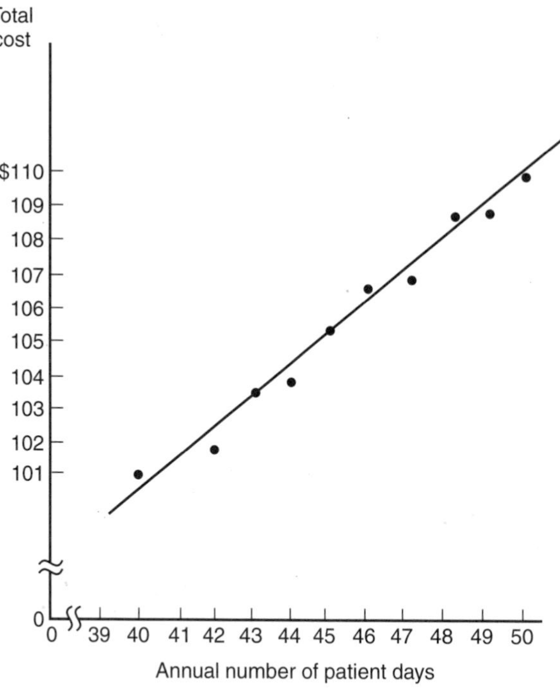

FIGURE 7–9. Simple linear regression of total costs for nursing (costs and patient days in thousands).

fixed costs of $59,970 and variable costs of $1.005. Recall that the fixed costs actually were $60,000 and the variable costs $1. As you can see, the input of judgment into the process can substantially improve the resulting estimates.

When regression analysis is performed, one statistic that is generally provided by the calculator or the computer is R squared (R^2). That value can range from a low of zero to a high of 1.0. If the value is close to zero, it means that the independent variable does not do a very good job of explaining the changes in the dependent variable. An R^2 value of .20, for example, might indicate that patient days are not a good predictor of nursing cost. On the other hand, an R^2 of .80 would indicate that it is a very good predictor. However, it is possible to become even more exact in estimating costs.

Multiple Regression Analysis

There is a type of regression analysis that is more sophisticated than simple linear regression. It is called *multiple regression* because it allows for use of multiple independent, or causal, variables. The use of simple linear regression can be a substantial aid in estimating future costs because it is so efficient at predicting the fixed cost and the variable cost per unit when there is one major independent variable. Sometimes, however, there are several key variables. For instance, suppose that the nursing costs vary with the number of patient days but also with the number of patients. That is most probably the case.

Certainly the costs vary with the number of patient days. The more patient days, the more temperatures to be taken, pulses to be checked, medications to be administered, and so on. Yet for each patient there is a health history to be recorded, a chart to be set up, a patient care plan to be established, valuables to be stored, orientation to be given, discharge planning to be done, discharge education, and so on. These costs are not fixed (the more patients, the more time spent on these activities), but they do not vary directly with the number of patient days. Several patients with a long length of stay will cost less than many patients with a short length of stay, even if the total patient days are the same. So it is likely that the cost of a nursing unit varies with both the number of patient days and the number of admissions.

Most hand-held business calculators cannot perform multiple regression. However, most statistical programs for personal computers can handle this easily. Instead of simply entering the X and Y values for each year into the calculator or computer, one enters an X value for the historical information for each of the independent variables as well as the Y value. Then to predict a future cost, provide the computer with, for example, the expected number of patient days and the expected number of patients to predict the expected costs.

Sometimes the multiple regression level of sophistication adds extra work and complexity without substantially changing the results. Recall that when all is said and done the result is just an estimate; all types of events can happen in the future that will throw off the estimate, no matter how finely tuned it is. It is not necessary to add complexity for its own sake. At times, however, multiple regression can produce information that would not otherwise be available.

For example, there has been more and more attention placed on measures of patient acuity, or the level of intensity of required nursing services. It certainly is clear that the amount of nursing services varies not just with the number of patient days but also with the severity of the patients' illnesses. If data about the number of patient days and the average acuity level are used as independent variables, the accuracy of estimated costs might improve substantially.

Another use for multiple regression is in investigatory work with respect to costs. Suppose that there is a strong feeling by the nursing staff that the way a particular physician practices medicine is extremely costly. This is common in the operating room, where particular surgeons often exhibit out-of-the-ordinary behavior. The number of operations by a specific physician each year can be used as an independent variable. Costs increasing as a result of more cases by that physician will show up as a positive coefficient for that independent variable. The nurse manager will then have evidence to support the more general feelings of the staff that the physician is an unusually high resource consumer.

The reader of this book is encouraged to pursue the topic of regression analysis further. This should be done on both a conceptual basis, reviewing the underlying principles and theories of regression analysis, and on a practical basis, using a computer software package to perform some regression analyses.

⋇ BREAK-EVEN ANALYSIS

To this point the general behavior of costs (fixed *vs* variable) has been discussed, as well as the techniques for cost estimation (high-low and regression). Attention will now be focused on using cost information for understanding whether a particular unit or service will lose money, make money, or just break even. This technique is useful for the evaluation of both new and continuing projects or services. It is often used in developing a business plan. Business plans are discussed in Chapter 20.

Nurse managers in many instances find it necessary to be able to determine whether a program or service will be profitable. One key to profitability is volume. Prices are often fixed. Average cost, however, is not fixed. As the number of patients rises, the cost per patient falls because of the sharing of fixed costs. One cannot simply compare price and average cost and determine that a program or unit will make a profit or a loss. To determine whether something will be profitable, it is critical to know the volume of patients.

Break-even analysis is a technique to find the specific volume at which a program or service neither makes nor loses money. Forecast information about the likely volume of the service can be compared with break-even volume to predict whether there will be profits or losses.

Break-even analysis is based on the following formula:

$$\text{Break-even quantity (Q)} = \frac{\text{Fixed costs (FC)}}{\text{Price (P)} - \text{Variable cost per patient (VC)}}$$

or

$$Q = \frac{FC}{P - VC}$$

where Q is the number of patients needed to just break even, FC is the total fixed cost, P is the price for each patient, and VC is the variable cost per patient. At a quantity lower than Q there will be a loss; at a quantity higher than Q there will be a profit.

The basis for the formula is the underlying relationship between revenues and expenses.[5] If total revenues are greater than expenses, there is a profit. If total revenues are less than expenses, there is a loss. If revenues are just equal to expenses, there is neither profit nor loss, and the service is said to just break even. Expenses are the sum of total fixed costs and total variable costs.

Example of Break-even Analysis

Suppose that a new home health agency opens in a rural area. It charges, on average, $50 per visit. The agency has fixed costs of $10,000 and variable costs of $30 per patient visit. If there are no patients at all, there is no revenue, but there are fixed costs of $10,000, and there is a $10,000 loss. If there were 100 patients, there would be $5,000 of revenue ($50 × 100 patients), $10,000 of fixed cost, and $3,000 of variable cost ($30 × 100 patients). Total costs would be $13,000 ($10,000 of fixed cost + $3,000 of variable cost), while revenues would be $5,000 and the loss $8,000. These data are hypothetical.

Each additional patient brings in $50 of revenue but causes the agency to spend only $30 more. The difference between the $50 price and the $30 variable cost, $20, is called the *contribution margin*. If the contribution margin is positive, it means that each extra unit of activity makes the organization better off by that amount. The contribution margin from each patient can be used to cover fixed costs; if all fixed costs have been covered, it represents a profit.

In this example, when there are 100 patients, there is $20 of contribution margin for each of the 100 patients, or a total contribution margin of $2,000. Note that the loss with zero patients was $10,000, while it was only $8,000 when there were 100 patients. The loss decreased by $2,000, exactly the amount of the total contribution margin for those 100 patients.

How many visits would the agency need to break even? The answer is 500. If each additional patient generates $20 of contribution margin, then 500 patients

---

[5]The formula may be derived as follows:

1. Profit = Revenues − Costs, or Profit = Revenues − Fixed costs − Total variable costs
2. At the break-even quantity, profit is zero, so: 0 = Revenues (R) − Fixed costs (FC) − Total variable costs (TVC)
3. Moving revenue to the left side of the equation and multiplying the equation by −1 yields: R = FC + TVC
4. Revenue is the price per unit (P) multiplied by the quantity of units (Q), and total variable costs are the variable costs per unit (VC) multiplied by the quantity of units (Q): (P × Q) = FC + (VC × Q)
5. Moving VC to the other side of the equation: (P × Q) − (VC × Q) = FC
6. Factor out Q from the left side of the equation: Q × (P − VC) = FC
7. Divide both sides of the equation by (P − VC) to yield the formula: Q = FC/(P − VC)

would generate $10,000 of contribution margin (500 patients × $20 = $10,000), exactly enough to cover the fixed costs of $10,000. If the agency has 500 patients, it will just break even.

This could have been calculated using the formula:

$$Q = \frac{FC}{P - VC}$$

or

$$Q = \frac{\$10,000}{\$50 - \$30} = \frac{\$10,000}{\$20} = 500 \text{ visits}$$

Break-even analysis can also be viewed from a graphic perspective, as shown in Figure 7–10. The total cost line starts at $10,000 because of the fixed costs. The total revenue line starts at zero because there is no revenue if there are zero patients. Where the revenue line and the cost line intersect, they are equal, and the agency just breaks even. Note that with fewer patients than the break-even point, the cost line is higher than the revenue line; with more patients than the break-even point, the revenue line is higher than the costs, and a profit is made.

Prior to the introduction of Diagnosis Related Groups (DRGs), most break-even analyses in hospitals focused on the number of patient days needed to break even. Hospitals do not get paid for extra patient days under the DRG prospective payment system. Therefore there is now attention on the total number of patients needed to break even, rather than patient days. Break-even analysis can also be performed based on the number of surgeries, clinic visits, or other appropriate service unit volume measure.

When there are different types of patients, break-even analysis becomes somewhat more complicated. The formula presented at the beginning of this section assumes that there is only one price and one variable cost and therefore one contribution margin. If there are different types of patients with different prices and different variable costs, it is necessary to find a weighted average contribution

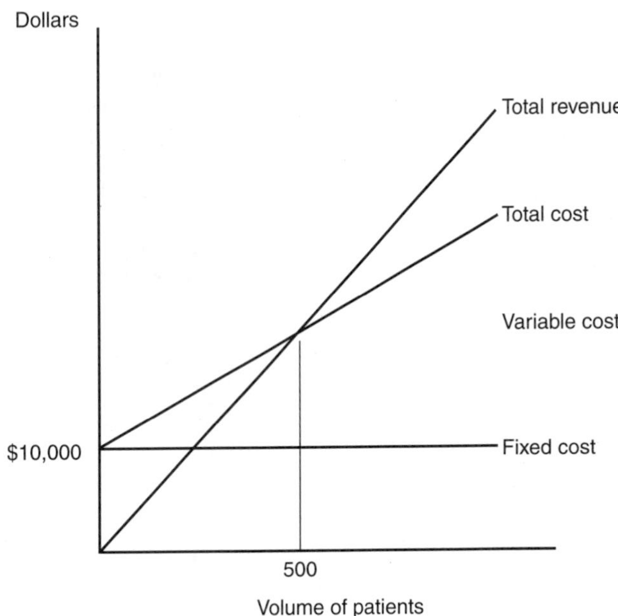

FIGURE 7–10. Break-even analysis.

※ TABLE 7–6. *Contribution Margin by Type of Patient Home Visit*

	Price (A)	Variable Cost (B)	Contribution Margin (C = A − B)
Complex	$80	$55	$25
Moderate	50	30	20
Simple	30	20	10

margin. That weighted average can be divided into the fixed costs to find the break-even volume for all patients.

For example, suppose that there are three classes of home care visits, referred to here as complex, moderate, and simple. The price for the visits is $80, $50, and $30, and the variable costs for the visits are $55, $30, and $20, respectively. The contribution margin for each type of visit can be calculated by subtracting the variable cost from the price, as shown in Table 7–6.

The crucial piece of information for calculating the break-even point is the relative proportion of each type of visit. Management of the home health agency expects that 20% of all visits are complex, 30% are moderate, and 50% are simple. This information can be used to determine a weighted average contribution margin. This requires multiplying the individual contribution margin for each type of visit by the percentage of patients that are that type of visit. The results are added together to get an overall weighted contribution margin, as shown in Table 7–7.

This $16 weighted contribution margin (CM) represents the average contribution margin for all types of visits. It can be used to calculate the break-even quantity. Assume that fixed costs are $10,000. The break-even quantity of visits is:

$$Q = \frac{FC}{P - VC} = \frac{FC}{CM}$$

or

$$Q = \frac{\$10{,}000}{\$16} = 625 \text{ visits}$$

Of the total of 625 visits needed to break even, 20%, or 125, are complex; 30%, or 188, are moderate; and 50%, or 312, are simple.

This method works for three different kinds of patients. What if there are more than three kinds? The same weighted average approach that can be used to find the break-even volume when there are three different types of patients can be used even if there are hundreds of different types of patients, as is the case with the DRG system.

What if there is more than one price for each type of visit? Medicaid pays one price, Medicare another, HMOs another, and self-pay yet another. This still can work

※ TABLE 7–7. *Calculation of Weighted Average Contribution Margin*

Visit Type	Percentage of Visits		Contribution Margin		Weighted Average Contribution Margin
Complex	20	×	$25	=	$ 5
Moderate	30	×	20	=	6
Simple	50	×	10	=	5
Total	100				$16

※ **TABLE 7–8.** *Contribution Margin by Type of Patient Home Visit and by Payer*

Visit Type	Price (A)	Variable Cost (B)	Contribution Margin (C = A − B)
Complex Medicaid	$40	$55	($15)
Complex other	80	55	25
Moderate Medicaid	40	30	10
Moderate other	50	30	20
Simple Medicaid	40	20	20
Simple other	30	20	10

within the same framework as has been presented. It will be necessary to calculate a weighted average contribution margin, treating each payer for each type of visit as a separate group. For example, if Medicaid pays $40 per visit regardless of the type of visit and the other payment rates are the same as indicated earlier, the contribution margin by type of visit by payer will be as shown in Table 7–8.

If it is possible to anticipate the percentage of each type of visit, a weighted average contribution margin can be estimated. Assume that 10% of all visits are Medicaid complex visits and 10% are other complex visits. Assume that 20% of all visits are Medicaid moderate visits and 10% are other moderate visits. Assume that 30% of all visits are Medicaid simple visits and that 20% are other simple visits. The weighted contribution margin will be as shown in Table 7–9.

The break-even volume can then be calculated as follows:

$$Q = \frac{FC}{P - VC} = \frac{FC}{CM}$$

or

$$Q = \frac{\$10{,}000}{\$13} = 769 \text{ visits}$$

The number of visits of any type can be determined by multiplying the 769 break-even volume times the percentage of visits in any given class. For example, since 30% of the visits are Medicaid simple, 30% of 769, or 231, Medicaid simple visits can be expected at the break-even level.

Some managed care organizations pay homecare agencies on a case rather than visit basis. With some patients paid on a case basis and others on a visit basis, these calculations become complex.

※ **TABLE 7–9.** *Calculation of Weighted Average Contribution Margin with Multiple Payers*

Visit Type	Percentage of Visits		Contribution Margin		Weighted Average Contribution Margin
Complex Medicaid	10	×	($15)	=	($ 1.5)
Complex other	10	×	25	=	2.5
Moderate Medicaid	20	×	10	=	2.0
Moderate other	10	×	20	=	2.0
Simple Medicaid	30	×	20	=	6.0
Simple other	20	×	10	=	2.0
Total	100				$13.0

Using Break-even Analysis for Decision Making

If a particular service is expected to have a volume of activity well in excess of the break-even point, managers have a clear-cut decision to start or continue the service. If the volume is too low to break even, several options exist.

One approach is to lower the volume needed to break even. There are three ways to reduce the required break-even level. One approach is to lower the fixed costs. In some cases it might be possible to do that. Another alternative is to increase prices. Price increases will increase the contribution margin per patient. That will also have the effect of lowering the break-even point. However, price increases might reduce the expected volume. In that case the price increases will defeat their purpose. Also, prices are sometimes regulated and beyond the control of the organization. Finally, one can try to reduce the variable cost per unit. This might be accomplished by increased efforts toward improved efficiency.

If it is not feasible to change fixed costs, price, or variable costs, an organization can try to attract more patients so that volume will rise above the break-even point. In the example presented, what type of visits would be desirable? The most desirable type of visit is a complex, non-Medicaid visit. That visit yields a contribution margin of $25. The least desirable is a Medicaid complex visit. The contribution margin is negative. For each additional Medicaid complex visit the agency loses money. In this particular example the most attractive visit brings the highest revenue. However, the focus should not be on revenue. If the highest-revenue visit also has extremely high variable costs, that visit might not be so attractive as one with lower revenue and much lower variable costs. The attractiveness of additional visits is determined by how much contribution margin they provide to the organization.

Break-even and Capitation

As managed care has become more and more prevalent, many negotiated contracts call for capitated payments. In such an arrangement the managed care organization pays the health care provider a set amount for each member for each month. This is called the per member per month (PMPM) payment. Under capitation, an increase in the amount of services provided to patients will not cause revenues to increase at all. On the other hand, an increase in the number of members will increase revenues.

Suppose that an HMO were to offer a home health agency $1 per member per month to provide all home care services for all of its members. Over the course of a year revenue would be $12 per member ($1 PMPM × 12 months = $12). Assume that the agency's variable costs are $30 per visit. Furthermore, the agency will have increased fixed costs of $10,000 if it takes the HMO members. How many members will the HMO need to have for the home health agency to break even on the contract?

We can use break-even analysis to calculate the break-even number of members. The fixed costs are $10,000. The variable costs are $30 per visit. The price is $12 per member per year. However, we do not have enough information to calculate the break-even point, because we know only the variable cost per visit. We need to know the variable cost per member per year. To find the break-even volume of members, it is necessary to predict the utilization levels, that is, how many home visits each member will have.

Most individuals will not need any visits in a typical year. Suppose that the average person consumes .3 visits in a given year. The variable cost for .3 visits per year is $9 (the $30 variable cost per visit multiplied by .3 visits per year). That $9 represents the variable cost per member per year. We can now calculate the break-even point as follows:

$$Q = \frac{FC}{P - VC}$$

$$Q = \frac{\$10,000}{\$12 - \$9} = 3,333 \text{ members}$$

Both the price and the variable costs in the calculation are per member per year. The quantity calculated represents the number of members needed to break even. If the HMO guarantees 5,000 members, the agency will likely make a profit. If there are only 2,000 members, it will lose money.

What if the agency has other fixed costs as well. Are they needed for the calculation? No. The determination of whether the HMO contract is profitable depends only on the marginal costs of the contract. Fixed costs that exist whether the agency contracts with the HMO or not are not relevant to the decision or the calculation. What if the HMO contract did not cause fixed costs to rise at all? Then the contract would be profitable for the agency as long as the revenue per member per year exceeded the variable cost per member per year.

Break-even Analysis Cautions

A few words of caution are advisable when working with break-even analysis. First of all, once a break-even point is calculated, one must decide whether it is likely that actual volume will be sufficient to exceed that point. That requires a volume forecast (see Chapter 18). To the extent that the forecast of volume is incorrect, the decision to go ahead with a new service may turn out to be a bad one, even if the break-even analysis is perfect.

Another potential problem is that break-even analysis assumes that prices and costs are constant. If it can be reasonably expected that prices will fall over time, then a higher volume will be needed to keep a service viable, unless variable or fixed costs fall as well. On the other hand, if prices are expected to rise faster than costs, then a marginal service today may become profitable over time, even without an increase in volume.

Another consideration is that there is an assumption that the mix of patients will stay constant. Suppose that in the above example, over time there are more and more Medicaid complex visits. The contribution margin for such visits is negative. If the demographics of the population are such that a shift in mix in that direction is likely, then the results of the break-even analysis require close scrutiny. Will there be enough of those visits to shift a profitable service over to a loss?

As with all budgeting tools, judgment is essential. The nurse manager must through experience, insight, and thought examine the assumptions of any modeling technique and consider the reasonableness of the results. If a result does not seem to make sense, often that is because it does not make sense. However, break-even analysis is a tool that can help give a manager a firm starting point in understanding whether a project or service is likely to be financially viable.

⋇ IMPLICATIONS FOR NURSE MANAGERS

Assessing costs is complex. In general, costs do not increase in direct proportion with volume. The implications of this are that if money is lost on a particular program, the solution may be to increase patient volume for that program. More patients do not necessarily mean greater losses. It is possible that volume increases can turn a loss into a profit. Understanding how that can happen requires an understanding of cost behavior. Some costs are fixed; others are variable. The result of that basic nature of costs is that the cost per patient will decline with increasing volume. The greater the number of patients who share the fixed costs, the lower the average cost per patient. Costing is further complicated by the fact that additional patients do not cause costs to increase by the average cost per patient. Decisions that are in the organization's best interests often require marginal cost analysis.

An important part of the budgeting process is the prediction of costs. Estimated costs can be based upon historical cost information. Some estimation relies upon using the historical information to isolate variable costs from fixed costs. To make such calculations, it is first necessary to convert historical cost information into common or constant dollars. This requires *indexation* of costs for the impact of inflation. Indexation is a process that adjusts a dollar value for the impact of inflation over a period of time by using a *price index,* such as the CPI. A price index is a tool that indicates year-to-year changes in prices. Using indexed historical costs, the results of the cost estimation process will be in constant dollars. In preparing next year's budget, the cost estimate has to be adjusted upward by the anticipated inflation rate over the next year.

Once constant-dollar information is available, cost can be estimated using the high-low method, simple linear regression, or multiple regression analysis. Being able to estimate fixed and variable costs is potentially a valuable tool. To apply the results, however, projections of the estimated number of patients, patient days, acuity level, and so forth are needed. Chapter 18 focuses on the process of forecasting such data.

Break-even analysis is a tool that allows one to focus specifically on the quantity of patients needed for a program, project, or service to be financially viable. Its foundations are in fixed and variable costs. At low volumes of patients, the average cost may surpass the revenue per patient. As the number of patients increases, the cost per patient falls because fixed costs are shared by more patients. Eventually the cost per patient falls below the revenue. Break-even analysis allows the manager to determine what the break-even quantity is so that a reasonable decision can be made about the likely financial viability of a program, project, or service.

From the nurse manager's standpoint, the topics of this chapter have critical implications. At the most basic level, falling volume will mean rising cost per patient. In such cases it is likely that a revenue crisis will exist, and actions to restrain costs should be immediately contemplated. On the other hand, rising volumes represent an opportunity. They not only bring in more revenue but also decrease average cost per patient. Therefore there is the opportunity for profit from more patients and for more profit from each patient. Profits ultimately allow the organization to replace buildings and equipment, add services, add staff, improve quality, and raise salaries.

Additionally, in preparing budgets nurse managers should take into account the behavior of costs. The fact that certain costs vary in proportion while others are fixed may reorient a manager's thinking from the notion that a 10% increase in volume requires 10% more resources. This in turn can allow a manager to prepare budgets in a more sophisticated and exact manner.

Finally, managers should remember that decisions to begin, continue, or stop a program are not made solely on the basis of profit-and-loss projections. Some programs are continued as a community service, and the institution makes a conscious decision to subsidize them from other sources of revenues. However, such decisions require as much information about anticipated profits or losses as possible.

KEY CONCEPTS

Service unit Basic measure of the product or service being produced by the organization, such as discharged patients, patient days, home care visits, ambulatory care visits, emergency room treatments, or hours of operations.

Direct costs Costs that are incurred within the organizational unit for which the manager has responsibility, or costs that are directly related to patient care.

Indirect costs Costs that are assigned to an organizational unit from elsewhere in the organization, or unit costs that do not directly relate to patient care.

Full cost Total of all costs associated with an organizational unit or activity. This includes direct and indirect costs.

Average cost Full cost divided by the volume of service units.

Fixed costs Costs that do not change in total as the volume of service units changes.

Variable cost Costs that vary directly with changes in the volume of service units.

Relevant range Normal range of expected activity for the cost center or organization.

Marginal costs Extra costs incurred as a result of providing care to one more service unit, such as for one extra patient day. If one considers the full or total costs incurred by an organization before it makes a change and the total costs after it makes the change, the difference in costs represents the marginal costs of that change.

Mixed costs Costs that contain both fixed and variable cost elements.

Impact of volume on cost per patient Average cost declines as the volume of patients increases because more patients are sharing the fixed costs. Therefore health care organizations almost always find higher volume preferable to lower volume.

Marginal cost analysis Decisions about changes should be based on the marginal costs of the change, not on full or average costs.

Cost estimation Prediction of costs. This process is complicated by the necessity to divide historical mixed costs into their fixed and variable cost components and by the necessity to adjust historical costs for the impact of inflation to use them for predicting future costs.

Adjusting costs for inflation Part of the change in costs over time is a result of volume changes, but part is due to inflation. To adjust for the impact of inflation, a historical cost must be multiplied by the current value of an appropriate price index divided by the value of that index when the cost was incurred.

Regression analysis Once historical costs have been adjusted for the impact of inflation, regression analysis can be used to estimate the fixed and variable costs. Costs are the dependent variable, and service units are the independent variable. The constant term of the regression represents fixed costs, and the coefficient of the independent variable represents the variable costs.

Multiple regression analysis and cost estimation This technique allows superior cost estimates by incorporating information from several independent variables rather than just one.

Break-even analysis Technique that allows the user to determine the volume of patients required for a program or service to be financially self-sufficient. At volumes above the break-even point a profit is made, and below that point a loss occurs. Break-even analysis is based on the following formula:

$$\text{Break-even quantity (Q)} = \frac{\text{Fixed costs (FC)}}{\text{Price (P)} - \text{Variable cost per patient (VC)}}$$

Contribution margin Price minus the variable cost per service unit. This represents the additional financial benefit to the organization from each additional service unit. This benefit can be used to cover fixed costs or provide a profit. A weighted average contribution margin is used for break-even analysis when there is more than one type of service unit or more than one price for each type service unit.

SUGGESTED READINGS

Anderson, Lane, and Donald Clancy, *Cost Accounting,* 2nd edition, Dame Publications, Houston, Tex., 1998.

Cleverley, William O., *Essentials of Health Care Finance,* Aspen Publishers, Gaithersburg, Md., February 1997.

Crockett, M. J., et al., "Activity-Based Resource Allocation: A System for Predicting Nursing Costs," *Rehabilitation Nursing,* Vol. 22, No. 6, November 1997, pp. 293–298, 302.

Finkler, Steven A., and David R. Ward, *Cost Accounting for Health Care Organizations: Concepts and Applications,* 2nd edition, Aspen Publishers, Gaithersburg, Md., 1999.

Gapenski, Louis C., *Financial Analysis and Decision Making for Healthcare Organizations: A Guide for the Healthcare Professional,* Irwin Professional Publishers, Burr Ridge, Ill., January 1997.

Garber, A. M., and C. E. Phelps., "Economic Foundations of Cost-Effectiveness Analysis," *Journal of Health Economics,* Vol. 16, No. 1, February 1997, pp. 1–31.

Hansen, Don, and Maryanne Mowen, *Cost Management,* 2nd edition, South-Western Publishing, Cincinnati, Ohio, 1997.

Jegers, M., "Cost Accounting in ICUs: Beneficial for Management and Research," *Clinical Therapeutics,* Vol. 19, No. 3, June 1997, pp. 570–581.

Jones, K. R., "Standard Cost Accounting," *Seminars for Nurse Managers,* Vol. 3, No. 3, September 1995, pp. 111–112.

Levy, V. M., *Financial Management of Hospitals,* Wm Gaunt & Sons, Holmes Beach, Fla., January 1998.

McKeon, Tad, *Home Health Financial Management,* Aspen Publishers, Gaithersburg, Md., January 1996.

McLean, Robert A., *Financial Management in Health Care Organizations,* Delmar, Albany, N.Y., 1996.

Neumann, Bruce R., Jan P. Clement, and Jean C. Cooper, *Financial Management: Concepts and Applications for Health Care Organizations,* Kendall/Hunt Publishing, Dubuque, Iowa, May 1997.

Pelfrey, S., "Cost-Accounting Techniques for Health Care Providers," *Health Care Supervisor,* Vol. 14, No. 2, December 1995, pp. 33–42.

Prince, Thomas R., *Financial Reporting and Cost Control for Health Care Entities,* Health Administration Press, Ann Arbor, Mich., June 1992.

Ward, William J., Jr., *Health Care Budgeting and Financial Management for Non-Financial Managers: A New England Healthcare Assembly Book,* Auburn House Publishers, Westport, Conn., January 1994.

Warner, K. E., and B. R. Luce., *Cost-Benefit and Cost-Effectiveness Analysis in Health Care: Principles, Practice, and Potential,* Health Administration Press, Ann Arbor, Mich., 1983.

Zelman, William N., Michael J. McCue, and Alan R. Milikan, *Financial Management of Health Care Organizations: An Introduction to Fundamental Tools, Concepts, and Applications,* Blackwell Publishers, Malden, Mass., January 1998.

CHAPTER

8

Determining Health Care Costs and Prices

CHAPTER GOALS

The goals of this chapter are to:

- Clarify the difference between the types of cost information needed for external reporting and the information useful to managers
- Explain the traditional cost-finding methods as required in Medicare cost reports
- Describe approaches to assessing the cost of nursing care and provide examples of specific approaches to determining the cost of nursing care
- Define productivity and describe measures of nursing productivity
- Describe the issues related to determining the costs of different patient product lines
- Introduce the concept of standard cost and discuss approaches designed to yield more accurate cost information
- Explain the various approaches to rate setting
- Discuss variable billing for nursing services

※ INTRODUCTION

Chapter 7 discussed the foundations of cost analysis, including fixed, variable, average, and marginal costs, and explained which costs to use for different types of management decisions. In addition, methods were discussed for estimating future costs and for calculating whether a program or service would be financially self-sufficient. All these elements are essential tools in routine management activities. One can think of that material as representing the trees. Now that the reader can identify each different type of tree, it is necessary to step back and look at the forest. This chapter looks at some broader, organization-wide costing issues as well as issues related to setting rates or prices for health care services.

The first section of this chapter considers the difference between cost information generated by the organization to help managers to manage the health care organization and cost information needed for reports provided to persons outside the organization. This is an important distinction because the needs of internal and external users of information differ significantly.

The requirements for external cost reporting are complex. Traditionally, health care institutions have calculated their costs in what is called a *cost-finding* process, which finds the costs of units of service such as laboratory tests, x-rays, or routine patient days based on an allocation of *nonrevenue cost center* costs to *revenue centers*. That process generates the information needed to complete Medicare cost reports. Virtually all health care organizations that receive some revenue from Medicare are required to submit such reports. Historically these reports formed the basis for cost accounting in health care organizations. The information generated by such reports was used to determine department and patient costs.

However, such reports do not provide particularly useful information about the cost of nursing services. To understand the costs of caring for any specific type of patient, one must know the resources consumed by that type of patient and the cost of those resources. One of the most significant elements in that calculation is an understanding of the nursing resources consumed by each type of patient. In recent years the nursing profession has placed an ever greater stress on improving the ability to make such calculations. Understanding the costs of nursing services provides the manager with valuable information for decision making.

The chapter next turns to the issue of productivity. *Productivity* has simply been described as the ratio of *outputs* to *inputs.* To determine this ratio, managers must first decide the appropriate outputs and inputs. The largest component of inputs for most health care organizations is nursing personnel. Determining outputs is more complicated. It has been traditionally defined as a unit of service such as a patient day of care or patient encounter such as a visit. More recently, however, outputs are being considered episodes of care or even patient outcomes defined as some level of health. Determining productivity ratios will depend on how inputs and outputs are defined.

After addressing productivity, the chapter discusses product-line costing. In the highly competitive health care marketplace, managers have found that to remain competitive, they must have information about the costs not only of departments or units but also of treating different types of patients. This has led to a growing emphasis on what is called *product-line costing.* In product-line costing an attempt is made to find the average costs for a given type of patient or group of similar patients. This is done for all costs, not just nursing service costs.

In recent years health care organizations have started to develop various *standard cost* approaches to provide improved cost information for managers, especially with respect to the cost of various types of patients. Product-line and standard costing are discussed in this chapter.

Setting prices and planning total revenues are also discussed. In the health care setting, pricing is often referred to as rate setting. Cost information is the most essential ingredient in the pricing decisions that health care organizations make. When an organization sets prices for its services, it wants to be sure they are at least as high as the cost of providing those services. If they are not, losses will be incurred. The amount of revenue received in relation to the costs of providing care is critical to the continued existence of the organization.

Revenues are no longer the sole domain of the financial officer. In the last twenty years there has been a shift in responsibility from finance to nursing for the planning and control of nursing costs. More recently this shift in financial responsibility has included responsibility for revenues. Nurse managers need to become knowledgeable about the revenue process in health care organizations. In some cases revenues are set outside the organization. For example, the federal government sets Medicare Diagnosis Related Groups (DRG) rates. More often prices are negotiated by the purchaser (often the insurer) and the organization. Managers must be able to determine whether the revenue received in such cases will be sufficient to cover all the costs of providing care.

In addition to general rate-setting issues, nurses are starting to focus on direct charging for nursing services. In home health care, for example, agencies are primarily charging for nursing care. Accurate information on the cost of nursing services can be used as a basis for charging for nursing services. Nursing historically has not been a revenue center in hospitals, because of lack of accurate data about the nursing cost for different patient types. With improved information, nursing can be a revenue department, similar to laboratory or radiology. This issue is also discussed in this chapter.

※ COSTS FOR REPORTING *vs* COSTS FOR MANAGEMENT CONTROL

Managers need to have cost information to manage their responsibility centers within large organizations or the entire operation of smaller organizations. Many decisions that managers must make require information about the costs their units incur. The correctness of the decisions depends to a great extent on the accuracy of the cost information available. Therefore cost data collection for use by managers should have a high priority.

At the same time, health care organizations are required to comply with a number of external reporting requirements. The financial statements for external reporting are discussed in Chapters 5 and 6. In addition to producing financial statements, most health care organizations also are required to complete other reports that focus on the organization's costs. These reports are most commonly prepared for Medicare, Medicaid, and other governmental agencies and for some insurance companies. Some health maintenance organizations (HMOs) now also require cost reports from hospitals.

External reports are generally required by law or to comply with contractual arrangements. Publicly traded organizations complete reports as required by the Securities Exchange Commission. It is important to keep in mind that historically many payments to health care organizations have been based on costs incurred. As a result, payers often needed to know the hospital's costs. For example, for outpatients at hospitals and for some other types of health care organizations, Medicare payments are still cost based.

Most health care organizations spend a great deal of energy generating reports that contain mandated cost information. Unfortunately, in some cases the information contained in the external reports is used for internal management without careful thought to how the needs of internal information users differ from those of external users.

What types of information are inappropriately used for internal management purposes? Many types. Some of the problems are relatively easy to deal with; others are much more complex and are built into the underlying cost-accounting calculations used throughout the organization.

Consider an example of an easily solvable problem. Suppose you are a hospital or nursing home unit manager and that nurses float from their home unit to others, depending on which units are slow and which are busy. In some organizations the nurse continues to be charged to the home unit, even when shifted temporarily to another unit. That results in charges to the home unit for more resources than it consumed, and it undercharges the unit that borrowed the float nurse.

For external reporting purposes it may be adequate to simply show the total cost for the nursing staff. However, the organization needs its managers to control their costs. When it is time to contrast budgeted costs with actual costs, the actual costs should reflect the resources actually consumed on the unit.

How can this problem be solved? A system needs to be put into place that tracks which units nurses are assigned to each day and charges float costs to the unit that actually had the use of the nurses. Such systems are widely, although not universally, used.

A much more difficult problem concerns the use of cost reports for determining the costs of treating different types of patients. Cost reports are complex and difficult to complete. There are a number of problems with the information they contain. However, those problems become buried in the calculations, and many managers treat the cost report information as if it were more accurate than it really is. The next section explains the cost-finding process used to develop cost reports. The problems with the process that make its resulting information less than optimal for management use are discussed. Later sections of the chapter discuss alternatives that provide managers with more accurate information.

⁘ TRADITIONAL COST-FINDING METHODS

Health care organizations consume a variety of resources in providing their services. Labor, supplies, and equipment are needed to provide care to each patient. The challenge faced by accountants in health care organizations is both to accumulate cost information relating to all resources used and to find an efficient, economical way to accurately associate with each patient the costs incurred to treat that patient.

Practically speaking, it is unrealistic to believe that assignment of perfectly accurate costs to each patient is a reasonable expectation. To keep track perfectly would require constant observation of each patient to see how many towels are used, exactly how many minutes of nurse time and technician time are expended, and so on. Cost information costs money to collect. All organizations use accounting shortcuts to save money. However, there is a clear trade-off between how much is spent on cost information and how accurate it is. The more accurate the information, the more it costs. Each organization must decide when the level of information is "good enough." Expanded use of bar coding and computers make it possible to collect more detailed and accurate information without substantially increasing the cost of data collection.

The simplest cost-finding approach is to simply divide the total dollars spent over a period of time by the number of patients treated over that period. The result is the average cost per patient. That average will be the same for all patients. Clearly, however, such an approach is not good enough. It would be impossible for managers to begin to determine which patients are profitable and which generate losses if such a method were used. If managers worked hard to treat a certain type of patient more efficiently, they would not have any sense of whether that goal were accomplished if the same cost were assigned to all patients regardless of resources consumed. The approach must be more sophisticated.

The Medicare Step-down Approach

The approach most health care organizations use for cost finding is the one mandated for Medicare cost reports. With that approach, all resource consumption is first associated with a cost center. Housekeeping, finance, medical records, pharmacy, intensive care, operating room (OR), and coronary care are examples of cost centers. Each cost center accumulates direct costs, such as labor and supplies used in the center.

The next step is to allocate all the costs of the nonrevenue cost centers to the revenue centers. Revenue centers are the parts of the organization that specifically charge for their services. For example, patients are generally charged a specific amount for an operation but not for security. Revenue center managers are responsible not only for the costs incurred in their unit or department but also for the revenues. While this creates the burden of additional responsibility, it also adds benefits. If a unit or department is a revenue center, it can point to an explicit measure of the financial contribution that it earns for the organization. The revenue it generates can be used as an argument for giving additional resources to the center. If given the choice, most managers would want their departments to be classified as revenue centers.

How do health care organizations distinguish between cost centers that are revenue centers and cost centers that are not? The key requirement for a revenue center is that it must be possible to measure different consumption of that center's services by different patients.

For example, each day each patient benefits equally from the presence of a security guard at the front door of the organization. Therefore there can be one catchall charge per patient per day, called the *per diem*. It will include costs such as the security guard. However, if patients consume different amounts of a resource, specific charges are needed to reflect those differences. For example, if one patient has surgery and one does not, we need to be able to charge only the one who had surgery. And we need to be able to charge a greater amount to someone who had a more expensive operation than to someone who had a less expensive operation. Therefore, security is not a revenue center, but the OR is.

Examples of revenue centers in hospitals include pharmacy, radiology, OR, respiratory therapy, central supply, and the laboratory. Examples of nonrevenue centers include dietary, administration, housekeeping, and medical records.

Why must the nonrevenue center costs be allocated to the revenue centers? Health care organizations get their revenues by charging for the services provided. When the prices or rates are set, the organization must consider all its costs. Laundry is not a revenue center. It does not charge patients a fee for its services. Operating rooms consume large amounts of scrubs and sheets, which must be laundered. If a hospital were to set its OR prices high enough to recover the cost of OR nurses but did not consider the cost of the laundry, its prices might not be set high enough to recover all costs incurred by the organization. Therefore, to ensure that the organization sets prices high enough to recover all its costs, the costs of the revenue centers must include all the costs of the nonrevenue cost centers.

Once all the nonrevenue center costs have been assigned to the revenue centers, each revenue center can in turn assign its total direct and indirect costs to the units of service that have been provided to the patients it has treated. The costs assigned to a specific patient by each of the revenue centers can be aggregated to determine the total cost of treating that patient.

Even though Medicare now pays hospitals on the basis of DRGs rather than based on cost reimbursement, the Medicare cost report is still completed by hospitals. The cost information from the report is used by the federal government in its process of setting national payment rates for each DRG.

A Detailed Look at the Cost-Finding Approach

Accumulate Direct Costs for Each Cost Center

The first step in the cost-finding process is to accumulate the direct costs of the cost center. For example, consider an OR, which is a revenue center.

Direct costs in the OR include salaries and wages for regular staff. This includes all supervisory and staff personnel that work in the OR and are included in the OR budget. The OR manager, the scrub and circulating nurses, technicians, orderlies, clerks, and secretaries are all included. Employee benefits are also included in direct costs.

Other direct costs include the costs for supplies, seminars, agency per diem nurses, and all other items under the direct control of the OR that are normally considered its direct costs.

Determine Bases for Allocation

The laundry department is an example of a nonrevenue cost center. Once its direct costs have been accumulated, they must be assigned to revenue centers. Each center that uses laundry should be charged for a portion of the costs of the laundry. To do this, the manager must first decide upon the basis for the allocation.

The cost of the laundry could be charged in equal shares to each department that uses it. However, that would be unfair to departments that use relatively little laundry. Such an allocation would not be good enough.

Other approaches to allocating the cost of laundry would be on the basis of pounds of laundry or pieces of laundry. In fact, most health care organizations that have a laundry department assign laundry costs on the basis of the number of pounds of laundry. All dirty laundry is placed in a laundry cart, which is weighed. Then total laundry costs can be allocated based on the share of total pounds of laundry consumed by each department.

Is that an appropriate basis for the allocation? It is not the best basis. A lab jacket may be more complicated to sort and fold than a sheet. Although four lab jackets together may weigh the same amount as one sheet, they no doubt require more labor than one sheet. Labor is one of the greatest expenses of the laundry department. Therefore cost accuracy would improve if costing were done on the basis of the number of each type of laundry item. However, it would cost more to keep track of pieces than pounds.

Most health care organizations have decided that pounds of laundry is a good enough measure. It effectively assigns all the costs of the laundry to the revenue centers, and it uses an allocation basis that takes some, if not perfect, account of relative usage by different cost centers. In any event, the only perfectly accurate measurement would require one staff member to constantly observe each patient to see exactly what laundry that patient used. The cost of that approach would obviously be prohibitive.

The problem of the specific basis to choose is not limited to the laundry. Other cost centers also have had to make choices. For example, any health care organization that has a building must allocate its annual depreciation to the various cost centers. That is usually done on the basis of square feet. A cost center that physically occupies many square feet would be charged more than one that has fewer square feet.

Actually, it costs more to build certain parts of a facility than other parts. For example, an OR costs much more per square foot than a patient room. By allocating an equal amount of depreciation per square foot, too little is assigned to the OR and too much to medical and surgical rooms. Ultimately this means that medical patients are overcharged, relative to their resource consumption, and surgical patients are undercharged. However, hospitals have generally decided that an equal depreciation charge per square foot is good enough.

Allocate from Cost Centers to Revenue Centers

All costs of the nonrevenue cost centers are allocated to the revenue centers using the allocating bases discussed above. Figure 8–1 provides a simplified example of what this type of allocation attempts. In the figure, housekeeping and laundry are nonrevenue centers. Coronary care and pharmacy are revenue centers. Each nonrevenue center must ultimately allocate all its costs to the revenue centers.

Table 8–1 provides a simplified numerical example. As in Figure 8–1, housekeeping and laundry are nonrevenue centers and the coronary care unit (CCU) and pharmacy are revenue centers. The first line in the table shows the direct cost incurred in each of the four centers; the next two lines show the allocation base and how much of the base is related to each department.

Housekeeping cost will be allocated on the basis of square feet, and laundry on

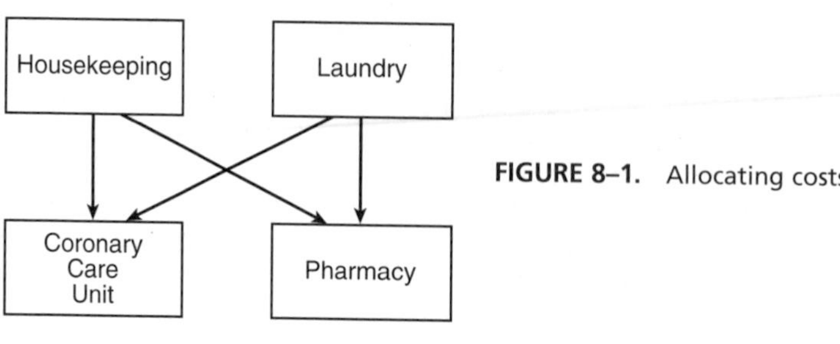

FIGURE 8–1. Allocating costs.

※ **TABLE 8–1.** *Cost-base Information for Allocation*

	Nonrevenue Cost Centers		Revenue Cost Centers		
	Housekeeping	**Laundry**	**Coronary Care Unit**	**Pharmacy**	**Total Cost**
Direct cost	$40,000	$60,000	$500,000	$500,000	$1,100,000
Allocation statistics:					
Housekeeping (square feet)	—	70%	25%	5%	100%
Laundry (pounds)	20%	—	10%	70%	100%

the basis of pounds. The table shows the percentage of all square feet that each cost center has and the percentage of all pounds of laundry used by each cost center. The square feet in the housekeeping department and the pounds of laundry done by the laundry for the laundry are excluded because no cost center allocates its own costs to itself. Thus housekeeping services are used 70% by the laundry, 25% by the CCU, and 5% by the pharmacy. Laundry services are used 20% by housekeeping, 10% by the CCU, and 70% by the pharmacy in this hypothetical example.

Table 8–2 shows an allocation of the direct costs to the revenue centers. The allocation in this table is called a *direct distribution*. In the direct distribution method nonrevenue center costs are allocated only to revenue centers. In making the allocation, a problem arises. Although 25% of the square feet are in the CCU and 5% are in the pharmacy (see Table 8–1), if those percentages are used for the allocation, the full $40,000 of housekeeping cost would not be allocated. This is because 70% of the square feet are in the laundry, and no cost is being allocated to the laundry. This problem is resolved by allocating to the revenue centers based on the remaining square feet after eliminating the nonrevenue centers. Thirty percent of the square feet is in all the revenue centers combined, and 25% is in the CCU. Thus 25% divided by 30% gives the proportion of the housekeeping cost allocated to the CCU. Similarly, 5% divided by 30% gives the housekeeping cost allocated to the pharmacy; 10% divided by 80% gives the laundry cost allocated to the CCU; and 70% divided by 80% gives the portion of the laundry cost allocated to the pharmacy. For example, 25% divided by 30% multiplied by the $40,000 housekeeping cost results in the $33,333 of cost allocated to the CCU.

There is an additional complexity because direct distribution fails to take into account the fact that some nonrevenue cost centers provide service to other nonrevenue centers. Housekeeping cleans the laundry. If all housekeeping costs went directly to revenue centers, none would be allocated to the laundry, and costs would be distorted. The possible distortion is so great that a direct allocation to revenue centers only is not considered good enough.

Instead an allocation approach is used called the *step-down method*, shown in Figure 8–2 and Table 8–3. The step-down method requires the organization to allocate all the cost of a nonrevenue cost center to *all* other cost centers (both revenue and nonrevenue). First one nonrevenue center's costs are allocated to every cost

※ **TABLE 8–2.** *Direct Distribution*

	Nonrevenue Cost Centers		Revenue Cost Centers		
	Housekeeping	**Laundry**	**Coronary Care Unit**	**Pharmacy**	**Total Cost**
Direct cost	$ 40,000	$ 60,000	$500,000	$500,000	$1,100,000
Allocation:					
Housekeeping (square feet)	–40,000	0	33,333	6,667	0
Laundry (pounds)	0	–60,000	7,500	52,500	0
Totals	$ 0	$ 0	$540,833	$559,167	$1,100,000

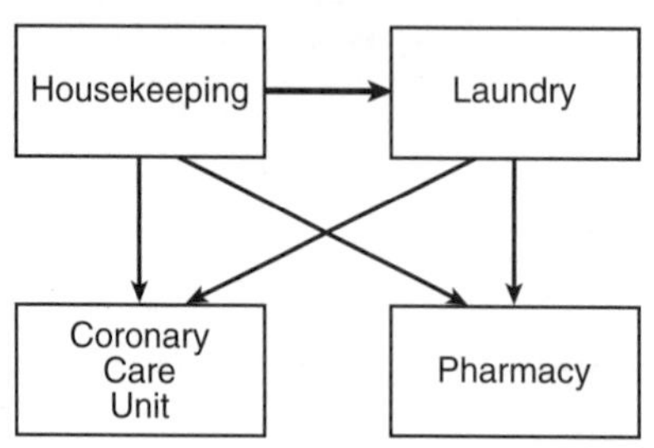

FIGURE 8–2. Allocating costs by step-down method.

center. Then another nonrevenue center is allocated. As each center is allocated, its cost balance becomes zero and it no longer is part of the process. In other words, no costs can be allocated to a cost center once it has allocated its costs. Note in Figure 8–2 that housekeeping now would allocate costs to coronary care, pharmacy, and laundry. The laundry, however, would allocate costs only to coronary care and pharmacy. Therefore some distortion still remains in the allocation process.

Other more elaborate allocation approaches eliminate most or all of the remaining distortion. These are called the *double distribution* and the *algebraic* or *matrix distribution* approaches. The algebraic or matrix distribution approaches are based on solving a set of simultaneous equations. While the allocation that results from use of such methods is more accurate, it is also more complicated to understand and implement. The hospital industry generally considers step-down allocation good enough.

The use of step-down allocation creates another problem: Should housekeeping be allocated before or after laundry? The order of the allocation may affect the ultimate outcome. Table 8–4 changes the order of allocation. Laundry is now allocated using the step-down method before housekeeping is allocated. Look at what happened to the ultimate cost in each revenue center. The total CCU cost has risen by $28,333, from $521,000 in Table 8–3 to $549,333 in Table 8–4. The pharmacy cost has fallen by $28,333, from $579,000 to $550,667. This is an extreme example, but it demonstrates the distortion possible by changing the order of allocation. In a perfect allocation system the ultimate cost in each revenue center would remain the same regardless of the order in which the nonrevenue center costs are allocated.

Are the actual resources consumed by the organization any different because the order of allocation of nonrevenue centers changed? No. The same total amount of money was spent. The same resources were used. However, the cost of the CCU and the pharmacy can vary because of the accounting method used. With the more sophisticated algebraic approach, such variation in costs does not occur. However, the step-down method, as noted, has been considered good enough.

※ **TABLE 8–3.** *Step-down Distribution*

	Nonrevenue Cost Centers		**Revenue Cost Centers**		
	Housekeeping	**Laundry**	**Coronary Care Unit**	**Pharmacy**	**Total Cost**
Direct cost	$ 40,000	$ 60,000	$500,000	$500,000	$1,100,000
Allocation:					
Housekeeping (square feet)	–40,000	28,000	10,000	2,000	0
Subtotal	$ 0	$ 88,000	$510,000	$502,000	$1,100,000
Laundry (pounds)		–88,000	11,000	77,000	0
Totals		$ 0	$521,000	$579,000	$1,100,000

※ **TABLE 8–4.** *Step-down Distribution with Altered Order of Step-down Allocation*

	Nonrevenue Cost Centers		Revenue Cost Centers		
	Laundry	**Housekeeping**	**Coronary Care Unit**	**Pharmacy**	**Total Cost**
Direct cost	$ 60,000	$ 40,000	$500,000	$500,000	$1,100,000
Allocation:					
Laundry (pounds)	–60,000	12,000	6,000	42,000	0
Subtotal	$ 0	$ 52,000	$506,000	$542,000	$1,100,000
Housekeeping (square feet)		–52,000	43,333	8,667	0
Totals		$ 0	$549,333	$550,667	$1,100,000

It is possible that the step-down method has allowed health care organizations to manipulate their cost reporting in an attempt to shift costs between revenue centers in an effort to increase reimbursement. For example, many hospitals have both inpatients and outpatients. Medicare inpatients are paid on a fixed DRG payment scale. Although it may change, currently outpatient payments for Medicare patients are not based on fixed DRG-type rates. If the order of the step-down allocation causes more costs to be allocated to the outpatient areas and fewer costs to departments that treat predominately inpatients, total reimbursement will rise.

Part of an institutional cost report is reproduced in the appendix to this chapter. This is from the type of report typically submitted to Medicare, Medicaid, and Blue Cross. It shows how the step-down allocation method is used in a real organization.

Allocate Costs to Units of Service

Up to this point the discussion has centered on allocating all costs of the organization into the cost centers that are revenue centers. The next part of the cost-finding process centers on assigning each revenue center's costs to the units of service that it provides. For example, a laboratory assigns its costs to the various lab tests it performs; an OR assigns its costs to the surgical procedures that take place. There are four approaches to allocating a revenue center's costs to units of service: the per diem or per visit, surcharge, hourly rate, and weighted procedure methods.

The per diem method is used if none of the other three methods reasonably applies. The per diem method divides the total costs of the center by the number of patient days, generating a uniform cost per patient day. Although some nursing cost centers do qualify for treatment using the other methods, that tends to be the exception rather than the rule. Most nursing costs are assigned ultimately to per diem categories. There are often different per diems for routine care as opposed to intensive care or coronary care. The major problem with such an approach is that it assumes that each patient consumes exactly the same amount of nursing (or other) resources per patient day. It takes no account of patient severity of illness or nursing requirements. However, the cost-finding process has treated this approach as being good enough.

The surcharge method is commonly used in the pharmacy and medical supplies cost centers. The revenue center compares its costs excluding inventory to the inventory cost and determines a surcharge. For example, if a pharmacy spends $10,000 on all costs except pharmaceuticals and $100,000 on pharmaceuticals, the surcharge would be 10% (i.e., $10,000 ÷ $100,000). As each prescription is filled, the cost would be calculated as the cost of the drug itself, plus 10%. The problem with this approach is that in reality, just because a drug costs ten times as much to buy as another drug does not mean that it requires ten times as much pharmacist time to process. Some organizations overcome this problem partly by using a minimum charge applied to all drugs dispensed. The proverbial hospital $10 aspirin is partly the result of charging a standard minimum amount for processing the aspirin order, storing the aspirin, and dispensing it.

The hourly rate approach measures the amount of service a revenue center provides by time. This method is used by respiratory therapy, physical therapy, ORs, and recovery rooms. For example, an OR would divide its total cost (after the step-down allocation) by the total number of hours of procedures to determine a cost per hour. Sometimes the calculations are done in minutes, yielding a cost per surgical minute. The logic of this method is that longer operations consume more resources.

This method is accurate for a service such as physical therapy, where generally only one therapist works with the patient. A problem with this approach in the OR is that an operation may require just one nurse, two nurses, or two nurses and a technician. Also, the supplies and equipment used may not bear a direct relationship to time. It is possible that a 2-hour operation might consume far more resources than a 3-hour operation. This method, while not very good, had traditionally been considered good enough. In recent years, however, ORs are trying alternative approaches. For example, many ORs keep track of person hours, rather than just surgical hours, to account for the number of staff members in the surgical suite.

The weighted procedure method (sometimes called the relative value unit method) is based upon a special study of the center's costs, which establishes a relative costliness of each type of service the center performs. This method is commonly used in departments such as laboratory or radiology, where there is a specific limited number of services provided, and they are provided in a similar fashion each time. A base value is assigned to one type of procedure, and all other procedures are assigned a relative value. Thus if blood gas analysis is twice as costly as a complete blood cell count (CBC), the CBC might be assigned a value of 1.0 unit of work and the blood gas a value of 2.0 units of work. In any given month, the values assigned to all the services provided can be summed and divided into the total cost of the revenue center. This yields a cost per unit of work.

For example, suppose that the total costs of the laboratory revenue center after the step-down allocation of nonrevenue centers costs is $5,000. If the laboratory performs 300 blood gas analyses and 400 CBCs, it performs a total of 1,000 units of work (300 blood gasses × 2 units of work + 400 CBCs × 1 unit of work). $5,000 divided by 1,000 units of work is $5 per unit of work. Therefore the $5,000 total laboratory costs would be assigned at a rate of $10 per blood gas analysis (2 units of work × $5 per unit) and $5 per CBC (1 unit of work × $5 per unit).

A problem with this approach is that it relies heavily on the assumption that a blood gas analysis is always twice as costly to perform as a CBC. This problem is exacerbated by the fact that many health care organizations use standard relationships based on a survey of institutions rather than measuring the relative costs in their own facility. Since the personnel pay rates and the equipment used will vary from one organization to another, the relative relationships are not likely to be exactly the same at all institutions. However, compared with having an accountant observe the resources used each time a lab test is performed, it is considered good enough.

Is Good-enough Cost Finding Good Enough?

For the first two decades under Medicare and Medicaid, the good-enough approximations that resulted from the above cost-finding system were considered acceptable. Most large third-party payers, such as Medicare, Medicaid, Blue Cross, and private for-profit insurers, have a large mix of patients. If they are overcharged for one patient, they are likely to be undercharged for another. As long as the total costs are not overstated, overcharges and undercharges are likely to average out for large groups of patients. It would not be sensible for them to require health care organizations to spend substantially more money on improved cost accounting. They would then have to bear the cost of the improved cost accounting in addition to the costs of patient care.

With the introduction of DRGs, however, incentives changed. Hospitals, in particular, are now at risk for the costs they incur. If patients cost more to care for than the DRG payment rate, the hospital suffers a loss. The growth of managed care has made it even more important for all health care providers to measure patient costs more accurately.

This means that to the extent possible, still being mindful of the cost of collecting more accurate information, managers of health care organizations would like to improve on the good-enough approximations. They would like to eliminate the inaccuracies of using pounds of laundry instead of pieces or using square feet instead of construction cost for depreciation. They would like to eliminate the distortions created by the order of allocation in the step-down process. They would like to remove the inaccuracies generated by weighted procedure and hourly, surcharge, and per diem assignments of cost.

Can this be done? Probably there will never be a 100% accurate costing system. As computer use in health care organizations increases, the potential exists to make great strides in accurate assignment of patient resource consumption. In the interim, many health care organizations are taking at least intermediate steps to improve their costing. Some of the approaches used are discussed in the remaining sections of this chapter.

⁜ COSTING OUT NURSING SERVICES

The essence of the costing problem is that often nursing costs are charged to patients as part of a general per diem charge rather than being charged separately on the patient's bill. As a result, all patients in the same level of care (e.g., CCU or general unit) receive the same charge for nursing care services. In terms of providing management with an understanding of the cost implications for different patients, this provides extremely poor information. It implicitly assumes that all patients consume exactly the same amount of nursing care, even though different patients have different nursing care requirements.

Until the 1980s, measurement of differential consumption was, if not impossible, at least too costly to consider. Hospitals are faced with two extreme alternatives. One choice is to divide the total annual costs of nursing care by the number of patients treated for the year to determine the average cost per patient. At the other extreme, the hospital could hire a data collector to follow each nurse and determine exactly how much of the nurse's time was used by each patient. Figure 8–3 reflects this extreme choice: alternative A is simple and inexpensive; alternative Z is extremely detailed and expensive.

What hospital could afford to assign a data collector to each nurse to observe how much time was devoted to each patient? The value of information should always justify its cost. Alternative Z in Figure 8–3 is just too costly to undertake. Figure 8–4 adds a compromise. In most cases a patient with a three-day stay would consume less nursing care than a patient with a fifteen-day stay. If total nursing care costs are divided by total patient days, patients who are in the hospital for more days can be assigned more nursing cost than patients in the hospital for fewer days. This is alternative B. It is still not nearly so precise and accurate an approach as alternative Z; however, it is not much more expensive than alternative A and gives a much better approximation of the nursing care cost for different patients.

However, under alternative B, which is the approach most hospitals use, the nursing cost is assumed to be the same for all patient days. More days imply more cost, but for the same number of patient days, all patients are assumed to use the same amount of nursing care. Although this is much better than alternative A, it is still a poor measure of nursing cost.

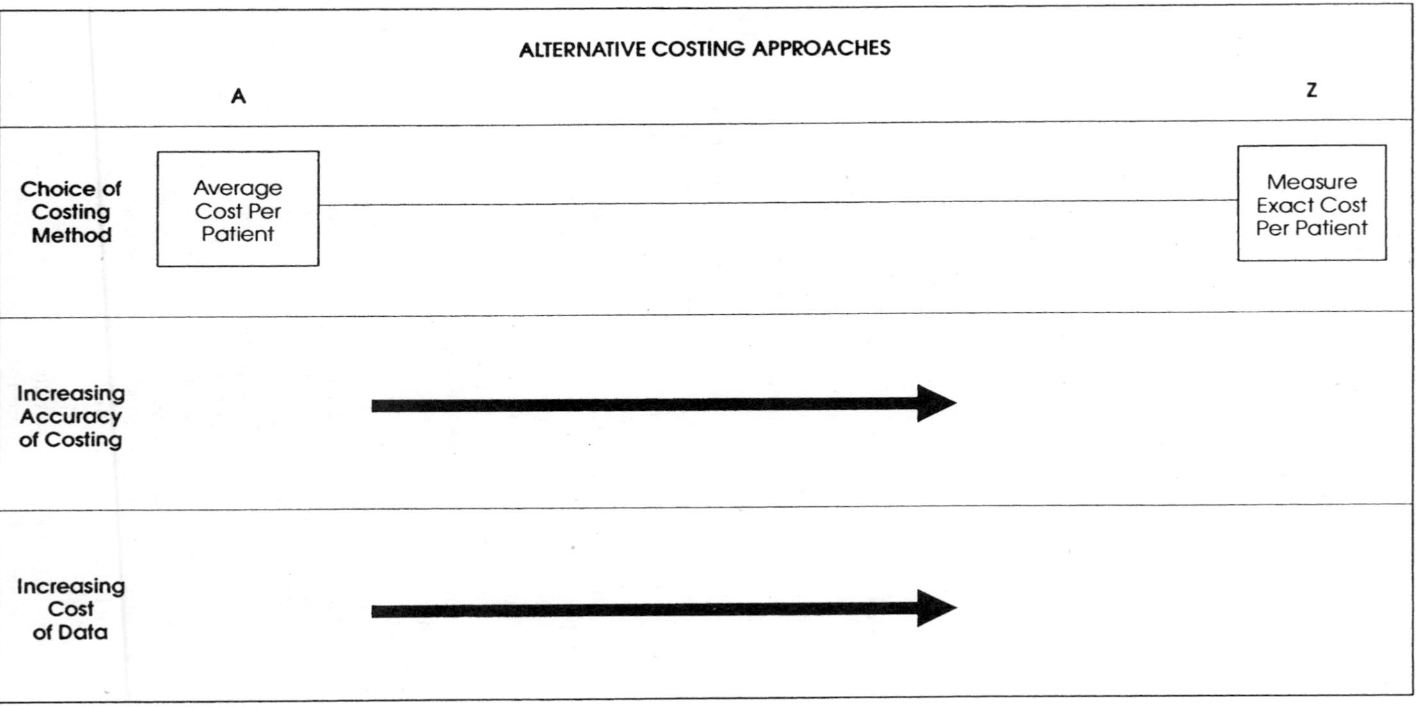

FIGURE 8–3. The A *vs* Z extremes.

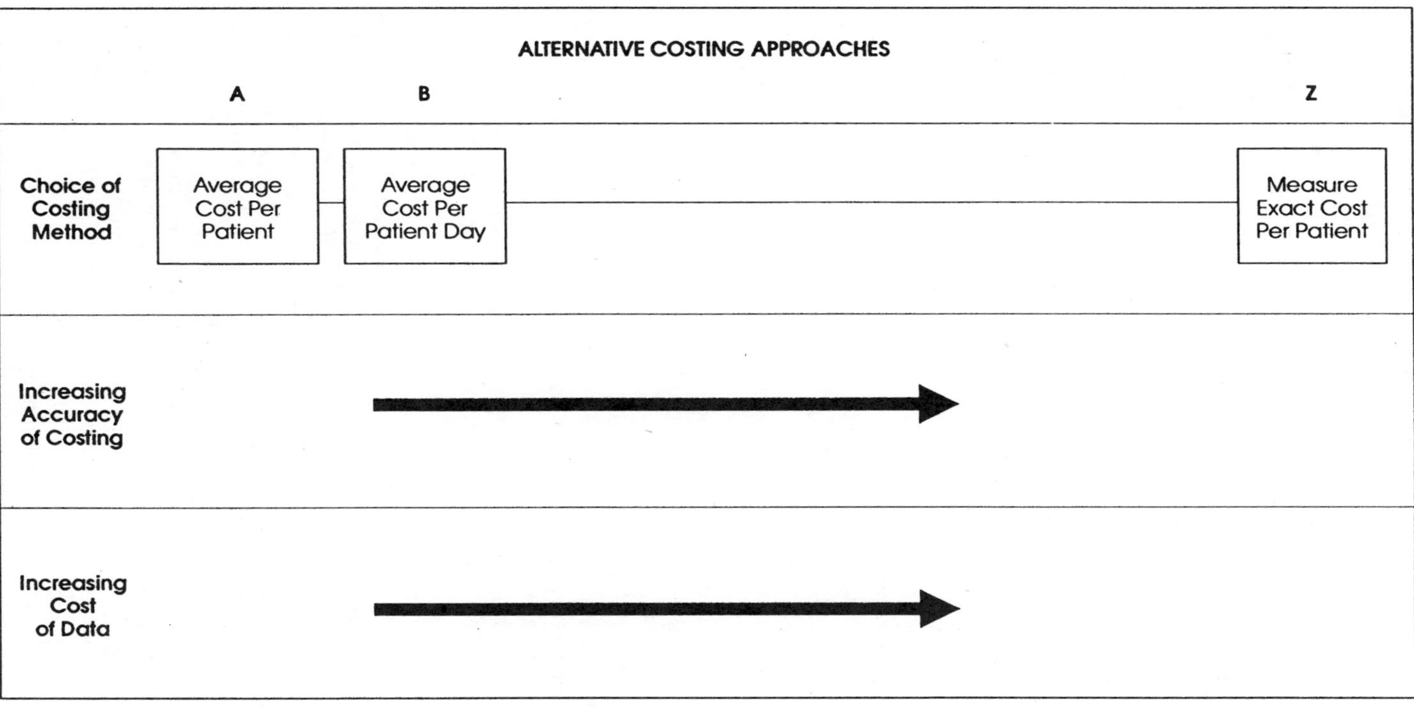

FIGURE 8–4. Alternative B.

Solutions to the Costing Problem

How can the cost of each individual patient be better measured without having an accountant follow every nurse? One solution that many hospitals are beginning to examine is computerization. The addition of computers not only at nursing stations but also by each bedside is seen by many nurses to be the future for all hospitals. Many hospitals have installed bedside computer terminals.

One use of bedside computer systems is to better track nursing costs. In Figure 8–5 computers have been added to the continuum from low-accuracy, low-cost information to high-accuracy, high-cost information. This is alternative Y. Nurses record on the computer when they are with each patient and what they are doing for that patient. The computer multiplies the time spent by the salary of the particular nurse providing the care to determine the specific cost of nursing care for a particular patient. When nurses are doing some indirect activities, such as documenting a patient's record, the computer can also assign that cost to the appropriate patient.

Substantial progress is currently being made in a variety of areas to ease the input of data into the computer. Uniform price codes (bar coding) are becoming more widely used on a variety of supplies consumed by hospitals. In some hospitals, employee identification cards are being issued with magnetic strips containing the employee number in computer-readable form. This allows nurses to just slide their card into the computer to identify themselves. Light pens have been replaced with touch-sensitive screens that allow the user to simply touch a particular item on the screen to select menu choices and enter data.

The result of progress in the computer area is that there will probably soon be bedside terminals widely available that can accurately capture most of the costs (direct and many indirect costs) of providing nursing care to specific patients.

Note that alternative Y is close to alternative Z in several respects. The data to be gained is potentially quite accurate and clearly can be made patient specific. It would enable the hospital to assign costs (and ultimately charges) to patients based on their differing consumption of nursing resources.

Another approach to estimating the cost of nursing care is a *patient classification system*. Patient classification systems require rating patients based on the likely nursing resource requirements resulting from the acuity of their illness. Sicker patients requiring more nursing care are assigned higher acuity or higher classification levels. Many hospitals have developed their own systems, and several commercial systems are widely used in hospitals throughout the United States. Patients are rated on scales such as 1 to 5.

Patient classification generally will not be perfectly accurate measures of the resources needed for each patient. Some patients classified as level 2 will require more care than level 2 calls for, and some level 2 patients will require less care than would be expected based on that classification. If the system is functioning reasonably well, however, average patient resource consumption will match what is expected based on the classification system. And certainly it would generally be expected that a level 2 patient will consume resources closer to the level 2 average than to the level 1 average or the level 3 average.

If a mechanism to determine patients' costs based on their patient classification can be established, it will not provide the precise accuracy of alternative Z. It will not even provide the alternative Y accuracy that a computer system can generate. However, it can create a new alternative, X, as shown in Figure 8–6. Alternative X is inaccurate in that all patients are assigned the same nursing cost for a day at the same classification level. If two patients are both level 2 on a given day, their cost is assumed to be the same, even though it is known that they will probably not consume exactly the same nursing resources. However, alternative X is much more accurate than alternatives A and B. Alternative B assumes that the cost is the same per patient day for all patients regardless of acuity.

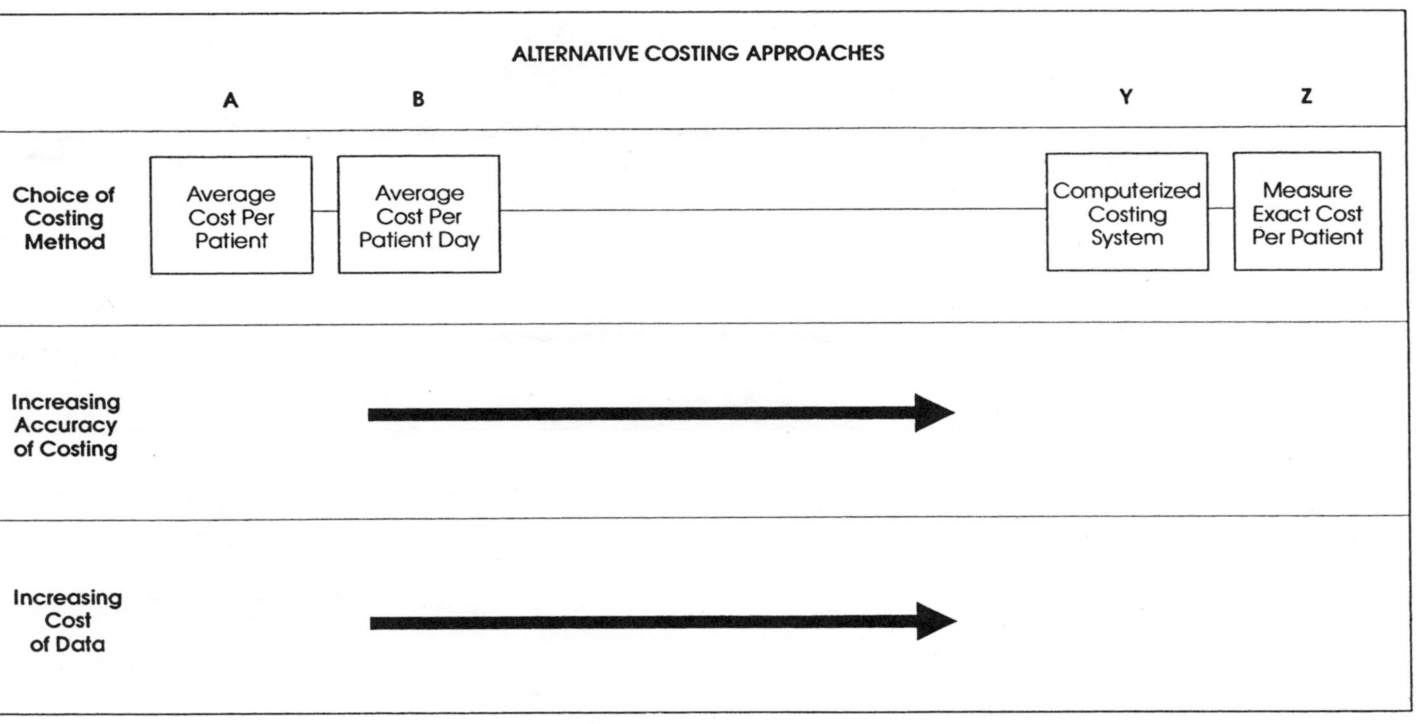

FIGURE 8–5. Alternative Y.

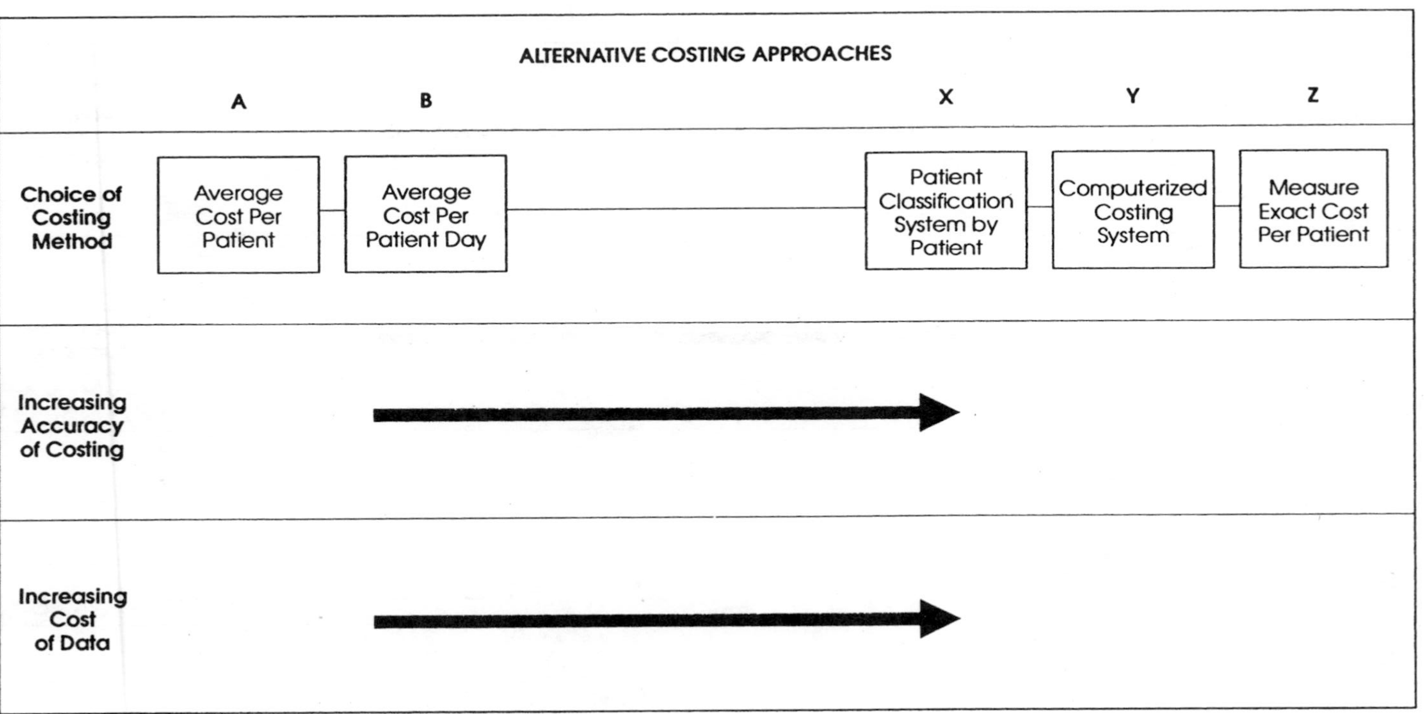

FIGURE 8–6. Alternative X.

Alternative X is an improvement because the cost is considered the same per patient day only for patients at the same acuity level. Different costs are assigned to patient days at different acuity levels. Users of alternative X must recognize that the information has some degree of inaccuracy. However, the system may be accurate enough, given the current high costs of using either alternative Y or Z. Therefore, patient classification systems can be the basis for a system that allows more accurate estimates of the cost a hospital incurs for nursing care for different types of patients.

Somewhere between X and Y on the scale from A to Z, one could place work-load measurement tools. These are variants of patient classification. Work-load measurement tools attempt to determine the nursing care time required for each individual patient each day. The approach is to identify the time required for each of the types of nursing interventions that take up most of the nurses' time. Each patient is evaluated each day to determine which interventions will be needed. Such tools can track required care hours specific to each patient. This is contrasted with patient classification systems that use an average hour figure for all patients within a broad category or level of care.

Such an approach is not as sophisticated as alternative Y, where the actual care hours are entered into the computer as the patient receives the care. It is likely that some interventions will take longer than typical for some patients, and less time for others. Therefore the cost ultimately assigned to the patient will be based on average time, not actual time. However, the work-load measurement approach is more sophisticated than alternative X, which uses average nursing care hours for all patients in a given patient classification category.

Although patient classification and work measurement systems can be used to determine the cost of nursing, these systems were initially developed to predict staffing needs, not to determine costs. The nurse managers should be aware that although patients require a designated amount of care, this does not mean that they receive it.

Why Change the Costing Approach?

The mere fact that the ability to improve costing now exists does not in itself explain why a nurse manager would want to more accurately identify costs. What is to be gained from having a more accurate measure of the different costs for nursing care for different types of patients?

A critical benefit from improved costing of nursing services is that the organization can generate information for better management decisions. Is a particular service too costly? What price can be bid for an HMO or preferred provider organization (PPO) contract? Hospital costing has long been based on averages and cross subsidizations. In the current environment, errors in calculations of costs become more serious as negotiations for discounted prices become more intense. Managers are being pushed along the increasing accuracy of the costing line in Figure 8–6, even though this also moves in the direction of increased cost of data.

In addition, as costing becomes more specific and more accurate, managers not only can deal better with pricing problems but also can be more efficient in the management of costs. Control of budgets improves as another measure of expected cost becomes available. Flexible budget systems can provide better analysis and control of costs, and productivity can be monitored better if more is known about costs. Not only is it possible to assess how costs should change based on changing numbers of patient days, but information about the cost per patient in a given DRG can also be used to assess costs as the number of patients in each DRG changes.

Should Costing Be Linked to DRGs?

If health care organizations are going to move in the direction of more accurate costing of nursing services, one of the critical questions is how to categorize the cost.

Should there be one nursing cost for medical patients and another for surgical patients? Should the cost for men as opposed to women be determined, or for young people as opposed to old people? Should there be one nursing cost for each type of patient based on International Classification of Diseases (ICD) code? Should the cost be found by DRG?

The problem managers face is the definition of the product of nursing care. What does nursing produce? If a nurse changes a dressing or gives a patient a medication, are those the products of nursing care? Probably most people would consider those activities to represent only intermediate products. The ultimate product is the health of the patient, not the care provided.

However, health care organizations treat many different kinds of patients. They do not have only one final product: a healthy patient. They have many final products represented by the different patients to whom nurses give care. Yet currently all patients are costed for nursing care as if they were the same. That needs to change. Final products need to be defined so that nurse managers can assess the cost of each. Patients could be divided into categories called *nursing resource groupings* (NRGs), perhaps based on nursing diagnoses. Ideally, patients should be divided into homogeneous NRGs based on nursing care consumed. Any patient in one NRG would consume a similar set of nursing resources as any other patient in that grouping.

What should be the basis for costing nursing services in the interim until a NRG type system is in use? One approach is to fall back on alternative X. A patient classification system can be used to determine how many days a given patient is at each classification level. If the cost of each day at each classification level (discussed later in this chapter) can be determined, the manager can add up the costs to determine the patient's total nursing care cost.

However, this requires determination of the patient classification for every patient for every day. Some hospitals will find the advantages of being at alternative X on the costing accuracy scale sufficient to warrant this investment in data collection. Doing this will not only improve costing but will also collect information that can be used for calculating acuity variances.[1]

However, many hospitals will not want to spend the resources needed to classify every patient every day. The alternative is to take a sample of patients from each DRG and determine the average nursing cost for patients in each DRG based on a sampling approach. All patients within a specific DRG will not consume the same nursing resources for each day at a specific patient classification level. Nor will all patients in one DRG have the same number of patient days at each classification level or even the same total number of patient days. This approach is based on average length of stay, average number of days at each patient classification level, and average nurse resource consumption within each patient classification level. However, the average amount of nursing resources for each type of DRG can be found.

For example, if a hospital uses a nursing patient classification system with a scale from 1 to 5, a group of patients from each DRG can be sampled to find out, on average, how many days of the patients' stay were at level 1, how many at level 2, and so on. Averaging all patients in a given DRG at a given hospital will not give a measurement alternative accurate enough to be labeled W on the scale from A to Z. Such an estimate of cost would probably be considered R on such a scale. It would not be nearly as accurate as X, but it would be substantially more accurate than A and B. This new alternative, R (see Fig. 8–7), would be substantially less expensive than alternatives X, Y, or Z.

DRGs, although perhaps not ideal for the purpose of costing nursing care, are

[1]See Chapter 13 and Steven A. Finkler, *Budgeting Concepts for Nurse Managers,* W.B. Saunders, Philadelphia, 1992, pp. 292–294.

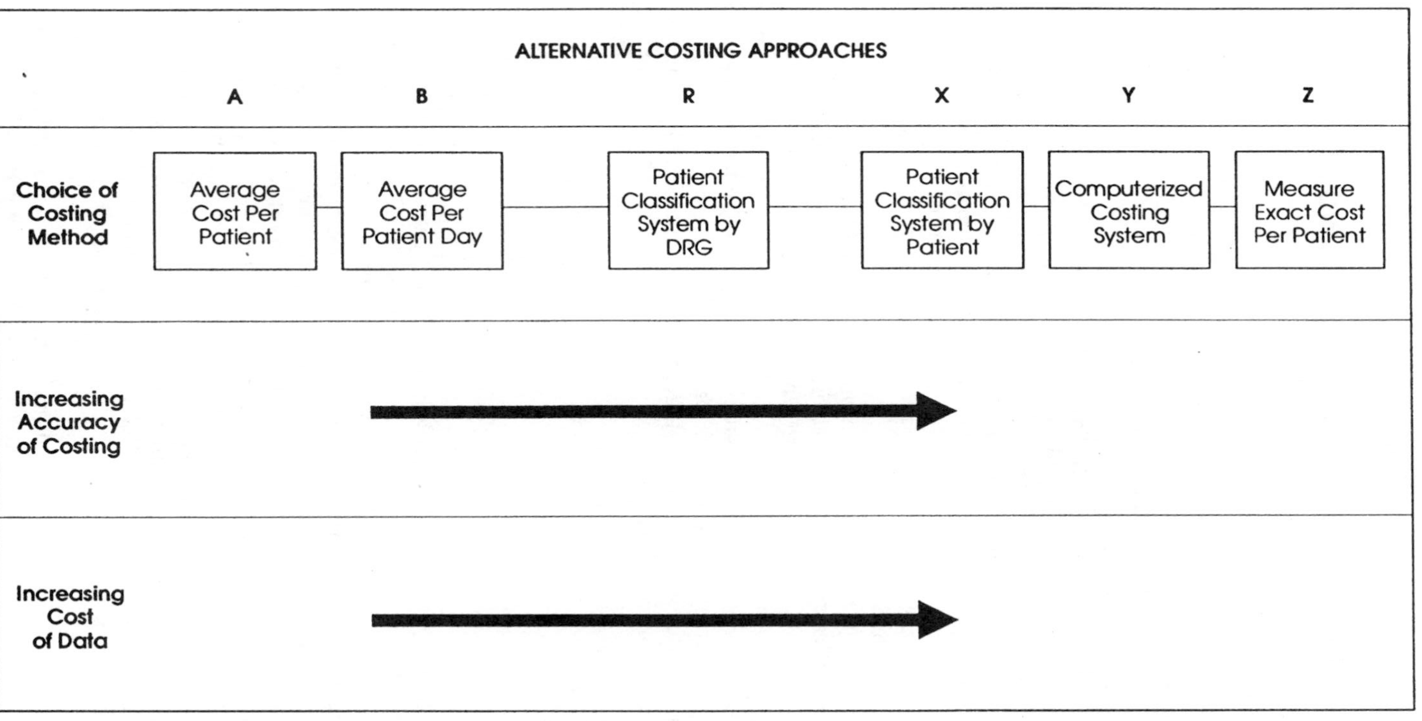

FIGURE 8–7. Alternative R.

an adequate categorization for the assignment of average differential nursing costs. Many hospital decisions are based on particular DRGs or clusters of DRGs, so the DRG-based cost information generated will be of considerable management value.

⁂ SPECIFIC APPROACH TO COSTING NURSING SERVICES

Nursing care costs consist of the following:

- Direct patient care (staff)
- Indirect patient care (e.g., staff, supervisors, secretaries)
- Patient care–related costs (e.g., patient and unit supplies)
- Overhead (allocated from other departments)

Note that the cost of nursing care is more than just the hourly salary and benefits for the nurse giving care at the bedside. Nursing management, assessment, planning, evaluating, teaching, and discharge planning are also critical elements of nursing care. In addition, supplies, secretaries, and overhead are elements of overall nursing care cost. A manager could try to determine the costs of each of these elements separately for each category of patient or do the costing in some more aggregate fashion. Start with the assumption that all nursing department costs are aggregated.

The key element that allows for improved costing of nursing services is the fact that nursing patient classification systems are currently in place in almost every hospital. Without such systems different patients consume different amounts of resources, but the manager has no way to measure the differential consumption. With a classification system, once a patient has been classified, the manager has some idea about the nursing resources that patient consumes.

For example, suppose that a nursing unit has the following hypothetical patient classification resource guidelines:

Acuity Level	Hours of Care
1	3.0
2	4.0
3	4.8
4	6.6
5	9.0

In developing the patient classification system, various clinical indicators are used to determine if a patient should be classified as 1, 2, 3, 4, or 5. Once the patient has been classified, the classification system tells how many hours of nursing care should be required to treat that patient. In the above example, a patient classified as a 4 would typically require an average of 6.6 hours of care.

Note that the scale is not proportional. A patient classified as a 2 does not require exactly twice as many hours as a patient classified as a 1. While a level 1 needs three hours of care, a level 2 needs four hours. Rather than double, this is only 33% more care. A level 3 patient needs 4.8 hours, that is, 20% more than a level 2. A level 4 patient requires 38% more care than a level 3. As one moves from level to level, the amount of additional care does not change in proportion. It changes based on the specific classification system and the clinical needs of a patient at each level in that system.

This complicates the cost calculation. If the scale were strictly linear (i.e., a ratio scale with zero the lowest score and a score of 2 requiring twice as much care as a score of 1), one could add up all the patient days at each level and divide into total nursing cost to get a cost per unit of patient classification. However, since the scale is not linear, it is necessary to create a relative value unit (RVU) scale. This scale will allow determination of how much care each level requires relative to the care needed for a typical level 1 patient. A patient classified as a 1 will be given a value of 1 on the *relative value scale*. Each other classification level would then be calculated in relative proportion. This can be accomplished by dividing the required hours of care for each level by the number of hours required for level 1. For example:

$$\frac{\text{Level 2}}{\text{Level 1}} = \frac{4.0 \text{ hours}}{3.0 \text{ hours}} = 1.33$$

Therefore the relative value assigned to classification level 2 is 1.33. This value of 1.33 represents the fact that a level 2 patient consumes .33 more nursing care hours than a level 1 patient. Continuing for all classification (acuity) levels:

Acuity Level	Hours of Care	RVU
1	3.0	1.00
2	4.0	1.33
3	4.8	1.60
4	6.6	2.20
5	9.0	3.00

Assuming the following information, the reader will be able to see how the RVU system can be used to develop cost information:

Total nursing costs:		$250,000
Number of patient days at each acuity level:	1	100 days
	2	220 days
	3	350 days
	4	110 days
	5	40 days

The first step is to determine the total amount of work performed by the nursing department. This is done by multiplying the RVUs for each acuity classification level by the number of days at that level. Using the number of patient days and the RVUs calculated above, the total RVUs would be:

Acuity Level	Patient Days	×	RVUs	=	Total RVUs
1	100	×	1.00	=	100.00
2	220	×	1.33	=	292.60
3	350	×	1.60	=	560.00
4	110	×	2.20	=	242.00
5	40	×	3.00	=	120.00
	820				1,314.60

There were 1,314.6 units of nursing work performed. We can divide this into the total nursing cost to find the cost for each RVU of nursing work.

$$\frac{\text{Total nursing costs}}{\text{Total RVUs}} = \text{Cost per RVU}$$

$$\frac{\$250{,}000}{1{,}314.60} = \$190.17 \text{ per RVU}$$

Here one can see that the nursing cost for a patient for one day with classification 1 would be $190.17. The cost for a patient with classification 4 would be $190.17 multiplied by 2.20 (the RVU for classification level 4).

How would a manager calculate the nursing cost for a patient from admission to discharge? Suppose that the average DRG 128 patient had a length of stay of seven days, with two days classed as a 1, four days classed as a 2, and one day classed as a 4. The nursing cost for DRG 128 then would be:

Acuity Level	Patient Days	×	RVUs	×	Cost per RVU	=	Total Cost
1	2	×	1.00	×	$190.17	=	$ 380.34
2	4	×	1.33	×	190.17	=	1,011.70
3	0	×	1.60	×	190.17	=	0.00
4	1	×	2.20	×	190.17	=	418.37
5	0	×	3.00	×	190.17	=	0.00
	7						$1,810.41

Would all patients in a given DRG be expected to consume the same resources? Not really, but the manager can still be confident that an approach such as this on average for any given DRG will give a much more accurate assignment of cost than simply assigning to every patient in a nursing unit the same daily cost for nursing care.

LIMITATIONS OF THE RVU APPROACH

Patient Classification *vs* Other Work-load Measurement

The purpose of the RVU patient classification approach is to provide a workable costing approach accessible to the majority of health care organizations in the country. However, it does not generate perfectly accurate measures of cost and is subject to a variety of limitations.

The idea of an alternative to patient classification was discussed earlier. If a work-load measurement tool is in place in a hospital and is being used on an ongoing basis to categorize resource needs of each patient each day, it can be used to provide cost information that is potentially more accurate. Rather than being limited to perhaps five patient classification levels for a given medical or surgical unit, such an approach collects indicators of hours of resource consumption for each patient. It is more patient specific than the RVU approach. Putting such an approach in place and following through with it on a continuous basis may be a considerable undertaking. However, if it is used, costing is made potentially easier.

Under such an approach the required interventions for each patient are translated into required hours of care. Total nursing care costs for direct and indirect expenses must be calculated as with the RVU system. Dividing total nursing costs by total hours of care generates a cost per hour of care. This cost per hour can be multiplied by the required hours of care for each patient for each day as determined by the system. This will give the cost per patient for each day in the hospital. If aggregate information is desired by DRG, it can be obtained by averaging the costs of each patient in that DRG. However, the majority of hospitals do not have patient-specific work measurement systems in place.

Indirect Nursing Costs

A problem with both the RVU and more detailed work measurement systems as described so far is the implicit assumption that all nursing costs vary in proportion to the hours of nursing care. Does that make sense for indirect costs? For example, will a sicker patient who requires more direct nursing care also require more indirect nursing care? More charting time? More supplies? More overhead? The answer to these questions depends on the specific situation of your institution.

Is it true that secretarial costs will be greater for more acutely ill patients? It may well be that a simple per diem allocation is a more appropriate way to allocate such costs. Costing could therefore be improved by dividing total nursing costs among those costs that vary with nursing care hours (e.g., RN staff and LPN staff and perhaps clinical supplies) and those costs that do not vary with nursing care hours (e.g., office supplies, nurse manager time, and secretarial time). Costs that vary with nursing care hours would be allocated by the RVU or work measurement approaches described above. The other costs could be divided by total patient days and assigned to patients based on their number of patient days.

Staffing Mix

A significant problem is the fact that most hospital nursing classification systems provide required hours of care but do not specify the mix of care. If 30% of all nursing care hours are provided by LPNs, it is assumed that 30% of the care for each patient is provided by LPNs.

It is possible that one patient at level 2 might require four hours of RN care, while another might require three hours of LPN care and only one hour of RN care. Obviously both of these patients do not consume the same amount of nursing care resources, even if they consume the same number of hours of care. Therefore there will be some distortion of costs unless the hospital uses a system that indicates not only how many hours of care are needed but also how many hours of care by staff type.

This problem is not unique to costing, however. It represents a weakness of patient classification systems. If the hospital does not know the required mix of care providers, the classification system is not going to be useful for staffing decisions. Part of this problem stems from the fact that different hospitals have different views on which functions can be done by different types of staff. However, over time one can expect that classification systems will improve. As they do, this mix problem should become less serious.

In the meantime, managers could attempt to separate the cost of RNs from LPNs and aides and assign those costs separately to patients. Special studies could be undertaken for each DRG to determine whether their care was biased toward more than an average amount of RN care or toward more than an average amount of LPN care. Then the cost of nursing care for that DRG could be adjusted accordingly. Other approaches to handling this problem are discussed in the following section, which deals with productivity.

How complex are managers willing to make the costing system? Each health care organization must decide how much it is willing to refine its costing system, realizing that generally the more accurate the costing system, the more expensive it is. Some managers believe that the historical average nursing cost per patient day is so inaccurate that an RVU-based system is a tremendous improvement, even with the problems cited here.

We have used a hospital as an example. The same principles apply whether the cost determination is for nursing care delivered in a hospital, nursing home, outpatient setting, or patient's home. However, for home care the costing is simplified because patient records explicitly indicate the level of staff that provided the care.

⁜ MEASURING PRODUCTIVITY

As the pressure to contain costs in health care continues, nurse managers are under increasing pressure to improve productivity. It is not enough to know nursing costs for different patient types. Managers hear the CEO saying "The staff must be more productive," "We've got to use fewer resources," and "Do something to improve efficiency." Productivity is defined as the ratio of outputs to inputs and is often notated as an algebraic equation:

$$\text{Productivity} = \frac{\text{Output}}{\text{Input}}$$

Productivity is a ratio and therefore affected by changes in output or input. If output increases and input stays the same, productivity is said to increase. If output stays the same and input decreases, productivity increases. To increase productivity the nurse manager must increase output while decreasing or not changing input, or provide the same output with fewer inputs.

Why must health organizations be more productive? Increasing productivity means getting more output for the same cost or the same output at a lower cost. Increasing productivity gives an organization the resources with which to develop and grow. Managed care organizations have put tremendous pressure on health care providers to reduce prices. This can be done only if productivity rises.

Although improving productivity is not a simple task in any industry, aspects of nursing care make it particularly complicated. The first step in measuring productivity is to define input and output. Inputs are the resources needed to produce the product. For nursing, inputs usually include nursing staff, equipment, supplies, and the organizational support needed to keep the nursing staff available, such as personnel and recruiting.

Nursing's output, or product, is more difficult to define. McHugh discusses many of the problems in measuring nursing productivity. She states that a patient day of care, the traditional measure of nursing output, is "really not a nursing output; it is an institutional output and relatively insensitive to nursing productivity."[2]

Although most nurses agree that a healthy patient is the goal of nursing and therefore nursing's output, most nurses recognize that there is wide disagreement on the definition of health. Further, there is wide agreement that the health of a patient is related not only to nursing care but also to the care of other health providers and a myriad of patient characteristics. Thus far, nurse managers (and CEOs) have been satisfied defining nursing output as some measure of what economists call throughput, i.e., what the nurse does for the patient.

For purposes of this chapter, we will discuss productivity as it has been traditionally defined, with output defined as units of service provided. Additionally one must consider how the health care organization is paid. It is critical to consider whether the outcome measure used by payers is the same as that used by the productivity system. If nurses reduce the time spent per visit in home care but increase the number of visits and the total number of hours of care, is that good or bad? Financially it would likely be good for the organization if it is paid for nurse visits, but bad if it is paid for the patient on a fixed basis regardless of the number of hours of care or nurse visits. Under the cost-based reimbursement systems, health care organizations are reimbursed on a per diem or per visit basis. Thus for each nurse visit provided, the organization charges the patient and receives a negotiated reimbursement rate or a regulated rate from a third-party payer or the charge from the patient. If an organization can produce a day of care or a visit with less input, productivity improves. Although this approach to productivity may be appropriate in a reimbursement system that pays based on visits, the approach is not appropriate for a reimbursement system that reimburses organizations for an episode of care. Thus as reimbursement moves to an episodic basis, nurse managers need to rethink the unit of output.

For example, assume that average hours of nursing care per patient day (HPPD) on a hospital unit were 4. A new nurse manager arrives and decreases the HPPD to 3.5 HPPD with no change in quality. The manager might be considered efficient. However, using this same case, assume that when HPPD were 4 the patient stayed in the hospital for six days, thus consuming 24 hours for the entire stay. Under the new efficient manager the HPPD decreased to 3.5, but the length of stay increased to seven days and the patient therefore used 24.5 hours of nursing care. Is the second nurse manager really more efficient? Clearly, the second manager is less efficient

---

[2]Mary L. McHugh, "Productivity Measurement in Nursing," *Applied Nursing Research,* Vol. 2, No. 2, 1989, p. 100.

than the first. However, under a per diem reimbursement system that pays a fixed amount per patient day, the hospital would receive more income from care provided when the patient received 3.5 hours of care per day and stayed for seven days. Thus, from the hospital's financial point of view, the less efficient manager would be the better manager. However, as payment systems increasingly are based on an episode of care (e.g., DRGs), a productivity measure based on an episode is necessary.

Most organizations have or should have a standard for the ratio of output to input. These standards are often developed based on the historical activities of the organization, industry standards developed by provider organizations, and collective bargaining contracts.

For hospitals the usual standard is an identified number of hours per patient day, while in home health care agencies the standard is usually nurse visits per day. Standards may be for direct care hours or some combination of direct care and indirect care.

In the simplest case, if the hospital's standard is to provide 4 hours of direct nursing care per day and 1,000 days of care are provided, it is expected that 4,000 hours (4 hours × 1,000 days) of care were needed. Assume that 3,000 hours of direct care are actually provided. The unit would be considered 133% productive (4,000 hours required/3,000 hours actual = 133%). Assume, however, that 4,500 hours of direct care were actually provided. The unit would then be considered 88% productive (4,000 hours required/4,500 hours actual = 88%). Note that this measure of productivity ignores quality of care. Being "more productive" could result from understaffing and thus potentially have a negative impact on quality of care.

Another factor relates to patient mix. A change in the mix of patients could affect required care hours. Nurse managers recognize that not all patients require the same amount of nursing care per day. Thus required care is usually adjusted for a measure of acuity. For example, suppose that a unit has two acuity levels. Based on hospital direct care standards, patients at acuity level 2 require six HPPD, and acuity level 1 patients require three HPPD. For one day the unit provides care for fifteen acuity 2 patients and twenty acuity 1 patients; therefore the required hours are calculated as follows:

15 acuity 2 patients × 6 HPPD =	90
20 acuity 1 patients × 3 HPPD =	60
Total hours required for the unit =	150

By determining the actual hours worked, the ratio of hours required to hours worked can be determined. Determining the actual hours worked requires identifying those staff who worked and the hours worked. Some financial managers suggest that all nursing staff are interchangeable. Therefore when calculating productivity they consider all nursing hours equally, whether they are provided by a professional nurse or a nursing assistant. Most nurses would agree that hours of professional nursing care cannot be equated with hours of nursing assistant or even LPN hours; thus some adjustment must be made.

One approach is to develop a standard based on the usual staffing mix on the unit and assume the differentiation in level of staff is consistent. Given the variation in staffing both among units and within units on particular days, this approach is usually not meaningful.

Determining output for an episode of care is far more complicated than determining productivity if the output is patient day of care. In the above example it is assumed that patients can be grouped in categories of care required for each day of care. Although nurse managers agree that these groups are not exact, they are precise enough to be adequate in most cases.

To determine productivity for an episode of care it is necessary to determine standards for episodes. No widely accepted systems have been developed to group patients into categories of nursing care required for their entire stay. The following section outlines some approaches to product-line costing, a variation on episode of care.

※ PRODUCT-LINE COSTING

One result of the work done on costing nursing services is that it is possible to group all patients of one type and find an average cost for that type of patient. In other words, *product-line* costing is feasible with this method. A product line is a group of patients with some commonality that allows them to be grouped together, such as a common diagnosis. In a similar approach, it is now common for organizations to focus on one disease, so-called disease management. Often an organization cannot eliminate one product in a product line without eliminating the entire product line. For example, if a hospital sells its bypass pump because it is losing money on bypass surgery, it will no longer be able to do heart valve surgery. They are both part of the open-heart surgery product line.

Many people believe that managers should be given hospital-wide responsibility for both the revenues and expenses related to specific patient product lines. For example, a manager might be responsible for the revenues related to the obstetrics product line. The manager is accountable for both the variance in the number of discharges and the revenue per discharge. Of course the manager would be responsible for the budgeted and actual costs of the product line as well.

Before one takes the step of costing by product line or budgeting by product line, it is necessary to question what the information will be used for. In terms of running a nursing unit, will knowledge of the cost for all patients in a given DRG be useful? The answer to that question depends a great deal on the types of decisions that a manager or organization faces.

Some authors envision use of cost information by DRG as a way to promote efficiency. For example, consider Table 8–5. In that table the treatment patterns of two physicians' patients are examined to see if one physician is inefficient.

※ TABLE 8–5. *Analysis of DRG 152**

	Dr. Getwell				Dr. Severe	
Description of Services	**Patient 1**	**Patient 2**	**Patient 3**	**Patient 4**	**Patient 1**	**Patient 2**
Medical surgical bed	$ 460	$ 460	$ 460	$ 460	$ 460	$ 460
Intensive care bed	720	1,440	720	720	720	720
Operating room	420	360	300	300	850	360
Anesthesia	300	300	300	300	425	150
Laboratory:						
Blood work	75	125	50	50	50	50
Tissue test	25	—	75	75	100	100
Urine analysis	35	35	35	—	70	70
Radiology:						
Chest 4 views	45	45	45	—	90	45
Spine, cervical	65	—	65	65	65	65
Nuclear medicine:						
Thyroid washout	95	95	95	210	210	95
Urinary recovery	105	105	105	—	105	105
T-3 uptake	85	85	85	85	85	85
Red-cell survival	40	40	40	40	40	40
Total	$2,470	$3,090	$2,375	$2,305	$3,270	$2,345

*Broken out by physician and hospital services ordered for minor small and large bowel procedures.

Reprinted from John Tselepis, "Refined Cost Accounting Produces Better Information," *Healthcare Financial Management*, May 1989, p. 34, with permission of Healthcare Financial Management Association.

TABLE 8–6. *Product-line Budgeting for Direct Care Hours*

	Forecast Volume of Patients	×	Forecast Average Length of Stay	=	Expected Patient Days	×	Expected Hours per Patient Day	=	Total Hours of Direct Care
Product line 1	200		3		600		5		3,000
Product line 2	50		5		250		6		1,500
Product line 3	100		4		400		3		1,200
Product line 4	300		7		2,100		6		12,600
Product line 5	500		3		1,500		4		6,000
									24,300

Alternately, suppose that a hospital is trying to decide whether to accept a group of cardiac patients from an HMO at a discounted price. Knowing the costs for that type of patient would certainly be advantageous in the negotiating process. Often product-line calculations include nursing costs simply as part of the overall per diem cost. The organization can have much better information about different types of patients if it relies on nurse costing approaches, discussed earlier in this chapter.

Direct Care Hours

Product-line information can be used not only for negotiations but also for budgeting. The direct care hours approach to product-line budgeting consists of dividing the patients for a given nursing unit into product lines, determining the number of hours of care required for each product line, and aggregating that information to find the total hours of care needed in the budget. This is a straightforward approach to using product-line information to improve budgeting capability. It represents an alternative to using acuity-adjusted patient days for determining nurse staff requirements (as will be discussed in Chapter 12).

In this approach, the first step is to separate all patients for a unit into specific groups. These groups, or product lines, could conform to DRGs but do not have to. The next step is to determine how many patients are expected in the coming period in each group. That information can be generated using the forecasting techniques discussed in Chapter 18. Using historical information, forecasting can also be used to predict the average length of stay of the patients in each group.

Once the manager has predictions of the number of patient days in each group and the average length of stay, those two numbers can be multiplied to determine the total number of patient days expected in each product line. The number of patient days can be multiplied by the expected average direct care HPPD for patients in the product line to generate the total hours of direct care needed for each specific product line. The total direct care hours for each product line can then be aggregated to determine the total direct care hours needed for the unit for the coming year. Based on that information the unit's budget for staff can be prepared. Table 8–6 presents a simplistic example of this process. In this example sufficient staff must be budgeted to provide 24,300 direct care hours. The benefit of this process is that it has the potential to accurately provide information on the resources needed by the unit.

The major difficulty with this process is the determination of an accurate measure of average direct care HPPD by product line. If that information is inaccurate, the resulting total direct care hours needed will be inaccurate as well. Planning the budget based on a forecast of the number of patients in each product line may be helpful to the manager.

An alternate approach is to determine the total number of days at each patient classification level for all patients in each product line. Using information from the patient classification system, the nursing staff requirements for that product line can be determined. If this is done for all product lines, the total nursing requirements can be determined.

Standard Costs

Most industrial organizations establish standard costs against which performance can be measured. Standard costs represent expectations of what it should cost to produce a good or service, usually on a per unit basis. They are targets, often established based on industrial engineering studies of the resources that should be consumed in the production of the good or service. Standard costing breaks the costs of each product down into its parts. These include direct and indirect costs, divided into their fixed and variable cost components.

It is important to isolate fixed and variable costs in standard costing so that the information can be used for decision making. By dividing costs in that manner the manager can determine the likely change in costs resulting from changes in the number of patients treated. Historically, health care organizations have not done much standard costing because providers have considered each patient to be unique, requiring a somewhat customized treatment.

If we could overcome that uniqueness, a number of benefits could be realized from the use of standard costs. They present a basis for comparing actual results with the predetermined standard. They can be used for decisions on HMO contracts, on expanding or contracting services, and on other revisions in the way services are offered. Even though patients are unique, there are standard approaches for most patients with specific problems. Those approaches can form the basis for development of standard costs. Table 8–7 presents an example of a standard cost for a pacemaker implant in a patient with acute myocardial infarction. The table accumulates costs per procedure for all types of procedures and for the quantity of each to arrive at a total cost of $11,710 per patient in this product line. Since revenues are estimated at $7,739, there is a projected loss of $3,971.

A central article on product-line standard costing overcomes much of the obstacle to standard costing by focusing on the idea that hospitals treat patients by providing them with a large number of intermediate products.[3] By carefully examining each department, one can make a list of the various intermediate products produced by that department.

For example, a laboratory produces different types of tests. Based on this approach, the set of intermediate products consumed by the average patient in a specific product line can be used to determine the standard costs of that product line. The set of intermediate products consumed by a patient in each product line is referred to as the standard treatment protocol (STP) for that product line.

In this system, each intermediate product line is called a service unit (SU). A chest x-ray would be one type of SU produced by the radiology department. A patient who has three chest x-rays receives three of that SU. A standard cost profile (SCP) must be established for each SU that indicates the cost of producing that SU. The profile would include direct and indirect costs, and would identify fixed and variable costs.

Conceptually this seems straightforward. The patient care provided by each department is broken down into intermediate products called SUs. The cost of each SU is determined. The average number of each SU from each department is found for each product line. Then the SUs consumed for a product line are multiplied by their cost to determine the total costs for patients in that product line.

A difficulty with the approach is determining SUs for nursing units. One could try to break down nursing care into the various specific activities and relate those to

---

[3]William O. Cleverley, "Product-Costing for Health Care Firms," *Health Care Management Review*, Vol. 12, No. 4, Fall 1987, pp. 39–48.

※ **TABLE 8–7.** *Product Resource Consumption and Cost Profile Report*

Procedure			Standard per Procedure			Standard in Total			Margin	
			Gross	Cost		Gross	Cost			
Number	Name	Usage	Revenue	Variable	Total	Revenue	Variable	Total	Gross	Net
12001110	Acuity class I	1	$ 190	$ 57.89	$ 199.32	$ 190	$ 58	$ 199	$ 132	$ (9)
12001111	Acuity class I (surgical)	1	202	62.30	203.01	202	62	203	140	(1)
12001112	Acuity class II (surgical)	1	258	79.96	260.55	258	80	261	178	(3)
12001113	Acuity class III (surgical)	1	314	97.62	318.11	314	98	318	216	(4)
14001000	Recovery base	1	38	7.58	25.89	38	8	26	30	12
14002000	Recovery less than 60 minutes	1	40	8.53	29.89	40	9	30	31	10
14006000	Recovery 61–90 minutes	1	76	22.76	77.94	76	23	78	53	(2)
31004000	Cardiac output monitor	2	437	222.53	361.27	874	445	723	429	151
31005670	OR time major per hour	1	47	96.82	201.71	47	97	202	(50)	(155)
31005000	Pacemaker	1	4,985	4,353.52	9,013.56	4,985	4,354	9,014	631	(4,029)
31000500	Pacemaker view	3	119	21.32	169.87	357	64	510	293	(153)
33752500	CBC	3	18	3.28	21.93	54	10	66	44	(12)
33754000	Platelet count	1	13	.71	4.74	13	1	5	12	8
35003000	Prothrombin time	1	13	1.16	7.72	13	1	8	12	5
35005000	Cell count differential fluids	1	13	4.22	28.15	13	4	28	9	(15)
35005500	IV service fee	3	3	.35	1.35	9	1	4	8	5
35509000	Demerol 100 MG Ing	8	4	.35	1.35	32	3	11	29	21
35505555	MA CL 0.9 100 MLS	9	11	.24	.91	99	2	8	97	91
35507500	Dex 5 R/L 1000CC	6	11	1.00	1.50	66	6	9	60	57
35508700	Gloves dispense	5	11	.14	1.24	55	1	6	54	49
35509870	Admission kit	1	4	.14	1.24	4	0	1	4	3
	Totals					$7,739	$5,327	$11,710	$2,412	$(3,971)

Source: Ernst & Young.

Reprinted from George Kis and George Bodenger, "Cost Management Information Improves Financial Performance," *Healthcare Financial Management,* May 1989, p. 42, with permission of Healthcare Financial Management Association and with permission of Ernst & Young.

SUs. Administering a medication could be an SU. Taking a patient's vital signs could be an SU. Charting information about a patient could be an SU. Using hospital computer information systems, it is possible to disaggregate nursing care and assign it to patients in this manner.

Current work in this area focuses on developing critical paths for a patient's hospital stay. Using this approach, the standard care required for patients (usually by DRGs) is determined. During the course of the stay, variances from this standard are noted. Some variances are acceptable, for example, a patient's health status, which is beyond the control of nursing. Other variances are not acceptable, for example, if a patient is not ambulating because nurses did not provide care as outlined in the standard plan. With these data it is possible to determine the ratio of outputs to inputs required (as determined by the standard) and actual (as determined by the actual care provided). Because of the amount of data required to assess productivity in this way, successfully determining productivity for an episode of care usually requires the use of a computer.

For organizations with sufficiently sophisticated information systems in place, it is possible to determine the average number of vital signs taken for a patient in a specific product line. For most hospitals, such a detailed level of information is not currently cost effective to collect. However, nursing SUs could be based on patient classification. Thus a patient day at level 3 could be one SU, and a day at level 4 would be a different SU. When the STP is established, it would consider which nursing SUs are typically consumed and how many of each. The costs for those SUs could be determined using the RVU method.

The RVU method is an ambitious approach to product costing, but it is used in more health care organizations each year. It creates an ability to have very detailed information about each product line from all parts of the organization, including nursing. The management implications of such information are significant. By examining all the SUs consumed in each department, a team of clinicians might be able to find ways to more efficiently provide care. SUs with a lower SCP might be substituted for more expensive ones. Ways might be found to reduce the number of SUs in various departments. If one considers product-line costing broadly as a tool in the case management of the organization's product lines, the potential benefits of product-line standard costing are significant.

ACTIVITY-BASED COSTING

Activity-based costing (ABC) is a relatively new approach to determining costs. In the last half of the 1990s, ABC became widely used in health care organizations. The approach is based on the observation that costs are incurred because of specific activities. In most costing methods, costs are assigned to cost centers and patients based on some measure of volume, such as patient days or visits or hours. For example, OR costs are assigned to patients based on minutes in the OR. From an ABC perspective, it is not necessarily the amount of time but the specific activities that generate costs. Based on this notion, managers need to focus on the actions that drive costs higher. The activities of an organization that cause it to incur costs are referred to as *cost drivers.*

The use of cost drivers to assign costs has the effect of improving accuracy by focusing cost measurement more on a cause-and-effect basis. For example, suppose a health care organization purchasing department orders many items on a routine basis and some items on a special order basis. The activity is placing orders. However, it is quite possible that a special order will be more costly than a routine order.

Purchasing departments are nonrevenue cost centers. Their costs must be allocated to patients in order for the organization to recover its full costs. One common approach to such allocation is based on the number of purchase orders.

Departments that generate a lot of purchase orders are assigned a greater share of the cost of the purchasing department. In turn, those costs are allocated to patients that use the department. This seems quite reasonable.

However, if a rush order is an activity that causes purchasing to spend extra money (e.g., time of the personnel in the department, express freight costs), then from an ABC perspective one would argue that the departments that generate a large number of rush orders should be charged more than departments that do not, other things being equal. In other words, costs should not be assigned simply based on the number of purchase orders generated by each department. Within purchasing, the activity of placing a rush order is more costly than the activity of placing a regular order. Rush orders drive costs higher.

The ABC approach requires the manager to analyze the activities of each cost center or department in an organization. The various activities that are cost drivers must be identified. Then costs can be assigned to departments and ultimately to patients based on the amount of the cost-driving activities they require.

For example, suppose that an OR has traditionally assigned its costs based on minutes of surgery. A patient with a two-hour surgery is charged twice as much as a patient with a one-hour surgery. However, one of the costs of surgery is cleaning and preparing the room after every surgery. Suppose that those costs are the same for each surgery, regardless of the length of the surgery. The activity of cleaning and preparing the room should then be charged equally to each surgical patient.

This probably means that more allocation bases will be needed. The depreciation cost of the surgical suite may be charged to patients based on the length of the procedure. The cost of cleaning the room may be charged equally per patient. The cost of supplies consumed during the surgery should include the extra cost of any rush orders that were required for the procedure. This will complicate the costing process but will produce substantially more accurate information. ABC proponents argue that most industries really do not have a good sense of which of their products or services are profitable and which lose money. Further, employees may be more cost conscious if they use ABC information.

Consider the purchasing department and OR examples above. Surgical patients who require special-order items are subsidized under the old costing system because costs of the rush orders are spread out over all departments that order supplies. This could cause a particular type of surgery to appear more profitable than it is, since the true costs of the rush orders are not assigned to the departments and patients that caused the special orders.

However, once the ABC system is in place, that will change. The OR will be directly charged for each special order. It can then assign the order to specific patients who required the rush order items. This in turn will provide more accurate information about the cost of care for each type of patient. Further, seeing the higher costs resulting from rush orders the manager of the OR may plan more carefully, avoiding the need for many of the rush orders. This will reduce the total costs for the patient, department, and organization.

In terms of routine medical or surgical nursing, using ABC requires an examination of what nurses do and why they do it. ABC works well with the concept of value-added costs. By examining everything we do, to try to determine the cost drivers, we can also assess whether each activity adds value to the patient. If it does not, perhaps it can be eliminated. If it does add value, the cost of the activity should be assigned to the patient who directly benefits from it.

One problem with ABC is deciding how minutely to define activities. Is taking a pulse or blood pressure an activity? Certainly. However, should we determine the cost of that activity and track how many times it is done for each patient? This is not an easy question. From a clinical perspective, we already track such activities in the patient chart. However, until costing and clinical systems are fully linked, it would require additional data input to track the activity for costing purposes. And what about activities that are necessary but that are never entered in the clinical chart. With ABC, as with any approach to costing, we must always balance the value of more accurate information against the extra cost of collecting that information.

※ SETTING PRICES

In the last decade nurse managers have started to become directly involved in the revenue process of health care organizations. It is no longer sufficient to simply control costs. For health care organizations to prosper, their managers must have an understanding of the processes by which they receive their revenues. Rate setting is the element of financial management that focuses on setting the prices the organization charges for the services it provides.

Historically, rate setting has been outside the control of health care organizations. The federal government sets hospital DRG rates for Medicare patients. In addition, many other rates of health care organizations are mandated by governmental bodies, such as state-controlled Medicaid rates. With the proliferation of managed care this process is changing. As Medicare and Medicaid recipients enroll in managed care organizations, hospital, home health care, and ambulatory care rates are more and more being determined on the basis of negotiation. Nevertheless, the process of developing a *charge master*, that is, a list of the organization's prices for each of its services, remains a critical element of the management process. Some patients still pay the prices set by the provider. And many negotiated rates are set as a percent of the organization's prices as listed in its charge master list.

Total Financial Requirements

Health care organizations strive to obtain the financial resources needed to meet their *total financial requirements* (TFR). These requirements are the financial resources needed to provide for the health care needs of the population served by the organization. Clearly, the financial requirements of any organization include sufficient money to cover the current costs of operations. On a broader perspective, however, the financial needs of the organization encompass the ability to replace facilities as they become obsolete and to adopt new technologies as they become available.

The total financial requirements of health care organizations have been defined to include five categories[4]:

1. Costs of doing business
2. Costs of staying in business
3. Costs of changing business
4. Returns to capital sources
5. Costs of uncertainty

The costs of doing business are the routine operating costs of the organization, including salaries and expenses. If the organization provides education or research, it must recover enough to pay for those services in addition to patient care. If some payers pay less than the full costs generated on their behalf, other payers must be charged more if the organization is to recover the full costs of doing business.

Costs of staying in business relate to having financial resources needed to operate, to replace assets, and to acquire new technology. Most patients do not pay for their care until after they are discharged. However, the organization must acquire supplies before the patient arrives and must pay salaries concurrent with the patient

---

[4]Bruce R. Neumann, James D. Suver, and William N. Zelman, *Financial Management: Concepts and Applications for Health Care Providers*, National Health Publishing, USA, 1984, p. 313.

stay. To stay in business, the organization must therefore have a reserve of cash available to tide itself over until revenues are received.

Costs of changing business relate to the modification of existing services and the addition of new services. Health care services do not remain stagnant over time. As the practice of nursing and medicine changes, health care organizations must be flexible enough to delete outmoded services and to add new ones.

Return to capital refers to repaying those who provide the organization with the basic resources to be in business. This includes the money needed to establish the organization, as well as additional monies to allow the organization to acquire buildings and equipment over time. Some of this money is borrowed. In that case return on capital refers to interest on the loan, as well as repaying the principal of the loan. For-profit entities have owners who have invested money. A return to those owners is generally in the form of dividends. In some cases the organization is either community owned or voluntary, and its original resources came from tax dollars or philanthropic sources or both. In such cases the return on capital may come in the form of subsidized health care services.

Costs of uncertainty refer to the fact that organizations may find themselves with unexpected and unplanned expenses. These include the impact of adverse legal decisions, political decisions, regulatory changes, and similar occurrences.

A stable entity must set rates in such a manner that all these financial requirements are considered. Some payers (such as Medicare) can dictate their prices to the organization. The rates the organization charges the remaining payers must be adequate so that in total the organization has the financial resources it needs. This means that if the organization loses money on Medicare patients, it must attempt to charge a higher price to non-Medicare patients to offset the loss. This is sometimes referred to as a "plug-figure" approach. The organization decides the amount of revenue it needs. It determines how much revenue it will receive from sources over which it has no ability to set prices. Then it plugs in the charges for the remaining patients to achieve the desired revenue.

Unfortunately, this may require the organization to charge a high price for its services. Charging a high price is likely to result in increased bad debts as prices become higher than patients can afford. Increased bad debts mean that charges to the remaining payers must be even higher to offset that loss. This can create a vicious circle, with the organization unable to collect enough to remain financially viable.

Rate-setting Approaches

Neumann, Suver, and Zelman[5] identify three approaches to rate-setting: cost-based prices, negotiated prices, and market prices.

Cost-Based Prices

Cost-based reimbursement generally relies upon the traditional cost-finding analysis, discussed earlier. Often cost-based payers, such as Medicaid, dictate that they will pay the lower of cost or charges. If for some reason the organization were to set its charges less than its costs, they would pay the lower amount.

The cost-based approach requires knowledge of the cost of treating each patient. If one is to reimburse the organization for the cost of treating the patient, one must know that cost. However, rather than actually trying to capture the cost of treating any one patient, cost-based payers generally use what is known as the ratio of charges to charges applied to costs, often referred to as the *ratio of cost to charges* (RCC). In this approach it is assumed that a given payer's costs and charges in any

[5]Ibid. p. 314.

revenue center will be approximately the same. Thus, if 30% of all surgical charges are for Medicaid patients, then Medicaid is responsible for 30% of all OR costs. That 30% can be applied to the total OR revenue center costs to determine the amount Medicaid must pay.

Looking at this calculation another way, suppose that the OR had total charges of $1 million and that 30% of those charges, or $300,000, were to Medicaid patients. Since Medicaid pays costs rather than charges, the costs of treating those patients must be determined. Suppose that the total costs of the operating room were $800,000. Costs are 20% lower than charges (i.e., $800,000 is only 80% of $1 million). Therefore Medicaid costs must be only 80% of the $300,000 of charges, or $240,000.

Negotiated Prices

Negotiated prices or rates are commonplace in the health care industry. HMOs, insurance companies, and even large employers actively negotiate directly with hospitals and other health care providers. Generally, guaranteed patient volume is offered in exchange for discounted prices. Based on the discussions of Chapter 7, negotiated prices should provide a positive contribution margin to the organization.

Market Prices

The market approach is based on the concepts of supply and demand introduced in Chapter 4. This commonly is how practitioners in private practice set prices. For example, suppose a nurse practitioner sets up a private practice. The nurse might charge less than other practitioners in the area and initially not make a profit. However, if volume increases, the practitioner may begin to make a profit. The organization can set any price it wishes. However, if its price is high enough to earn a large profit, that would encourage additional competitors to enter the market and underbid the organization. If the price set is too low, the organization will lose money and eventually go out of business. Health care organizations therefore must walk a tightrope in setting prices.

Furthermore, there are times when competition may cause the organization to lower some prices and raise others so as not to be perceived as being an expensive provider. For example, suppose that two hospitals in the same area offer open heart surgery but that one performs 500 per year while the other performs 50 per year. The charge at the hospital with the higher volume might be significantly less than at the one with low volume because of economies of scale. The low-volume hospital has fewer patients to share the fixed costs of doing open heart surgery (such as the expensive equipment required). It is not unreasonable to expect that the low-volume hospital will lower its charges to match the competition, even if this means that it is charging less than cost.

How will the low-volume hospital survive in that case? It would probably raise charges on a low-cost high-volume item for all patients. For example, it might add a charge of $1 per test for all lab tests done for all patients to offset the reduced charge to open heart surgery patients for their surgery. In this way it would avoid the possibility of being labeled as very expensive for a high-visibility program such as open heart surgery. If a policymaker were to question the wisdom of allowing a low-volume open heart surgery program to exist, the hospital could counter that it is so efficient that its charges are no higher than those of the high-volume program.

Major payers are aware of such influences on hospital rate setting. That is why cost-based payers often mandate that they pay only the lesser of cost or charges. This allows them to take advantage of competitive situations that result in prices below cost.

Rate setting is a critical area of health care management. Managers must take into account their total financial requirements, the patient mix by type of patient, and the patient mix by type of payer. Balancing these factors is often essential to organizational viability. It is particularly important for nurses in private practice.

⁂ FINANCIAL REIMBURSEMENT FOR NURSING SERVICES

Despite the limitations of costing systems, great progress has been made in costing out nursing services. It is now possible to recognize different nursing costs for different patients. That means that it is feasible for nursing to become a revenue center that charges directly for its services. The ability to recognize different consumption of resources by different patients and to charge accordingly is the essential ingredient for a revenue center. Establishment of nursing as a revenue center is feasible as long as different patient classification levels can be assigned different costs.

Clearly, nurses who work in home health are in a revenue center. Nurses in private practice, whether alone or in a group with physician providers, are revenue generators.

If an organization's patients are all fixed-fee patients, revenue centers make little sense. For example, a fixed DRG payment to a hospital will not vary if nursing, lab, or radiology varies its charges. If all patients were paid on a DRG basis, eventually there would be no revenue centers.

However, at present most health care organizations still have some patients who pay charges. Therefore, there are potential benefits if nursing is treated as a revenue center. First, it does charge patients more fairly by charging on a closer approximation of their actual consumption of resources. Second, for hospitals it clearly segregates nursing from room and board. Third, it can help to alleviate the "nursing as a burden" misconception.

As health care organizations find an ever increasing need to manage themselves in a businesslike manner, a clearer understanding of both revenues and expenses will be required. The movement toward recasting the nursing function as a revenue center in hospitals can help in that evolution. Separate costing for different types of patients allows for *variable billing;* that is, the amount billed to each patient per patient day or per visit varies. Instead of simply charging all patients the same amount per day or per visit for nursing care, different patients are charged different amounts based on their differing resource consumption. Once the different costs of caring for different patients are known, they can be charged accordingly. For example, in ambulatory care it is common to charge more for a new patient visit than for a follow-up visit.

Variable billing may be a way to better justify hospital bills and in some cases increase overall revenues to the hospital. Variable billing may be beneficial to nursing because it shows dramatically the specific contribution that nursing makes to the overall revenue structure of the hospital.

Home health agencies generally charge on a per visit basis, although nurse managers recognize that different patients require different amounts of care. For example, the patient who requires an insulin injection requires much less care than the HIV patient with opportunistic infections. Most managers assume that the variation will balance. For each visit requiring a substantial amount of time, there will be an "in-and-out" visit to offset it. This approach was adequate in the past when most nurses were paid on a salaried basis. As more and more home health agencies are paying nurses on a per visit basis, this approach may no longer prove workable. Billing may move to a variable basis depending on nursing resources consumed.

⁂ IMPLICATIONS FOR NURSE MANAGERS

Nurse managers not only have a responsibility to units and departments but also a broader responsibility to the organization. It is imperative for nurse managers to understand the organization's perspective on cost finding and rate setting. It is particularly important for nurses in private practice.

However, that does not mean that all accounting methods and procedures will always be correct or appropriate. By understanding how the organization conducts its cost accounting, nurse managers can identify situations in which the accounting data are inadequate for their needs. Perhaps all supplies are charged to the nursing department when paid for rather than when consumed. While that would have little impact on external reporting of costs, it makes monthly evaluation of performance difficult. Are the right amounts of supplies being used for the number of patients actually being cared for? That question cannot be answered without cost information related to monthly consumption of resources. Information about how much was paid in a given month for supplies is not useful to the nurse manager.

Once such problems are identified, the organization's accountants must be informed of the inadequacy of the existing information. Nurse managers and financial managers can then work together to generate and use relevant information to improve the organization's overall management capabilities and results.

Nurse managers cannot lose sight of the fact that a great deal of the organization's revenues depend on following the cost-finding requirements of external payers and providing them with external reports. The reasons for the cost-finding techniques should be understood lest they be condemned for their lack of perfection. At the same time, recognition of their limitations makes clear the need for the nursing profession to step forward and develop its own approaches for costing out nursing services.

This need is made more critical by the introduction of fixed-payment systems such as DRGs, by capitation payments, and by insurer-negotiated rates for episodes of care. The shift away from cost reimbursement makes knowledge about the cost of treating different types of patients essential. Improved costing of nursing services is a vital step toward getting a more accurate cost for each of the organization's product lines.

Whether this will in turn lead to variable billing for nursing services in hospitals on a universal basis is still unclear. Accurate costing information for nursing does, however, remove the roadblocks to variable billing.

Improving the costing of nursing services has become important to nurse managers for several reasons. One reason is that improved cost information can be used to get an improved understanding of the contribution that nursing makes to the organization as a whole. A second reason is that the information generated by improved costing can be used to help managers make effective decisions and better control the costs of providing nursing services. Third, it is important to understand the nursing resources needed by patients. Costing information is also useful for examining changes in the way nursing care is provided. For example, the cost impact of various skill mixes on inpatient units or in ambulatory care centers can be examined.

The most accurate costing system requires continuous observation of all nurses by data collectors. The cost of such highly accurate costing is prohibitive. However, one can think of a continuum of costing methods. In general, less expensive methods provide less accurate data; more expensive methods provide more accurate data.

Fully integrated computer systems have been introduced in most hospitals, and over time software programs have been developed and perfected to make using the computers easy and efficient. Many organizations are experimenting with various software programs to integrate clinical and financial systems.

In the meantime, activity-based costing and patient classification systems can be used to substantially improve the assignment of nursing costs to patients in an economical way.

Costing out nursing services is an extremely useful tool for product-line costing and budgeting. Information about product-line costs can show management where profits are being made and where losses are accruing. Product-line information can aid managers substantially in understanding which patients place the greatest burden on the unit and in helping the organization make appropriate decisions regarding changes in its patient mix.

KEY CONCEPTS

Cost information for reporting *vs* for management Managers must be careful to use information appropriate to their needs. Cost information generated for external reports may provide managers with information that will lead to poor managerial decisions.

Traditional cost finding Allocating the direct costs of nonrevenue centers to other nonrevenue centers and to revenue centers with the goal of ultimately allocating all the organization's costs to its revenue centers. The total direct and indirect costs of the revenue centers are then allocated to units of service. Revenue centers are cost centers that charge for their services. To be a revenue center, the cost center must be able to distinguish the different amount of resources consumed by different patients. The steps in cost finding are:

1. **Accumulation of direct costs for each cost center:** Costs directly incurred within the cost center.
2. **Determine basis for allocation:** Costs must be allocated on some measurement basis such as pounds or square feet.
3. **Allocate to revenue centers:** The step-down method is widely used to assign nonrevenue center costs to revenue centers.
4. **Allocate revenue center costs to units of service:** Using the weighted procedure, hourly rate, surcharge, and per diem methods.

Costing out nursing services Process of determining the cost of providing nursing care for different patients. This cost has traditionally been included in the room and board charge.

Prospective payment Patients are classified into a variety of categories. The health organization is paid a predetermined amount for patients in these various categories. The payment is not based on the amount of resources a patient uses.

Patient classification system Scheme for grouping patients into categories. Each category contains patients who require similar amounts of nursing care. Some systems are commercially available; others are developed by individual health care organizations.

Acuity How acutely ill patients are. Usually used in conjunction with the nursing resources required to care for patients. The higher the acuity, generally the more resources needed for care.

Variable billing Amount billed to each patient reflects the amount of resources consumed by that patient. Rather than billing a patient for a patient day of care, patients are billed an amount based on the nursing care hours and supplies actually used.

Productivity Ratio of outputs to inputs.

Inputs Those resources required to produce outputs. In nursing, inputs usually include personnel, supplies, and equipment necessary to care for clients.

Outputs Products produced by nursing. Traditionally these are identified as patient days of care, visits, and episodes of care. More recently outputs are being defined as patient outcomes such as health or wellness.

Product-line costing Determination of the cost of providing care to specific types of patients. This approach is sometimes aided by the use of standard cost techniques such as Cleverley's model of standard treatment protocols.

Activity-based costing An approach to costing based on cost drivers and measurement of the cost of activities rather than the cost of patients.

Rate setting Process of assigning prices to the units of service of the revenue centers. Prices must be set high enough to recover the organization's total financial requirements.

SUGGESTED READINGS

Alvarez, C.A., "Setting Fees for Service: Are the Dilemmas More Acute for Nurses?," *Clinical Nurse Specialist,* Vol. 10, No. 6, 1996, p. 309.

Anderson, L., and D. Clancy, *Cost Accounting,* 2nd edition, Dame Publications, Houston, Tex., 1998.

Baker, J.J., and G.F. Boyd, "Activity Based Costing in the Operating Room at Valley View Hospital," *Journal of Health Care Finance,* Vol. 24, No. 1, Fall 1997, pp. 1–9.

Barfield, J., et al., *Cost Accounting: Tradition and Innovations,* West Publishing, Minneapolis, Minn., 1997.

Brannon, Robert L., "Restructuring Hospital Nursing," *International Journal of Health Services,* Vol. 26, No. 4, 1996, pp. 643–654.

Bruttomesso, K.A., "Variable Hospital Accounting Practices: Are They Fair for the Nursing Department?" *Journal of Nursing Administration,* Vol. 25, No. 1, January 1995, p. 6.

Cleverley, William O., *Essentials of Health Care Finance,* Aspen Publishers, Gaithersburg, Md., February 1997.

Crockett, M.J., M. DiBlasi, P. Flaherty, and K. Sampson, "Activity-Based Resource Allocation: A System for Predicting Nursing Costs," *Rehabilitation Nursing,* Vol. 22, No. 6, November 1997, pp. 293–298, 302.

Doyle, John J., "Full Cost Determination of Different Levels of Care in the Intensive Care Unit: An Activity-Based Costing Approach," *PharmacoEconomics,* Vol. 10, No. 4, October 1996, pp. 395–408.

Eastaugh, Steven R., *Health Care Finance,* Aspen Publishers, Gaithersburg, Md., 1998.

Edwardson, Sandra R., and Patricia Nardone, "Resource Use in Home Care Agencies," *Applied Nursing Research,* Vol. 4, No. 1, February 1991, pp. 25–30.

Finkler, Steven A., *Budgeting Concepts for Nurse Managers,* 3rd edition, W.B. Saunders, Philadelphia, Penn., 2000.

Finkler, Steven A., and David R. Ward, *Cost Accounting for Health Care Organizations: Concepts and Applications,* 2nd edition, Aspen Publishers, Gaithersburg, Md., 1999.

Finkler, Steven A., "Costing Out Nursing Services," *Hospital Cost Management and Accounting,* Vol. 1., No. 12, March 1990, pp. 1–5.

Finkler, Steven A., "The Distinction Between Cost and Charges," *Annals of Internal Medicine,* Vol. 96, No. 1, January 1982, pp. 102–109.

Gapenski, Louis C., *Financial Analysis and Decision Making for Healthcare Organizations: A Guide for the Healthcare Professional,* Irwin Professional Publishers, Burr Ridge, Ill., January 1997.

Garber, A.M., and C.E. Phelps, "Economic Foundations of Cost-Effectiveness Analysis," *Journal of Health Economics,* Vol. 16, No. 1, February 1997, pp. 1–31.

Gardner, K., J. Tobin, J. Kamm, and J. Allhusen, "Determining the Cost of Care Through Clinical Pathways," *Nursing Economic$,* Vol. 15, No. 4, July-August 1997, pp. 213–217.

Hansen, Don, and Maryanne Mowen, *Cost Management,* 2nd edition, South-Western Publishing, Cincinnati, Ohio, 1997.

Hendrickson, Gerry, Theresa M. Doddato, and Christine T. Kovner, "How Do Nurses Spend Their Time?" *Journal of Nursing Administration,* Vol. 20, No. 3, March 1990, pp. 31–37.

Heshmat, S., "Managed Care and the Relevant Costs for Pricing," *Health Care Management Revue,* Vol. 22, No. 1, Winter 1997, pp. 82–85.

Horngren, C.T., G. Foster, and S.M. Datar, *Cost Accounting: A Managerial Emphasis,* 9th edition, Prentice Hall, Upper Saddle River, N.J., 1996.

Jegers, M., "Cost Accounting in ICUs: Beneficial for Management and Research," *Clinical Therapeutics,* Vol. 19, No. 3, June 1997, pp. 570–581.

Jones, K.R., "Standard Cost Accounting," *Seminars for Nurse Managers,* Vol. 3, No. 3, September 1995, pp. 111–112.

Kovner, Christine T., "Public Health Nursing Costs in Home Care," *Public Health Nursing,* Vol. 6, No. 1, March 1989, pp. 3–7.

Kovner, Christine T., "Measuring Indirect Nursing Costs," *Hospital Cost Accounting Advisor,* Vol. 1, No. 3, June 1989, pp. 6–7.

Levy, V.M., *Financial Management of Hospitals,* Wm Gaunt & Sons, Holmes Beach, Fla., January 1998.

McLean, Robert A., *Financial Management in Health Care Organizations,* Delmar, Albany, N.Y., 1996.

Neumann, Bruce R., Jan P. Clement, and Jean C. Cooper, *Financial Management: Concepts and Applications for Health Care Organizations,* Kendall/Hunt Publishing, Dubuque, Iowa, May 1997.

Nyman, John A., and Robert A. Connor, "Do Case-Mix Adjusted Nursing Home Reimbursements Actually Reflect Costs? Minnesota's Experience," *Journal of Health Economics,* Vol. 13, No. 2, July 1994, pp. 145–162.

Pelfrey, S., "Cost-Accounting Techniques for Health Care Providers," *Health Care Supervisor,* Vol. 14, No. 2, December 1995, pp. 33–42.

Pelletier, K.R., W.L. Haskell, M. Krasner, and A. Marie, "Current Trends in the Integration and Reimbursement of Complementary and Alternative Medicine by Managed Care, Insurance Carriers, and Hospital Providers," *American Journal of Health Promotions,* Vol. 12, No. 2, November-December 1997, pp. 112–122.

Prince, Thomas R., *Financial Reporting and Cost Control for Health Care Entities,* Health Administration Press, Ann Arbor, Mich., June 1992.

Robinson, James C., "Administered Pricing and Vertical Integration in the Hospital Industry," *Journal of Law and Economics,* Vol. 39, No. 1, April 1996, pp. 3, 5, 7–78.

Strasen, Leann, "Implementing Salary Cost Per Unit of Service Productivity Standards," *Journal of Nursing Administration,* Vol. 20, No. 3, March 1990, pp. 6–10.

Swindle, Ralph, Martha C. Beattie, and Paul G. Barnett, "The Quality of Cost Data: A Caution from the Department of Veterans Affairs Experience," *Medical Care,* Vol. 34, No. 3, March 1996, pp. 83–90.

Warner, K.E., and B.R. Luce, *Cost-Benefit and Cost-Effectiveness Analysis in Health Care: Principles, Practice, and Potential,* Health Administration Press, Ann Arbor, Mich., 1983.

West, D.A., T.D. West, E.A. Balas, and L.L. Mcks, "Profitable Capitation Requires Accurate Costing," *Nursing Economic$,* Vol. 14, No. 3, May-June 1996, pp. 150, 162–170.

Zelman, William N., Michael J. McCue, and Alan R. Milikan, *Financial Management of Health Care Organizations: An Introduction to Fundamental Tools, Concepts, and Applications,* Blackwell, New York, N.Y., January 1998.

Institutional Cost Report

This appendix presents and discusses several pages from a real institutional cost report. Exhibits 8A–1 through 8A–3 present just a small portion of an institutional cost report form; the actual report was nearly 2 inches thick. This form was submitted to Empire Blue Cross and Blue Shield, which acts as an agent for the Health Care Financing Administration (HCFA), the federal government agency in charge of Medicare. The institution's cost report is a public document. Exhibit 8A–1 is the cover page of the report, for the year ending December 31, 1997.

Exhibit 8A–2 shows a portion of Worksheet B, Part I of the report. This provides the allocation of general services costs. This part of the report, although much more complex and set up somewhat differently, parallels the allocation process made in Table 8–3. In Table 8–3 all cost centers and revenue centers are shown across the top of the table, and the allocation proceeds row by row. In the official cost report, all cost centers and revenue centers are shown as rows; the allocation proceeds column by column.

Notice that in the 0 column on the first page of this exhibit there are $3,471,343 of costs in Row 19.03 for "nursing administration." These costs must be allocated. However, there are no costs in rows 19.04 or 19.05. Those costs have already been reclassified in an earlier section of the report. That reclassification placed the costs of nursing units directly into departments for which the hospital makes a per diem charge. This includes line 25 "adults & pediatrics," line 26 "intensive care unit," line 27 "coronary care unit," and a number of other departments. The hospital has more than fifty-five departments; the rest of the departments appeared on additional pages not shown here.

Looking across all four pages of Exhibit 8A–2, one can see the pattern created by the process from which it earned the name step-down report. On the third page of Exhibit 8A–2, Worksheet B, Part I, you can see in column 19.03 that $5,847,895 is being taken out of "nursing administration" and allocated to the departments on lines 25 through 39. Note that the $5,847,895 is greater than the original $3,471,343 of direct costs of nursing administration. That is because nursing administration has received allocations of costs for depreciation, employee benefits, administrative services (other than nursing), plant operations, laundry, housekeeping, and cafeteria on the previous two pages. For example, there is a $78,175 allocation from laundry & linen service (column 9) into nursing administration.

What is the basis for each cost allocation? Exhibit 8A–3 provides the statistical basis for each allocation. This is Worksheet B-1 of the report. Notice in the headings for each column that the basis is given. For example, in column 1 the basis for allocating the building depreciation is square feet. On the second page of the exhibit, laundry & linen service is allocated based on pounds of laundry and dietary is allocated based on meals served. On the third page of the exhibit note that nursing administration is allocated based on time spent on supervision of nurses. A total of 74,909,473 nursing minutes have been worked, and the amount of work by nurses in each of the departments is shown lower in that column. For example, the nurses in the adults and pediatrics department used 32,193,061 nursing minutes.

Worksheet B-1 (i.e., Exhibit 8A–3) parallels the information shown in Table 8–1. However, in Table 8–1 percentages were used. In Exhibit 8A–3 the raw numbers are shown. To determine what portion of nursing administration costs to allocate to subsequent departments in the step down, one would have to determine what portion of nursing time was consumed by each department. For example, since 32,193,061 minutes of the total 74,909,473 (both numbers are from column 19.03 on the third page of Exhibit 8A-3) were consumed by adults & pediatrics, 43% of

Text continued on page 202

Medicare Cost Report Excerpts

※ EXHIBIT 8A–1. *Institutional Cost Reports—Certification*

Provider No.	Empire Blue Cross and Blue Shield	Version: 97.12
Period from 01/01/1997 to 12/31/1997	In lieu of Form HCFA-2552-96 (9/96)	06/01/1998 09:54:13

Hospital and Health Care Complex Cost Report
Certification and Settlement Summary

Worksheet S
Parts I & II

Intermediary	[ ] Audited	Date Received ____	[XX] Initial	[ ] Re-opening
Use Only	[ ] Desk Reviewed	Intermediary No. ____	[ ] Final	

Part I—Certification

Check	__ Electronically Filed Cost Report	Date: ________
Applicable Box	__ Manually Submitted Cost Report	Time: ________

Misrepresentation or falsification of any information contained in this cost report may be punishable by criminal, civil and administrative action, fine and/or imprisonment under federal law. Furthermore, if services identified in this report were provided or procured through the payment directly or indirectly of a kickback or where otherwise illegal, criminal, civil and administrative action, fines and/or imprisonment may result.

Certification by Officer or Administrator of Provider(s)

I hereby certify that I have read the above statement and that I have examined the accompanying electronically filed or manually submitted cost report and the balance sheet and statement of revenue and expenses prepared by ____________________ ______________(Provider Name(s) and Number(s)) for the cost report period beginning 01-01-1997 and ending 12-31-1997, and that to the best of my knowledge and belief, it is a true, correct and complete statement prepared from the books and records of the provider in accordance with applicable instructions, except as noted. I further certify that I am familiar with the laws and regulations regarding the provision of health care services and that the services identified in this cost report were provided in compliance with such laws and regulations.

(Signed) ____
Officer or Administrator of Provider(s)

____
Title

____
Date

Part II—Settlement Summary

		Title V	Title XVIII		Title XIX	
			Part A	Part B		
		1	2	3	4	
1	Hospital		8833178	3209534		1
2	Subprovider I		849605	−72569		2
3	Swing Bed—SNF					3
4	Swing Bed—NF					4
5	Skilled Nursing Facility					5
6	Other Nursing Facility					6
7	Home Health Agency					7
8	Outpatient Rehabilitation Provider					8
100	Total		9682783	3136965		100

The above amounts represent 'due to' or 'due from' the applicable program for the element of the above complex indicated.

※ EXHIBIT 8A–2. *Institutional Cost Reports—Cost Allocation—General Service Costs*

PROVIDER NO.
PERIOD FROM 01/01/1997 TO 12/31/1997

EMPIRE BLUE CROSS AND BLUE SHIELD
IN LIEU OF FORM HCFA-2552-96 (9/97)

VERSION: 97.12
06/01/1998 09:54.13

COST ALLOCATION - GENERAL SERVICE COSTS

WORKSHEET B
PART I

	COST CENTER DESCRIPTION	NET EXP FOR COST ALLOCATION 0	OLD CAP BLDGS & FIXTURES 1	OLD CAP MOVABLE EQUIPMENT 2	NEW CAP BLDGS & FIXTURES 3	NEW CAP MOVABLE EQUIPMENT 4	EMPLOYEE BENEFITS 5	SUBTOTAL 5A	ADMINIS-TRATIVE & GENERAL 6	
	GENERAL SERVICE COST CENTERS									
1	OLD CAP REL COSTS-BLDG & FIXT	3499179	3499179							1
2	OLD CAP REL COSTS-MVBLE EQUIP	689061		689061						2
3	NEW CAP REL COSTS-BLDG & FIXT	14158662			14158662					3
4	NEW CAP REL COSTS-MVBLE EQUIP	16014216				16014216				4
5	EMPLOYEE BENEFITS	44618444	25929	23858	101541	45188	44814960			5
6	ADMINISTRATIVE & GENERAL	56415228	631099	35967	2556217	5586391	5153152	70378054	70378054	6
7	MAINTENANCE & REPAIRS									7
8	OPERATION OF PLANT	7524814	304523	123478	1192568	743944	678237	10567564	2513590	8
9	LAUNDRY & LINEN SERVICE	1906168	39014	16254	152786	81222	258530	2453974	583700	9
10	HOUSEKEEPING	6315841	28007	6623	109682	286626	1247210	7993989	1901442	10
11.01	DIETARY - RAW FOOD	2071719						2071719	492777	11.01
11.02	DIETARY - OTHER	3725241	65509	8741	256544	474563	841595	5372193	1277824	11.02
12	CAFETERIA	-506128	17459		68371			-420298		12
13	MAINTENANCE OF PERSONNEL	560799					179	560978	133434	13
17	MEDICAL RECORDS & LIBRARY	3299617	48504	429	189950	28045	549526	4116071	979045	17
18	SOCIAL SERVICE	933292	10371		40617		2268112	1212392	288378	18
19	MEDICAL SUPPLIES AND EXPENSE	1249241		5892		116906		1372039	326352	19
19.01	CENTRAL SERVICES & SUPPLY	917411	23725	5530	92910	589173	119047	1747796	415729	19.01
19.02	PHARMACY	13448740	23677	27887	92724	86716	1173354	14853098	3532943	19.02
19.03	NURSING ADMINISTRATION	3471343	39558	46204	154918	185791	594032	4491846	1068426	19.03
19.04	INTENSIVE NURSING CARE									19.04
19.05	GENERAL NURSING SERVICE									19.05
19.06	SUPERVISING PHYSICIANS-OTHER	19725739						19725739	4691945	19.06
22	I&R SERVICES-SALARY & FRINGES A	15386912					3818022	19204934	4568066	22
23	I&R SERVICES-OTHER PRGM COSTS A	1153124	20743	6906	81233	3829		1265835	301090	23
23.01	SPRVSNG PHYSICIANS-TEACHING	14650379						14650379	3484724	23.01
	INPATIENT ROUTINE SERV COST CENTERS									
25	ADULTS & PEDIATRICS	35111893	947485	112520	3710520	2697833	12362646	54942897	13068553	25
26	INTENSIVE CARE UNIT	4372081	31050		121596	166741	952890	5644358	1342561	26
27	CORONARY CARE UNIT	1903194	13621		53343		418663	2388821	568203	27
29	SURGICAL INTENSIVE CARE UNIT	4698609	3868		15147		963295	5681919	1351496	29
	NEONATAL INTENSIVE CARE UNIT	3403972	14779		57879		724616	4201246	999304	30
	SUBPROVIDER	4790697	109816	3298	407519	44377	1237720	6593427	1568306	31
33	NURSERY	1289571	10665		41767		274014	1616017	384384	33
	ANCILLARY SERVICE COST CENTERS									
37	OPERATING ROOM	21879215	86433	41955	338488	867908	1855258	25069257	5962948	37
39	DELIVERY ROOM & LABOR ROOM	4349524	53335		395029		811197	5609085	1334171	39
40	ANESTHESIOLOGY	1298966	16396	27242	64208	125596	122618	1655026	393663	40
41	RADIOLOGY-DIAGNOSTIC	6097235	99817	31932	390900	1326753	899178	8845815	2104057	41
42	RADIOLOGY-THERAPEUTIC									42
43	RADIOISOTOPE	7801	8600		33678			50079	11912	43
43.01	CAT SCAN	1088717	11806	4461	46235	41502	150968	1343689	319609	43.01
44	LABORATORY	4760950	164405	52695	643839	727916	1367795	7717600	1835701	44
47	BLOOD STORING, PROCESSING & TRA	3970192	22234	3008	87072	108675	378782	4569963	1067007	47

※ **EXHIBIT 8A–2.** *Institutional Cost Reports—Cost Allocation—General Service Costs* Continued

	COST CENTER DESCRIPTION	OPERATION OF PLANT 8	LAUNDRY & LINEN SERVICE 9	HOUSE-KEEPING 10	DIETARY RAW FOOD 11.01	DIETARY-OTHER 11.02	CAFETERIA 12	MAIN-TENANCE OF PERSONNEL 13	MEDICAL RECORDS & LIBRARY 17	
	GENERAL SERVICE COST CENTERS									
1	OLD CAP REL COSTS-BLDG & FIXT									1
2	OLD CAP REL COSTS-MVBLE EQUIP									2
3	NEW CAP REL COSTS-BLDG & FIXT									3
4	NEW CAP REL COSTS-MVBLE EQUIP									4
5	EMPLOYEE BENEFITS									5
6	ADMINISTRATIVE & GENERAL									6
7	MAINTENANCE & REPAIRS									7
8	OPERATION OF PLANT	13081154								8
9	LAUNDRY & LINEN SERVICE	193883	3231557							9
10	HOUSEKEEPING	139185	62871	10097487						10
11.01	DIETARY - RAW FOOD				2564496					11.01
11.02	DIETARY - OTHER	325551	7032			6982600				11.02
12	CAFETERIA	86762					-333536			12
13	MAINTENANCE OF PERSONNEL							694412		13
17	MEDICAL RECORDS & LIBRARY	241044							5336160	17
18	SOCIAL SERVICE	51542								18
19	MEDICAL SUPPLIES AND EXPENSE		44120							19
19.01	CENTRAL SERVICES & SUPPLY	117902								19.01
19.02	PHARMACY	117666								19.02
19.03	NURSING ADMINISTRATION	196589	78175					12859		19.03
19.04	INTENSIVE NURSING CARE									19.04
19.05	GENERAL NURSING SERVICE									19.05
19.06	SUPERVISING PHYSICIANS-OTHER									19.06
22	I&R SERVICES-SALARY & FRINGES A									22
23	I&R SERVICES-OTHER PRGM COSTS A	103084						375498		23
23.01	SPRVSNG PHYSICIANS-TEACHING									23.01
	INPATIENT ROUTINE SERV COST CENTERS									
25	ADULTS & PEDIATRICS	4708608	1376579	4888542	1648017	4487213		172317	2490386	25
26	INTENSIVE CARE UNIT	154303	193604	1036678				15431	104589	26
27	CORONARY CARE UNIT	67692	50186					5144	48559	27
29	SURGICAL INTENSIVE CARE UNIT	19221	88019					7716	114727	29
30	NEONATAL INTENSIVE CARE UNIT	73447	69296	290277				12859	124866	30
31	SUBPROVIDER	517137	83966	622016	230906	628710		18003	133404	31
33	NURSERY	53002	118718	290277				7716	149412	33
	ANCILLARY SERVICE COST CENTERS									
37	OPERATING ROOM	429537	495337		16620	45254		41150		37
39	DELIVERY ROOM & LABOR ROOM	501288	166192	435416	13711	37331		15431		39
40	ANESTHESIOLOGY	81479								40
41	RADIOLOGY-DIAGNOSTIC	496048	38881	154921						41
42	RADIOLOGY-THERAPEUTIC									42
43	RADIOISOTOPE	42737								43
43.01	CAT SCAN	58672								43.01
44	LABORATORY	817024	59148	154921						44
47	BLOOD STORING, PROCESSING & TRA	110493								47

Exhibit continued on following page

※ EXHIBIT 8A–2. *Institutional Cost Reports—Cost Allocation—General Service Costs* Continued

	COST CENTER DESCRIPTION	SOCIAL SERVICE 18	MEDICAL SUPPLIES & EXPENSE 19	CENTRAL SERVICES & SUPPLY 19.01	PHARMACY 19.02	NURSING ADMINI-STRATION 19.03	SUPERVIS-ING PHYSI-CIANS-OTHER 19.06	I&R SALARY & FRINGES 22	I&R PROGRAM COSTS 23	
	GENERAL SERVICE COST CENTERS									
1	OLD CAP REL COSTS-BLDG & FIXT									1
2	OLD CAP REL COSTS-MVBLE EQUIP									2
3	NEW CAP REL COSTS-BLDG & FIXT									3
4	NEW CAP REL COSTS-MVBLE EQUIP									4
5	EMPLOYEE BENEFITS									5
6	ADMINISTRATIVE & GENERAL									6
7	MAINTENANCE & REPAIRS									7
8	OPERATION OF PLANT									8
9	LAUNDRY & LINEN SERVICE									9
10	HOUSEKEEPING									10
11.01	DIETARY - RAW FOOD									11.01
11.02	DIETARY - OTHER									11.02
12	CAFETERIA									12
13	MAINTENANCE OF PERSONNEL									13
17	MEDICAL RECORDS & LIBRARY									17
19	SOCIAL SERVICE	1552312								18
19	MEDICAL SUPPLIES AND EXPENSE		1742511							19
19.01	CENTRAL SERVICES & SUPPLY			2281427						19.01
19.02	PHARMACY				18503707					19.02
19.03	NURSING ADMINISTRATION					5847895				19.03
19.04	INTENSIVE NURSING CARE									19.04
19.05	GENERAL NURSING SERVICE									19.05
19.06	SUPERVISING PHYSICIANS-OTHER						24417684			19.06
22	I&R SERVICES-SALARY & FRINGES A						57862	23830862		22
23	I&R SERVICES-OTHER PRGM COSTS A				2425				2047932	23
23.01	SPRVSNG PHYSICIANS-TEACHING									23.01
	INPATIENT ROUTINE SERV COST CENTERS									
25	ADULTS & PEDIATRICS	1037875	1089661	896896	15032933	2513196	16569484	10766958	925270	25
26	INTENSIVE CARE UNIT	11332	102671	215786	583862	309732		1292035	111032	26
27	CORONARY CARE UNIT	5278	35819	72888	55481	136084		861356	74022	27
30	SURGICAL INTENSIVE CARE UNIT	105402	82224	304934	538476	313114				29
31	NEONATAL INTENSIVE CARE UNIT	40671	35964	87185	33434	235533		1579154	135706	30
31	SUBPROVIDER		55092		1721751	283773		430678	37011	31
33	NURSERY		6236		11756	89067		143559	12337	33
	ANCILLARY SERVICE COST CENTERS									
37	OPERATING ROOM			153888	42893	604896				37
39	DELIVERY ROOM & LABOR ROOM		95566	13672	19878	263675		1148475	98696	39
40	ANESTHESIOLOGY		42780		158454		52071	1363814	117201	40
41	RADIOLOGY-DIAGNOSTIC	46725	5801	30240	107684			789577	67853	41
42	RADIOLOGY-THERAPEUTIC									42
43	RADIOISOTOPE									43
43.01	CAT SCAN									43.01
44	LABORATORY		16242		125		2012036	143559	12337	44
47	BLOOD STORING, PROCESSING & TRA		4641		27					47

※ EXHIBIT 8A–2. *Institutional Cost Reports—Cost Allocation—General Service Costs* Continued

	COST CENTER DESCRIPTION	SPRVSNG PHYSICIANS TEACHING 23.01	SUBTOTAL 25	I&R COST & POST STEP-DOWN ADJS 26	TOTAL 27	
	GENERAL SERVICE COST CENTERS					
1	OLD CAP REL COSTS-BLDG & FIXT					1
2	OLD CAP REL COSTS-MVBLE EQUIP					2
3	NEW CAP REL COSTS-BLDG & FIXT					3
4	NEW CAP REL COSTS-MVBLE EQUIP					4
5	EMPLOYEE BENEFITS					5
6	ADMINISTRATIVE & GENERAL					6
7	MAINTENANCE & REPAIRS					7
8	OPERATION OF PLANT					8
9	LAUNDRY & LINEN SERVICE					9
10	HOUSEKEEPING					10
11.01	DIETARY - RAW FOOD					11.01
11.02	DIETARY - OTHER					11.02
12	CAFETERIA					12
13	MAINTENANCE OF PERSONNEL					13
17	MEDICAL RECORDS & LIBRARY					17
18	SOCIAL SERVICE					18
19	MEDICAL SUPPLIES AND EXPENSE					19
19.01	CENTRAL SERVICES & SUPPLY					19.01
19.02	PHARMACY					19.02
19.03	NURSING ADMINISTRATION					19.03
19.04	INTENSIVE NURSING CARE					19.04
19.05	GENERAL NURSING SERVICE					19.05
19.06	SUPERVISING PHYSICIANS-OTHER					19.06
22	I &R SERVICES-SALARY & FRINGES A					22
23	I&R SERVICES-OTHER PRGM COSTS A					23
23.01	SPRVSNG PHYSICIANS-TEACHING	18135103				23.01
	INPATIENT ROUTINE SERV COST CENTERS					
25	ADULTS & PEDIATRICS	11838058	148453443	-23530286	124923157	25
26	INTENSIVE CARE UNIT		11117974	-1403067	9714907	26
27	CORONARY CARE UNIT		4369533	-935378	3434155	27
29	SURGICAL INTENSIVE CARE UNIT		8607248		8607248	29
30	NEONATAL INTENSIVE CARE UNIT		7918942	-1714860	6204082	30
31	SUBPROVIDER	247715	13171895	-715404	12456491	31
33	NURSERY		2882481	-155896	2726585	33
	ANCILLARY SERVICE COST CENTERS					
37	OPERATING ROOM		32861780		32861780	37
39	DELIVERY ROOM & LABOR ROOM		9752587	-1247171	8505416	39
40	ANESTHESIOLOGY	40642	3905130	-1521657	2383473	40
41	RADIOLOGY-DIAGNOSTIC		12687602	-857430	11830172	41
42	RADIOLOGY-THERAPEUTIC					42
43	RADIOISOTOPE		104728		104728	43
43.01	CAT SCAN		1721970		1721970	43.01
44	LABORATORY	1602523	14371216	-1758419	12612797	44
47	BLOOD STORING, PROCESSING & TRA		5772131		5772131	47

※ EXHIBIT 8A–3. *Institutional Cost Reports—Cost Allocation—Statistical Basis*

PROVIDER NO. 33-0194 — EMPIRE BLUE CROSS AND BLUE SHIELD — VERSION: 97.12
PERIOD FROM 01/01/1997 TO 12/31/1997 — IN LIEU OF FORM HCFA-2552-96 (9/97) — 06/01/1998 09:54.13

COST ALLOCATION - STATISTICAL BASIS — WORKSHEET B-1

	COST CENTER DESCRIPTION	OLD CAP BLDGS & FIXTURES SQUARE FEET 1	OLD CAP MOVABLE EQUIPMENT DOLLAR VALUE 2	NEW CAP BLDGS & FIXTURES SQUARE FEET 3	NEW CAP MOVABLE EQUIPMENT DOLLAR VALUE 4	EMPLOYEE BENEFITS GROSS SALARIES 5	RECON-CILIATION 6A	ADMINIS-TRATIVE GENERAL ACCUM COST 6	
	GENERAL SERVICE COST CENTERS								
1	OLD CAP REL COSTS-BLDG & FIXT	809725							1
2	OLD CAP REL COSTS-MVBLE EQUIP		645802						2
3	NEW CAP REL COSTS-BLDG & FIXT			836625					3
4	NEW CAP REL COSTS-MVBLE EQUIP				13869437				4
5	EMPLOYEE BENEFITS	6000	22360	6000	39136	186596992			5
6	ADMINISTRATIVE & GENERAL	146039	33709	151045	4838210	21456269	– 70378054	295881851	6
7	MAINTENANCE & RE PAIRS								7
8	OPERATION OF PLANT	70468	115728	70468	644308	2823988		10567564	8
9	LAUNDRY & LINEN SERVICE	9028	15234	9028	70344	1076444		2453974	9
10	HOUSEKEEPING	6481	6207	6481	248238	5193029		7993989	10
11.01	DIETARY - RAW FOOD							2071719	11.01
11.02	DIETARY - OTHER	15159	8192	15159	411005	3504165		5372193	11.02
12	CAFETERIA	4040		4040			420298		12
13	MAINTENANCE OF PERSONNEL					745		560978	13
17	MEDICAL RECORDS & LIBRARY	11224	402	11224	24289	2288072		4116071	17
18	SOCIAL SERVICE	2400		2400		949795		1212392	18
19	MEDICAL SUPPLIES AND EXPENSE		5522		101249			1372039	19
19.01	CENTRAL SERVICES & SUPPLY	5490	5163	5490	510265	495676		1747796	19.01
19.02	PHARMACY	5479	26136	5479	75102	4885515		14953098	19.02
19.03	NURSING ADMINISTRATION	9154	43303	9154	160908	2473381		4491846	19.03
19.04	INTENSIVE NURSING CARE								19.04
19.05	GENERAL NURSING SERVICE								19.05
19.06	SUPERVISING PHYSICIANS-OTHER							19725739	19.06
22	I&R SERVICES-SALARY & FRINGES					15897164		19204934	22
23	I&R SERVICES-OTHER PROM COSTS	4800	6472	4800	3316			1265835	23
23.01	SPRVSNG PHYSICIANS-TEACHING							14650379	23.01
	INPATIENT ROUTINE SERV COST CENTERS								
25	ADULTS & PEDIATRICS	219252	105456	219252	2336512	51474743		54942897	25
26	INTENSIVE CARE UNIT	7185		7185	144409	3967564		5644358	26
27	CORONARY CARE UNIT	3152		3152		1743194		2388821	27
29	SURGICAL INTENSIVE CARE UNIT	895		895		4010887		5681919	29
30	NEONATAL INTENSIVE CARE UNIT	3420		3420		3017097		4201246	30
31	SUBPROVIDER	25412	3091	24080	39434	5153515		6593427	31
33	NURSERY	2468		2468		1140916		1616017	33
	ANCILLARY SERVICE COST CENTERS								
37	OPERATING ROOM	20001	39321	20001	751669	7724769		25069257	37
39	DELIVERY ROOM & LABOR ROOM	12342		23342		3377597		5609085	39
40	ANESTHESIOLOGY	3794	25532	3794	108775	510545		1655026	40
41	RADIOLOGY-DIAGNOSTIC	23098	29927	23098	1149061	3743923		8845815	41
42	RADIOLOGY-THERAPEUTIC								42
43	RADIOISOTOPE	1990		1990				50079	43
43.01	CAT SCAN	2732	4181	2732	35944	628588		1343689	43.01

※ EXHIBIT 8A–3. *Institutional Cost Reports—Cost Allocation—Statistical Basis* Continued

	COST CENTER DESCRIPTION	MAIN-TENANCE+ REPAIRS SQUARE FEET 7	OPERATION OF PLANT SQUARE FEET 8	LAUNDRY & LINEN SERVICE POUNDS OF LAUNDRY 9	HOUSE-KEEPING HOURS OF SERVICE 10	DIETARY-RAW FOOD MEALS SERVED 11.01	DIETARY-OTHER MEALS SERVED 11.02	CAFETERIA AVG NO OF EMPLOYEES 12	MAIN-TENANCE OF PERSONNEL NUMBER HOUSED 13	
	GENERAL SERVICE COST CENTERS									
1	OLD CAP REL COSTS-BLDG & FIXT									1
2	OLD CAP REL COSTS-MVBLE EQUIP									2
3	NEW CAP REL COSTS-BLDG & FIXT									3
4	NEW CAP REL COSTS-MVBLE EQUIP									4
5	EMPLOYEE BENEFITS									5
6	ADMINISTRATIVE & GENERAL									6
7	MAINTENANCE & REPAIRS	679580								7
8	OPERATION OF PLANT	70468	609112							8
9	LAUNDRY & LINEN SERVICE	9028	9028	6093973						9
10	HOUSEKEEPING	6481	6491	118560	220889					10
11.01	DIETARY - RAW FOOD					817008				11.01
11.02	DIETARY - OTHER	15159	15159	13260			817008			11.02
12	CAFETERIA	4040	4040					2251		12
13	MAINTENANCE OF PERSONNEL								270	13
17	MEDICAL RECORDS & LIBRARY	11224	11224					84		17
18	SOCIAL SERVICE	2400	2400					7		18
19	MEDICAL SUPPLIES AND EXPENSE			83200						19
19.01	CENTRAL SERVICES & SUPPLY	5490	5490					16		19.01
19.02	PHARMACY	5479	5479					96		19.02
19.03	NURSING ADMINISTRATION	9154	9154	147420				20	5	19.03
19.04	INTENSIVE NURSING CARE									19.04
19.05	GENERAL NURSING SERVICE									19.05
19.06	SUPERVISING PHYSICIANS-OTHER									19.06
22	I &R SERVICES-SALARY & FRINGES									22
23	I&R SERVICES-OTHER PRGM COSTS	4800	4800					374	146	23
23.01	SPRVSNG PHYSICIANS-TEACHING									23.01
	INPATIENT ROUTINE SERV COST CENTERS									
25	ADULTS & PEDIATRICS	219252	219252	2595911	106940	525032	525032	527	67	25
26	INTENSIVE CARE UNIT	7185	7185	365092	22678			18	6	26
27	CORONARY CARE UNIT	3152	3152	94640				8	2	27
29	SURGICAL INTENSIVE CARE UNIT	895	895	165984				17	3	29
30	NEONATAL INTENSIVE CARE UNIT	3420	3420	130676	6350			30	5	30
31	SUBPROVIDER	24080	24080	158340	13607	73563	73563	59	7	31
33	NURSERY	2468	2468	223875	6350			15	3	33
ANCILLARY SERVICE COST CENTERS										
37	OPERATING ROOM	20001	20001	934092		5295	5295	64	16	37
39	DELIVERY ROOM & LABOR ROOM	23342	23342	313400	9525	4368	4368	28	6	39
40	ANESTHESIOLOGY	3794	3794					16		40
41	RADIOLOGY-DIAGNOSTIC	23098	23096	73320	3389			105		41
42	RADIOLOGY-THERAPEUTIC									42
43	RADIOISOTOPE	1990	1990							43
43.01	CAT SCAN	2732	2732					16		43.01

Exhibit continued on following page

※ EXHIBIT 8A–3. *Institutional Cost Reports—Cost Allocation—Statistical Basis* Continued

PROVIDER NO.
PERIOD FROM 01/01/1997 TO 12/31/1997

EMPIRE BLUE CROSS AND BLUE SHIELD
IN LIEU OF FORM HCFA-2552-96 (9/97)

VERSION: 97.12
06/01/1998 09:54:13

WORKSHEET B-1

COST ALLOCATION - STATISTICAL BASIS

	COST CENTER DESCRIPTION	MEDICAL RECORDS & LIBRARY % TIME SPENT 17	SOCIAL SERVICE TIME SPENT 18	MEDICAL SUPPLIES & EXPENSE COSTED REQUIS 19	CENTRAL SERVICES & SUPPLY COSTED REQUIS 19.01	PHARMACY COSTED REQUIS 19.02	NURSING ADMINI-STRATION SPVSN OF NURSTIME 19.03	SUPERVIS-ING PHYSI-CIANS-OTHR HOURS OF SERVICE 19.06	I&R SALARY & FRINGES ASSIGNED TIME 22	
	GENERAL SERVICE COST CENTERS									
1	OLD CAP REL COSTS-BLDG & FIXT									1
2	OLD CAP REL COSTS-MVBLE EQUIP									2
3	NEW CAP REL COSTS-BLDG & FIXT									3
4	NEW CAP REL COSTS-MVBLE EQUIP									4
5	EMPLOYEE BENEFITS									5
6	ADMINISTRATIVE & GENERAL									6
7	MAINTENANCE & REPAIRS									7
8	OPERATION OF PLANT									8
9	LAUNDRY & LINEN SERVICE									9
10	HOUSEKEEPING									10
11.01	DIETARY - RAW FOOD									11.01
11.02	DIETARY - OTHER									11.02
12	CAFETERIA									12
13	MAINTENANCE OF PERSONNEL									13
17	MEDICAL RECORDS & LIBRARY	10000								17
18	SOCIAL SERVICE		10000							18
19	MEDICAL SUPPLIES AND EXPENSE			3975488						19
19.01	CENTRAL SERVICES & SUPPLY				835534					19.01
19.02	PHARMACY					9025540				19.02
19.03	NURSING ADMINISTRATION						74909473			19.03
19.04	INTENSIVE NURSING CARE									19.04
19.05	GENERAL NURSING SERVICE									19.05
19.06	SUPERVISING PHYSICIANS-OTHER							19219616		19.06
22	I&R SERVICES-SALARY & FRINGES							45544	13280	22
23	I&R SERVICES-OTHER PRGM COSTS					1183				23
23.01	SPRVSNG PHYSICIANS-TEACHING									23.01
	INPATIENT ROUTINE SERV COST CENTERS									
25	ADULTS & PEDIATRICS	4667	6686	2486034	329473	7332603	32193061	13042149	6000	25
26	INTENSIVE CARE UNIT	196	73	234240	79028	294790	3967564		720	26
27	CORONARY CARE UNIT	91	34	81720	26694	27062	1743194		480	27
29	SURGICAL INTENSIVE CARE UNIT	215	679	187591	111677	262652	4010887			29
30	NEONATAL INTENSIVE CARE UNIT	234	262	82051	31930	16308	3017097		880	30
31	SUBPROVIDER	250		125690		839817	3635036		240	31
33	NURSERY	280		14228		5734	1140916		80	33
	ANCILLARY SERVICE COST CENTERS									
37	OPERATING ROOM				56359	20922	7748523			37
39	DELIVERY ROOM & LABOR ROOM			218031	5007	9696	3377597		640	39
40	ANESTHESIOLOGY			97601		77289		40986	760	40
41	RADIOLOGY-DIAGNOSTIC		301	13235	11075	52525			440	41
42	RADIOLOGY-THERAPEUTIC									42
43	RADIOISOTOPE									43
43.01	CAT SCAN									43.01

※ **EXHIBIT 8A–3.** *Institutional Cost Reports—Cost Allocation—Statistical Basis* Continued

	COST CENTER DESCRIPTION		I&R PROGRAM COSTS ASSIGNED TIME 23	SPRVSNG PHYSICIANS TEACHING HOURS OF SERVICE 23.01	
	GENERAL SERVICE COST CENTERS				
1	OLD CAP REL COSTS-BLDG & FIXT				1
2	OLD CAP REL COSTS-MVBLE EQUIP				2
3	NEW CAP REL COSTS-BLDG & FIXT				3
4	NEW CAP REL COSTS-MVBLE EQUIP				4
5	EMPLOYEE BENEFITS				5
6	ADMINISTRATIVE & GENERAL				6
7	MAINTENANCE & REPAIRS				7
8	OPERATION OF PLANT				8
9	LAUNDRY & LINEN SERVICE				9
10	HOUSEKEEPING				10
11.01	DIETARY - RAW FOOD				11.01
11.02	DIETARY - OTHER				11.02
12	CAFETERIA				12
13	MAINTENANCE OF PERSONNEL				13
17	MEDICAL RECORDS & LIBRARY				17
18	SOCIAL SERVICE				18
19	MEDICAL SUPPLIES AND EXPENSE				19
19.01	CENTRAL SERVICES & SUPPLY				19.01
19.02	PHARMACY				19.02
19.03	NURSING ADMINISTRATION				19.03
19.04	INTENSIVE NURSING CARE				19.04
19.05	GENERAL NURSING SERVICE				19.05
19.06	SUPERVISING PHYSICIANS-OTHER				19.06
22	I &R SERVICES-SALARY & FRINGES				22
23	I&R SERVICES-OTHER PROGM COSTS	13280			23
23.01	SPRVSNG PHYSICIANS-TEACHING		14369643		23.01
	INPATIENT ROUTINE SERV COST CENTERS				
25	ADULTS & PEDIATRICS	6000	9380079		25
	INTENSIVE CARE UNIT	720			26
27	CORONARY CARE UNIT	480			27
29	SURGICAL INTENSIVE CARE UNIT				29
30	NEONATAL INTENSIVE CARE UNIT	880			30
31	SUBPROVIDER	240	196281		31
33	NURSERY	80			33
	ANCILLARY SERVICE COST CENTERS				
37	OPERATING ROOM				37
39	DELIVERY ROOM & LABOR ROOM	640			39
40	ANESTHESIOLOGY	760	32203		40
41	RADIOLOGY-DIAGNOSTIC	440			41
42	RADIOLOGY-THERAPEUTIC				42
43	RADIOISOTOPE				43
43.01	CAT SCAN				43.01

the nursing administration costs should be allocated to adults & pediatrics ($32,193,061/74,909,473 \times 100\% = 43\%$).

Looking back at the third page of Exhibit 8A–2, we find that of the $5,847,895 in nursing administration when it gets its turn to allocate, $2,513,196 has been allocated to adults & pediatrics (line 25). If we divide $2,513,196 by the total of $5,847,895, we find that it is 43%. The portion of nursing administration that was consumed by adults & pediatrics has in fact been allocated to adults & pediatrics in the step-down process.

CHAPTER

9

Costs and Other Issues Related to Recruiting and Retaining Staff

CHAPTER GOALS

The goals of this chapter are to:

- Describe the relationship between the availability of nursing staff and budgeting
- Explain how to plan for variations in the availability of nursing staff
- Discuss retention as a strategy to maintain cost-effective nursing staff
- Analyze the costs of retention programs
- Discuss recruitment as a strategy to maintain cost-effective nursing staff
- Identify some alternative solutions when nursing staff are in short supply

✲ INTRODUCTION

The largest part of most operating budgets for nursing departments and organizations consists of *personnel* costs. Justifying the need for a given level of staff requires careful calculations and a lucid argument. However, in the preparation of an operating budget it is often assumed that hiring the amount of labor approved in the final budget is not a problem. That is not necessarily the case in nursing. Nursing shortages have occurred on and off in recent decades. Sometimes the shortages are nationwide; other times only certain geographic areas are affected. To staff adequately in the face of a shortage substantially increases the costs of recruiting and retaining nurses. Even when there is no shortage these costs are significant. Nurse managers must be aware of the substantial resources that should be devoted to this area.

Recruitment of staff is a critical element in the overall management process. If positions are left unstaffed throughout the year, two potentially serious side effects occur. The first is that the nurses working on a unit begin to suffer burnout from being overburdened. Shortages of staff lead to overwork, poor morale, increased sick leave, and other stress-related problems. This in turn tends to lead to loss of staff, exacerbating the shortage on the unit.

The second side effect is that the health care organization starts to assume that less money will be spent than has been put into the budget. Positions are approved with the expectation that they will never be filled. Eventually, if staff is finally available to be hired, the organization may resist filling the positions because it has made its overall plans based on the expectation that the money allocated for those positions would never be spent. The approved but vacant positions provide top management with a cushion to ease the impact of other unexpected financial problems throughout the year. Essentially, the budgeted but unfilled positions may be permanently lost. This effectively lowers the nursing care hours per patient day per procedure, or per visit on a permanent basis.

The costs of these two side effects on the quality of patient care and on staff satisfaction are almost never measured and rarely considered. However, their existence stresses the importance of attempting to understand and explicitly measure the costs of staff recruitment and retention.

Furthermore, an attempt must be made to make financial decisions based on the expected *actual* staffing pattern. If twelve full-time equivalent positions (FTEs) are authorized in a budget, the dollars in the budget should be based on the best expectation of how those twelve FTEs will be staffed. Suppose that because of recruitment difficulties it is most likely that the unit will be able to have eleven FTEs filled with regular full-time or part-time employees; the twelfth position will be filled with overtime or agency staff. In that case the excess cost of overtime or an agency nurse, as compared with a full-time employee, is a cost related to retention and recruitment.

Another approach to the problem of retention and recruitment that was used in the 1990s was to revise the manner in which nursing care was offered to use fewer professional staff. Nursing units were reorganized to make greater use of alternative types of workers. Computers were acquired in an effort to reduce the number of nursing hours needed for documentation. Introduction of shared governance, case management, alternative workers, or computers may have had an impact on the actual staffing of a nursing unit. These changes and their costs are in a sense costs related to retention and recruitment in that they represent money spent to achieve and maintain an appropriate staffing level.

This chapter is confined to the actions that individual nurse managers can take, or should be aware of, in their management of recruitment and retention of nursing staff within their organizations. When shortages occur, a given organization may be relatively helpless when it comes to overcoming the entire national or regional shortage in the supply of nurses. However, organizations have a great degree of control over recruitment and retention for their own organizations. Recruitment and retention are important management concerns regardless of whether there is a shortage.

※ RETAINING STAFF

Although some degree of *turnover* will keep an organization "healthy" by bringing new blood into the organization, the most effective personnel strategy a health care organization can take is to work at retaining the staff it already has. An organization may not want to retain all staff. The goal should be to decrease undesired turnover. It is often the case that every nurse hired must be hired away from somebody else or recruited from nonworking nurses. Therefore it should be clear that recruiting nurses may require a costly level of competition. Major efforts should be made in an attempt to reduce turnover. Both individual characteristics and organizational factors are postulated to be related to nurse *retention*. One key to staff retention is to have a high level of nurse satisfaction.

Nurse Satisfaction

Surprisingly, little is definitively known about what leads to nurse satisfaction. Many factors are believed to be relevant to keeping a nursing staff happy. Studies have not consistently shown any one factor or any unique set of factors that are always present in satisfied staffs, or whose absence will necessarily lead to a dissatisfied staff. Nevertheless, a number of elements are generally accepted as being related to nursing satisfaction. These elements are discussed here.

One primary element of nursing satisfaction is the development of professionalism in the delivery of health care services through a combination of increased autonomy and the availability of resource personnel for consultation. Nurses must feel like professionals and be treated like professionals to be satisfied in their employment. Time cards, for example, are often thought to be demeaning for nurses and can lead to dissatisfaction. Similarly, working as hourly workers does not generally result in the same level of satisfaction as working as salaried employees.

A positive attitude toward nursing and professional treatment by the physician staff and the administration can be critical factors in having a satisfied staff. Negative attitudes by these groups can cause staff dissatisfaction. This ties in with the overall issue of nursing image. The institution has little control over the national image of nursing. However, it can take strides toward creating a positive image internally. The way nurses are treated and the way nursing is presented to patients can make a substantial difference in the attitudes of nurses as well as the rest of the organization's staff. Image building begins with actions taken by nursing to create a positive image. Programs with physicians and administration can be suggested by nursing administration, if they are not forthcoming otherwise.

The issue of financial payment is, of course, relevant. Nurses report that pay is important to them in determining their level of satisfaction. High salaries and good benefits will help keep staff from looking elsewhere. This also requires that there be ample opportunity for advancement, either into management or on a clinical track.

Flexible hours have also become a key to retaining staff. A wide variety of alternative working hours have been developed by organizations attempting to recruit new nurses. These flexible arrangements must be made available to existing staff as well, or they may become dissatisfied and move to an organization that offers such hours.

From a budgeting perspective, this can become quite complex. The use of four ten-hour shifts to create a four-day work week is not a major budgeting problem. Although it may create a complicated staffing pattern for coverage, it still results in forty hours of pay for forty hours of work, the same as five days of eight hours each. On the other hand, innovations such as three twelve-hour shifts, or two twelve-hour weekend shifts, for forty hours of pay can create a variety of budgeting complications. Clear decisions must be made as to how many hours equals an FTE position. (See Chapter 12 for further discussion.)

Fringe Benefits

Clearly, one element of nursing satisfaction is related to the organization's employee benefits, commonly referred to as *fringe benefits*. How many weeks of vacation do staff get each year? How many paid holidays are there? Is free life insurance provided to employees? These are some of the most obvious employee benefits. Some benefits are required by law. For example, the employer must pay for "FICA," a tax for Social Security, which eventually will provide the employee with a Social Security pension. Most benefits, however, are voluntary or the result of labor negotiations.

Other critical benefits concern the quality of the health insurance package offered to employees. Do nurses have to contribute to the cost of their health insurance? If so, how much? Are their family members covered? If so, is there additional cost to the nurse? Are staff members subject to *coinsurance* and *deductibles* on their health insurance? Coinsurance means that the insurer bears a portion of the cost (often 70% or 80%) and the employee bears the remainder (usually 30% or 20%). A deductible means that 100% of some amount (often $200 to $2,000 per year) must first be paid by the employee before there are any health benefits.

Most employers also offer a variety of other benefits that are somewhat less obvious and are more responsible for the term "fringe benefits," as opposed to employee benefits. For example, if the CEO belongs to a golf club and the membership is paid for by the organization, that is a fringe benefit. If the CEO drives a hospital-owned car, that is another fringe benefit.

In terms of the budget, fringe benefits really represent several different types of cost. The vacation and holiday time for each employee is already built into the annual salary cost for that individual. There is no need to budget for that fringe benefit, except for making sure that there is adequate staff coverage for all days off. That is accounted for by budgeting additional personnel (see Chapter 12). On the other hand, the cost of life insurance, pension payments, Social Security taxes, health insurance, child care, and other fringe benefits that require cash outlays must be budgeted for explicitly.

In most organizations the specific costs of the fringe benefits are calculated by the finance office and are assigned to departments based on salaries, usually as a percentage. For example, a nursing unit might be charged 22% for fringe benefits for every dollar of salary paid to any staff member. Certainly, not all employees have the same cost to the organization per dollar of salary. That is simply an average. Is it fair? It might well be that certain fringe benefits are worth more to members of some departments than employees of other departments. However, over the years it has been decided that it is not worth the effort to get a more refined measure of costs. Therefore budgeting for fringe benefits generally requires only the addition of a set percentage (provided by the finance office) to the budgeted salary amounts.

Many organizations are now offering a *cafeteria* approach to fringe benefits. The organization determines the amount of money it will contribute to fringe benefits. The cost of each fringe benefit is determined, and employees choose from a list, much as food is chosen in a cafeteria. Employee wants for fringe benefits vary. The young new graduate might not care about life insurance but might prefer a low deductible on health insurance. The young mother might prefer child care and have no need for health insurance because her spouse has family coverage from his employer.

Retention Programs

The problem of turnover is significant enough to warrant specific attention and direct programs aimed at staff retention. This should go beyond the basic notions of having competent managers, physicians who work on a collegial professional basis with nurses, autonomy in work, and the other elements of nurse satisfaction. Such programs should work toward making the institution one that shows caring for its staff and creates a loyalty bond that is hard to break. Some such programs involve significant financial investment; others take relatively little. Prior to the development of a retention program, the manager should determine the desired retention goal and the actual retention level at the organization. It is also important to differentiate involuntary turnover from employees who leave because the organization no longer needs or wants them.

The first step in a retention program is to determine the retention level goal for an organization or unit. Most organizations would be unhappy with 100% retention. Unless the organization expands, this level of retention would leave no room for new staff. New staff are desired both because they provide new ideas to an organization and because new staff nurses are generally paid a lower wage than experienced nurses. On the other hand, most managers would agree that 70% retention is perhaps too low. Orienting 30% of the staff each year is likely to be too costly and disruptive.

The second step is to determine the historical level of retention. Most nurse managers determine turnover. This is defined as the number of employees terminating during a period of time. The converse of turnover is then considered retention. If 10% of the staff terminate each year, retention is considered 90%. However, this approach tells the manager little about the retention pattern of the nursing staff. Do most people leave within the first three months? Is there an even distribution among staff with all levels of tenure? Using a "life tables" approach actual retention rates can be determined.[1]

With this method actual patterns of retention are determined. All staff are identified, and a determination is made about how long staff stay. For example, how many of the staff stay more than six months? More than three years? More than ten years? If 50% of the staff leave within the first year and less than 5% of those who have been there more than five years leave, efforts can be directed at the former group rather than at the nurses who have been at the institution for more than five years. It could also be the case that nurses who have been at the organization for more than five years are now leaving because the organization raised salaries of entry level staff, whereas a competing organization instituted a policy for increases in salary for every year of experience. After determining the organization's retention goal and the historical retention rate, a retention program can be developed.

First of all, employees should have a way of being recognized. There should be a formal mechanism that allows a pattern of exemplary work, or even one good deed, to gain recognition. There are a variety of ways that employee behavior can be recognized. The first is in the form of performance evaluations with interviews. Such evaluations are a two-edged sword. They need to be firm enough to make clear that poor performance will not be ignored or rewarded. However, there should be a strong focus on positive aspects. This may be in terms of recognizing good performance or even in terms of offering training in areas where performance should be improved. Rather than dwelling on poor past performance, a greater amount of time should be spent on discussing ways to accomplish more and to improve future performance.

Performance evaluation meetings are often uncomfortable for both the evaluator and the one being evaluated. However, such meetings should not be given short shrift. Employees should leave the meeting with a feeling that they understand what is expected of them, with a sense that their individual efforts make a difference in the overall performance of the unit, and with a clear sense that their positive contributions have been noted and specifically recognized by the organization.

Another key element of performance conferences should be to elicit input. What is going on that the employee likes, and what is going on that the employee objects to? Open lines of communication—with honest follow-up on suggestions and complaints—are likely to win over support and loyalty. A refusal to budge from the way things are is more likely to result in resentment and, in some cases, resignations.

In addition to meetings, specific actions may warrant letters of commendation. Such letters could be the result of favorable patient comments on a form supplied to patients for that purpose. Or they could be based on recommendations from other staff. Commendations should be presented in appropriate ceremonies and noted in organizational newsletters so that as many people as possible are made aware of them. This provides further psychological benefit to the recipient and perhaps serves notice to other workers that it is possible they too can gain such recognition. Achievement of such recognition should be within the reach of most staff members.

In providing motivation, the carrot or the stick can be used. Some schools of thought argue that the stick is more appropriate than the carrot. Poor performance is unacceptable, and that fact should be conveyed to workers. Other schools of thought argue that in the long run the carrot will have more positive results. Accentuating the positive and decentuating the negative results in a happier and psychologically healthier work environment. In many cases a combination of the carrot and the stick is probably optimal.

Another program for retention involves financial remuneration. Money is not a solution to all problems. One study has shown that having adequate numbers of

---

[1]For a more detailed description of this process, see M. Beth Benedict, Jay H. Glasser, and Eun Sul Lee, "Assessing Hospital Nursing Staff Retention and Turnover: A Life Table Approach," *Evaluation & The Health Professions*, Vol. 12, No. 1, March 1989, pp. 73–96.

staff, nursing management support, alternate weekends off, support of administration, and permanent shift assignments all rank ahead of benefits and salary in terms of importance to nurses. On the other hand, benefits and salary rank ahead of general staffing patterns, support of physicians, opportunity for advancement, location, and staff development programs.[2] Nursing departments should attempt to deal with all these factors. However, while money is not the solution to all problems, financial incentives have become a major competitive factor.

Higher wages are one type of financial incentive. They can be very costly to health care organizations. Other types of financial incentives can be achieved without substantially higher cost to the institution. One example is annual salaries instead of hourly wages. This approach may make nurses feel better about themselves and their institutions. Another financial approach is bonuses. Bonuses generally are paid only out of cost savings. Thus the institution can afford to pay for them because the payment is only part of a larger amount that would otherwise have been spent anyway. Bonuses had little use just a decade ago but are becoming more and more widespread.

Innovative employee benefits are another area that can be used to help retain nurses. For example, child-care centers at the health care organization (perhaps with discounted or subsidized rates) can help in employee retention. Additionally, such centers have the capacity to reduce sick leave substantially. Much sick leave is the result of a nurse staying home to take care of a sick child. Sick leave can therefore be reduced if the child-care center has facilities for mildly ill children.

The above approaches to retention are already in the nursing literature. However, to be truly competitive an organization must be innovative. For example, suppose that a nurses' dramatics group were formed and each six months it staged a dramatic or musical play with performances for the staff and patients. A club of that type provides an excellent release from the routine work pressures. In that way it reduces the burnout syndrome. Over the years such a "club" develops intense loyalties. Nurses might not leave the organization because they don't want to be left out of the show. Bridge clubs and other organization-sponsored activities such as annual picnics and trips to the ballpark result in development of a sense of family and community rather than strictly a workplace. And when times get tough, families and communities hang together.

Clinical Ladders

A frequent complaint of staff nurses is that there is little room for advancement within the clinical ranks. Nurses can go into management. However, if they choose to pursue a bedside hands-on clinical career, there is little difference in reward for a nurse with thirty years of experience compared with one with five years. The concept of clinical ladders is one suggestion for overcoming that deterrent to nurse retention.

There are a wide variety of clinical ladder models. Some are completely distinct from administrative career paths. Others allow for branching off from a clinical ladder into an administrative path after a certain point. Some clinical ladders require on-the-job experience for promotions, while others require additional education including advanced degrees. In some models, moving up the ladder requires community or professional service and publication. Another distinction among models is the amount of additional responsibility that must be assumed as one moves up the ladder.

There is a widespread belief that clinical ladders do improve nurse retention. Such an approach improves the professional identity of the nurse and generates loyalty. Another perspective is that if nurses with more experience with a given

[2]"What Nurses Want Most from a Job," *Nursing 88*, Vol. 18, No. 2, February 1988, p. 38.

institution earn substantially more than those with fewer years at the specific organization, it becomes more costly to move. It becomes expensive to give up seniority. If that is the case, retention of the more experienced, expensive personnel becomes easier, but higher turnover rates may occur among nurses at the lower, less expensive rungs of the ladder. Over time this may lead to an organization with a large proportion of its staff near the higher compensation end of the ladder.

Determining the Cost

What does it cost to retain staff? As with any decision in a health organization, the cost-benefit ratio of a retention program should be estimated in advance and also evaluated after the program has been implemented. Having accurate data on current retention patterns and knowing the organization's goal provide the first step in determining the costs of the program. Although it is often difficult to associate a particular program with overall retention, some estimates can be made. If a new program such as free parking is instituted, its cost can easily be determined. Often, however, new programs have several goals and potential benefits. A hand-held computer system for home visits may be intended to retain nurses who want to work in a "high tech" environment where charting is easier. However, the computer system is also expected to improve the quality of patient care and to decrease the time nurses spend on documentation. Other programs aimed at improving retention may have additional benefits as well. Shared governance may be instituted to improve retention, and it may also improve patient care. Increasing salaries may retain staff in the short run, but as soon as the competitor across town increases its salaries, the benefits of such a program may disappear.

Determining the costs of turnover and therefore the benefits of decreasing turnover is somewhat more straightforward. What is important to remember is that the costs of turnover do not include just the costs of advertising for staff and the nurse recruiter's salary. Costs include the effect short staffing has on the remaining staff and the decreased productivity of new staff. Jones[3] describes a detailed approach to determine the costs of turnover. She suggests that the following costs be included:

- Advertising/recruiting
- Costs of unfilled positions
- Hiring costs
- Termination costs
- Orientation/training
- Decreased new RN productivity

For the hospitals studied by Jones the mean cost per RN turnover was $10,198 (range $6,886–$15,152).

Blaufuss, Maynard, and Schollars[4] present an alternative approach to evaluating turnover costs in response to a specific incentive. They do not include general advertising and recruiting costs in their calculations because, they argue, hospitals must advertise regardless of turnover rates, since there will naturally be some turnover in all organizations.

They include interviewing, preparing for orientation, the orientation itself, and a learning period. Using a zero-base approach, they identify the individual cost of hiring each new staff member. In addition, they include estimated revenue enhancements as an offset to the recruiting cost. This is particularly important when

---

[3]For a complete description of this approach see Cheryl Bland Jones, "Staff Nurse Turnover Costs: Part II, Measurements and Results," *Journal of Nursing Administration,* Vol. 20, No. 4, May 1990, pp. 27–31.

[4]Judy Blaufuss, Jan Maynard, and Gail Schollars, "Methods of Evaluating Turnover Costs," *Nursing Management,* Vol. 23, No. 5, May 1992, pp. 52–61.

increases in staff can lead to providing more home health care visits or in some other way increasing the number of patients cared for. Essentially, if you look at the cost of attracting new staff, you must also consider the extra revenue the organization will earn if it has those new staff members.

※ RECRUITING STAFF

No matter how effectively an organization works to retain its existing staff, some turnover must be expected. Some staff members will retire; others will move to another health care organization or a different part of the country. Some replacement of staff will always be occurring. Concurrent with the nursing department's setting retention goals and working toward achieving them, there should be a *recruitment* effort. Recruitment is an ongoing process, not something that is done just at a time of staff shortage. Recruitment strategies may change during shortages, but the successful organization continually works on recruitment.

Identifying the existing level of recruitment is the first step in developing a recruitment strategy. What is the current level of recruitment? Is this acceptable? Do you anticipate any changes in the organization (e.g., addition of a new unit) that will require changes in that level or an improvement in retention due to new initiatives in the organization?

The second step is to assess the external environment. What changes are occurring that will affect the level of recruiting? Are enrollments increasing in nursing schools, thus making recruitment easier? Is the increase likely to continue? What specific factors in the environment may affect the organization's ability to recruit? Have there been salary increases in competing organizations? After assessing the external environment and determining a desired level of recruitment, a specific recruitment plan can be developed.

Marketing

A key element of recruiting is an effective marketing strategy. As long as a limited supply of talented nurses exists, there will be a winner and a loser in the effort to recruit qualified personnel. Therefore a plan must be developed to address the recruiting issue.

The essence of marketing is that the needs and desires of a group are determined on the basis of market research, and then an effort is made to satisfy them. Notice that this definition does not revolve around advertising, which may or may not be part of a marketing effort. The first step is to find out what nurses want from their employment. Next, efforts must be made to ensure that the hospital meets those needs to the extent possible. Finally, it is necessary to be able to convey the fact that the needs have been met.

In performing market research, a decision should first be made concerning whom the organization wants to recruit. New nurses, right out of school? Experienced nurses? Nurse managers? Specialists? Local nurses? Out-of-state nurses? In trying to determine what the potential employee wants and needs, it is critically important to correctly evaluate the group that is to be the target of the marketing effort.

Since most health care organizations already have some staff, the organization must have some attractive characteristics. In relative terms, all existing organizations have some strengths. Therefore, there should not be a hopeless attitude of "how can we compete with the rich research-oriented medical center in town?" Perhaps many nurses would prefer to provide care in a patient-oriented rather than research-oriented setting. It is important to identify the existing strengths of the organization so that the information can be conveyed to a target group.

At the same time, weaknesses must be identified and a long-term plan designed to overcome as many of them as possible. Perhaps lack of convenient parking is the one overwhelming negative the organization has. In that case, replacing expensive advertising with a major fund-raising campaign to finance the building of an enclosed parking garage may be an appropriate marketing strategy. That is an example of a one-shot, expensive solution to a recruiting problem, but one that helps recruitment over many years.

In other cases solutions may be less expensive but require ongoing efforts. For example, a hospital could distinguish itself through a concerted effort to develop a system of shared governance. Such efforts are not necessarily expensive. They do, however, require tremendous cooperation and commitment. The potential result is that expensive newspaper ads can be replaced with free news stories on the change at the hospital. Nursing schools can be encouraged to have the organization's staff give lectures on the shared governance approach used by the organization. If the new system really provides something that nurses value, the word will eventually get out, even without advertising. Advertising may be used to speed the communication process if desired.

Note, however, that marketing does not start with advertising but with identification of the need or desire and the filling of that need or desire. These elements must precede advertising. Only then can a specific plan be developed regarding the communication of what strengths the organization has to offer. Advertising in newspapers, on television or radio, or by direct mail is one approach to that communication. Another is college visits. Bonuses to existing employees who bring in new employees is another.

Each of these approaches often results in inquiries by potential employees. The package of material that the organization develops to respond to those inquiries is a critical element of the overall marketing strategy. The marketing strategy should take into account all the steps in the recruiting process. Generating inquiries without a strategy to follow up effectively is one critical mistake often made by those who view marketing only in terms of advertising. If a strategy is likely to generate inquiries, the organization should not appear unorganized or uncaring when it receives them. That is the point when the organization has the chance to reaffirm the feeling that caused the nurse to inquire about the position.

Suppose a hospital runs a newspaper ad that says, "Join the nursing staff at ABC Hospital, where nurses work in an environment of shared governance and shared commitment to the highest level of patient care." Some carefully planned literature must be available for the person who asks for more information about the shared governance program. Its history, how it works, and the hospital's commitment should be included.

If the response to the inquiry leads to an interview, the interviewer should be aware that the candidate has inquired about the hospital's shared governance program. The interview should include at least some specific discussion that emphasizes or highlights the shared governance system.

Marketing is a critical element of recruiting. That does not mean that the organization has to sell someone something that he or she doesn't want or need. Rather, having researched the wants and needs of a targeted nursing group, marketing should allow the hospital to effectively convey to the target group the extent to which the organization has made efforts to meet those desires and needs.

Although advertising is not the first part of a marketing plan, in many instances it is an effective mechanism for speeding the word-of-mouth process. Targeted advertising can reach a potential group of employees very effectively. This is particularly important in a competitive marketplace. If competing organizations are effectively communicating what they have to offer, your organization must be prepared to get its message to that group of potential employees as well.

One important element of advertising is that only a part of current advertising should be aimed at current recruitment. Another part, equally substantial, should be aimed at long-term image building. Often people associate with an organization because of its "well-known" reputation. Such reputations are built over a period of years. They are built through an effort of getting the message out year in and year out. When there is a staffing shortage the institution advertises why it is a good place to work. It should also do so when there is no shortage of personnel. Image building is not a short-term response to shortages. By laying the groundwork over a long period of time, when the need for personnel occurs, the organization will have a head start over its competition.

In budgeting for a marketing plan, it is necessary to include the costs of advertising. However, any other costs related to the overall marketing plan should also be included in the budget. These might include consulting costs and the costs of doing market research.

Determining the Cost

Recruitment and replacement of staff is inherently costly. The costs of replacing staff include:

- Overtime and agency nurse costs while the position is vacant
- Advertising
- Interviewing potential employees
- Travel for recruiters
- Entertainment
- Moving
- Signing bonuses
- Administrative processing
- New employee training

Other costs related to the replacement of personnel should also be budgeted. The average duration of the vacancies should be anticipated, and the extra cost of overtime and agency nurses should be included in the coming year's operating budget. Newly hired employees are often less productive than experienced staff. This may require extra hours of nursing care per patient day, often in the form of overtime. An effort should be made to anticipate turnover and to anticipate the costs related to turnover. Sufficient nursing care hours should be budgeted to allow for the lower productivity of new staff. If relocation costs are charged directly to the unit, those costs should be included in the budget as well.

Recent years have seen increasing use of signing bonuses. For positions that are particularly difficult to fill, bonuses of $10,000 or more are not uncommon.

⋇ USE OF ALTERNATIVE HEALTH CARE EMPLOYEES

Despite the efforts of organizations to retain nurses, nurse retention will be unable to solve all health care organizations' nursing needs. Recruitment more often results in shifting the staff from one organization to another (particularly if recruitment is for experienced nurses) rather than increasing the overall supply. Thus, despite the best efforts to retain and recruit nurses, there will probably be at least some organizations with inadequate staffing. Decreasing the demand for nurses will decrease the need to both retain and recruit staff. One suggested approach to solving this shortage is the use of alternative health care employees.

A variety of alternative health care employees are sometimes used. One is foreign nurses. This approach attempts to retain the concept of using RNs to the extent possible. It comes to grips with a national nursing shortage by looking outside the United States. A very different approach is to use non-RNs to perform activities that in the past were performed by RNs.

Foreign Nurse Recruitment

Foreign nurses are one possible alternative for staffing a health care institution. However, this solution involves a number of difficulties ranging from regulatory to language barriers. On the other hand, many foreign nurses welcome the chance to come to the United States on either a temporary or permanent basis, and this approach can be used to fill a large gap in the nursing staff.

Because of language problems, most foreign recruitment takes place in English-speaking countries such as Canada, the British Isles, and Australia. The Philippines and India are also common places for recruitment. Northern states may be able to recruit in Canada relatively easily compared with other alternatives. For recruiting outside the continent, expenses of travel and relocation can become substantial. An alternative to an organization doing it all by itself is to use an agency and pay a flat fee for each nurse hired. The more nurses hired, the more likely it is to be cost effective to undertake the entire recruiting project yourself.

If a strategy of foreign recruiting is chosen, careful budgeting becomes essential. The choice between using a recruiting agency and doing it yourself can have a dramatic financial impact. A budget allows considering the costs of each alternative. For example, suppose an agency charges one month's salary for recruiting an individual plus one month's salary for relocation expenses. It could easily cost in excess of $10,000 for each nurse recruited.

There are other recruiting costs as well. One cost of recruiting foreign nurses is the time between their arrival and the time when they have completed all examinations and other requirements necessary to practice as an RN. During this period they are being paid but are not fully productive. Other costs include providing convenient housing and helping the nurses settle in. Another cost is related to loss of recruits between their recruitment and their arrival. Since a fairly lengthy period is required to meet various visa and other requirements, there is a dropout rate.

Alternative Care Givers

A drastically different approach to the use of foreign nurses is the alteration of the model of care within a health care organization to assign more activities to non-RNs. While this was a movement away from the goal of all-RN staffs, it was based on recognition of the realities of nursing shortages.

The many types of alternate care givers include, but are not limited to, the traditional alternate providers, that is, LPNs and unlicensed assistive personnel (UAP) such as nurses' aides. A variety of new positions such as hosts or hostesses were also developed to help organizations cope. Such a person introduces patients to the unit and responds to many of the nonclinical needs and questions of patients and their families. There is little controversy about the use of alternative care givers to perform nonnursing functions such as transport and clerical activities.

There is substantial controversy about using UAPs to perform nursing activities. In some cases the RN is placed in a position of greater direct supervision of UAPs, who provide more of the care. In other cases, "partnerships" are developed between the nurse and the UAPs. In many cases the ultimate impact of the use of UAPs is less bedside time for the RN and more supervisory responsibility.

No single approach has emerged as the dominant path for providing nursing care in the future. There is little information about the costs of these alternative models. The main conflict seems to be between a model that would have RNs serving as supervisors of UAPs and a model in which nursing activities are divided into an RN subset and a UAP subset. In the former, RNs have a decreasing bedside role but greater authority and responsibility for patient care. In the latter alternative, RNs may spend as much time as usual giving bedside care but perform only activities that require the clinical skills of an RN.

⁜ THE USE OF COMPUTERS

Changing how nursing care is provided because of a staff shortage is a less than ideal way for a profession to evolve. The changes are not the result primarily of an impetus to find better ways to give care; rather, they represent recognition of personnel availability constraints. If nursing shortages could be permanently eliminated, the approach to the delivery of nursing care might be substantially different. The computerization of nursing units has been put forth as a potential solution.

Some claims have been made that as much as half of all nursing time is spent on documentation and that bedside computer terminals could save half that time. If true, as much as one quarter of all required nursing time could be eliminated without taking any time away from nursing care provided to patients.

Although highly touted for their timesaving potential throughout the 1990s, computer systems have yet to live up to that glowing potential. The *hardware* (equipment) capacity exists. Technological advances have reached a point at which terminals by each bedside are used in some hospitals. In fact, it would be surprising to see a new hospital without computer wiring to each room as part of the electrical blueprints. Gaining nurse acceptance for the use of unit or bedside computers has not turned out to be the problem that many predicted. On the other hand, developing the *software* (computer programs) has been a complicated process.

Each health care institution tends to be unique in its procedures. This lack of industry standardization creates difficulties in the development of software. Furthermore, the process of recording the activities surrounding patient care and integrating patient care clinical and financial information with those activities is highly complicated.

It is likely that computer software advances will be made and that computer usage by staff nurses will become commonplace in most health care organizations. In the long run this will likely increase the quality of patient care due to more accurate and timely information, while at the same time creating at least some efficiencies in the use of nursing time. This should release more RN time for patient care. To the extent that computers reduce time spent on documentation relative to time spent in providing patient care, computerization should work both to reduce nursing shortages and to increase nursing satisfaction.

⁜ IMPLICATIONS FOR NURSE MANAGERS

Retention and recruitment of staff will be ongoing issues for organizations that employ nurses. A certain amount of turnover is expected and is in fact healthy for an organization. Historically there have been national and local shortages of nurses. This cyclical pattern will likely continue. Organizations should be concerned with recruitment and retention regardless of shortages.

The issue of retention and recruitment of staff members—whether RNs, LPNs, UAPs, or other staff—is significant. There should be careful enumeration of all the costs related to recruitment and retention. These include market research, consulting, advertising, travel, and relocation. They also include the costs necessary to make an organization attractive, such as training costs related to implementing a system of shared governance.

One fundamental point in this process is that for a specific organization to have an adequate staff, it must recognize a need to change over time. The environment of health care organizations is in a constant state of change. Other career opportunities exist for potential staff. If a hospital job is not adequately attractive, a nurse can go into home health care or work in a physician's office. It is important to remain current in understanding what nurses desire from their employment in addition to a salary.

Successful organizations will be aware of the desires of the work force, respond to those desires, and effectively communicate to potential employees the ways in which they meet those needs and desires.

KEY CONCEPTS

Retention Continued employment of personnel. This is often measured as the converse of turnover or staff leaving an organization.

Fringe benefits Compensation in addition to wages; also called employee benefits. This usually includes such things as health insurance, life insurance, and disability insurance. Some organizations provide child care, free parking, and other benefits as a way to recruit and retain staff. Fringe benefits often cost as much as 20% to 25% of a worker's wages.

Cafeteria plan Method of providing fringe benefits in which the employee chooses from a variety of options those fringe benefits that the employee wants.

Retention programs Variety of approaches used by organizations to retain staff. These include clinical ladders, reorganization of the way care is provided, and a variety of compensation plans.

Clinical ladders Approach to promotion and compensation based on clinical excellence.

Recruitment Effort directed at getting potential employees to become employees. This process should be ongoing and not just developed in times of shortages of key workers.

Unlicensed assistive personnel Employees who are less skilled than professional nurses but who may be able to assume some activities traditionally performed by RNs.

SUGGESTED READINGS

Ames, Adrienne, Sharon Adkins, Dana Rutledge, et al., "Assessing Work Retention Issues," *Journal of Nursing Administration,* Vol. 22, No. 4, April 1992, pp. 37–41.

Blaufuss, Judy, Jan Maynard, and Gail Schollars, "Methods of Evaluating Turnover Costs," *Nursing Management,* Vol. 23, No. 5, May 1992, pp. 52–61.

Blegen, M., "Nurses' Job Satisfaction: A Meta-Analysis of Related Variables," *Nursing Research,* Vol. 42, No. 1, 1993, pp. 36–41.

Corcoran, Nora M., Lesley A. Meyer, and Bonnie L. Magliaro, "Retention: The Key to the 21st Century for Health Care Institutions," *Nursing Administration Quarterly,* Vol. 14, No. 4, Summer 1990, pp. 23–31.

Davidson, H., P. Folcarelli, S. Crawford, L. Duprat, and J. Clifford, "The Effects of Health Care Reforms on Job Satisfaction and Voluntary Turnover Among Hospital-Based Nurses," *Medical Care,* Vol. 35, No. 6, 1997, pp. 634–645.

de Savorgnani, A., R. Haring, and S. Galloway, "Recruiting and Retaining Registered Nurses in Home Healthcare," *Journal of Nursing Administration,* Vol. 23, No. 6, 1993, pp. 42–46.

Gillies, Dee Ann, Martha Franklin, and David A. Child, "Relationship Between Organizational Climate and Job Satisfaction of Nursing Personnel," *Nursing Administration Quarterly,* Vol. 14, No. 4, Summer 1990, pp. 15–22.

Goodell, T., and H. Coeling, "Outcomes of Nurses' Job Satisfaction," *Journal of Nursing Administration,* Vol. 24, No. 11, 1994, pp. 36–41.

Hendrikson, Gerry, and Christine T. Kovner, "Effects of Computers on Nursing Resource Use: Do Computers Save Nurses Time?" *Computers in Nursing,* Vol. 8, No. 1, January-February 1990, pp. 16–22.

Hendrikson, Gerry, Theresa M. Doddato, and Christine T. Kovner, "How Do Nurses Use Their Time?" *Journal of Nursing Administration,* Vol. 20, No. 3, March 1990, pp. 31–37.

Herrick, Linda, Diane Newman, Julianne Hass, et al., "Job Satisfaction in the Head Nurse Role," *Nursing Management,* Vol. 23, No. 3, March 1992, pp. 27–29.

Hesterly, Sandra C., and Margaret Robinson, "Alternative Caregivers: Cost-Effective Utilization of RN's," *Nursing Administration Quarterly,* Vol. 14, No. 3, Spring 1990, pp. 18–23.

Irvine, D., and M. Evans, "Job Satisfaction and Turnover Among Nurses: Integrating Research Findings Across Studies," *Nursing Research,* Vol. 44, No. 4, 1995, pp. 246–253.

Irvine, D., and M. Evans, "Job Satisfaction and Turnover Among Nurses: A Review and Meta-Analysis," *Quality of Nursing Worklife Research Unit Monograph 1, University of Toronto Faculty of Nursing Monograph Series,* Toronto, Ontario, 1992.

Jones, Cheryl Bland, "Staff Nurse Turnover Costs: Part II, Measurements and Results," *Journal of Nursing Administration,* Vol. 20, No. 5, May 1990, pp. 27–32.

Kersten, Joanne, and Jeanne Johnson, "Recruitment: What Are the New Grads Looking For?" *Nursing Management,* Vol. 23, No. 3, March 1992, pp. 44–48.

Klemm, R., and Schreiber, E., "Paid and Unpaid Benefits: Strategies for Nurse Recruitment and Retention," *Journal of Nursing Administration,* Vol. 22, No. 3, 1992, pp. 52–56.

Lucas, M., J. Atwood, and R. Hagaman, "Replication and Validation of Anticipated Turnover Model for Urban Registered Nurses," *Nursing Research,* Vol. 42, No. 1, 1993, pp. 29–35.

MacRobert, M., J. Schmele, and R. Henson, "An Analysis of Job Morale Factors of Community Health Nurses Who Report a Low Turnover Rate," *Journal of Nursing Administration,* Vol. 23, No. 6, 1993, pp. 22–28.

McClure, Margaret, Muriel A. Poulin, Margaret D. Sovie, et al., *Magnet Hospitals: Attraction and Retention of Professional Nurses,* ANA Publishing, Kansas City, Kan., 1983.

Morse, Gwen Goetz, "Resurgence of Nurse Assistants in Acute Care," *Nursing Management,* Vol. 21, No. 3, March 1990, pp. 34–36.

Mottaz, Clifford J., "Work Satisfaction Among Hospital Nurses," *Health Services Management: Readings and Commentary,* Anthony R. Kovner and Duncan Neuhauser, eds., Health Administration Press, Ann Arbor, Mich., 1990, pp. 298–315.

Mueller, Charles W., and Joanne Comi McCloskey, "Nurses; Job Satisfaction: A Proposed Measure," *Nursing Research,* Vol. 39, No. 2, March-April 1990, pp. 113–117.

Muus, K., T. Stratton, J. Dunkin, and N. Juhl, "Retaining Registered Nurses in Rural Community Hospitals," *Journal of Nursing Administration,* Vol. 23, No. 3, 1993, pp. 38–43.

Pattan, John, "Developing a Nurse Recruitment Plan," *Journal of Nursing Administration,* Vol. 22, No. 1, January 1992, pp. 33–39.

Pooyan, Abdullah, Bruce J. Eberhardt, and Elvira Szigeti, "Work-related Variables and Turnover Intention Among Registered Nurses," *Nursing and Health Care,* Vol. 11, No. 5, May 1990, pp. 255–258.

Powers, Patricia Harrison, and Carol A. Dickey, "Evaluation of an RN/Co-Worker Model," *Journal of Nursing Administration,* Vol. 20, No. 3, March 1990, pp. 11–15.

Prescott, Patricia, "Forecasting Requirements for Health Care Personnel," *Nursing Economic$,* Vol. 9, No. 1, January-February 1991, pp. 60–66.

Robertson, J.F., K.A. Herth, and C.C. Cummings, "Long-Term Care: Retention of Nurses," *Journal of Gerontological Nursing,* Vol. 20, No. 11, 1994, pp. 4–10.

Spitzer-Lehmann, Roxanne, "Recruitment and Retention of Our Greatest Asset," *Nursing Administration Quarterly,* Vol. 14, No. 4, Summer 1990, pp. 66–69.

Stamps, P., *Nurses and Work Satisfaction: New Perspective,* Health Administration Press, Chicago, Ill., 1997.

Stratton, T., J. Dunkin, N. Juhl, and J. Gellar, "Recruiting Registered Nurses to Rural Practice Settings," *Applied Nursing Research,* Vol. 6, No. 2, 1993, pp. 64–70.

Warren, Margaret Townsend, "SUN Program: An Approach to the Health Care Personnel Shortage," *Nurse Educator,* Vol. 15, No. 4, July-August 1990, pp. 38–39.

Winkler, J.B., D.L. Flarey, and M.L. Cameron, "The Nursing Human Resource Budget: Design for Success," *Health Care Supervisor,* Vol. 13, No. 4, June 1995, pp. 61–69.

Yoder, L., "Staff Nurses' Career Development Relationships and Self-Reports of Professionalism, Job Satisfaction, and Intent to Stay," *Nursing Research,* Vol. 44, No. 5, 1995, pp. 290–297.

PART

IV

PLANNING AND CONTROL

Planning and control are central to the success of any organization. Planning helps the organization know where it wants to go and develop a plan to get there. Control helps to ensure that the adopted plan is carried out.

A long-standing definition of planning is "an analytical process which involves an assessment of the future, the determination of desired objectives in the context of that future, the development of alternative courses of action to achieve such objectives and the selection of a course (or courses) of action from among those alternatives."[1] Control has been defined as a "process that involves measurement and evaluation of the performance of organizational units, the identification of deviations from planned performance, the initiation of appropriate responses to these deviations, and the monitoring of remedial actions, all done with the intent of ensuring that managers' decisions and actions are consistent with planned organizational objectives."[2] Planning and control together have developed into a strategic management process for the organization, operational budgeting, and control of the activities of an organization, department, or unit.

Strategic management is an emerging field that is an outgrowth of the long-range planning of the 1950s. However, it goes beyond long-range planning, integrating strategic thought throughout the management process. Organizational success largely depends on the care with which the organization acts strategically. Knowing its strengths and weaknesses and being aware of its opportunities and threats are the critical elements upon which the field of strategic management has developed.

Strategic management is discussed in Chapter 10. How are strategic plans defined? Why are they prepared? What benefits can the organization hope to achieve from strategic management? The chapter also discusses some specific elements of strategic management, namely, long-range plans, program budgets, and business plans.

The budgeting aspect of planning is explored in the next two chapters of this part of the book. Chapter 11 provides an overview of the various types of organizational budgets and of the budget process. Chapter 12 provides greater depth on the preparation of the operating budget.

Plans are of only limited usefulness unless actions are taken to ensure that the plans are followed to the extent possible. Chapter 13 discusses the issue of control. That discussion includes the provision of specific tools of variance analysis, which

[1]Brian Scott, "Some Aspects of Long-range Planning in American Corporations with Special Attention to Strategic Planning," Ph.D. dissertation, Harvard University, 1963, p. 8.

[2]John Camillus, *Strategic Planning and Management Control*, Lexington Books, Lexington, MA, 1986, p. 11.

are used to help managers discover variations from the original plan and keep outcomes as close to the plan as possible.

Chapter 14 looks at performance budgeting. This approach allows the manager to plan for the amount of resources to be devoted to each of the major objectives of each unit or department of the organization. ※

CHAPTER

10

Strategic Management

CHAPTER GOALS

The goals of this chapter are to:

- Define strategic management, its importance to health care organizations, and the benefits of the strategic planning process
- Describe the evolution of strategic management from long-range planning to strategic planning to strategic management
- Distinguish between broad, long-term goals and time-oriented, specific, measurable objectives
- Introduce the concepts of total quality management and continuous quality improvement
- Discuss each element of a strategic plan, including a mission statement or nursing philosophy, a statement of long-term goals, a statement of competitive strategy, a statement of organizational policies, a statement of needed resources, and a statement of key assumptions
- Stress the importance of strategic thought by all managers in carrying out all elements of their managerial responsibilities
- Explain the role of the long-range budget and strategic plan in the planning process
- Define program budgeting and discuss the zero-base budgeting technique, stressing the importance of examining alternatives
- Outline the elements of a business plan
- Introduce the concept of pro forma financial statements

※ INTRODUCTION

Strategic management is the process of setting *goals* and *objectives* for the organization, determining the resources to be allocated to achieving those goals and objectives, and establishing policies for getting and using those resources.[1] This process includes an environmental assessment and depends heavily on data concerning the organization's external environment. The strategic management process is critical to the organization's success. Managers and their staffs must not only do the things they do well but also carefully decide what must be done.

One planning text quotes Henry Thoreau: "It is not enough to be busy—the question is, what are we busy about?"[2] This simple question should cause nurse managers to pause and consider their role in the management process. Day-to-day routine activities often cause nurse managers to become overloaded. Managers become so busy that they have little time to plan for the future or to introduce

[1] John C. Camillus, *Strategic Planning and Management Control*, Lexington Books, Lexington, Mass., 1986, p. 18.

[2] Darryl J. Ellis and Pekar, Peter P. Jr., *Planning for Nonplanners*, Amacom, New York, N.Y., 1980, p. 24.

innovations. It is important for all managers to structure their jobs so that planning is not pushed aside by the pressing day-in and day-out issues.

Planning theory indicates that the higher a manager is in the organization's chain of command, the greater the portion of time that should be spent on planning. Planning should not be simply a rote process repeated each year. It should focus on change. It should focus on improvement. It has been suggested that at least two thirds of the chief executive officer's (CEO) time be spent on planning and one third or less on day-to-day operations.[3] Chief nurse executives should probably spend between half and two thirds of their time on planning and innovation. The proportion of time spent on planning becomes less as one moves down through the ranks of nursing management, but it should never become an insignificant amount.

Strategy applied in managing organizations is still a developing field. In the middle of the twentieth century, businesses began to place growing reliance on *long-range planning*. Long-range plans focus on general objectives to be achieved by the organization, typically over three to five years. By the 1960s the term *strategy* became commonplace, and long-range planning began to be referred to as *strategic planning*. It was contrasted with operational planning, the development of a detailed plan for the coming year.

When strategic planning was introduced, the concept of strategy was that operational planning is tactical, whereas long-range planning is strategic. Under strategic or long-range planning an organization prepares a set of goals, and a strategy is developed for accomplishing them. That strategy is formalized into a plan of action generally covering a horizon of three to five years.

In the late 1980s and early 1990s, experts in the area began to use the more generic term *strategic management* to better define the role of strategic thought in organizations.[4] Such experts argue for a broad view of strategic planning. The primary focus remains the identification of broad, long-term goals and the creation of plans to achieve them. However, the current view of strategic management or strategic planning relies on the use of strategic thought in guiding all plans and actions in an organization. This relates to short-term operational plans as well as long-range plans.

Strategic planning is no longer simply long-range planning with a new name, as it was in the 1970s and 1980s and into the 1990s. Strategic management "stresses three points: that the strategic planner is clearly the advisor and facilitator to line management decision-makers; that the program executive, not the strategic planner, is the key strategist; and that strategic planning is always integrated with other functions of the program management process—program design, organizing, budgeting, staffing, controlling, and evaluating."[5] Long-range planning is still a part of strategic planning, but it is no longer the only feature.

The current philosophy is that thinking strategically should not be the sole domain of the strategic planners of the organization. Planning by planners is important but insufficient. Strategic thought should be an element of the job description of all managers throughout the organization. Nurse managers have a central role in strategic planning in this new philosophical approach. The way a nursing unit is organized to provide care, the way it establishes patterns of staff to provide care, and the financial budgets it develops to gain authorization of needed resources to provide care should all be outcomes of a strategic process managed at the unit level. The principal change from earlier views of strategic planning is the emphasis on bringing all managers into the direct process of working to achieve the

---

[3]Ibid. p. 25.

[4]Jack Koteen, *Strategic Management in Public and Nonprofit Organizations*, Praeger, New York, N.Y., 1989, pp. 19–21.

[5]Ibid. p. 21.

organization's primary goals rather than focusing narrowly on specific short-term objectives.

This chapter first discusses total quality management and then moves on to the definition, aims, and benefits of strategic planning and strategic thought. It then focuses on several specific aspects of strategic management, namely, long-range plans, program budgets, and business plans.

※ TOTAL QUALITY MANAGEMENT

A theme for the provision of health services in the twenty-first century is improved quality of care at decreased cost. Two prominent methods to achieve this are total quality management (TQM) and continuous quality improvement (CQI). These represent philosophies concerning the production of an organization's goods and services. Arikian notes that "TQM emphasizes a preventive approach to management, one that addresses problems before they arise, and handles concerns with a studied, long-term commitment to continuous improvement in product and service."[6] From a strategic management perspective, production in America has been dominated by an attitude of getting it done and then fixing it if it is wrong. Observations of the Japanese production process, however, have taught us that if more time is spent on planning, less will be wrong and less will have to be fixed.

Many U.S. corporations learned this lesson throughout the 1990s as they lost some of their competitive edge. To regain that edge, corporations have adopted procedures that focus on avoiding the costs associated with poor quality. Examples of the change in attitude are apparent in the slogans adopted by corporations. For example, Ethicon, a manufacturer of sutures, adopted the policy, "Get it right the first time, every time."

Quality costs money. However, so does lack of quality. TQM focuses on the issue of being responsive to the needs of customers while reducing waste. Kirk notes in examinations of Japanese firms, "The most significant discovery related to their determination to *build quality into the product (or service)* rather than to inspect for errors and assume that error removal would lead to quality. Many Japanese managers bought into the concept of planning and followed through on it—unlike many American managers who avoid this concept like the plague, in preference to the ready-fire-aim approach. 'We don't have time to plan,' some American managers say. Contrarily, many Japanese businessmen say 'We don't have time *not* to plan.' "[7]

Various authors have identified different elements of TQM and CQI. Deming, the pathbreaker in the field, established 14 points related to TQM.[8] These include such factors as a focus on education and training of employees, viewing employees not only as providers but also as customers, quality insurance, and a constant focus on finding ways to continuously improve quality.

TQM and CQI are not financial management tools per se. We will not go into a detailed analysis of the methods here[9]; however, TQM and CQI have tremendous financial implications. Historically, health care organizations have minimized planning and maximized control over day-to-day operations. The lesson of TQM and CQI is that managers will more likely achieve their objectives if they can redesign their work to allow much more time for planning and innovating. Such activities are not occasional but should be viewed as a major element of the

---

[6]Veronica Arikian, "Total Quality Management: Applications to Nursing Service," *Journal of Nursing Administration,* Vol. 21, No. 6, June 1991, p. 46.

[7]Roey Kirk, "The Big Picture: Total Quality Management and Continuous Quality Improvement," *Journal of Nursing Administration,* Vol. 22, No. 4, April 1992, p. 24.

[8]T. Gillem, "Deming's 14 Points and Hospital Quality: Responding to the Consumer's Demand for the Best Value in Health Care," *Nursing Quality Assurance,* Vol. 2, No. 3, 1988, p. 70.

[9]The interested reader is referred to the readings on the topic listed at the end of this chapter.

management function. We must learn to focus on improving the service we provide rather than on simply making sure we provide it. We must spend money only on activities that add value. All non-value-added functions represent wasted resources. In the long run, increased focus on improvement of quality may well lead to more satisfied staff and patients, higher quality of care, and lower costs.

⁂ STRATEGIC PLANNING

Strategic management calls for setting objectives, allocating resources, and establishing policies concerning those resources. With this strategic planning approach, all managers become involved in this process.

To establish and achieve goals, strategic planners have found it useful for the managers of an organization to focus on a series of key questions. The following questions are the most essential an organization must consider:

- Why does the organization exist?
- What is the organization currently?
- What would it like to be?
- How can we make the transformation to what it wants to be?
- How will it know when it is done?

These questions in turn lead to many other questions. What are the organization's strengths? Its weaknesses? Its opportunities? Its threats? Who are the organization's primary customers? Are they being well served? Does the organization learn from its mistakes? Does the organization have a vision for the future? These questions are related to the organization as a whole, but they also relate to each department and unit within the organization.

Managers need to step aside from the current day-to-day activities and assess the nature of the existing organization. Has the organization over the years lost track of its reason for existence? Is the current status of the organization the desired one? If not, the organization needs to formally address the issue of how it can change things to become the type of organization it believes it should be. Again, this is true for departments and units as well as for entire organizations.

Strategic planning asserts that the way to become the type of organization you want to be is to establish a set of clear goals and objectives and then a plan for achieving them. Goals are defined as the broad aims of the organization; objectives are specific targets to be achieved to attain those goals.[10]

Once goals and objectives are identified, specific tactics can be designed to move the organization toward those goals. Tactical plans require resources. Often in the segregation of strategic planning as the long-range plan *vs* operational planning for the short run, operating resource allocations fail to match the allocation needed to reach strategic goals. That is one reason that strategic management now takes a more global perspective.

In developing a short-term operating budget for the coming year, the unit manager must decide whether to place more emphasis on short-run profits or long-term growth. Spending extra money on quality improvements now will generate expenses not offset by revenues. But the reputation for quality will generate more revenues in the future. The dichotomizing of strategic plans and operating budgets forces managers with responsibility for operating expenses to focus on reducing short-run expenses. That tends to be exactly counter to the long-run strategic goals of the organization as designed by preparers of the strategic plan.

[10]The planning literature is inconsistent in the definition of goals and objectives. In some instances the definition used here for goals is assigned to objectives, and vice versa.

Therefore managers must balance the short-term objectives of their units or departments with a long-range vision for the organization.

It is not clear whether any organization will ever get to where it wants to be. The target goals tend to be modified over time in reaction to changes both inside and outside the organization. However, to make progress toward goals, the organization should constantly attempt to answer the questions asked earlier and to take necessary actions based on the answers to the questions.

The Elements of a Strategic Plan

Strategic plans must be adapted to specific situations. The elements of a plan for one organization may not be perfectly suited to another. Flexibility is a positive attribute in the strategic planning process. For most organizations, however, the basic elements of a strategic plan include:

- Mission statement or philosophy
- Statement of long-term goals
- Statement of competitive strategy
- Statement of organizational policies
- Statement of needed resources
- Statement of key assumptions

The Mission Statement or Philosophy

The first step in strategic management is the development of a *mission statement* for the organization, department, or unit. What is the purpose of the organization or unit? An organization cannot begin to plan goals effectively and allocate resources sensibly until it first clearly determines its reason for existence. Strategic planners refer to an organization-wide statement of purpose or focus as the mission statement. In the department of nursing this is often referred to as the philosophical statement.

A great deal of care should be taken in developing a mission statement. The mission statement should focus the organization by defining what it does. Some health care organizations set their mission statement either too broadly or too narrowly. At one extreme they wind up running restaurants or other nonhealth facilities that sap time and energy and often fail because the organization lacks expertise in that area. At the other extreme, growth and change are not encouraged by the statement, and the organization stagnates.

Some degree of limitation in the mission statement is beneficial, forcing the organization to concentrate on what it knows how to do. At the same time, the mission statement should allow growth and diversification. The mission statement should be defined in such a way as to prevent the organization from exceeding its manageable boundaries but to encourage exploration within those boundaries. Camillus notes that a

> health care organization engaged in providing eye-care services can describe itself as fulfilling the mission of examining eyes and writing prescriptions for corrective lenses or the mission of protecting and improving human vision. The first statement is essentially a description of activities in which the organization is engaged. The second statement, in contrast, identifies consequences rather than activities and thus leads to the identification of such possibilities as opening clinics where eye surgery is carried out, engaging in the development and possibly the manufacture of devices for rectifying faulty vision, and running programs for educating the public about the proper care of eyes.[11]

The key to designing the mission statement is to focus not on what the organization does right now as much as to think about the range of possible types

---

[11]John Camillus, *op. cit.*, p. 47.

※ EXHIBIT 10–1. *Examples of Simplified Mission Statements*

Hospital

Narrowly defined mission To provide short-term acute hospital care to the community in the area immediately surrounding the hospital.

Broadly defined mission To improve the health of members of the community.

Overly broadly defined mission To provide health care and other services and products to all potential patients and customers.

Hospital Nursing Department

Narrowly defined mission To deliver high-quality care to the hospital's patients.

Broadly defined mission To deliver high-quality nursing care at a reasonable cost to the citizens of the community.

Overly broadly defined mission To promote the well-being of the organization by undertaking such activities as might be in the organization's interests.

of activities one would see as a logical extension for the organization over time. Several examples of mission statements are shown in Exhibits 10–1 to 10–4.

Statement of Long-term Goals

Goal setting is the organization's attempt to set the direction for itself as it tries to meet its mission. Often an organization will have both quantitative and qualitative goals. Quantitative goals may relate to financial outcomes, such as rates of growth in the number of patients served and in revenues. Qualitative goals may relate to patient satisfaction and general reputation.

In developing the long-term goals of the organization, their timeless nature should be kept in mind. Objectives are intended to be attained within a specific time frame. Goals tend to stay in force over long periods. Providing the needs of an increasing percentage of the community's citizens is a long-term goal. Increasing the number of patients by 8% in the coming year is a specific measurable objective.

While statements of objectives are necessary, the statement of goals is of greater concern in strategic management. As managers attempt to respond in their operations to specific, time-oriented objectives, they should bear in mind the overriding goals that the organization wants to achieve. Innovations that allow the organization to make major steps toward achieving its long-range goals should constantly be sought by all managers.

Statement of Competitive Strategy

The organization's competitive strategy is its plan for achieving its goals, specifically, what services will be provided and to whom. The development of this

※ EXHIBIT 10–2. *Mission Statement of Beth Israel Medical Center*

Since its founding, over 100 years ago, as a medical dispensary to serve the Jewish community of the Lower East Side, Beth Israel Medical Center has been committed to serving and caring for the health and well-being of persons of all races, religions and creeds. Now a major health care provider of specialized, tertiary services, the Medical Center remains proud of its heritage and reaffirms the original mission of Beth Israel Hospital: to provide the highest quality patient care, with compassion and with concern for patient well-being.

To this end, we pledge all our available resources. We will continue to maintain the highest standards of professionalism and dedication. Through our training of physicians, nurses and other health care professionals, as well as our clinical and research programs, we remain committed to attracting and retaining outstanding staff at all levels. We will also continue to seek innovative and cost effective ways to deliver the finest and highest quality of health care services possible.

Reprinted with permission of Beth Israel Medical Center, New York, New York.

※ EXHIBIT 10–3. *Mission Statement of Lutheran Medical Center*

LUTHERAN MEDICAL CENTER
Board of Trustees
Statement of Mission
Adopted October 24, 1990

Preface

Lutheran Medical Center, founded in 1883 by a Norwegian Lutheran Deaconess-nurse, Sister Elisabeth Fedde, gratefully affirms both its Christian heritage exemplified by her Christ-like compassion and dedicated care for struggling new immigrants and its contemporary call to enhance the health and well being of its neighbors throughout a diverse urban area. For 80 years Lutheran Medical Center grew and declined with other neighborhood institutions as a function of an economy based on the Brooklyn waterfront. In recent decades, however, Lutheran Medical Center aggressively volunteered to be the corporate stimulus for community renewal, the catalyst for constructive change, and the advocate for the health and well being of an entire urban area.

Principles and Point of View

Lutheran Medical Center has no reason for being of its own; it exists only to serve the needs of its neighbors.

Lutheran Medical Center defines health as the total well being of the community and its residents. Beyond the absence of individual physical illness, this includes, at least, decent housing, the ability to speak English, employment and educational opportunities, and civic participation.

Lutheran Medical Center understands a hospital not as a collection of buildings, machines and beds, but a staff of talented, creative and committed people who serve the community as they are needed.

Lutheran Medical Center works in partnership with its neighbors, each relying on the other as friends who care about and assist each other.

Program

Guided by these principles, Lutheran Medical Center serves the communities of Bay Ridge, Sunset Park and Park Slope and adjacent areas of southwest Brooklyn. As an acute general community hospital Lutheran Medical Center endeavors to bring the benefits of scientific research and academic medicine to the people of southwest Brooklyn. Through its Family Health Center, Lutheran Medical Center operates an extensive ambulatory care network to provide primary care for the ethnically and economically diverse population of southwest Brooklyn. Lutheran Medical Center also provides home care and other innovative programs for the frail and elderly as well as other educational and human services in response to specific current needs within the community. In addition to its total reimbursement income Lutheran Medical Center devotes other financial resources and seeks major grants to sustain its comprehensive spectrum of health and human services.

Motivated to serve by its own history within the biblical tradition of faith and teaching, and organized as a not-for-profit organization according to the uniquely American heritage of democratic voluntary associations, Lutheran Medical Center's purpose is to serve as the corporate vehicle for its trustees, medical and dental staff, nurses, employees, volunteers and others to care for the needs of our neighbors.

※ EXHIBIT 10–4. *Mission Statement for Family Home Care Services*

The mission of *Family Home Care* is to be an excellent provider of home care services to clients with a commitment to improving their quality of life.

Family Home Care will enable clients to be cared for safely and with dignity;

Family Home Care will respond to changing health care needs;

Family Home Care will provide an atmosphere of mutual respect and growth for every employee; and

Family Home Care will ensure long-term financial viability for the Agency in order to continue to provide quality services in the future.

strategy relies to a great extent on a thorough internal and external review. What are the organization's strengths and weaknesses, its opportunities and threats?

Competitive strategy is the planning of what care will be provided and to whom. To develop such a plan the organization must consider what competitors are or are not doing and what expertise the organization does or does not possess. On the basis of that information the organization can decide where it should expand and perhaps where it should pull back.

Essentially the organization must evaluate its mission and goals in light of its particular strengths and weaknesses and in light of the demand for services and competition in the external environment. Based on that evaluation it can make a plan that will take advantage of opportunities that present themselves and plan a reaction to threats that exist.

Statement of Organizational Policies

The role of policies is to specify what practices are and are not acceptable for the organization. The establishment of a mission and objectives incorporates a set of values. It integrates the values of the organization's founders, the values of its management and staff, and the values of the community. Those values should be incorporated in the decisions made by the organization.

In most organizations no single person can review each and every decision and decide if it is appropriate. A set of policies that clearly indicates what actions are appropriate and what actions are not removes an unreasonable burden from managers throughout the organization. It removes the necessity for guesswork by individual managers in many specific situations.

Policy statements are substantially different from mission statements, statements of goals, and statements of competitive strategy. In each of those earlier statements there is a need to encourage creativity. Each one leaves room for the organization to innovate or grow. In contrast, policy statements are generally limiting. They provide the constraints that the organization wants to place on managerial discretion.

Surprisingly, such constraints can ultimately enhance organizational growth. Without specific policies, managers may find that they are chastised for specific actions without any rhyme or reason. They become uncertain as to when it is okay to take initiative and make changes and when higher levels of management want things done just the way they always have been done. This high degree of uncertainty will lead managers over time to become reluctant to innovate in any respect. The availability of specific procedures clearly delineates where innovation is not allowed. However, that also provides the manager a sense of where innovation is allowed and welcomed.

Statement of Needed Resources

Strategic planning cannot be held apart from the reality of the resources needed to carry out the plan. These include resources in terms of personnel, the facilities for the personnel to work in and with, and the other requirements for accomplishing the goals of the organization. Without linkage between the plan and the resources to carry it out, there can be little hope of achieving the organization's goals.

Statement of Key Assumptions

Part of the planning process is development of a statement of key assumptions. Since strategic management calls for decentralization of the planning process, there must be a set of guidelines that all managers use in common. If management expects to have additional contracts with managed care organizations, that will affect the entire organization. The same assumption about such contracts should be used consistently by all managers. This will make plans consistent and will improve coordination of plans throughout the organization. It will also help in determining whether variations from the plan are due to carrying out the plan or the accuracy of the underlying assumptions.

Benefits of the Strategic Planning Process

One can think of a number of benefits that result from having a strategic planning system. One of the predominant benefits is that it forces the organization to determine its long-run goals and come up with an approach to accomplish them. Establishing long-run goals forces managers to decide what the organization's purpose is and to formalize that purpose. Many health care organizations were established long before any of the current employees worked for the organization. The original goals of the organization can easily become lost among the personal needs and desires of the current management and staff. The process of establishing a formalized mission and goals gives a sense of direction to the organization.

A strategic planning system also promotes efficiency. Managers working toward clear goals are less likely to be inefficient. When everyone clearly knows what the organization is trying to achieve, there is a likelihood that less effort will be spent on unnecessary activities.

The strategic planning process provides a means of communication among the various hierarchical levels of the organization. In large organizations (and sometimes even in relatively small ones) communication between organizational levels becomes difficult. The managers on the lower rungs may know that things are not being done efficiently. The managers on the upper rungs may believe that the systems they have in place do generate efficiency. Inadequate channels exist for moving information up or down through the ranks. Innovation in such cases is expected to be dictated from the higher levels of the organization. In fact, often the need for and opportunities for improvements are most visible at the lower levels. A strategic management process should allow new ideas to flow smoothly down or up.

Lower-level managers will learn more about why changes are taking place if they share the strategic plan and can see how changes relate to achieving the plan's goals. Higher level managers will receive better information if lower level managers focus some of their attention on factors that affect the organization's long-run goals.

The strategic planning process develops management skills at levels throughout the organization. Management skills are developed primarily by giving managers the opportunity to make decisions and to handle things that are not part of the routine. Out-of-the-ordinary activity requires skilled management even more than repetitive tasks. By working at the planning process managers develop skills needed to deal with change and with unusual events.

The strategic planning process provides managers with an improved sense of the needs of the organization and of its environmental constraints. It has often been found that a partnership approach to management works better than a dictatorial approach. Managers who are told they must live within constraints resist them. Managers who are asked to become part of the team to solve the problem of constraints learn to understand the difficulty in the constraints and are more willing to work cooperatively instead of adversarially.

The strategic planning process increases the level of organizational creativity in addressing problems. Successful organizations encourage rather than resist change. Things are done differently now than they were twenty years ago. Change, however, does not occur at some arbitrary point every twenty years. It occurs gradually in an evolutionary process. The fact that most organizations do things a certain way now that they did not do twenty years ago indicates that someone tried a new approach and found it superior. Who is that someone? Is it the lucky one who accidentally fell upon an improved approach?

Generally, this is one area where organizations make their own luck. Creativity cannot be forced from people. One cannot tell employees to be creative and to develop innovative improvements. However, creativity can be either fostered or stifled. A strong commitment to strategic management throughout the organization will convey the organization's view of creativity as positive rather than negative.

One can summarize strategic management as the process that adds creative vision to all the other processes of the organization. Strasen defines vision as "the ability to set goals that are not limited to what is presently inevitable. In order to be meaningful, goals must stretch the imagination and efforts of the individual or organization setting them. If goals are inevitable occurrences in the future, they are set too low and are no real measure of progress or accomplishment."[12] Once the vision of the future is in place and is clearly communicated, the organization's managers can creatively work on changes to bring that vision to fruition.

Implementing a Strategic Management Process

This chapter has alternatively referred to the strategic plan and to the strategic planning or management process.

The specific development of a strategic plan is discussed in the next section of this chapter. However, strategic management relies not just on a plan but on a broad planning process. That process is one of making managers aware of the need to think strategically as they carry out all their management activities. In developing the long-range plan, managers must relate the plan to the mission. In designing specific program budgets or business plans, the manager must consider how the program will help the organization achieve its goals. In developing the specific details of the operating budget, again the manager should be trying to link the details with how they help the organization reach its long-term aims.

The remainder of this chapter focuses on some long-range elements of strategic planning, specifically, long-range planning, program budgets, and business plans. As the reader proceeds to the remaining four chapters in Part IV of this book, the notion of trying to link operational activities with strategic thought should be kept in mind.

※ LONG-RANGE PLANNING

In developing the long-range budget the organization begins the process of translating its general goals and objectives into a specific action plan. Long-range budgets or long-range plans are often referred to as the organization's strategic plan. Such plans generally cover a period of three to five years.

Given a strategic management process that calls on managers to focus on the organization's goals, is a strategic plan essential? The answer is clearly yes. Long-range planning is critical to the vitality of an organization. For organizations to thrive, they must move forward. The staff of an organization should be able to look back and see the progress that has been made over an extended period. Budgeting for one year at a time does not allow for the major types of changes that would take years to plan and implement. Yet that lengthy process is needed for the efforts that will substantially move the organization forward.

For example, suppose that one goal of the organization is to move from being a primary care community hospital to a regional tertiary care center. This cannot be accomplished by having each department attempt to modify its operating budget. An overall organizational plan is needed. Which of the new tertiary services can or should be added in the next five years? Which programs already exist but need to be expanded in the next five years to accommodate the changing role of the organization? These questions are specifically addressed in the strategic plan or long-range budget.

Nursing should be involved in this planning process. The success of the plan will depend on how well it is carried out. If the plan does not have adequate nursing input when it is prepared, it is unlikely that the nursing staff will fully support it. Nurses must push their organizations to incorporate nursing leadership into the

---

[12]Leann Strasen, *Key Business Skills for Nurses*, J. B. Lippincott, Philadelphia, 1987, p. 208.

planning process, not only for the good of nurses and nursing but also for the ultimate success of the organization.

The strategic plan may lay the groundwork for a fund-raising campaign to precede and parallel expansion of services. Or the plan may indicate that each year for five years growth in specified existing profitable areas must be undertaken to offset start-up losses on the introduction of major new programs. Specific dollar amounts of additional revenue and new program cost may be projected only as an extremely rough estimate. Although general, such a plan does give the organization enough specific information about the implications and requirements for expansion into a tertiary care center to allow for development of specific programs to move the organization toward that ultimate goal.

The strategic plan may be somewhat more detailed, showing projections of the dollar amounts expected to be available (and their sources) as well as which specific programs will be adopted and what their approximate costs will be. Since a strategic or long-range plan projects at least three, and up to ten, years into the future, it is unlikely that revenue and cost estimates will be highly accurate. Therefore, while rough estimates are often included in such plans, they are generally not overly detailed or refined.

The plan should not focus only on major program additions. The services and programs that already exist are equally important to an organization. Expanding a service, downsizing one, or even eliminating a program or service requires the same consideration and planning as adding a program or service. A part of the planning process should be to explicitly address whether those services and programs that make up the majority of operations of the organization are being retained at a steady-state level or whether they are to be contracted or expanded in scope.

One serious potential problem arises if this issue is ignored in preparing strategic plans. If existing programs are implicitly assumed to continue unchanged, a plan that includes a number of new programs may appear feasible. However, it may not be feasible when technological and other changing factors are explicitly considered for the ongoing operations of the organization. Therefore, expectations regarding existing programs should be explicitly reviewed and included as part of the plan.

Once the plan has been finalized and formalized, it serves as a guide for a number of years. Long-range plans are typically prepared only once every three or five years. Creating a new plan each year would only lead to constant changes in the organization's direction. This would lead to wasted efforts and frustrated managers. However, such plans should be reviewed each year. Assumptions may turn out to be wrong. A cure for cancer could change patient volume. The external environment can change dramatically. An influx of refugees could change the demand for services. Annual reviews allow the organization to adjust the strategic plan to react to current events.

Each year elements of the plan are brought into the current activities of the organization. To make the transition from the plan into operations, many proposed additions or changes require thorough evaluation. This may be accomplished through the development of a program budget.

※ PROGRAM BUDGETING AND ZERO-BASE BUDGETING

Program budgeting is the part of the overall strategic planning process that focuses on all the costs and benefits associated with a specific program. The program may be an existing one that the organization is considering expanding, downsizing, or eliminating, or it may be a new program that the organization is thinking of adding. Program budgeting examines alternative programs to meet the organization's objectives and examines feasible alternative ways to accomplish each program.

Some program budgeting is done within a nursing unit or department. Often, however, the program changes generated by a strategic plan have interdepartmental impact. Such program changes are much more complicated because of the need for coordination between departments. It is vital that nursing participate fully in such interdepartmental planning. Working on key committees is essential not only to protect the interests of nursing but also to ensure that any plans developed make sense from a nursing perspective and can be supported by the nursing staff.

In most cases program budgets relate directly to the strategic planning of the organization. The projects being evaluated are under consideration because they relate directly to moving the organization toward achievement of its long-term goals.

Program budgets are substantially different from other types of budgets. Long-range budgets or strategic plans look in general terms at the entire organization over a period of years. Their information is based on rough approximations rather than on details. Operating and cash budgets look in great detail, but only at the coming year. A program budget combines a great amount of detailed information for a long period for one specific program. Further, while most budgets focus on a given department's revenues and costs, program budgets compare revenues and expenses for an entire program, cutting across departments or cost centers.

A program budget compares all its costs and benefits to evaluate the entire program's effect on the organization over its lifetime. In doing this the program budgeting methods identify costs and benefits of different programs aimed at the same purpose or of different approaches to one program. Because resources are limited, program budgeting often focuses on trade-offs; that is, program budgeting considers the extra benefit to be gained by spending additional money on a program. Alternatively, program budgeting considers how much of the benefit of a program would be lost if less money were spent on the program.

Zero-base Budgeting

Zero-base budgeting (ZBB) is a popular program budgeting technique that gained fame for its strong push toward analysis of all costs. All costs from a base of zero must be justified. Until the introduction of ZBB, it was common for budget negotiations to revolve around the appropriate amount of increase in a budget. How much more should be spent next year than was spent in the current year? Implicitly, such an approach assumes that all current-year spending continues to be reasonable and justified for the next year. Only the amount of the increment is subject to examination and discussion.

In reality, as technology and diseases change, some departments have growing financial needs, while other departments can get by with decreasing resources. The concept of requiring zero-base evaluation is attractive because it means that budgets are not allowed to become "fat" over time. Many organizations use ZBB analysis to see exactly how money is being spent within a unit or department. Such an approach requires existing programs to justify their continued existence. Rather than basing the future budget on the past budget, the program must demonstrate why all expenditures in the proposed budget are needed.

Additionally, the ZBB approach pays great attention to the alternative ways that any one given program can be offered. ZBB collects information regarding a program into a *decision package.* A decision package contains documentation in support of the program and summaries of the analyses performed. In that sense, the decision package is just a mechanism to ensure a formal, systematic review of each budget.

Each package (Fig. 10–1) contains a statement of the purpose of the program, the

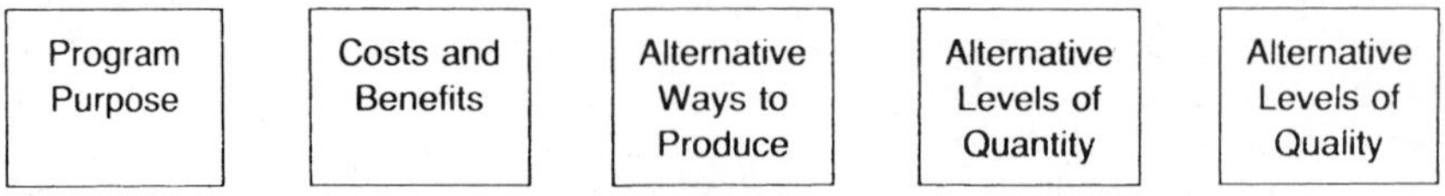

Program Purpose	Costs and Benefits	Alternative Ways to Produce	Alternative Levels of Quantity	Alternative Levels of Quality

FIGURE 10–1. Elements of a ZBB decision package.

consequences of not performing the program, and the ways that the costs and benefits of the program can be measured. More interestingly, the package also includes statements of alternatives. These statements are the heart of ZBB.

ZBB provides a great degree of sophistication in the analysis of alternatives. ZBB not only compares different programs with separate decision packages but also compares three major types of alternatives within the decision package for each individual program. The first alternative involves ways to produce the treatment, service, or other output. The second set of alternatives relates to the quantity of treatments, service, or output to be provided. The third set of alternatives considers varying levels of quality.

For many nurses, considering trade-offs such as these is counter to their traditional education. Nurses, as health care professionals, are trained to provide the best possible care to each patient. At the larger level of organizational planning, however, it must be acknowledged that no health care provider can provide everything to everyone. There simply are limited resources. ZBB forces recognition of the need to determine the greatest overall good that can be provided to the entire population served by an organization, in contrast to the view of providing care to a specific individual.

Perhaps the best way to understand how these alternatives are examined is to work through a potential program budget problem.

ZBB Case Study: Hemodialysis

Suppose that the hypothetical Wagner Hospital has decided on the basis of its environmental review that there is a pressing need for additional hemodialysis services in the community. In Wagner's long-range plan the introduction of a hemodialysis program has been included, although the plan does not include much in the way of specifics other than to note that within the next five years some form of hemodialysis program should be fully instituted. This program was highly placed when priorities were established, although it would have to vie for funds with several other important new programs that were also included in the long-range plan, such as a new primary care center.

Wagner has compiled a decision package for the hemodialysis program. The formal documentation in the package first notes the name of the program (hemodialysis) and the sponsoring department within the hospital (internal medicine). The stated purpose of the program is to reduce levels of mortality and morbidity currently experienced in the community due to insufficient hemodialysis facilities. The resources needed for the program are stated in general terms. They include dialysis machines, physicians, nurses, technicians, supplies, and overhead items such as electrical power and physical space.

If Wagner were not a user of ZBB, it is likely that the renal specialists in the hospital would have designed a first-class hemodialysis center, perhaps as a new hospital wing, with five machines to satisfy all community needs. The proposal would have been a take-it-or-leave-it package, with strong political emphasis on its acceptance.

There is nothing wrong with wanting everything to be first class. It is not wasteful to provide top-quality care. However, that does not mean that an organization can afford to provide that care. Having a first-class hemodialysis center may mean that there will not be enough resources left for adequate cancer treatment.

Because Wagner Hospital uses ZBB, the hemodialysis plan cannot be approved until an analysis is performed that examines a number of alternatives. The first issue concerns the level of output. How much treatment will be provided? Suppose that five machines would take care of the entire community demand now and for the foreseeable future. Suppose that the estimated annual cost of this alternative were $2 million including depreciation, supplies, personnel, overhead, maintenance, and so on. A second alternative may be to purchase only four machines. Suppose that at this level it would still be possible to eliminate mortality and morbidity, but some of the machines might have to operate two or three shifts per day, causing some inconvenience for nurses and physicians.

Four machines might cost a total of $1,700,000. Note that while the number of machines would decrease 20%, from five to four, the costs would fall only 15%. That is possible because some costs associated with the program are likely to be fixed. As discussed in Chapter 7, fixed costs do not change as the output level increases. Does this mean that five machines would be better than four, since the hospital would get 20% more machines for only 15% more cost? Not necessarily. That is the wrong comparison. The goal is to provide cost-effective, high-quality health care to the community; the goal is not to buy unnecessary equipment to minimize the cost per machine.

The alternative of four machines instead of five would save $300,000. Although there would be some inconvenience, the reduced cost would not result in higher mortality or morbidity. The extra convenience gained by having five machines must be compared with the benefits from spending $300,000 for some other program. Would the extra machine generate additional revenue? Or would it affect only scheduling?

Other alternative levels of output might be the use of three machines, which would eliminate 100% of mortality and 50% of morbidity for a cost of $1,400,000; two machines, which would eliminate only 80% of mortality at a cost of $1,100,000; and one machine, which would eliminate only 40% of mortality at a cost of $800,000.

Itemizing the costs and benefits of the alternative output levels is informative. Unlike the usual all-or-nothing presentation for a new program, either five machines or no program at all ("We don't practice second-class medicine here!"), the choice is not that dramatic. In fact, in a constrained environment it may well be that after seeing all the alternatives the choice will be between three machines or four machines. Less than three may be considered inadequate to accomplish the long-run objectives; more than four may raise questions of priorities.

It is not only the amount of output that is a question here. The ZBB system requires that alternative ways to produce the output also be considered. Is there a choice? Is it hemodialysis machines or nothing? Perhaps the answer is yes, but one of the major roles of ZBB is to ask questions such as that. The next question might be, does hemodialysis have to be performed in the hospital? The answer is no. While one alternative would be to perform all dialysis in the hospital, another alternative would be to perform all dialysis in one clinic location. Another alternative would be to have a series of external locations spread throughout the community, one location for each machine. It is also possible to use one mobile van for each machine, allowing dialysis to be performed at many locations. Each of these alternatives would be matched with one, two, three, four, and five machines.

Other alternative options must also be considered. Can a patient be on the machine for a shorter period, thus increasing the number of patients who have access to it? Can money be saved by buying machines with fewer accessories? Such questions almost certainly hit upon issues of quality. However, the trade-offs between quality and cost must be examined.

Trade-offs are always made, and they sometimes affect the quality of care. If one person dies of heart disease, it may be because not enough resources were devoted to having the very latest open-heart surgery equipment. That person suffered from a lack of high-quality care. More resources devoted to heart surgery equipment might have saved that individual. Perhaps the hospital should cut back in another area and pursue the very best in heart surgery. In the vast majority of cases, that would simply result in other people dying in another area. The program budgeting system must attempt to select a set of projects that are carried out in a way that minimizes the overall negative impact on quality. That may mean undertaking two new services, each at less than the optimal level of care, rather than totally sacrificing either service so the remaining one can be run on an optimal basis. Table 10–1

⁜ TABLE 10–1. *ZBB Decision Package—Hemodialysis*

1. Name of program: Hemodialysis
2. Department: Internal Medicine
3. Purpose: Reduce mortality and morbidity due to lack of hemodialysis facilities
4. Resources required: Dialysis machines, physicians, nurses, technicians, supplies, overhead
5. Quantity or level of output alternatives

Level	Health Implications	Cost
Five machines	Eliminates all mortality and morbidity; no inconvenience to staff	$2,000,000
Four machines	Eliminates all mortality and morbidity; some inconvenience to staff	1,700,000
Three machines	Eliminates all mortality and 50% of all morbidity	1,400,000
Two machines	Eliminates 80% of mortality	1,100,000
One machine	Eliminates 40% of mortality	800,000

6. Alternative ways to produce output: This section should consider the various approaches to providing the product and the cost of each. For instance, it should consider providing the care in the hospital, in clinics, or in mobile vans. For each way of providing the output, each output level (i.e., one machine, two machines, etc.) should be considered.
7. Alternative levels of quality of care: This should consider the cost of using different types of machines and/or changing the amount of time each patient is on the machine for each way of producing the output and for each level of output in terms of numbers of machines.

provides a summary of the hemodialysis decision package and its focus on trade-offs in this hypothetical example.

The difficult part of the analysis is to explicitly and creatively seek and examine trade-offs from alternatives. Specifically, it is necessary to ask whether more lives could be saved by the organization if it spent $300,000 less on hemodialysis and got four machines instead of five. Could even more lives be saved in some other program if dialysis was cut to three machines and $600,000 less was spent on this? Three machines might mean less care and lower quality care—less time on the machine for each noncritical patient. What could $600,000 do elsewhere in the organization? Would $600,000 spent elsewhere provide enough benefit to justify less care and lower-quality of care in this area?

Suppose that in addition to hemodialysis a primary care center has also been proposed. A first-class primary care center might cost $1 million per year (the numbers here are hypothetical). This primary care center would provide access to care for 50,000 visits per year (or about 12,000 patients). However, a ZBB review of primary care indicates that for $600,000 a total of 35,000 visits could be handled. All children in the community could get immunizations, but some older patients would have to travel extra minutes to go to an existing clinic.

Because of the large capital investment, the Wagner Hospital does not have sufficient cash to establish both a primary care center and a hemodialysis service at the ideal first-class levels. It is highly likely that without a ZBB review the hospital might well select either hemodialysis or primary care, and the choice would likely depend largely on politics. The well-being of the community can get lost in the struggle between vested interest groups within an organization.

There might, however, be enough resources to provide both hemodialysis and primary care at slightly reduced levels of care. The hospital could add three dialysis machines and a primary care unit.

The ZBB review forces the examination of alternatives. It forces recognition of the fact that more lives would be saved by scaling back the levels of hemodialysis and primary care and providing both services. Given the explicit information contained in the ZBB reviews, both vested interest groups are likely to be more willing to accept the resulting compromise.

Ranking Decision Packages

Since the resources of the organization are always limited, it is rare that all proposed packages can be accepted. Therefore ZBB requires each manager to rank the alternative decision packages. The best alternative is ranked number 1.

During the process of budget review and negotiation, managers at higher levels of the organization will receive ranked decision packages from a number of subordinate managers. For example, a nurse manager with responsibility for a number of units might receive packages from each unit nurse manager. The packages from all these different units must be ranked in order of importance by the manager responsible for the group of units. Then the packages will continue up through the organization. The chief nurse executive and the administrative staff will rank all the packages received from all the different nursing areas.

In large organizations the ranking process can become quite tedious. However, it is a necessary evil if the goal of the program budgeting process is to compare all the alternatives available to the organization and to ultimately allocate the organization's resources to those projects that best lead to attainment of the organization's goals.

⁜ BUSINESS PLANS

One approach to program budgeting that first became widely used in the 1980s is the business plan. This technique, widely used in industry, became popular in health care as it became clear that health care organizations would have to take a more businesslike approach to providing their services in an ever more difficult financial environment. It is a method that is still gaining support in all types of health care organizations.

What Is a Business Plan?

A *business plan* is a detailed plan for a proposed program, project, or service, including information to be used to assess the venture's financial feasibility. Often the plan is used as a sales document that makes the case for undertaking a new project. However, despite its advocacy role, the plan should provide an honest appraisal of the project. If in fact the proposed project is not good for the organization, that should be determined at the planning stage rather than after a large financial investment has been made to implement it.

The first step in planning a new program should be to understand which goals of the organization the program promotes. Does the proposed project fit with the organization's mission statement? In developing the plan, sufficient information must be gathered to indicate whether the proposed program will move the organization closer to its goals. In evaluating the plan, it is important not to lose sight of the original organizational goal to which the project relates.

For example, one business plan might relate to the development of a community education program for patients with diabetes; another plan might focus on providing home health care. Both of these new programs might fit nicely within a mission of providing health care services to the community. It is possible, however, that the program on community education would not be expected to be financially self-sufficient. It fits into the element of mission that concerns providing important services on a charitable basis. On the other hand, the home care plan may be based on the notion of earning profits to be used to subsidize the charitable elements of the organization's mission. The organization cannot provide some services at a loss unless it provides some at a profit.

Even the program aimed at the charitable mission would require a business plan. The fact that it is not expected to earn a profit does not remove the need to understand just how large a subsidy it might require. At the same time, if home care is being proposed to earn profits to subsidize the other operations of the organization, we should not lose sight of that fact during the planning process. Business plans are discussed in Chapter 20.

※ IMPLICATIONS FOR NURSE MANAGERS

Often nurse managers at all levels of the organization have insights that can result in significant operational changes that will move the organization closer to its strategic goals. That is why strategic management takes the view that strategic planning is not limited to the development of the long-range plan and program budgets. Strategic management must exhibit itself through strategic thought by managers throughout the organization. All nurse managers should make themselves aware of their organization's mission and goals as well as its specific objectives and policies. Knowing the philosophical statement of the nursing department alone is too narrow a view.

The organization-wide goals developed in the strategic management process are used as a point of reference in assessing where the organization has been, where it is going, and what it hopes to accomplish in the coming years.

Strategic management requires a significant effort from managers at all levels. However, that effort is rewarded. Careful planning reduces the extent to which managers move from crisis to crisis. It promotes the efficient use of resources and the financial health of the organization. It results in goal setting and the establishment of a vision for the organization. Strategic planning helps ensure that managers will identify opportunities and take reasonable risks to take advantage of those opportunities. Strategic management promotes organizational change within a stable framework of constant mission and goals.

The strategic plan or long-range budget indicates which programs are to remain at a steady state, which are to be downsized or eliminated entirely, which are to be expanded, and which are to be added. This gives impetus to specific program budgets in which a unit, department, or program undergoes a complete assessment.

Using a method such as ZBB, the organization's managers can systematically examine all the implications of a program over its lifetime. The program can be compared with others that would achieve the same end. The program can also be assessed in terms of alternative ways to produce the output, alternative levels of quality, and alternative levels of quantity of output.

Program budget analyses can uncover unneeded costs in existing programs. There is waste in health care organizations, as in virtually all organizations. Further, program budgeting can help the organization to make effective choices as to how best to use limited resources. Trade-offs among various alternatives can be more clearly assessed with the increased information program budgets provide about the impact of different available options.

The organization can settle for a less-than-first-class bedside computer system but can also have new unit-based videocassette recorders (VCRs) for patient education. Alternatively, it can have a new first-rate bedside computer system and forgo having unit-based VCRs. This book cannot say which of the choices would be best. However, there should be an awareness that the alternatives do exist. The organization should not blindly get a first-rate bedside computer system because of internal political pressure and then simply accede that there is no money for VCRs. The alternatives should be considered and an explicit choice made.

Program budgeting techniques are equally as effective for reviewing the operations of an ongoing unit as for evaluating a new program. The way a nursing unit performs its tasks may go unchanged from year to year. A ZBB review, however, can force the manager to consider whether there are alternative ways or levels of effort that could be used to accomplish the unit's goals.

Performing a ZBB review for a nursing unit is expensive. It takes a substantial amount of time to evaluate all the cost elements of a budget. It is much simpler to simply indicate that the next year's operating budget will be 5% more than the current year's. However, the chances of making a significant positive gain for the organization are much higher when a thorough justification of each and every expenditure is undertaken. Managers tend to accept the status quo. Instead, managers should spend less time on day-in and day-out routine activities and more time on innovation. Examining all aspects of a unit's operations can result in significant and lasting benefits for the unit and the entire organization.

Business plans are documents that are becoming essential for the introduction of new programs. Such plans help managers complete a comprehensive examination of a proposed program. By making such a thorough review, the manager and the organization gain an in-depth understanding of the program as well as its financial implications for the organization.

Strategic management has broader implications than just for use in specific areas such as ZBB reviews or business plans. Managers should be creative in their applications. For example, there are many models for the delivery of nursing services. Each has financial, quality, and other implications. A nurse manager who understands strategic management can apply its principles when the organization makes choices among alternative delivery care models. In this way the choice made will reflect consideration of the wide range of factors that relate to that decision.

KEY CONCEPTS

Strategic management Process of setting the goals and objectives of the organization, determining the resources to be allocated to achieving those goals and objectives, and establishing policies concerning getting and using those resources. The current view of strategic management or strategic planning relies on the use of strategic thought by all managers in guiding all plans and actions of an organization. Strategic thought requires managers to balance the short-term objectives of their units or departments with a long-range vision for the organization. Nurse managers have a central role in strategic management under this new planning philosophy.

Goals and objectives Goals are the broad, timeless ends of the organization meant to aid the organization in accomplishing its mission. Objectives are specific targets to be achieved to attain goals. Planning calls on each organization to establish a set of clear goals and objectives and a plan for achieving them.

Elements of a strategic plan Basic elements of a strategic plan include:

- Mission statement
- Statement of long-term goals
- Statement of competitive strategy
- Statement of organizational policies
- Statement of needed resources
- Statement of key assumptions

Mission statement Statement of the unit's, department's, or organization's purpose or reason for existence. The mission statement should be defined in such a way as to prevent the organization from exceeding its manageable boundaries but encouraging exploration within those boundaries.

Competitive strategy Organization's plan for achieving its goals, specifically, what services will be provided and to whom. The development of this strategy relies to a great extent on a thorough internal and external review. What are the organization's strengths and weaknesses, its opportunities and threats?

Policy statements Limiting statements indicating what managers can or cannot do as they work to carry out the organization's mission by attainment of goals and objectives.

Benefits of strategic planning

- Forces the organization to determine its long-run goals and devise an approach to accomplish them
- Promotes efficiency
- Provides a means of communication among the various hierarchical levels of the organization
- Develops management skills at all levels throughout the organization
- Provides managers with an improved sense of the needs of the organization and of its environmental constraints
- Increases the level of organizational creativity in addressing its problems
- Reduces the extent to which managers move from crisis to crisis
- Promotes the efficient use of resources and the financial health of the organization
- Results in goal setting and establishment of a vision for the organization
- Helps ensure that managers identify opportunities and take reasonable risks to take advantage of those opportunities
- Promotes organizational change within a stable framework of constant mission and goals

Long-range budgets (long-range plans) Often referred to as the organization's strategic plan. Such plans generally cover a period of three to five years.

Program budgeting Part of the overall strategic planning process that focuses on all costs and benefits associated with a specific program. A program budget combines a great amount of detailed information, cutting across departments, for a long-term period.

Zero-base budgeting (ZBB) Popular program budgeting technique that gained fame for its analysis and justification of all costs. From a program budgeting perspective, ZBB is especially useful because of its strong focus on an examination of alternatives.

Business plan Detailed plan for a proposed program, project, or service, including information to be used to assess the venture's financial feasibility. The plan should clearly state the objectives of the proposed project and provide a linkage that shows how the plan's objectives will lead to accomplishment of the organization's goal.

SUGGESTED READINGS

Abrams, Rhonda M., *The Successful Business Plan: Secrets and Strategies,* Oasis Press, Grant's Pass, Ore., 1993.

Arkebauer, James B., *Guide to Writing a High-Impact Business Plan,* McGraw-Hill, New York, N.Y., 1995.

Bobnet, N.L., J. Illcyn, P.S. Milanovich, M.A. Ream, and K. Wright, "Continuous Quality Improvement: Improving Quality in Your Home Care Organization," *Journal of Nursing Administration,* Vol. 23, No. 2, 1993, pp. 42–48.

Brent, N.J., "Setting Up Your Own Business: Facing the Future as an Entrepreneur," *AORN Journal,* Vol. 51, No. 1, January 1990, pp. 205, 208, 210–213.

Campbell, Sandy, "The Newest Gatekeepers: Nurses Take on the Duties of Primary Care Physicians," *Health Care Strategic Management,* Vol. 15, No. 3, March 1997, pp. 14–15.

Castaneda-Mendez, K., "Value-Based Cost Management: The Foundation of a Balanced Performance Measurement System," *Journal of Healthcare Quality,* Vol. 19, No. 4, 1997, pp. 6–9.

Cortes, T.A., "Zero-Based Budgeting for a Radiology Service: A Case Study in Outsourcing," *Hospital Cost Management and Accounting,* Vol. 8, No. 2, May 1996, pp. 1–6.

Crow, G.L., "The Business of Planning Your Practice: Success is No Accident," *Advances in Practical Nursing Quarterly,* Vol. 2, No. 1, Summer 1996, pp. 55–61.

Daigh, R.D., "Financial Implications of a Quality Improvement Process," *Topics in Health Care Financing,* Vol. 17, No. 3, 1991, pp. 42–52.

Dillon, R.D., *Zero-Base Budgeting for Health Care Institutions,* Aspen Publishers, Gaithersburg, Md., 1979.

Etinger, W.H., Jr., "Consumer-Perceived Value: The Key to a Successful Business Strategy in the Healthcare Marketplace," *Journal of the American Geriatric Society,* Vol. 46, No. 1, January 1998, pp. 111–113.

Finkler, Steven A., and David R. Ward, *Cost Accounting for Health Care Organizations: Concepts and Applications,* 2nd edition, Aspen Publishers, Gaithersburg, Md., 1999.

Fredrickson, James W., *Perspectives on Strategic Management,* Harper Business, New York, N.Y., 1990.

Gillem, T., "Deming's 14 Points and Hospital Quality: Responding to the Consumer's Demand for the Best Value in Health Care," *Nursing Quality Assurance,* Vol. 2, No. 3, 1988, pp. 70–78.

Gitlow, H., and S. Gitlow, *The Deming Guide to Quality and Competitive Position,* Prentice-Hall, Englewood Cliffs, N.J., 1987.

Hough, Douglas E., and James E. Bolinger, *Developing a Managed Care Business Plan,* American Medical Association, Chicago, Ill., 1998.

Hughes, G., "Budget Management," *Journal of Accidental (Emergency) Medicine,* Vol. 14, No. 3, May 1997, pp. 187–188.

Kirk, R., "The Big Picture: Total Quality Management and Continuous Quality Improvement," *Journal of Nursing Administration,* Vol. 22, No. 4, 1992, pp. 24–31.

Latzer, D.B., "Total Quality Management: An Application in a Biomedical Laboratory," *Hospital Cost Management and Accounting,* Vol. 9, No. 2, 1997, pp. 1–6.

Lynn, M.I., and D.P. Osborn, "Deming's Quality Principles: A Health Care Application," *Hospitals and Health Services Administration,* Vol. 36, No. 2, 1991, pp. 111–119.

Magiera F.T., and R.A. McLean, "Strategic Options in Capital Budgeting and Program Selection Under Fee-for-Service and Managed Care," *Health Care Management Review,* Vol. 21, No. 4, Fall 1996, pp. 7–17.

McKeon, T., "Performance Measurement: Integrating Quality Management and Activity-Based Cost Management," *Journal of Nursing Administration,* Vol. 26, No. 4, 1996, pp. 45–51.

McLaughlin, C.P., and A.D. Kaluzny, "Total Quality Management," *Health Care Management Review,* Vol. 15, No. 3, pp. 7–14.

McLaughlin, C.P., P. Kaluzny, and D. Arnold, "Total Quality Management Issues In Managed Care," *Journal of Health Care Finance,* Vol. 24, No. 1, Fall 1997, pp. 10–16.

Milakovich, M.E., "Creating a Total Quality Health Care Environment," *Health Care Management Review,* Vol. 16, No. 2, 1991, pp. 9–20.

Omachonu, V.K., *Total Quality and Productivity Management in Health Care Organizations,* Industrial Engineering and Management Press, Institute of Industrial Engineers, Norcross, Ga., 1991.

Pelfrey, S., "Managing Financial Data," *Seminars in Nurse Management,* Vol. 5, No. 1, March 1997, pp. 25–30.

Pyhrr, P.A., *Zero-Base Budgeting: A Practical Management Tool for Evaluating Expenses,* Wiley-Interscience, New York, N.Y., 1973.

Reinertsen, James L., "Outcomes Management and Continuous Quality Improvement: The Compass and the Rudder," *Quality Review Bulletin,* Vol. 19, No. 1, January 1993, pp. 5–7.

Seymour, D.W., and Guillett, W.V., "Connecting the Dots: Grounding Quality Improvement and Cost Cutting Initiatives in Strategic Planning," *Journal of Healthcare Resource Management,* Vol. 15, No. 7, September 1997, pp. 14–19.

Simpson, Roy L., "Take Advantage of Managed Care Opportunities," *Nursing Management,* Vol. 28, No. 3, March 1997, pp. 24–25.

Stahl, Dulcelina A., "The Phases of Managed Care: Where Does Subacute Care Fit?" *Nursing Management,* October 1996, pp. 8–9.

Stahl, Dulcelina A., "Business Strategies in Subacute Care," *Nurse Manager,* Vol. 28, No. 2, February 1997, pp. 27–28.

Stiles, R.A., and S.S. Mick, "Components of the Costs of Controlling Quality: A Transaction Cost Economics Approach," *Hospital and Health Services Administration,* Vol. 42, No. 2, Summer 1997, pp. 205–219.

Stodolak, F., and J. Carr, "Systems Must Be Compatible with Quality Efforts," *Healthcare Financial Management,* June 1992, pp. 72–77.

Suver, James D., Bruce R. Neumann, and Keith E. Boles, *Management Accounting for Healthcare Organizations,* 3rd edition, Pluribus Press, Westchester, Ill., 1992.

Turner, S.O., "Transitioning Yourself Into the New Health Care Business," *Turner Healthcare Associates, Inc.,* Vol. 17, No. 2, March-April 1998, pp. 30–32.

Winkler J.B., D.L. Flarey, and M.L. Cameron, "The Nursing Human Resource Budget: Design for Success," *Health Care Supervisor,* Vol. 13, No. 4, June 1995, pp. 61–69.

CHAPTER

11

Budgeting Concepts

CHAPTER GOALS

The goals of this chapter are to:

- Define budgeting and control
- Describe some benefits of budgeting
- Introduce and describe the various types of budgets, including master, operating, capital, long-range, program, and cash
- Discuss the generation, justification, and evaluation of capital budget proposals
- Introduce the concepts of the time value of money, discounting, net present value, and internal rate of return.
- Distinguish between revenue and expense and between cash inflows and outflows
- Outline the steps in cash budget preparation and provide a cash budget example
- Describe the budgeting process
- Provide an example of a budget timetable
- Discuss specific steps in the budgeting process
- In a technical appendix the chapter also discusses technical aspects of time-value-of-money computations.

※ INTRODUCTION

A *budget* is a plan. The plan is formalized (written down) and quantified (e.g., stated in dollar terms). It represents management's intentions or expectations. In financial terms, an organization-wide budget generally compares expected revenues with expected expenses to ascertain the organization's expected excess of revenues over expenses (i.e., profit or loss) for the coming year.

Preparation of a budget forces the organization's managers to plan ahead. Management experience has shown that, in general, actively managed organizations will do better than those that just let things happen. A budget forces managers to establish goals. Without goals, organizations tend to wander aimlessly, rarely improving the results of their operations or the services they offer.

By requiring managers to prepare a budget at least annually, organizations compel their management to forecast the future. Changes in nursing and medical practice, technology, and *demographics* can be anticipated and their impact predicted. This allows managers to anticipate changes that will affect the organization and to plan actions accordingly. When one responds to changes after the fact, alternatives may be limited. By looking at the impact of changes during the planning phase, the broadest possible range of alternative actions can be considered. Often the result of careful planning is that more cost-effective approaches can be found and put into place.

In the budget process, after plans are made an effort is made to meet or exceed the goals of the plans. This latter effort is referred to as the *control* process. Control of costs requires a concerted effort by both managers and staff. Control techniques such as variance analysis (discussed in Chapter 13) uncover problems that may have a negative financial impact on the organization and allow actions to be taken to correct those problems at an early stage.

Budgets can be used to provide both managers and staff with the motivation to work positively for the organization. They can also show how well both management and units or departments are performing. However, budgeting requires effort and commitment from all levels of management. Often a budget committee (which should include the chief nurse executive [CNE]) is formed to ensure maximum cooperation and coordination throughout the budget process.

Many organizations produce a "budget calendar" that indicates the various specific activities to be carried out in the budget process, identifies the responsible individuals (e.g., finance office, unit or department managers, board of trustees), and provides deadlines for completion of each budget activity. Larger organizations have budget manuals. These manuals include uniform instructions and forms to be used throughout the organization, a copy of the budget calendar, and a statement of organizational mission. They also generally include a variety of other pieces of information relevant to the process of budget preparation. For instance, inflation rates, specific measurable goals, and an environmental statement are often included. Budget manuals or packages are institution specific, differing substantially from one organization to another.

The budgeting process in any organization depends as much on the specific individuals working in that organization as it does on the formalized mechanical steps involved in budget preparation and use. The role of individuals in the budget process cannot be overemphasized. Organizations not only have their own forms and procedures, but also tend to have specific philosophies of fiscal affairs. The amount of participation that any individual manager has in the budget process depends on the approach or philosophy of the organization's top management. Some organizations are top-down, allowing unit managers very limited control over their budget. Other organizations delegate substantially all budget preparation and control duties to the unit level.

Teachers of budgeting often stress the importance of participation in the budget process by individuals at all levels in the organization. If the budget is expected to be a useful tool for managing, it must be realistic. It is often not possible for top-level managers to be aware of all the specific circumstances and conditions that exist in the day-to-day operations throughout the organization. Unit managers have experience, judgment, and specific information about their units that lets them provide valuable input to the budget.

※ TYPES OF BUDGETS

Many managers tend to think of the budget as simply a cap on expenses that instructs them regarding how much they may spend. This is a very limited view of just the *operating budget*. The operating budget, in turn, is only a small part of the overall budget of the organization. A well-managed organization has a *master budget*. The master budget is a set of all the major budgets in the organization. It generally includes the *operating budget*, a *long-range budget*, *program budgets*, a *capital budget*, and a *cash budget*. Many organizations are also starting to use *product-line* budgets. From time to time the organization will also need to budget for some additional special project that is not part of the organization's normal activities. In those cases it will prepare a *special purpose budget*.

An operating budget typically plans for the revenues and expenses of the organization for the coming year. A long-range budget covers a period of three to five years. Program budgets look at specific programs that cut across a number of departments. Such budgets take a multiyear perspective. Capital budgets look at proposed equipment and building acquisitions that will be used by the organization for more than one year. Cash budgets look specifically at the organization's cash inflows and cash outflows. Product-line budgets focus on groupings of specific types of patients rather than on budgets for cost centers. Special purpose budgets are used to develop a plan for any specific special purpose not covered by one of the other types of budgets.

Operating Budget

The operating budget is the plan for day-in and day-out operating revenues and expenses for the organization. It generally covers a period of one year. If the budget shows an excess of revenues over expenses, it means that the organization expects to make a *profit* from its activities for the year. If the organization is a *for-profit* company, some of the profits can be paid to the owners of the company in the form of a *dividend*. Even not-for-profit organizations need to earn profits. Profits can be used to replace worn-out equipment and old buildings or to expand the services available to the community. If any health care organization, for-profit or not-for-profit, consistently fails to earn profits, it will not be able to add new technologies and continue to provide high-quality care. Chapter 12 provides a detailed discussion of the operating budget and its preparation.

Long-range Budgets

Budgets help managers plan for the future. Operating budgets give a detailed plan, but just for the coming year. Many changes in an organization require a long lead time and take a number of years to be fully implemented. To avoid suffering from shortsightedness, many organizations employ a long-range plan or budget. Such a budget is often referred to as a strategic plan (strategic plans are defined and discussed in Chapter 10). Such three-, five-, or even ten-year plans allow management to temporarily ignore the trees and focus on the forest. Where is the organization relative to its peer group? What improvements can be made over the next three, five, or ten years? What must be done each year to move toward those goals?

In many organizations, managers tend to look at the current year, then add an increase for inflation and produce a budget for the next year. The problem with this approach is that it contains no vision. There is no way to make a major leap forward because what has been done in the past is simply being projected into the future. If one would like to be able to look back five years from now and say, "Look at how far we have come," it is necessary to have a way to make major strides forward. Otherwise five years from now the organization will have made little, if any, advancement.

That is where long-range or strategic plans are helpful. Their focus is not on how to get through next year but on the overriding organization goals and on the major changes that ought to be made over the coming years to achieve those goals. Long-range plans help to give the organization a sense of commitment to the future. Such plans serve a vital function in allowing the organization to prepare each year's detailed operating budget on the basis of an overall sense of purpose and direction. The operating budget becomes more than just next year's survival plan; it becomes a link between where the organization has been and where it is going. Long-range budgets are discussed as part of strategic management in Chapter 10.

Program Budgets

Program budgets are special budgeting efforts analyzing specific programs. Generally the orientation is toward evaluating a planned new program or closely examining an existing program, rather than merely planning the revenues and expenses for the program for the coming year. Often the program involved is in some way optional. The purpose of the program budget is to make a decision. Should the new program be undertaken or not?

Often program budgets are developed for specific programs as a result of the long-range budgeting process. The long-range budget or strategic plan may determine that three tertiary care services should be added over the next five years. Because new services often require a year to plan and sometimes more than a year to implement once the planning phase is complete, one result of the long-range plan may be to immediately select one new service to be added. Frequently new services involve labor and equipment from numerous departments. By setting up a program budget process for the new service, all the information related to the addition of that service can be considered and evaluated.

Since program budgets often cut across departments, they generally must be developed with committee input from at least the major departments that will be affected by the service. Program budgets also cut across years. The financial impact of the service needs to be assessed not just in the coming year but over a reasonably long period. Since the operating budget is a one-year budget, this is another reason for special budget treatment for new programs or services.

In recent years business plans have become a vital tool for program budgeting. The elements of such plans are discussed along with long-range budgets and other aspects of program budgeting in Chapter 10.

Capital Budgets

A capital budget is a plan for acquisition of long-term investments. These investments can range from investments as small as acquiring a new IV pole to projects as large as completely rebuilding a hospital at a new location. The key element in capital budgeting is that the building or piece of equipment being acquired has a lifetime that extends beyond the year of purchase. Capital budget items are often referred to as *capital assets, long-term investments, capital investments,* or *capital acquisitions.* The money used to purchase long-term investments is often referred to as *capital.*

These assets are treated separately from operating budget expenses because of their multiyear nature. They are only partly used up in any one year, and in any one year the organization earns only part of the revenues that the capital assets generate over their useful lifetimes. If these assets were included in the operating budget, their entire acquisition cost would be compared with revenues only in the year the asset was purchased. Many capital assets that are good financial investments over their entire useful lifetime would appear to lose money when only one year's worth of revenues is considered. By having a separate capital budget, multiyear assets can be evaluated based on their implications for the organization over their entire useful life.

Capital assets generally are purchased to replace older items of a similar nature, to improve productivity (substituting equipment for more expensive labor), to improve quality of care (often addition of newer technology), or to provide needed equipment for a new service or expansion of an existing service. A variety of other reasons to acquire capital assets will also arise from time to time, such as for equipment that will improve employee safety.

Capital assets are often quite expensive. However, high cost is not a required element for an asset to be classified and treated as a capital asset. The only requirement is that the capital asset must be able to provide useful service beyond the year it is first put into use. For pragmatic purposes, most organizations set a minimum dollar limit for inclusion in the capital budget. It is not worth the extra effort to analyze and track relatively inexpensive items over a period of years. Items that have a low cost will be treated as part of the operating budget even if they have a multiyear life. Most health care organizations have a minimum cost requirement of anywhere from $500 to $2,000 for an item to be included in the capital budget.

Generation of Capital Budget Proposals

The starting point in the capital budgeting process is the generation of proposed investments. The nurse manager in a home health agency may propose the acquisition of several company cars to reduce travel time between patients (assuming public transportation is currently being used). The nurse manager in the coronary care unit or the operating room of a hospital may suggest the acquisition of a particular piece of equipment.

Exhibit 11–1 presents an example of the type of worksheet a nurse manager would use to list capital proposals. The first column represents the manager's priority ranking for the request. The most important acquisition is ranked number 1. The second column indicates the type of capital item being requested. These include *c*onstruction or *r*emodeling (CR), *r*eplacement of an *e*xisting item (RE), *r*eplacement and *u*pgrading of an existing item (RU), an item that is an *a*ddition to *s*imilar existing items and adds to their capacity (AS), or an *a*dditional item that is *n*ot currently available in the unit (AN).

In proposing a capital acquisition, the manager must provide financial information with respect to the asset. A required piece of information is the likely cost of the asset. Additionally, to the extent possible, information must be collected about how much cash will be spent or received each year over the life of the investment or project. The difference between the cash received and the cash spent in any given year is referred to as the *net cash flow* for that year.

The nurse manager can generally seek the aid of financial managers of the organization for the specific estimates of annual cash inflows and outflows. Cash inflows can be particularly difficult, since the entire billing process is often handled outside the control of the nurse manager. On the other hand, with respect to estimating costs, the nurse manager is more likely than any financial manager to be able to estimate what resources will be needed and when. The payroll and purchasing departments can be a great aid in converting the raw resource information into dollars based on projected salaries and prices. This estimating process should be done separately for each year that the capital asset is expected to provide useful service. Having information on the annual cash flows as well as the acquisition cost will make it easier for the organization's managers to make a decision about whether to acquire the asset.

Justification of Capital Requests

Sufficient resources are not usually available to allow an organization to acquire all the items it desires. The capital budget facilitates choices that have to be made in deciding how to spend the organization's limited resources. In describing proposed capital expenditures the nurse manager provides a priority ranking. It is also appropriate to justify each requested purchase by giving a description of the item, its cost, its impact on operating expenses and revenues, and the justification for acquiring it. Exhibit 11–2 is an example of a justification form for a capital asset acquisition.

The justification should be thorough and should specifically indicate the consequences if funding for the item is not made available. Equipment costs include not only the purchase price but also shipping and installation. Construction costs should be reviewed by the planning and engineering departments. In all cases vendor estimates or proposals should be included if possible. The impact on operating costs should include salaries, fringe benefit costs, maintenance costs or maintenance contracts, utilities, supplies, and any interdepartmental impact. Incremental revenue to be generated by the capital asset, if any, should be described and estimated to the extent possible.

※ EXHIBIT 11–1

CAPITAL BUDGET WORKSHEET

FY______

COST CENTER______________________

PRIOR. #	TYPE CR/RE/RU AS/AN	EQUIP. QTY	DESCRIPTION	UNIT COST	EXTENDED COST	COMMENTS

※ EXHIBIT 11–2

CAPITAL JUSTIFICATION FORM

FY______

COST CENTER____________________ **PRIORITY ITEM #________**

Description of item or project:

Justification:

Construction Costs:		**Equipment Costs:**	
Fees	__________	Purchase Price	__________
Construction	__________	Installation	__________
Contingency	__________		
Total	__________		

Date of Estimate____________________ By__________________________________

Impact on Operational Expenses:

Impact on Revenues:

Evaluation of Capital Budget Proposals

The capital budgets for all departments are evaluated in light of available cash. An investment that seems to make a lot of sense to a clinical department manager may have to be deferred for a year, or indefinitely, simply because the organization does not have enough cash to make the purchase.

Even if sufficient cash is available to make a capital acquisition, the organization may choose not to acquire the item because of its financial evaluation of the asset. In recent years the financial analysis of capital assets has been growing more sophisticated. Organizations have started to adopt investment analysis techniques used in other industries.

One widely used approach is the payback method. The payback approach calculates how many years it takes for the profits from a capital expenditure to repay the initial cash outlay. The less time it takes to recover the initial investment, the better the project.

The payback method does have some severe weaknesses. First, it ignores what happens after the payback period is over. Thus one might fail to select a very profitable project that does not earn substantial profits until after the payback period in favor of a less profitable project with a shorter payback period. Second, it ignores the timing of cash flows within the payback period. Two projects would be considered equal if they both have a three-year payback period. However, if one pays back the bulk of the investment in the second year and the other pays back the bulk of the invested cash in the third year, they are not equally good.

The payback method is often used for a first appraisal of the project. If a proposed investment cannot pay back its cost within a reasonable period, it should be rejected to the extent the decision is based on financial merit. If an investment passes the payback test, more sophisticated evaluation is still needed to determine if a specific proposal is acceptable.

The more sophisticated methods used to overcome the problems of the payback method are called discounted cash flow methods. These methods consider the cash flow over the full life of the capital asset rather than just the payback period. They also consider the timing of cash flows or the time value of money. The time value of money is a concept based on the fact that money paid or received at different points in time is not equally valuable. One would always prefer to receive money sooner and to pay it later. By receiving money sooner, one can use the money for current needs or can invest it and earn interest.

When a nurse manager looks at alternative investment opportunities, there must be consideration of not only how much the organization will put in and how much it will get out but also of *when* money will be spent and received. Financial managers can calculate the economic viability of a project by using discounted cash flow techniques. *Discounting* is the reverse of compounding interest. One hundred dollars today would be worth $121 in two years with 10% compound interest. In the first year, $10 of interest is earned on the $100 investment (i.e., 10% of $100 = $10). In the second year the $10 of interest earned in the first year itself earns interest. Therefore the original $100 plus the $10 of interest earned in the first year equals a total of $110. Ten percent interest in the second year would be $11 (i.e., $110 × 10%). The $110 plus the $11 would total $121. When interest earns interest, it is referred to as compound interest. In just the reverse process, $121 received two years from now would be worth just $100 today if one were to *discount* the interest earned in the two intervening years.

Discounted cash flow techniques are designed to take future receipts and discount the interest to find out what those receipts would be worth today. The receipts can then be compared with current cash outlays to determine if a project is financially worthwhile. The two most common discounted cash flow models are *net present value* and *internal rate of return.*

The net present value approach requires the manager to indicate a specific interest rate, called the discount rate. It is sometimes called the required rate of return. Under this method the cash outlay to acquire an asset must be recovered, plus a return at least equal to the discount rate. The discount rate is usually set at the rate that the bank would charge the organization if it borrowed money. Thus the capital asset must recover not only its cost but also the interest the organization would have to pay the bank if it borrowed the money necessary to buy the asset. If the project earns a positive net present value, it is earning at more than its cost plus interest. Therefore it is profitable. If the net present value is negative, the project does not even recover the investment plus the interest cost, so it is unprofitable.

The internal rate of return method does not require the manager to indicate a specific discount rate. Instead, the method looks at how much cash is required to acquire the capital asset and how much cash will be received and determines the rate of return (called the internal rate of return, or *IRR*) the asset earns. If that rate is higher than the organization's discount rate, the asset should be acquired. The technical details of calculating net present value and IRR are discussed in the appendix to this chapter.

Many times health care organizations acquire capital assets that cannot be clearly connected to specific inflows of cash. Replacing old monitors in the intensive care unit with a newer type may improve quality of care rather than increasing revenues. The use of formalized, quantitative approaches to capital investment evaluation should not and does not rule out the acquisition of assets that cannot be evaluated on a profit basis, or even those that seem to result in losses. The evaluation of capital budget requests should consider both the quantitative and qualitative benefits that any asset provides the organization and its community.

Product-line Budgets

A product line is a group of patients with some commonality that allows them to be grouped together, such as a common diagnosis. Budgeting in health care organizations is largely focused on departments and units. In all hospitals, for example, radiology has a budget, dietary has a budget, nursing has a budget. It is less common for there to be a budget for heart attack patients or child-bearing women. However, the move toward managed care may result in a new focus on budgets for enrollees in a managed care plan.

The national introduction of *diagnosis related groups* (DRGs) by Medicare in 1983 has substantially reoriented the attention of hospital managers. Since the DRG system has a fixed payment for each group of patients, it becomes of great managerial interest to be able to budget for the planned revenues and expenses of specific patient groups. Such an approach has the potential to reveal the profitability of different types of patients.

The move toward product-line budgeting has also gained impetus from the active pressure by health maintenance organizations (HMOs) and preferred provider organizations (PPOs) in negotiating with hospitals for discounted rates for specific groups of patients. It is difficult to negotiate sensible revenue rates unless the related costs of the patients are known.

Health care organizations have therefore been moving in a product-line budgeting direction while not abandoning department budgets. However, the process is difficult. Product-line costing is discussed in Chapter 8.

Cash Budgets

Cash is the lifeblood of any organization. Survival depends on the ability to maintain an adequate supply of cash to meet monetary obligations of the organization as they become due. Operating budgets focus on the revenues and expenses of the organization. If the organization is expected to lose money, that will be reflected in the operating budget. It is possible, however, for the organization to have a cash crisis even if it is not losing money. Many expenses an organization incurs are paid currently. Wages are typically paid at least monthly and frequently biweekly or weekly. However, revenues may take several months to collect because of the internal lags in processing patient bills and the external lags before organizations such as Blue Cross or Medicare make payment. Thus an organization can literally run out of cash even though it is making a profit!

Another cash problem relates to major capital expenses. Suppose the organization budgets to add a wing for $10 million and it is expected to have a twenty-year life. The full $10 million will not be an operating budget expense in the budget year. However, the entire $10 million will have to be paid in cash in the coming year.

For these reasons, a cash budget is prepared. Cash budgets plan for the monthly receipt of cash and disbursement of cash from the organization. If a shortage is predicted for any given month, appropriate plans can be made for short-term bank financing or longer term bond financing (see Chapters 15 and 16).

Cash budgeting is as vital as program, capital, and operating budgets to the survival and well-being of the organization. For this reason the nurse manager should have a reasonable understanding of cash budgets and the cash budgeting process. Additionally, often cash budget constraints force a need for modifications in the budgets nurse managers prepare. While the organization's managers should pursue various ways to get the cash for worthwhile investments—whether they are worthwhile because they are profitable or simply because they are good for the patients—there is a responsibility to the well-being of the organization not to spend the money until it is first determined that there will be sufficient cash available.

Cash Budget Preparation

In health care organizations the cash budget is generally prepared for the entire coming year on a monthly basis. Each month begins with a starting cash balance. The expected cash receipts for the month are added to this. These receipts may be broken down into categories such as inpatient, outpatient, other operating, and nonoperating or by payer (e.g., Medicare, Medicaid, Blue Cross, other insurers, self-pay patients, donations, and cafeteria sales). The starting cash balance is added to the total receipts to get a subtotal of available cash.

Expected cash payments are subtracted from the available cash. The principal categories of payments include salaries, payments to suppliers, payments for capital acquisitions, and payments on loans. The result of subtracting total payments from the available cash is a tentative cash balance. This balance is considered tentative because the organization will generally have a minimum desired cash balance at the end of each month. That minimum balance is used for cash payments at the beginning of the next month and also serves as a safety net for any required but unexpected cash outlays.

If the tentative balance exceeds the minimum desired balance, the excess can be invested. If the tentative cash balance is less than the minimum desired balance, the organization will borrow funds to meet the minimum level, if its credit is good enough. The final cash balance is the tentative cash balance less any amounts invested or plus any amount borrowed. The ending cash balance for one month becomes the starting balance for the next month.

Cash Budget Example

An example of a cash budget for the first quarter of a year is presented in Table 11–1.

In the example, the beginning cash balance for January is $20,000. With the $385,000 expected in receipts during January, there is $405,000 available in cash. With expected disbursements of $375,000, the tentative cash balance is $30,000. Assuming that $20,000 is desired as a safety cushion, there is $10,000 available to invest. In February, cash payments have risen by $25,000 to a total of $400,000, but cash receipts have risen even more. The result is that an additional $18,000 is available for short-term investment.

In March cash receipts are down and cash payments are up. What could logically cause this result? Does it indicate a serious problem? Very possibly not. It is reasonable to assume that during December, substantially fewer elective procedures were done because of the Christmas holiday season. The March cash receipts from Medicaid, Medicare, and Blue Cross are likely to be influenced by what happened in December. On the other hand, because January, February, and March may have colder weather, they are quite possibly very busy months, with high salary payments for overtime and per diem agency nurses. Thus it is not surprising to see lower cash receipts in a given month and at the same time see cash payments rising during that month. Frequently health care organizations find that in any given month their

※ **TABLE 11–1.** *Cash Budget for One Quarter*

	January	February	March
Starting cash balance	$ 20,000	$ 20,000	$ 20,000
Expected receipts			
Medicare	$120,000	$140,000	$115,000
Medicaid	80,000	90,000	75,000
Blue Cross	90,000	90,000	85,000
Other insurers	42,000	40,000	45,000
Self-pay	40,000	38,000	41,000
Philanthropy	5,000	10,000	8,000
Other	8,000	10,000	9,000
Total receipts	$385,000	$418,000	$378,000
Available cash	$405,000	$438,000	$398,000
Less expected payments			
Labor costs	$170,000	$180,000	$190,000
Suppliers	25,000	30,000	40,000
Capital acquisitions	0	10,000	15,000
Payments on loans	180,000	180,000	180,000
Total payments	$375,000	$400,000	$425,000
Tentative cash balance	$ 30,000	$ 38,000	$(27,000)
Less amount invested	(10,000)	(18,000)	28,000
Plus amount borrowed			19,000
Final cash balance	$ 20,000	$ 20,000	$ 20,000

payments reflect that month's activity, but their receipts are more influenced by what happened in earlier months.

The March tentative balance indicates a cash deficit of $27,000. Additionally, there is a desired $20,000 ending balance. The organization needs $47,000 of additional cash for March. This need can be met in several ways. The organization could simply borrow $47,000. More likely, the $10,000 invested in January and the $18,000 invested in February will be used to reduce the amount needed to $19,000; then the $19,000 will be borrowed. In Table 11–1 the $28,000 in March in the "less amount invested" row indicates a use of money previously invested.

Planning for necessary borrowing should take place well in advance. The plan developed should also include a projection of when it will be possible to repay the loan. Bankers are much more receptive to an organization's needs if it has specific plans and projections than if it simply tries to borrow money when an immediate cash shortage becomes apparent. From the bank's perspective, an organization that can plan reasonably well is more likely to be able to repay a loan than one that does not even know several months in advance that a cash shortage is likely.

Special Purpose Budgets

A budget is a plan. There is not a great deal of rigidity in the definition of a budget. Therefore, there is also not a great limitation placed on the types of possible budgets. Any health care organization can prepare a budget for any activity for which it desires a plan.

In recent years a number of health care organizations have offered screening for high cholesterol, colon cancer, diabetes, and AIDS. In some cases these screenings have been free, and in others there has been a charge. What will it cost to provide the service for free (i.e., to help the community and at the same time get some favorable press)? How much would you have to charge to just cover the costs of such a program?

Often these programs are not part of the yearly operating budget. They are special programs, put together on the spur of the moment as a public relations effort or in response to a current need. A special purpose budget can be prepared any time a plan is needed for some activity that is not already budgeted as part of one of the ongoing budget processes. The budget does not have to have any formal system or set of forms. It is desirable, however, to know the impact on staffing and on the morale of the staff. One would want to know if a profit, loss, or neither is anticipated. The key to development of a special purpose budget is to try to rationally consider all the human and financial consequences of the proposed activity.

※ THE BUDGET PROCESS

Although a budget is simply a plan, the budgeting process in health care organizations has become quite complex. To compile all the information necessary for the organization to complete a master budget, most organizations require completion of a number of complicated documents. Often a budget timetable is developed that outlines the deadlines for completion of various parts of the budget process.

Throughout the budget process it is important to consider that the budget is carried out by all employees of the organization. Therefore it is essential to involve the nursing staff in all aspects of budgeting. Their input should be solicited as the budget is prepared, as it is implemented and carried out, and after the fact as well.

One of the first steps that must be taken in the annual budgeting process is the establishment of the foundations for budget preparation. The foundations of the budgeting process consist of an environmental scan; a statement of general goals, objectives, and policies; a list of organization-wide assumptions; specification of program priorities; and a set of specific, measurable operating objectives. The information developed in these foundations provides the direction needed by unit and department managers in preparing their own budgets. Additionally, strategic plans and program budgets must be developed early in the process to provide further input needed by managers in completing budgets for specific parts of the organization.

Once that information is available, unit and department managers prepare budgets for their individual areas. That information in turn is used to compile a cash budget. After the initial round of budget preparation, it is often found that budget requests exceed resources available to the organization. Negotiation and revisions follow in an attempt to arrive at an acceptable budget. Once a budget is approved, the organization must work to control results and keep to the plan as closely as possible.

Budget Timetable

It is important to have a plan for the planning process itself. Managers should have a road map that tells them what steps must be taken in the planning process and when they should be undertaken. Table 11–2 presents a sample budget calendar or timetable. Each organization will have its own timetable. In small organizations the entire process described by the timetable may take only several months. In large hospitals the budgeting process often takes more than six months from start to finish.

Just as the length of time to complete the budget process varies from organization to organization, so do the specific elements of the budget timetable. Table 11–2 assumes a budget process for an organization with a July 1 through June 30 fiscal year. As one reviews this sample timetable, it becomes clear why budgeting is a complex task and one constantly subject to deadlines.

The first step is the appointment of the supervisory budget committee. This committee is usually selected by the chief executive officer (CEO) but may be

※ **TABLE 11–2.** *Sample Budget Timetable*

Activity	Responsibility	Deadlines
1. Appointment of budget committee	CEO	December
2. First meeting of budget committee	Budget committee chair	January
3. Complete budget foundations activities and communicate to department heads	Budget committee	February 28
4. Complete long-range and program budgets	Budget committee and subcommittees	March 31
5. Unit capital and operating budgets	Unit managers	April 15
6. Negotiation between nursing units and nursing administration	Chief nurse executive	April 22
7. Compilation of all nursing unit budgets	Chief nurse executive	April 30
8. Development of cash budget	Chief financial officer	May 15
9. Negotiation and revision process	All managers	June 15
10. Approval and implementation	Board of trustees; all managers	June 16

appointed by the board. It is especially important for the CNE to be a member of this committee. This selection process should take place as early as feasible, and the committee should meet promptly. In this example it is assumed that the committee first meets no later than January, a full six months before the next fiscal year. The committee must ensure that department heads will have the information needed to prepare their budgets. In this example, two months are allowed for that process.

During the month of March the strategic plan must be reviewed and specific programs considered. The decisions regarding these programs must be known early in the budget process so that each department head can take the impact of new programs or of program changes into account in preparing their operating and capital budgets. In actuality, the strategic plan and new programs are generally considered at some length even before the budget process begins. The month of March in this example is used to finalize decisions based on months of consideration and data collection and analysis.

Unit managers will have started preparing their budgets in early March. However, the revisions to the strategic plan and the new program budgets may result in some changes. This leaves just two weeks for unit nurse managers to finish preparing a first draft of their unit's budget. This is followed by a brief but intense period of negotiation between the nursing administration and its units. In this example, only one week is available for this negotiation process. If this period of time can be expanded, there would be less likelihood of an atmosphere of crisis and more time for reasoned discussions.

The nursing department has one week in this timetable to compile all the unit budgets into a final nursing department budget. Finance has two weeks to take the information from all the hospital budgets and develop a cash budget. One month is then allowed for organization-wide negotiation and budget revision. If all goes well, the budget can be approved by the board at its June meeting so that it can be put into effect July 1. Even with this seven-month process, delays would not be unusual (especially in negotiation and revision), which prevent developing an acceptable budget by July 1. To avoid such a situation, the process could be started earlier.

However, to start the process any earlier would mean that the information collected at the very start of the budget process would be outdated by the start of the year.

Since many aspects of the budgeting process cannot be undertaken without information generated by one of the previous activities, the budget timetable becomes a crucial guide in the budget process. Failure to meet one deadline may have an impact on all the remaining deadlines.

Statement of Environmental Position

No organization exists in a vacuum. The community, its economy, shifting demographics, inflation, the roll of a key employer, the socioeconomic setting, and other external factors play a vital role in the organization's success or failure. Each organization must understand its position within the community and its relative strengths and weaknesses. Based on knowledge of the needs of the community, the characteristics of the population, the existing competition, and other similar factors, the organization can determine its relative strengths and weaknesses and set its overall goals and objectives.

The lessons of strategic management (see Chapter 10) tell us that it is inadequate to review the environment only when the strategic plan is being formulated once every three to five years. Each year the external environment must be evaluated, and changes in the environment must be factored into the planning process.

What data can a nurse manager collect to contribute to the organization's environmental review? Although much of the demographic data will be collected by marketing and other nonclinical staff, nurse managers can contribute some critical information. For example, they can get a sense about changing physician attitudes toward the use of the organization's facilities as opposed to a competitor's. Based on their industry contacts, they may be aware of changes taking place at other organizations that will affect the competitiveness of their facilities. These types of information form part of the overall picture that the organization requires to correctly assess its position in the community.

The annual environmental analysis serves as a good review of where the organization is and where it is feasible for it to go. Having done that review, it is more likely the budgets prepared by its managers will merge the organization's desired long-term direction with its range of reasonable possible actions. The result should be a plan that is within the organization's capabilities and strives to achieve the organization's strategic goals.

General Goals, Objectives, and Policies

Once the organization's position in the environment is understood, the overall goals of the organization can be established. These goals are broad, long-term objectives, reassessed in light of the organization's strengths and weaknesses. It is not likely that goals will change annually. Over time, however, factors may arise that will cause goals to change.

For example, based on the environmental review, a home health agency may decide that the adjacent communities are underserved and that it is consistent with its mission to initiate a five-year period of geographic expansion. A nursing home may set a goal of establishing a life-care community. A hospital may decide to phase out its maternity service.

The key to long-run goal setting is that it is basically more a qualitative direction-setting process than a quantitative exercise with specific numerical objectives. The detailed numbers can be worked out later. First, the overall direction must be set. The overall goals, objectives, and policies of the organization may not change each year. They should be reviewed annually, however, if only to place in the minds of budget preparers the picture of the forest before they start to plan for the individual trees.

Organization-wide Assumptions

Throughout the budget process it will be necessary for all managers to work on the basis of some explicit assumptions. How large will salary increases be during the next year? What will the impact of inflation be on the purchase price of supplies? Will the government change its policies with respect to reimbursement of Medicare and Medicaid patients? Probably the most crucial assumptions concern workload. What will the occupancy or patient volume be in the coming year? These assumptions must be prepared annually.

Specification of Program Priorities

The next step is to establish a set of priorities for the entire organization. It is not unusual for the strategic plan, program budget, and capital budget to contain proposed spending for more things than the organization will be able to afford. There is a tendency to want to achieve all elements of a long-range plan immediately. When it becomes clear that the organization cannot do everything, a choice must be made between what is done and what is postponed.

It is advisable to try to set a generalized hierarchy of priorities at an early stage before detailed program budgets are developed. When it is necessary to make choices, top management can use the formalized guidelines that have been developed from the perspective of long-term growth and development, as opposed to letting power politics rule the budgeting process. Prioritization should be designed so that resources are allocated to areas that best promote the organization's long-term goals.

Specific, Measurable Operating Objectives

One of the most frustrating elements of budgeting for unit and department managers occurs when they are expected to develop a budget, totally unaided by any communicated guidelines, and then find the budget rejected because it does not provide for adequate achievement of objectives such as improved efficiency or reduced cost per patient day.

Organizations should provide a set of specific, measurable objectives that the budget should accomplish. This set of objectives should be communicated before the units and departments prepare their budgets. Managers can then attempt to prepare a budget that achieves those objectives. If the objectives are unattainable, managers can be prepared to explain why they feel that is the case.

The established objectives should be consistent with the overall general policies and goals of the organization, but they should be much more specific. For example, staffing reductions of 5% or ceilings on spending increases of 3% provide firm, specific objectives.

Budget Preparation

Once the foundations have been laid, the organization can establish its various budgets. Strategic plans and program budgets must be completed first. Decisions made about new programs or changes in existing programs will have a specific impact on the capital and operating costs of the various departments throughout the institution. Once that information is available, the next step in the budget process is preparation of unit and departmental budgets. The operating and capital budgets are generally prepared at the same time. Decisions concerning one budget are also likely to affect the other. For example, if the capital budget includes computer equipment for the nursing station, there may be some impact on staffing.

Having completed an operating and capital budget, the next step in the budget process is preparation of a cash budget by the finance office. This is followed by budget negotiation and revision.

Budget Negotiation and Revision

As a result of limitations on the resources available to health care organizations, budgets often cannot be accepted as submitted. Some needs will be so critical that certain departments will have to receive larger-than-average increases. However, such increases may necessitate cuts in other departments. This results in a series of negotiations, with managers having to defend why their proposed budgets should not be cut. This creates substantial complexity because most of the budgets that constitute the organization's master budget are interrelated. Changes in one type of budget can have direct ramifications on the other budgets of the organization.

For example, the capital budget for the various units and departments of the organization cannot be finalized until all program budgets have been prepared. This is because a new program may require departments to purchase additional capital items. The operating budget, in turn, must contain revenues and expenses related to capital items to be purchased during the coming year. And the cash budget cannot be prepared until after the operating budget is established.

The cash budget may show an unacceptable cash shortfall. This will necessitate a reevaluation of which programs and capital budget items provide the most benefit and which can be postponed or disapproved. These changes may result in an acceptable set of budgets that constitute the master budget. On the other hand, there may be so many vital capital expenditures that it is preferable to go back and increase revenues or cut the operating budget expenses. Or perhaps more borrowing will be planned.

Eventually, negotiation with all departments, followed by budget revisions, will result in a budget that top management feels is acceptable. Such a budget may be far from optimal. However, it represents the overall management attempt to accomplish organizational goals to the extent possible, given the limited resources available to the organization. The completed budget is sent to the board for review and approval.

Control and Feedback

The last steps in the budget process are control and feedback. Control relates to actions taken to help the organization follow its plan. Feedback relates to using actual results to improve the accuracy and usefulness of future budgets.

The control process is one in which managers attempt to keep the organization operating in an efficient manner. Much of the control process centers around variance analysis, which is discussed in Chapter 13. Variances compare actual results with the budget. The underlying causes of differences between actual results and the budget are determined. If the cause is something managers can control, actions are taken to eliminate the variance in the coming months. If the causes are beyond the control of managers, that information goes into the feedback process.

Any information about actual results that is used to improve future plans is called feedback. During the year many things will not happen according to budgeted plans. Some variations from the budget will be due to random uncontrollable events that establish no pattern. Other actual results will indicate that certain factors were not adequately considered in making the current budget. Those factors must be given more weight in the preparation of the next budget. Other elements will simply change from past patterns. Those changes will also have to be accounted for in future budgets.

※ IMPLICATIONS FOR NURSE MANAGERS

Budgeting consists of planning and controlling. The planning phase of the budget process requires that managers think ahead, anticipate changes, establish goals, forecast the future, examine alternatives, communicate goals, and coordinate plans. The controlling phase of budgeting requires that managers work to keep actual results close to the plan, motivate employees, evaluate performance of staff and units, alert the organization to major variances, take corrective actions, and provide feedback for future planning.

Each organization has its own approach to budgeting and its own philosophies regarding the budget process. Some health care organizations treat budgeting as a highly centralized process. That approach tends to generate frustration by the managers asked to carry out the budget. Other organizations call for more participation by managers throughout the organization. Such budgets tend to gain more support by the staff and are more likely to result in targets that are achieved.

The actual budgeting process requires that the organization consider its environment, define goals and policies, make assumptions for use throughout the organization, specify priorities, and define specific, measurable objectives. Each of the various types of budgets in the master budget must be prepared, and they are generally not approved without a process of review, justification, and revision. Finally, once budgets have been approved and are in place, a system must be created to control the results of operations.

Often the approved budget is more constrained than one would like. However, it is necessary to balance the long-term financial needs of the organization with the short-term quality-of-care needs for patients and the needs of the organization's employees. The final budget is a result of a compromise of these and other factors that affect the organization.

KEY CONCEPTS

Budget plan The plan is formalized (written down) and quantified (e.g., stated in dollars). It represents management's intentions or expectations.

Control Effort to meet or exceed the goals of the plans.

Operating budget Plan for day-in and day-out operating revenues and expenses for the organization. It generally covers one year.

Long-range budget or strategic plan Covers a period of three, five, or ten years. Serves a vital function as a link between where the organization has been and where it is going.

Program budgets Special budgeting efforts analyzing specific programs. They cut across departments and look at programs over their expected lifetime rather than one year.

Capital budget Plan for the acquisition of investments that will be used by the organization beyond the year they are acquired. Such assets are excluded from the operating budget because of their multiyear nature.

Time value of money Any specific amount of money is worth more today than the same amount in the future. Capital assets often require large cash outlays in the budget year. To assess the financial impact of those outlays, one must consider the time value of money.

Discounted cash-flow techniques Capital investment analysis techniques that incorporate the time value of money. The two most common are net present value and internal rate of return.

> **Net present value** Method that determines whether a proposed investment earns at least a predetermined rate of return.
>
> **Internal rate of return** Method that determines the specific rate of return earned by a proposed investment.

Qualitative analysis Evaluation of capital budget requests should consider the qualitative benefits that the asset provides the organization and its community.

Product-line budget Budget for a group of patients with some commonality that allows them to be grouped together, such as a common diagnosis.

Cash budgets Budget for the cash receipts and cash payments of the organization. Since capital expenditures require large cash outlays and revenues often are received in cash after expenses are paid, it is vital for the organization to have a plan for its cash flows.

Budget process Organization develops a statement of environmental position, a statement of general goals, objectives, and policies, a list of organization-wide assumptions, specification of program priorities, and a set of specific, measurable operating objectives. Then long-range and program budgets are prepared. Next, unit and departmental budgets are compiled. Based on those budgets, a cash budget is prepared. Based on information from all these elements, a process of negotiation and revision generally precedes budget approval. A final essential element of the budget process is control of actual results and feedback.

SUGGESTED READINGS

Cavouras, C.A., and J. McKinley, "Variable Budgeting for Staffing Analysis and Evaluation," *Nursing Management,* Vol. 28, No. 5, May 1997, pp. 34–36, 39.

Esmond, T.H., *Budgeting for Effective Hospital Resource Management,* American Hospital Association, Chicago, Ill., 1990.

Finkler, Steven A., and David R. Ward, *Cost Accounting for Health Care Organizations: Concepts and Applications,* 2nd edition, Aspen Publishers, Gaithersburg, Md., 1999.

Finkler, S.A., *Budgeting Concepts for Nurse Managers,* 3rd edition, W.B. Saunders Co., Philadelphia, Penn., forthcoming 2000.

Hughes, G., "Budget Management," *Journal of Accidental (Emergency) Medicine,* Vol. 14, No. 3, May 1997, pp. 187–188.

Johns V., "Capturing the Activity Factor: Impact on Volume," *Nursing Management,* Vol. 24, No. 12, December 1993, pp. 26–29.

McLean, Robert A., *Financial Management in Health Care Organizations,* Delmar, Albany, N.Y., 1996.

Moss, M.T., and S. Shelver, "Practical Budgeting for the Operating Room Administrator," *Nursing Economic$,* Vol. 1, No. 1, January-February 1993, pp. 7–13.

Pelfrey S., "Financial Techniques for Evaluating Equipment Acquisitions," *Journal of Nursing Administration,* Vol. 21, No. 3, March 1991, pp. 15–20.

Pelfrey S., "Managing Financial Data," *Seminars for Nurse Managers,* Vol. 5, No. 1, March 1997, pp. 25–30.

Ratcliffe, J., C. Donaldson, and S. Macphee, "Programme Budgeting and Marginal Analysis: A Case Study of Maternity Services," *Journal of Public Health Medicine,* Vol. 18, No. 2, June 1996, pp. 175–182.

Samuels, David I., *The Healthcare Financial Management and Budgeting Toolkit,* Richard D. Irwin, Burr Ridge, Ill., December 1997.

Sengin, K.K., and A.M. Dreisbach, "Managing with Precision: A Budgetary Decision Support Model," *Journal of Nursing Administration,* Vol. 25, No. 2, February 1995, pp. 33–44.

Shelver, S.R., and M.T. Moss, "Operating Room Budget Factors: A Pocket Guide to OR Finance," *Nursing Economic$,* Vol. 12, No. 3, May-June 1994, pp. 146–152.

Suver, James D., Bruce R. Neumann, and Keith E. Boles, *Management Accounting for Healthcare Organizations,* 3rd edition, Pluribus Press, Westchester, Ill., 1992.

Swansburg, Russell C., *Budgeting and Financial Management for Nurse Managers,* Jones & Bartlett Publishers, Sudbury, Mass., March 1997.

Ward, William J., Jr., *Health Care Budgeting and Financial Management for Non-Financial Managers: A New England Healthcare Assembly Book,*" Auburn House Publishers, Westport, Conn., January 1994.

Wild, J., and L. Imbrogno, "Market Changes Create Need for Practice Budgets," *Healthcare Financial Management,* Vol. 50, No. 7, July 1996, pp. 77–78.

Time Value of Money

※ INTRODUCTION

The concept of the time value of money requires sophisticated analysis to calculate the profitability of a proposed investment. The critical issue is that money received at different points in time has a different value. One would much rather have $100 today than one year from now. If you have the money today, then at the very least the $100 could be put in a bank and earn interest. A year from now you would have more than $100.

Suppose that two investments are being considered. One investment requires an outlay of $10,000 today, whereas another requires an outlay of only $7,500. Over the life of the investment the operating costs will be $3,000 each year for five years for the first alternative but $3,600 per year for the second alternative over the same five years.

	Alternative 1	Alternative 2
Initial outlay	$10,000	$ 7,500
Year 1	3,000	3,600
Year 2	3,000	3,600
Year 3	3,000	3,600
Year 4	3,000	3,600
Year 5	3,000	3,600
Total cost	$25,000	$25,500

Which alternative is less expensive?

Note that there is no revenue in this example. Often in health care the focus is on cost-efficient ways to accomplish an objective. Suppose different types of air conditioners are being compared. Over the five-year life of the air conditioners the organization will spend $25,000 for the first alternative. The second type of air conditioner is less expensive but not so fuel efficient. It will cost a total of $25,500. Which alternative is cheaper? The first project requires the organization to spend $500 less over its lifetime. But it does require spending $2,500 more at the beginning. That $2,500 could have been earning interest, thus offsetting some of the extra operating costs.

A way is needed to compare dollars spent at different points in time. Then one would be able to consider not just how much cash is involved but also when it is received or spent. Rather than solve the problem of the air conditioners now, put it aside for the time being. Let us focus attention on the methods for dealing with cash flows at different points in time. Then it will be possible to solve the problem of the air conditioner investment later in this appendix.

※ TIME-VALUE-OF-MONEY CALCULATION MECHANICS

In time-value-of-money calculations, the amount of money spent or received today is referred to as the present value (PV). The interest rate is referred to as i%. The number of interest compounding periods is referred to as N. There are several time-value-of-money calculation formulas. The most fundamental is:

$$FV = PV\ (1 + i\%)^{N}$$

This formula allows a one-step determination of the future value (FV) of some amount of money invested today (PV) at an interest rate (i%) for a period of time equal to N. Many modern hand-held business calculators have this and other time-value-of-money formulas built in. Calculators are relatively simple to use for this process. One should be sure to coordinate N and i%. If N is years, then i% is the annual interest rate. If N is months, then the annual interest rate must be divided by 12 to get a monthly i%.

So far this discussion has focused on finding out how much an amount of money held today would grow to in the future. Discounting requires that one be able to take an amount of money to be received in the future and determine what it would be worth today. That requires reversal of the compounding process. The interest rate used in the calculation is called the *discount rate.*

What if it is expected that some money will be received or spent every year rather than all at one time in the future? For instance, what is the value today of receiving $100 every year for the next three years? One way to solve this problem would be to take the PV of $100 to be received one year from now, plus the PV of $100 to be received two years from now, plus the PV of $100 to be received three years from now.

Obviously this has the potential to be a rather tedious process. Anytime payments are to be made or received and the payments are exactly the same in amount and evenly spaced in time, those payments are referred to as an annuity payment (PMT). To calculate the PV of $100 received every year for three years, the PMT = $100, N = 3, and i% = 10. A calculator could be used to determine the PV, which is $248.69. Note that FV does not enter into this calculation because there is not one single future value but rather a series of payments, all considered by the term PMT.

THE PRESENT COST APPROACH

To return to the problem raised earlier, recall that there are two potential air conditioners. One will cost $10,000 and will have operating costs of $3,000 per year for five years. The other will cost $7,500 and will have operating costs of $3,600 per year for five years. The problem of choosing one or the other concerns the fact that the total cost of the first alternative is $25,000, while the second alternative costs $25,500, but the one with the lower total cost has the higher initial cash outlay.

In today's dollars, the first alternative is $10,000 plus the present value of an annuity of $3,000 per year for five years. The second alternative is $7,500 plus the present value of $3,600 per year for five years. Assume that the discount rate is 10%. At N = 5, i% = 10, and PMT = $3,000, the PV is $11,372. When the PMT = $3,600, the PV is $13,647. Combined with the initial outlays, the PV of the first alternative is $21,372, and for the second alternative it is $21,147. Therefore, other things being equal, the second alternative would be chosen because it is less expensive when one considers the time value of money.

This method is the present-cost approach. It considers the present value of the costs of alternative projects that accomplish the same end. Assuming that both projects are just as effective in terms of accomplishing the desired outcome, the alternative with the lower cost in present value is superior.

THE NET PRESENT VALUE APPROACH

The net present value (NPV) method of analysis determines whether a project earns more or less than a stated desired rate of return, which is used as the discount rate in the calculations.

It is reasonable to assume that any investment that can earn more than the rate for borrowing money should be accepted, assuming the organization has a good enough credit rating to be able to borrow the necessary funds. Therefore the interest rate that the organization would pay on a loan is often used as the discount rate.[1]

[1]In addition, assets that earn less than the rate for borrowing money might be acquired if they have strong social merit and there are sufficient funds available to the organization to acquire the asset.

The NPV method can be used to assess whether a project is acceptable. The NPV method compares the present value of a project's cash inflows to the present value of its cash outflows, as calculated at a particular hurdle rate. If the present value of the money coming in exceeds the present value of the money going out, then the project is earning a rate of return greater than the hurdle rate. In equation form, NPV can be defined as follows:

$$\text{NPV} = \text{PV inflows} - \text{PV outflows}$$

If the NPV is greater than zero, the inflows are greater than the outflows when evaluated at the hurdle rate. If the NPV is less than zero, then the organization is spending more than it is receiving. If the NPV is exactly zero, the inflows are equal to the outflows, and the project is earning exactly the hurdle rate. In most cases financial managers rather than nurse managers will perform the actual calculations. Nevertheless, nurse managers should understand the evaluation process capital projects are subjected to prior to approval.

To find the NPV, first sum the PVs of the cash received in each year. Then find the sum of the PVs of the cash spent each year. Then compare the sum of the PVs of the inflows to the sum of the PVs of the outflows.

For example, suppose that a hospital is considering adding a new wing. There is an initial cash outflow of $10 million. Assume that the money for the wing could be borrowed at 10%. Suppose that the operating cash expenses (including information about the costs relating to nursing, which you have contributed to the analysis) and the cash revenues for each of the 20 years of the useful life of the wing are as shown in Table 11A–1. Without considering the timing of the cash flows, a total of $16,570,000 is being spent and $35,435,192 is being received. The project appears to be very profitable. Note, however, that a large amount of money is spent at the beginning of the project, while revenues are earned gradually over the twenty years.

By using present value methods, the present value of each cash flow can be

TABLE 11A–1. *An Example of Project Cash Flows and Present Values*

	Cash Flow		Present Value (PV)	
	Cash Expenses	**Cash Revenues**	**Cash Expenses**	**Cash Revenues**
Start	$10,000,000		$10,000,000	
Year 1	200,000	$ 1,000,000	181,818	$ 909,091
2	230,000	1,020,000	190,083	842,975
3	250,000	1,081,200	187,829	812,322
4	270,000	1,146,072	184,414	782,783
5	270,000	1,214,836	167,649	754,318
6	280,000	1,287,726	158,053	726,888
7	290,000	1,364,990	148,816	700,456
8	310,000	1,446,889	144,617	674,985
9	310,000	1,533,703	131,470	650,440
10	320,000	1,625,725	123,374	626,787
11	330,000	1,723,269	115,663	603,995
12	345,000	1,826,665	109,928	582,032
13	355,000	1,936,265	102,831	560,866
14	370,000	2,052,440	97,433	540,472
15	380,000	2,175,587	90,969	520,818
16	390,000	2,306,122	84,875	501,879
17	400,000	2,444,489	79,137	483,628
18	410,000	2,591,159	73,742	466,043
19	420,000	2,746,628	68,673	449,096
20	440,000	2,911,426	65,403	432,765
Totals	$16,570,000	$35,435,192	$12,506,777	$12,622,639

calculated; then the present values of the inflows and the outflows can be summed. The result is that the total PV of the inflows is $12,622,639, while the PV of the outflows is $12,506,777. The NPV, equal to the PV of the inflows less the PV of the outflows, is $115,862. Since this is greater than zero, the project is earning more than 10% and is acceptable. However, it is not nearly so profitable as it appeared at first glance.

※ THE INTERNAL RATE OF RETURN APPROACH

The principal objection to the net present value approach is that it does not indicate the specific rate of return that a project is earning. This creates problems if several capital assets exceed the hurdle rate and the projects conflict, or if there are insufficient funds to undertake all the projects with a positive NPV. The internal rate of return (IRR) method is a mathematical formulation that sets the present value of the inflows equal to the present value of the outflows. That equation is true only at the exact interest rate that a project is earning. If the equation is solved for the interest rate that makes it hold true, that is the rate of return that the project is earning.

The mathematics for calculating the IRR are complex. This is particularly true when the cash flows are not the same from year to year. However, business calculators can be used to solve for the IRR with variable cash flows.

The IRRs calculated can be used to rank projects by profitability. The IRR method tells the specific interest rate that each project is expected to return. Even if the organization is not-for-profit, it must consider that the projects with the highest return on investment, or rate of return, will provide the largest amount of cash coming into the organization in the future. That cash in turn can be used to allow for additional projects to be undertaken. By listing projects in order from the highest rate of return to the lowest, this ranking makes the project selection process far easier.

Calculators that compute time value of money calculations can be purchased for a relatively small sum, around $30. The computations can also be performed easily using a spread sheet computer program, such as the Microsoft's Excel or LOTUS 1-2-3.[2]

※ SUMMARY

Discounted cash flow techniques—including net present cost, net present value, and internal rate of return—account for the time value of money. The present-cost approach is useful for comparing alternative ways to accomplish the same goal. The method does not evaluate revenues. Both the net present value and internal rate of return methods determine whether the cash inflows are adequate to justify the cash outflow from a strictly economic point of view. The internal rate of return method additionally allows for a ranking of projects by rate of return on investment.

[2]Excel is a registered trademark of Microsoft; LOTUS 1-2-3 is a registered trademark of the LOTUS Development Corp.

KEY CONCEPTS ※

Time-value-of-money calculation mechanics Amount of money spent or received today is the present value (PV), interest rate is i%, number of interest compounding periods is N, and

$$FV = PV\,(1 + i\%)^N$$

where FV is the future value (FV).

Net present value approach Comparing the present value of a project's cash inflows with the present value of its cash outflows, as calculated at a particular hurdle rate, determines whether a project earns more or less than a stated desired rate of return.

Internal rate of return approach Method sets the present value of the inflows equal to the present value of the outflows and solves for the interest rate at which that is true.

CHAPTER

12

Operating Budgets

CHAPTER GOALS

The goals of this chapter are to:

- Explain the various factors related to preparation of an operating budget
- Define the elements of workload
- Provide a technique for calculating personnel service requirements and costs
- Provide a technique for calculating other-than-personnel service requirements and costs
- Discuss the revenue element of the operating budget
- Describe the process of budget submission, negotiation, and approval
- Consider issues related to the implementation of the operating budget

⁜ INTRODUCTION

The operating budget is a plan for the organization's revenues and expenses. It generally covers a period of one year. Preparation and control of the operating budget is probably the single most time-consuming aspect of most nurse managers' involvement with financial management.

In most organizations the manager of each cost center is directly involved in preparation of the operating budget. The finance office of the organization provides support as needed throughout the budget process. The budgets for the costs centers are consolidated, and the executive management of the organization makes final decisions on a budget to be submitted to the board for approval.

For nurse managers to begin the process of preparing operating budgets for their cost centers, they need a variety of information. Much of this information is generated by the budgeting foundations process, discussed in Chapter 11. Specifically, the information generated by the organization's environmental review and by its development of general goals, objectives, policies, organization-wide assumptions, program priorities, and specific measurable objectives is essential to the manager in preparing a budget.

That information will accomplish two primary objectives: It will enable the manager to understand the forest before becoming immersed in the trees, and it will provide specific budget preparation guidance. The environmental review and the general goals, objectives, and policies allow the manager to understand what the organization wants to accomplish and what it believes it will be able to accomplish. Program priorities provide the manager with information about the level of importance that will likely be assigned to various types of budget requests. These pieces of background information will help the manager focus on what the specific cost center should be trying to accomplish.

The organization-wide assumptions and specific measurable objectives then provide the manager with information needed to start preparing the specific details of the budget. Inflation rates and likely changes in patient volume and mix are examples of assumptions that are critical for the manager in determining likely resource requirements and costs. Measurable objectives such as an overall 3% maximum increase in unit costs provide a target to aim for in the budget development process. They also serve notice to the manager that it will be necessary to justify any proposed budget expenses that exceed those specified in the objectives or revenue categories that fall short of stated objectives.

Within nursing administration, additional background data are needed before nurse managers can commence cost center budget preparation. Specifically, the organization's approach to delivering nursing care must be clearly understood by all nurse managers. To what extent does the organization rely on LPNs as opposed to RNs? What is the role of aides? What proportion of staff works on each of the three shifts of the day, and what variations are there between weekday and weekend shifts? Is the mix of staff different on different shifts and, if so, how? The answer to these questions may vary from unit to unit. Once resolved, these guidelines may remain unchanged for a number of years (although they should be reviewed annually for needed changes).

Information from long-range and program budgets (discussed in Chapter 11) should also be available to unit managers as they begin their budgeting process. The addition of new services or programs will have a direct bearing on the planning of the budget for each cost center affected, even if only indirectly. For example, the addition of certain types of esoteric surgery may result in increased demands upon the recovery room, postsurgical intensive care units (ICUs), or even the general medical/surgical units.

Similarly, if other units or departments of the organization are planning changes in procedures, that information must be communicated to all relevant cost centers. For example, if pharmacy plans to ask nursing units to reconstitute more drugs on the unit, this will save money in the pharmacy but will likely increase nurse staffing needs on the units. Coordination, cooperation, and communication are vital to arriving at an operational plan that is best for the organization as a whole and allows all cost centers to plan their budgets according to their work requirements.

Once the background information required to commence the budget process is available, nurse managers can move forward to prepare the three primary elements of the operating budget: the expense budget for personnel, the expense budget for costs other than personnel services, and the revenue budget. All nursing cost centers have expense responsibility. Many hospital nursing units are not required to prepare revenue budgets. However, some cost centers managed by nurses, such as the operating room (OR), do have revenue responsibility. The role of nursing with respect to revenue is growing and is discussed in this chapter. After the budget is prepared, it must be submitted and possibly negotiated prior to approval. Once it is approved, it must be implemented and controlled.

The development of the operating budget discussed in this chapter is one possible approach to calculating the elements of the budget. Various institutions will have specific forms and specific step-by-step procedures. Therefore the forms used in this chapter and the order of the steps taken in developing the budget should not be viewed as the focal points; rather, one should try to understand the elements of the budget—what items must be included and why. A conceptual understanding of the operating budget will allow the reader to adapt to a wide variety of types of organizations and to the specific procedures of any organization.

※ WORKLOAD BUDGET

To prepare the revenue or expense portions of the operating budget, the first step is to ascertain the volume of work for the coming year. The amount of work performed by a unit is referred to as its *workload.* Workload is often measured in terms of *units of service.* A unit of service is the measurement of the work performed by the cost center. Workload may be measured in a variety of ways, such as the number of patients, patient days, deliveries, visits, treatments, or procedures. Each cost center must determine the measure that is most appropriate for its unit of service.

Units of service can provide a meaningful basis for both revenue and expense calculations. For example, a patient may be charged based on the number of hours an operation takes. Hours of operations represent the unit of service. That measure may also be used as a starting point in developing the staffing needs for the OR.

Once a cost center defines its key unit or units of service, it must predict the number of units of service that will be provided in the coming year. This will allow development of the operating budget. In some organizations nurse managers may be told a specific number of units of service to use in their budget. In many cases, however, the nurse manager will have to forecast that number. In fact, given the specific knowledge a unit manager has about that specific cost center, probably the individual nurse manager is in the best position to forecast units of service for the cost center. (See Chapter 18 for specific forecasting techniques.)

In addition to units of service, it may be necessary to forecast things such as the average length of stay or the mix of patients by Diagnosis Related Group (DRG) or severity of illness. Once these forecasts are made, the nurse manager will translate the work that must be done into a set of personnel and other-than-personnel resource requirements.

Activity Report

One aid in forecasting the coming year budgeted workload is the *activity report.* This report measures key statistics concerning current activity. It centers on both the number of units of service and the relative proportion of the organization's capacity that is being used. For example, in a hospital or nursing home the most common measure of capacity is the number of beds available for patients in total. The *census* represents the number of these beds occupied each day at a certain point in time (usually midnight). The occupancy rate is the percentage of total beds filled. For example, if a nursing home has 120 beds and on average 108 of them are occupied, it has a 90% occupancy rate (i.e., 108 filled beds ÷ 120 total beds × 100%).

Two other statistics commonly found in an activity report are the *average daily census* (ADC) and the *average length of stay* (ALOS). The average daily census is the number of patients cared for per day on average over a period of time. One patient cared for, for one day, is a patient day. The ADC is found by dividing the number of patient days over the time period by the number of days in the period. The ALOS is the average number of days that each patient is in the hospital or nursing home. It is found by dividing the total number of patient days by the total number of admissions. Outpatient providers of health care collect similar data, such as the average number of visits or treatments.

The activity report is valuable, but it must be used with care. Patients tend not to be *homogeneous.* Knowing the number of patient days is inadequate for planning purposes. A more useful budget for a medical/surgical unit would be developed if the manager knew the type of patients and their severity of illness rather than just the number of patient days. An OR needs to know the types of different procedures rather than simply the number of hours of operations. The same total number of patients in two different years can have widely differing nursing care costs if they represent a different mix of patients. The unit of service often needs adjustment for patient mix in the budget process, whether we are considering inpatient surgery or home health visits.

Adjusting Units of Service

As a consequence of the heterogeneity of patients, whenever possible budgeting should be based on adjusted units of service. For example, in the case of a hospital, the number of medical/surgical patient days for a nursing unit can be adjusted using a system for classifying patients based on the resources they are expected to use; this is often referred to as patient acuity.

The most general approach to using patient classification is to determine workload based on required hours of nursing care. Suppose that a medical/surgical unit expects to have 9,000 patient days for the coming year. Rather than trying to determine a budget based solely on the number of patient days, an estimate can be made based on the acuity level of the 9,000 patient days. For example, assume that a unit classifies patients into one of five categories from 1 to 5. The 9,000 patient days might be expected to be as follows:

Patient Classification	Number of Patient Days
1	1,500
2	3,700
3	2,400
4	900
5	500
Total	9,000

Segregating the 9,000 patients into the five classifications allows the operating budget to be developed based on the resource requirements of the specific mix of patients expected for the unit.

Calculating Workload

For the separation of patient days or visits or treatments by classification level to be valuable for budgeting, there must be a way to differentiate resource consumption by patients in each category. Patient classification systems generally provide information on the average required care hours per patient day per twenty-four hours for each level or per visit or treatment. The number of hours of care are based on a specific staff mix. If the staff mix changes, the required hours of care at any patient classification level also change.

Using expected patient classification information, it is possible to determine the number of care hours for these 9,000 patient days. For example, assume the average care hours are as shown in Table 12–1.

In this case, the total care hours required for the year, based on the organization's patient classification system, is 60,820 for this unit. Based on 9,000 patient days, the care hours per patient day on average are 6.76 (60,820 care hours divided by 9,000 patient days).[1]

Note, however, that one cannot assume, based on the above, that for this particular nursing unit 6.76 care hours per patient day is a permanent standard. The

[1]An alternative approach to measuring workload is to use a relative value unit (RVU) system. In such an approach a specific level of patient classification is chosen to be assigned an acuity index value of 1. All other levels are assigned RVUs based on the amount of hours of care they require relative to the index level. For example, if classification level 2 were set to a relative value index of 1, and if classification level 5 required four times as many care hours as level 2, then level 5 would be assigned a relative value of 4. The advantage of the RVU scale over the average required hours scale is that the RVU scale describes the patient population, whereas the average required hours scale focuses on the resources required to treat the population. For a further discussion of using RVUs for acuity and staffing see Christina Graf, "The Operating Budget," in Steven A. Finkler, *Budgeting Concepts for Nurse Managers*, 2nd edition, W.B. Saunders, Philadelphia, Penn., 1992, Chapter 8.

※ **TABLE 12–1.** *Required Patient Care Hours*

Patient Classification	Number of Patient Days	×	Average Care Hours per 24-hour Period	=	Total Unit Workload
1	1,500		2.5		3,750
2	3,700		4.7		17,390
3	2,400		8.0		19,200
4	900		12.2		10,980
5	500		19.0		9,500
Total	9,000				60,820

6.76 care hours result is sensitive to the expected mix of patients each year. Suppose, for instance, that the original mix of patients had been:

Patient Classification	Number of Patient Days
1	1,100
2	3,000
3	2,600
4	1,400
5	900
Total	9,000

In that case the total work load is 71,830 care hours, calculated as in Table 12–2.

The total care hours of 71,830 divided by 9,000 patient days is 7.98 care hours per patient day. Without the total number of patient days having changed at all, the change in the mix of patients calls for an increase in nursing care hours of 18%, from 6.76 to 7.98! On average, patient resource requirements have risen from 6.76 hours of care per patient day to 7.98 hours. To accurately budget for expenses it is essential that the anticipated workload be specified as accurately as possible. That is the purpose of adjusting units of service for the specific anticipated mix of patients. Similar calculations can be made in ambulatory settings. All that is required is a method to classify patients into different categories and to estimate the average resource consumption for patients in each category.

※ EXPENSE BUDGET: PERSONNEL SERVICES

Once the manager has a workload forecast, the next step is to start the process of determining the staff requirements for the unit. These requirements include all personnel under the manager's direction, usually including RNs, LPNs, aides, and clerical staff. Additionally, other types of employees may be part of the unit, such as technicians, orderlies, and unit hostesses.

There are no universally accepted standards for staffing levels. Each institution

※ **TABLE 12–2.** *Required Patient Care Hours for Revised Patient Mix*

Patient Classification	Number of Patient Days	×	Average Care Hours per 24-hour Period	=	Total Unit Workload
1	1,100		2.5		2,750
2	3,000		4.7		14,100
3	2,600		8.0		20,800
4	1,400		12.2		17,080
5	900		19.0		17,100
Total	9,000				71,830

has unique physical plant characteristics, a unique mix of services offered and types of patients, and its own philosophy concerning the appropriate provision of care. Therefore the mix of staff and standard care hours deemed appropriate will vary from one health care organization to another. The patient classification system in place provides the institution's assessment of the care hours required per patient by classification level. It often does not address the mix of staff, which is discussed below.

Calculation of staffing requires more than simply knowing the total number of hours of care to be provided per patient day on average. To explain how staffing needs can be determined, we will use an example. Assume that the number of hours of care needed by a thirty-bed medical/surgical unit is 71,830. This number was calculated earlier for an expected workload of 9,000 patient days, spread across five different patient-classification levels.

Average Daily Census and Occupancy Rate

Assuming that the unit is open 365 days of the year, we can start by calculating the average daily census (ADC) and the occupancy rate.

$$\begin{aligned} \text{ADC} &= 9{,}000 \text{ patient days} \div 365 \text{ days per year} \\ &= 24.7 \text{ patients per day} \end{aligned}$$

$$\begin{aligned} \text{Occupancy} &= 24.7 \text{ patients per day} \div 30 \text{ beds} \times 100\% \\ &= 82\% \end{aligned}$$

This information is important to managers because it indicates the capacity of the unit to expand its service. Recall from Chapter 7 that since some costs are fixed and some are variable, volume is critical. As volume rises, revenues tend to rise in direct proportion. Costs also rise but less than proportionately. That means that increases in patient volume are especially profitable. The 82% occupancy rate seen here indicates that there is still substantial physical capacity for expansion of the services provided by this unit.

Outpatient providers can also calculate an "occupancy" or utilization type of statistic if they believe their capacity is limited. The volume of patients would be divided by the number of days per year the organization provides service. It might be closed Sundays and holidays. If so, those days are excluded in calculating average patients per day. The average patients per day is divided by the capacity to find the occupancy equivalent for the organization.

Staffing Requirements and Full-time Equivalents

Next we need to consider staffing requirements for the number of expected hours. In this case, 71,830 hours of care are required. How many staff members will be needed to provide that care? Some people work full-time; others part-time. We need a way to distinguish between those who are full-time workers and those who are not. The approach that has been developed is to distinguish between *positions* and *full-time equivalent* (FTE) employees. One person working for the organization for any number of hours per week occupies a position. One person who works full-time is a full-time employee. Any number of positions that combine to provide the hours of work of a full-time employee is an FTE.

Thus one employee working full-time is one FTE. So are two employees each working half-time. They occupy two positions but generate only one FTE of work. Staffing calculations must first determine how many FTEs are required. Then those FTEs can be provided by filling any number of positions that add up to that amount of FTEs.

One FTE gets paid for full-time work. That is most commonly pay for eight hours per day, five days per week, fifty-two weeks per year, or a total of 2,080 hours per year.[2] However, the staff needed to provide the 71,830 required care hours cannot be determined by dividing 71,830 by 2,080. That would assume that all 2,080 paid hours per FTE were productive hours. The 2,080 paid hours include "nonproductive" time. Vacations, sick leave, holidays, and any other nonworked time are nonproductive hours. The organization may also count time worked, but away from the nurse's unit, as nonproductive. For example, this would include things such as time spent at educational seminars. Since the 71,830 hours represent needed care hours, we must relate them to productive hours rather than paid hours.

Productive vs *Nonproductive Hours*

How can one distinguish between productive hours and nonproductive hours? This information is generally available from reports that payroll provides to each unit. The report shows the total paid hours as well as the number of nonworked hours or worked but nonproductive hours in each category. Based on paid and worked hours over the last twelve months, the nurse manager can determine an average number of productive hours per FTE. This requires dividing total worked hours by total paid hours and multiplying by 100% to arrive at a percentage of paid hours that are productive. For example, assume that for this unit for the previous twelve months:

Productive hours: 75,480
Paid hours: 94,350
$(75{,}480 \div 94{,}350) \times 100\% = 80\%$

This means that 80% of paid hours are productive. There are 0.8 productive hours for every paid hour.

Using a standard 2,080 paid hours per FTE, we could then determine how many productive hours one would expect from each FTE:

$$2{,}080 \text{ paid hours} \times 80\% = 1{,}664 \text{ worked or productive hours per FTE}$$

The total care hours, 71,830, can be divided by the 1,664 productive hours per FTE to find the number of FTEs needed.[3] In this example, the result of that division is 43.17 FTEs. Based on decisions made by the organization, that FTE total will be separated into different types of staff members (RN, LPN, aide) and assigned to different shifts. Those 43.17 FTEs will be responsible for providing direct and indirect care twenty-four hours per day, seven days per week, all year long.

Assignment of Staff by Type and Shift

One should not assume that there will be 43.17 staff members working each day. The 43.17 FTEs represent an adequate number to provide care seven days per week, every week. On any given day some people are sick or on vacation, taking a holiday, or taking one of their "weekend" days (not necessarily on the weekend). How many staff members will actually be working each day? The total hours of care required was 71,830 over a period of one year. Dividing the 71,830 by 365 days in a year produces the required care hours per day on average.

$$71{,}830 \text{ care hours} \div 365 \text{ days per year} = 197 \text{ hours of care per day}$$

---

[2]In some geographic areas it is common for employees to work a 7.5 hour day. This totals to 37.5 hours per week or 1,950 paid hours per year per FTE. Some organizations use seven ten-hour shifts per two-week period for an FTE. That adds up to 1,820 paid hours per year. Each organization can set its own standard number of paid hours per FTE.

[3]As noted in Footnote 2, not all organizations use 2,080 paid hours for one standard FTE. Regardless of the number of paid hours per FTE for a specific organization, the percentage of productive paid hours can be multiplied by the total paid hours per FTE to find how many productive hours are provided per FTE. That can be divided into the total hours of care needed to determine the number of FTEs needed.

※ TABLE 12–3. *Allocation of Staff by Type and Shift*

Staff Type	Staff Allocation	7–3 Shift	3–11 Shift	11–7 Shift	Total
	100%	45%	35%	20%	
Staff nurse	65%	7.2	5.6	3.2	16.0
LPN	25%	2.7	2.2	1.2	6.1
Aide	10%	1.1	.9	.5	2.5
Total		11.0	8.7	4.9	24.6

Assuming that employees work eight-hour shifts, that results in 24.6 person-shifts per day (197 hours per day divided by eight hours per shift = 24.6 shifts).[4] These 24.6 person-shifts per twenty-four hours must be allocated by shift and by type of employee. Suppose that this medical/surgical unit has a predetermined pattern that requires approximately 65% RN staff, 25% LPN, and 10% aides. Assume further that the scheduling standard is 45% days, 35% evenings, and 20% nights. These numbers, like the others in this chapter, are hypothetical. In practice, these standards must be established by the nursing department based on its decisions about the most appropriate division of staff for this specific unit.

Table 12–3 spreads the available 24.6 person-shifts across the various staff categories and shifts. First, the total number is calculated for each type of staff. Since 65% of shifts are to be covered by staff nurses, 65% of the 24.6 is allocated to the staff nurse category, generating the 16.0 in the total column for the staff nurse row. Then 25% and 10% are used to allocate 6.1 total LPNs and 2.5 total aides.

The next step is to take 45% of the total for each type of staff and allocate that to the 7–3 shift. Of 16 staff nurses, 45% is 7.2, so there will be 7.2 staff nurses on the 7–3 shift each day. Continuing, 45% of 6.1 is 2.7, and 45% of 2.5 is 1.1. This step is repeated for the 3–11 shift and 11–7 shift using 35% and 20%, respectively. The results of these calculations fill in the numbers of staff on each shift, by type of staff, as shown in Table 12–3.

This provides a basic guideline for the manager. However, the manager will next want to make some minor modifications to determine the actual number of people to be on duty on each shift (Table 12–4). In this case, the manager might decide to decrease the number of staff nurses on the 7–3 day shift to an even 7, instead of using the exact 7.2 that had been calculated. The number of RNs (staff nurses) on the 3–11 shift was increased to 6, while the number on the 11–7 shift was decreased to 3. This leaves the total of staff nurses at 16 per day. The LPN category, on the other hand, is increased somewhat on the day shift and reduced on the other two shifts. The total coverage has also been reduced by 0.1. Similar changes are made in the aide category. The total number of shifts per day has been reduced from 24.6 to 24.5.

After the manager modified the categories, the percentages are recalculated. This allows the manager to see how far from the guidelines the actual proposed staffing pattern has varied as a result of the adjustments. The new total for each shift is divided by the new total shifts, and the new total for each type of staff is divided by the new total for all shifts to get the updated percentages. For example, in Table 12–4 there are now 4.5 total employees on the night shift. Dividing 4.5 by 24.5 total shifts gives 18.4%, as compared to the guideline of 20%. Most of the percentage changes for

[4]Alternately, 197 divided by 10 equals 19.7 ten-hour shifts per day. Use of ten- or twelve-hour shifts instead of eight-hour shifts does not create a problem for finding the number of persons needed on duty each day. However, if the length of shift creates overlapping shifts (the second shift comes on duty before the first shift goes off duty), then the manager must plan work activities with care to ensure that patients receive all required care and productivity levels are maintained.

※ TABLE 12–4 *Final Allocation of Staff by Type and Shift*

Staff Type	Staff Allocation	7–3 Shift	3–11 Shift	11–7 Shift	Total
	100.0%	44.9%	36.7%	18.4%	
Staff nurse	65.3%	7.0	6.0	3.0	16.0
LPN	24.5%	3.0	2.0	1.0	6.0
Aide	10.2%	1.0	1.0	.5	2.5
Total		11.0	9.0	4.5	24.5

both shift and staff type were reasonably small in this example; large variations from the guidelines would require specific justifications.

It is important to bear in mind that the required total staffing hours are based on the hours needed per patient at differing patient classification levels. However, the hours per patient are established based on a specific staff mix. If the staff mix changes substantially, then the required hours might change as well. In this example, the changes in actual staff mix from that pre-established are minor and would not require any adjustment.

The patterns developed here also assume that staffing is the same throughout the week. If some days are particularly busy or slow, it would be possible to have a daily staffing guide. In that case the total number of shifts per week would be kept at approximately the target level (i.e., 24.6 shifts per day × 7 days per week = 170.2 shifts per week). However, these 170.2 shifts per week could be allocated so that there would be more than 24.6 shifts on some days of the week and less on others.

Fixed Staff

In addition to the staff calculated above, there are employees who do not vary with patient volume. This includes the unit manager, perhaps clinical specialists, and clerical staff. Such staff members are budgeted in addition to the staff retained to directly fill the 71,830 required hours of care. Often such staff members are not replaced when they are sick or on vacation. In those cases there is no need to calculate sufficient hours to provide coverage when they are out, as was done with the staff FTEs.

Table 12–5 adds fixed staff to the patient care staff in the example. In the table a nurse manager, a clinical specialist, three secretaries (one per shift), and one clerk

※ TABLE 12–5. *Staff by Type and Shift (Including Fixed Staff)*

Staff Type	7–3 Shift	3–11 Shift	11–7 Shift	Total
Fixed Staff				
Nurse manager	1.0			1.0
Clinical specialist	1.0			1.0
Clerk	1.0			1.0
Secretary	1.0	1.0	1.0	3.0
Subtotal	4.0	1.0	1.0	6.0
Variable Staff				
Staff nurse	7.0	6.0	3.0	16.0
LPN	3.0	2.0	1.0	6.0
Aide	1.0	1.0	.5	2.5
Subtotal	11.0	9.0	4.5	24.5
Total	15.0	10.0	5.5	30.5

have been added. Note that it is assumed that there is only one manager, with no coverage when that manager is not present on the unit. This clearly represents fixed staffing. On the other hand, a secretary is required during all three shifts, every day. Therefore, enough FTEs will have to be hired to ensure that the secretarial position is filled every single day. Nevertheless, the secretaries are still fixed staff, because they do not vary with the number of patients. Were the expected 9,000 patient days to increase or decrease by 5%, 10%, or 15%, the unit would not employ more or fewer secretaries.

Converting Staff and FTEs to Positions

At this point the number of shifts per day and the number of FTEs needed have been calculated. The next step is to convert this information into the specific positions that will be needed to provide that care. Specifically it is necessary to determine how many full-time and part-time employees will be needed, how much overtime, and how much per diem agency time.

Calculating FTEs by Type and Shift

To establish staff positions, it is necessary to calculate the relationship between shifts per day and FTEs. If the manager divides the 43.17 required FTEs by the 24.5 daily staff shifts, it turns out that each person-shift calls for employing 1.76 FTEs. Recall that one FTE will provide coverage one shift per day, five days per week, fifty-two weeks per year, less vacation, holiday, and other nonproductive time. An adequate number of FTEs are needed to provide for the other two days out of seven per week plus the vacations, holidays, and so on. It is important to note that the staff who were hired to fill in two days per week, plus vacation, holidays, and other nonproductive time, will *themselves* be taking vacations, holidays, and so on. Therefore, it is not unreasonable to find that coverage of one shift for 365 days per year would require the organization to employ 1.76 FTEs.

Table 12–6 converts the number of staff who are needed to the number of FTEs to be employed. For those employees for whom coverage is not provided when they are on vacation or are otherwise being paid for nonproductive time, the number of person-shifts from Table 12–5 is identical to the number of FTEs in Table 12–6. For example, the one nurse manager shown in Table 12–5 remains as one FTE in Table 12–6.

For each position that must be covered 365 days per year, the number of

TABLE 12–6. *FTEs by Type and Shift (Including Fixed Staff)*

Staff Type	7–3 Shift	3–11 Shift	11–7 Shift	Total
Fixed Staff				
Nurse manager	1.0			1.0
Clinical specialist	1.0			1.0
Clerk	1.0			1.0
Secretary	1.8	1.8	1.8	5.4
Subtotal	4.8	1.8	1.8	8.4
Variable Staff				
Staff nurse	12.3	10.6	5.3	28.2
LPN	5.3	3.5	1.8	10.6
Aide	1.8	1.8	.9	4.5
Subtotal	19.4	15.9	8.0	43.3
Total	24.2	17.7	9.8	51.7

※ **TABLE 12–7.** *FTEs Divided by Straight Time (ST) and Overtime (OT)*

	7–3 Shift			3–11 Shift			11–7 Shift			Total		
Staff Type	**ST**	**OT**	**Total**	**ST**	**OT**	**Total**	**ST**	**OT**	**Total**	**ST**	**OT**	**Total**
Fixed Staff												
Nurse manager	1.0		1.0							1.0		1.0
Clinical specialist	1.0		1.0							1.0		1.0
Clerk	1.0		1.0							1.0		1.0
Secretary	1.8	—	1.8	1.8	—	1.8	1.8	—	1.8	5.4	—	5.4
Subtotal	4.8	—	4.8	1.8	—	1.8	1.8	—	1.8	8.4	—	8.4
Variable Staff												
Staff nurse	12.0	.3	12.3	10.5	.1	10.6	5.0	.3	5.3	27.5	.7	28.2
LPN	5.0	.3	5.3	3.5		3.5	1.5	.3	1.8	10.0	.6	10.6
Aide	1.8	—	1.8	1.8	—	1.8	.9	—	.9	4.5	—	4.5
Subtotal	18.8	.6	17.6	15.8	.1	15.9	7.4	.6	8.0	42.0	1.3	43.3
Total	23.6	.6	22.4	17.6	.1	17.7	9.2	.6	9.8	50.4	1.3	51.7

person-shifts from Table 12–5 is multiplied by 1.76.[5] For example, the 7 person-shifts for staff nurses from 7 AM to 3 PM (see Table 12–5) when multiplied by 1.76 becomes 12.3. This procedure is carried out for each type of staff member for each shift.

Establishing Positions

The 12.3 FTE staff nurses could be provided by hiring twelve full-time staff nurses and having those twelve nurses additionally share a total of 0.3 FTEs of overtime. Or it could be staffed with twenty-four half-time nurses and 0.3 FTEs of per diem agency nurses. Or it could be staffed by any of a wide variety of other combinations.

Once the manager knows how many FTEs are needed for each shift for each type of employee, the next step is to divide the FTEs into straight time (ST) and overtime (OT), as is shown in Table 12–7. This division will depend on organizational policy and on practical realities. In this example the policy of the organization is to never use overtime for more than 0.5 FTE for any type of employee on any shift. It is assumed that if more than 0.5 FTE is needed, it can be supplied by hiring a half-time employee, which would be less costly than paying an overtime premium to a full-time employee. For example, a total of 1.8 FTEs are needed for LPNs on the 11–7 shift. It is assumed that 1.5 FTEs will be filled at straight time, probably by using one full-time employee and one half-time employee. The remaining 0.3 FTEs will be filled by overtime.

In some cases, it is assumed that there is even more flexibility that allows overtime to be avoided. For example, 1.8 FTEs are needed for secretaries on each shift. However, the straight-time *vs* overtime breakdown differs from that used for the LPN on the 11–7 shift. It is assumed by the organization in this example that secretaries are easier to hire on a part-time basis than clinical staff. Therefore, no overtime is planned. It must be expected that the organization can hire secretaries who will work part of an FTE as needed by the organization. A similar assumption is made about aides.

Once the separation of straight time and overtime is made, the FTEs shown in

[5]Note that 1.76 is not an industry standard. It depends on the portion of paid time that is productive at a specific institution. In this example we want to cover each position eight hours a day for 365 days per year. That means we need 2,920 productive hours (365 × 8). On the basis of our productive/total paid time ratio of 0.8, we determined that we get 1,664 productive hours/FTE (2,080 paid hours/FTE × 0.8). If we divide 2,920 required hours by 1,664 productive hours/FTE, we find that we need 1.76 FTEs for each position covered one shift for 365 days per year.

Table 12–7 can be converted into specific numbers of positions, as shown in Table 12–8. This budget is a link between resources required to care for patients and the cost of the resources. By converting FTEs into the specific number of full-time and part-time positions, the manager can start to assign specific individuals to positions to provide patient care. By determining the number of hours that each position will be paid for at straight time and overtime, the manager is beginning to develop the specific information that will be needed to determine the cost of the personnel resources. Often the current-year positions budget is used as a guide in preparing the positions budget for the coming year.

Table 12–8 is derived by taking the information from Table 12–7 that indicates the number of FTEs needed on each shift by type of employee. The FTEs are split between full-time and part-time employees according to the manager's perception of staffing needs. In some cases full-time employees are desired for continuity of care; in others part-time employees are desired because they allow the manager greater flexibility in filling in for vacations, holidays, and other nonproductive time.

According to the number of positions column of Table 12–8, a total of fifty-nine individuals will be hired by the unit, either full-time or half-time. However, that is not always the case. A variety of staffing patterns are observed. For example, under fixed staff in Table 12–8, note that it is assumed that one secretary can be hired to

※ TABLE 12–8. *Positions and Hours Budget*

Position Title	Shift	Number of Positions	ST FTEs	ST Hours	OT FTEs	OT Hours	Total FTEs	Total Hours
Fixed Staff								
Nurse manager	7–3	1	1.0	2,080	.0	0	1.0	2,080
Clinical specialist	7–3	1	1.0	2,080	.0	0	1.0	2,080
Clerk	7–3	1	1.0	2,080	.0	0	1.0	2,080
Secretary: full-time	7–3	1	1.0	2,080	.0	0	1.0	2,080
Secretary: part-time	7–3	1	.8	1,664	.0	0	.8	1,664
Secretary: full-time	3–11	1	1.0	2,080	.0	0	1.0	2,080
Secretary: part-time	3–11	2	.8	1,664	.0	0	.8	1,664
Secretary: full-time	11–7	1	1.0	2,080	.0	0	1.0	2,080
Secretary: part-time	11–7	4	.8	1,664	.0	0	.8	1,664
Subtotal		13	8.4	17,472	.0	0	8.4	17,472
Variable Staff								
Staff nurse: full-time	7–3	11	11.0	22,880	.3	624	11.2	23,296
Staff nurse: part-time	7–3	2	1.0	2,080	.0	0	1.1	2,288
Staff nurse: full-time	3–11	10	10.0	20,800	.1	208	10.1	21,008
Staff nurse: part-time	3–11	1	.5	1,040	.0	0	.5	1,040
Staff nurse: full-time	11–7	5	5.0	10,400	.3	624	5.3	11,024
Staff nurse: part-time	11–7	0	.0	0	.0	0	.0	0
LPN: full-time	7–3	5	5.0	10,400	.3	624	5.3	11,024
LPN: part-time	7–3	0	.0	0	.0	0	.0	0
LPN: full-time	3–11	3	3.0	6,240	.0	0	3.0	6,240
LPN: part-time	3–11	1	.5	1,040	.0	0	.5	1,040
LPN: full-time	11–7	1	1.0	2,080	.3	624	1.2	2,496
LPN: part-time	11–7	1	.5	1,040	.0	0	.6	1,248
Aide: full-time	7–3	1	1.0	2,080	.0	0	1.0	2,080
Aide: part-time	7–3	1	.8	1,664	.0	0	.8	1,664
Aide: full-time	3–11	1	1.0	2,080	.0	0	1.0	2,080
Aide: part-time	3–11	1	.8	1,664	.0	0	.8	1,664
Aide: full-time	11–7	0	.0	0	.0	0	.0	0
Aide: part-time	11–7	2	.9	1,872	.0	0	.9	1,872
Subtotal		46	42.0	87,360	1.3	2,704	43.3	90,064
Total		59	50.4	104,832	1.3	2,704	51.7	107,536

work 0.8 FTEs on the 7–3 shift. On the 3–11 shift, it is expected that two part-time employees will split 0.8 FTEs, and on the 11–7 shift four employees will make up 0.8 FTEs. Under variable staff it is noted that even though twelve full-time staff nurses could have been hired for the 7–3 shift, eleven full-time and two half-time positions are used. This may provide a greater degree of staffing flexibility for the manager.

Calculating Labor Cost

Once the positions have been identified, the next step is to determine the labor cost. This will include straight-time hours, overtime hours, differentials, premiums, and benefits.

Straight-time and Overtime Salaries

Table 12–8 indicates the paid hours related to the positions. These hours are calculated based on the number of FTEs for each position at a rate of 2,080 paid hours per FTE. For example, two part-time aide positions have been established on the 11–7 shift. Those two positions total 0.9 FTEs. Multiplying 0.9 by 2,080 hours results in a total of 1,872 paid straight-time hours for that employee type. It is important to know the paid hours for overtime separately from total paid hours because overtime is generally paid at a higher rate.

As a check in the process, it would be appropriate to determine if the number of care hours budgeted is approximately the number that had earlier been calculated as being required. Recall that for these 9,000 patients, it was determined that 71,830 care hours were needed. From Table 12–8 it is noted that the variable staff subtotal for total hours is 90,064. These represent paid hours. Since 80% of paid hours are productive, according to the earlier calculations, 80% of 90,064 is the budgeted number of care hours. Multiplying 80% by 90,064, the result is 72,051. This is almost exactly the required care hours.[6]

On the basis of hours by type of employee, a cost budget can be prepared. This can be done either by using an average wage rate by category or by listing each of the individuals who will fill the positions and specifying their exact pay rate. The latter approach is more time-consuming but also more accurate.[7] In Table 12–9 the straight-time (ST) and overtime (OT) hours are taken from Table 12–8, and an average wage is used for each class of employee for each shift. That average would generally be based on the manager's knowledge of the specific individuals making up each category.

The rates used in the budget should be based on the anticipated rates for the coming year. That rate includes any raises over current rates. In some cases raises are an across-the-board percentage; in other cases raises may differ by type of employee or even employee by employee.

In some cases, top management may change the amount of raises built into the operating budget. They may either raise or lower the amount of raises calculated in the initial preparation of the budget. This may require recalculation of the entire budget. It is advisable to prepare all budgets on computers, using a spreadsheet program such as the widely used Excel or LOTUS 1-2-3 programs.[8] If such a program is used, hourly rates used in the budget preparation can be changed and a new budget generated without the manager having to manually recompute the entire

---

[6]The difference of 221 care hours over the course of the year is a rounding error. We had originally expected to need 43.2 FTEs. The actual plan resulted in 43.3 FTEs, a minor difference.

[7]See Christina Graf, "The Operating Budget," in Steven A. Finkler, *Budgeting Concepts for Nurse Managers*, 2nd edition, W.B. Saunders, Philadelphia, Penn., 1992, p. 192, for an example of that detailed approach.

[8]Excel is a registered trademark of Microsoft; LOTUS 1-2-3 is a registered trademark of the LOTUS Development Corp.

※ **TABLE 12–9.** *Personnel Cost Budget*

Column:		A	B	C	D	E	F	G	H	I
Position Title	**Shift**	**ST Hours**	**Average Rate**	**Shift Premium**	**Total ST Rate (B + C)**	**Total ST $ (A × D)**	**OT Hours**	**OT Rate (D × 1.5)**	**Total OT $ (F × G)**	**Total $ (E + H)**
Fixed Staff										
Nurse manager	7–3	2,080	$28.00	$0.00	$28.00	$ 58,240	0	$ N/A	$ 0	$ 58,240
Clinical specialist	7–3	2,080	24.50	0.00	24.50	50,960	0	N/A	0	50,960
Clerk	7–3	2,080	6.50	0.00	6.50	13,520	0	9.75	0	13,520
Secretary: FT	7–3	2,080	11.00	0.00	11.00	22,880	0	16.50	0	22,880
Secretary: PT	7–3	1,664	10.00	0.00	10.00	16,640	0	15.00	0	16,640
Secretary: FT	3–11	2,080	11.00	1.00	12.00	24,960	0	18.00	0	24,960
Secretary: PT	3–11	1,664	10.00	1.00	11.00	18,304	0	16.50	0	18,304
Secretary: FT	11–7	2,080	11.00	2.00	13.00	27,040	0	19.50	0	27,040
Secretary: PT	11–7	1,664	10.00	2.00	12.00	19,968	0	18.00	0	19,968
Subtotal		17,472				$ 252,512	0		$ 0	$ 252,512
Variable Staff										
Staff nurse: FT	7–3	22,880	$21.50	$0.00	$21.50	$ 491,920	624	$32.25	$20,124	$ 512,044
Staff nurse: PT	7–3	2,080	24.00	0.00	24.00	49,920	0	36.00	0	49,920
Staff nurse: FT	3–11	20,800	20.00	2.00	22.00	457,600	208	33.00	6,864	464,464
Staff nurse: PT	3–11	1,040	22.00	2.20	24.20	25,168	0	36.30	0	25,168
Staff nurse: FT	11–7	10,400	18.50	2.78	21.28	221,260	624	31.91	19,913	241,173
Staff nurse: PT	11–7	0	20.00	3.00	23.00	0	0	34.50	0	0
LPN: full-time	7–3	10,400	14.00	0.00	14.00	145,600	624	21.00	13,104	158,704
LPN: part-time	7–3	0	15.00	0.00	15.00	0	0	22.50	0	0
LPN: full-time	3–11	6,240	13.50	1.35	14.85	92,664	0	22.28	0	92,664
LPN: part-time	3–11	1,040	14.00	1.40	15.40	16,016	0	23.10	0	16,016
LPN: full-time	11–7	2,080	13.00	1.95	14.95	31,096	624	22.43	13,993	45,089
LPN: part-time	11–7	1,040	14.00	2.10	16.10	16,744	0	24.15	0	16,744
Aide: full-time	7–3	2,080	8.00	0.00	8.00	16,640	0	12.00	0	16,640
Aide: part-time	7–3	1,664	8.00	0.00	8.00	13,312	0	12.00	0	13,312
Aide: full-time	3–11	2,080	8.00	.80	8.80	18,304	0	13.20	0	18,304
Aide: part-time	3–11	1,664	8.00	.80	8.80	14,643	0	13.20	0	14,643
Aide: full-time	11–7	0	8.00	1.20	9.20	0	0	13.80	0	0
Aide: part-time	11–7	1,872	8.00	1.20	9.20	17,222	0	13.80	0	17,222
Subtotal		87,360				$1,628,110	2,704		$73,999	$1,702,108
Total		104,832				$1,880,622	2,704		$73,999	$1,954,620

budget. Such a computerized approach is also advisable because it will ease the process of budget revision necessitated by any other changes in the budget as well.

Note that the wage rates for the same type of employee tend to vary by shift and by whether the employee is full-time or part-time. Since part-time employees may not receive the same benefits as full-time employees (perhaps no pension, life-insurance, etc.), it may be necessary to pay a higher hourly wage to attract sufficient numbers of part-time employees. In some cases the less desirable shifts may be staffed by less senior staff, and therefore their base rate is lower than for those working on the day shift.

Such rate differences tend to be highly idiosyncratic. For instance, in this example the base pay rate for aides is the same on all shifts for both full-time and part-time employees. Part-time secretaries receive a lower hourly base wage than full-time. Part-time RNs and LPNs receive a higher hourly wage.

If positions are vacant, care must be exercised in selecting an appropriate pay rate. Will those positions most likely be filled by entry-level employees at the lowest wage rates or by experienced employees at higher pay levels? Managers should try to assess who will be hired to keep the budget as accurate as possible.

That assumes that vacancies are filled. In some cases, positions may remain open for some time. According to Graf, "If float, per diem or agency staff are used only rarely to cover temporarily vacant positions, then the dollars allocated to the vacant positions can be assumed to cover the alternate staff and the nurse manager can be authorized to hire into all positions."[9]

If it is known that a fair amount of per diem agency time will be used even if positions are not vacant, then those hours should be converted to FTEs and budgeted for in addition to the staffing shown in Table 12–8.

Differentials and Premiums

Table 12–9 provides a calculation of personnel cost based on average wage rates. Average rates can be obtained from the personnel or payroll offices or by simply averaging the specific rates paid to current staff members. It is common for health care organizations to provide a higher wage for evening and night shifts and sometimes for weekend shifts. There are two common approaches for including these costs in the budget. One is to calculate the total lump-sum cost of the differentials to the unit. The other approach is to adjust the hourly wage of employees to include the differential.

To calculate differentials on a lump-sum basis it is necessary to calculate the number of evening and night hours by class of employee for all the days per year and multiply that by the differential for that class of employee. For example, in the shift premium column in Table 12–9 we note that secretaries on the night shift receive a $2 per hour differential. There are 2,080 and 1,664 total night hours scheduled for full-time and part-time secretaries, respectively. That adds up to 3,744 hours for the year. At $2 per hour differential, the night secretary differential will be $7,488 (i.e., $2 per hour × 3,744 hours). That amount and the differential for each other class of employee must be added into the total personnel cost. The lump-sum approach is especially useful if differentials are stated by the organization on an annual basis per FTE rather than on an hourly basis.

The alternative approach is to calculate the differentials as shown in Table 12–9. This figure specifically adjusts the straight-time hourly wage of each class of employee (column B) based on the appropriate shift differential (column C). This adjustment results in a total straight-time rate (column D) including the differential (i.e., column B + column C = column D).

In this example some differentials are a flat dollar amount and some are based on a percentage of base salary. In the case of secretaries, there is a $1 per hour premium

---

[9]Graf, *op. cit.*, p. 187.

for working the 3–11 shift and a $2 per hour premium for working the 11–7 shift. The clinical staff in this example receive a 10% differential for the 3–11 shift and a 15% differential for the 11–7 shift. For example, note in column C of Table 12–9 that a full-time 3–11 shift LPN, paid a base wage of $13.50, earns a shift differential of 10%, or $1.35 per hour, while a full-time 11–7 shift LPN, paid a base wage of $13.00, earns a shift differential of 15%, or $1.95 per hour. The ST rate from column D, which includes the differential, is multiplied by the straight-time hours from column A (taken from Table 12–8) to find the cost of straight-time wages (column E).

An overtime rate is calculated in column G by multiplying the column D straight-time rate by 1.5. The resulting overtime rate is multiplied by the column F overtime hours, which came from Table 12–8, to find total overtime dollars (column H). The column I combination of straight-time and overtime wages gives the total of these two cost elements.

Overtime in this example was calculated at time and a half. In some organizations the straight-time salary is increased by 50% for overtime, and then the shift differential is added. If the differential is added to the straight-time salary and then the rate is increased by 50%, the resulting wage is higher than if the differential is added after the salary has been multiplied by 150%.

Weekend differentials, holiday premiums, and on-call premiums create additional complexities in the calculations of personnel cost. A complete budget will consider all factors that affect the total salary received by each employee in each position. The specific approach to calculating these premiums differs from organization to organization. Effectively, however, the manager must determine the hourly differential or premium; the number of weekend, holiday, and on-call shifts per year; the number of employees on each of those shifts; and the total cost of those differentials. That total cost must be added into the budget for the unit.

Fringe Benefits

An additional element of personnel cost is fringe benefits. Fringe benefits are costs of employees in addition to their salary. Fringes typically include health and life insurance, pension costs, Social Security (FICA) payments, and other employee benefits. Generally, an average fringe benefit rate is calculated and applied on a uniform basis to payroll costs. The calculation of the fringe benefit rate itself is generally performed by the finance or payroll departments. In some organizations those departments adjust the budgets of each department or unit to include fringe benefits. In other cases they communicate the rate, and the unit or department managers increase their budgets by the amount of the fringe benefits.

For example, Table 12–10 shows the addition of fringe benefits to personnel cost in our example. In this organization, two different fringe benefits rates are used, one for full-time and one for part-time personnel. Frequently, part-time employees receive substantially fewer benefits than full-time employees. By calculating two rates to be used, the manager realizes the financial impact on the organization of the decision of using full-time *vs* part-time personnel to provide the needed FTEs. Keep in mind, however, that there is a trade-off, as noted earlier. While part-time employees have a lower fringe benefit cost to the organization, they may have a higher hourly base salary.

In Table 12–10, the total personnel costs before fringe benefits (column A) is from the last column in Table 12–9 (column I). Those costs (column A, Table 12–10) are multiplied by the appropriate fringe benefit rate to find fringe benefit costs (column C). The cost before fringe benefits (column A) plus the fringe benefit cost (column C) is the total personnel cost (column D).

Special Situations

A variety of specific situations may require that the manager make additional calculations. An important element of the budget process is for the manager to think

※ **TABLE 12–10.** *Personnel Cost Budget (Including Fringe Benefits)*

Column:		A	B	C	D
Position Title	**Shift**	**Total Cost before Fringes**	**Fringe Rate**	**Fringe $ (A × B)**	**Total Personnel Cost (A + C)**
Fixed Staff					
Nurse manager	7–3	$ 58,240	23.5%	$ 13,686	$ 71,926
Clinical specialist	7–3	50,960	23.5	11,976	62,936
Clerk	7–3	13,520	23.5	3,177	16,697
Secretary: FT	7–3	22,880	23.5	5,377	28,257
Secretary: PT	7–3	16,640	14.3	2,380	19,020
Secretary: FT	3–11	24,960	23.5	5,866	30,826
Secretary: PT	3–11	18,304	14.3	2,617	20,921
Secretary: FT	11–7	27,040	23.5	6,354	33,394
Secretary: PT	11–7	19,968	14.3	2,855	22,823
Subtotal		$ 252,512		$ 54,288	$ 306,800
Variable Staff					
Staff nurse: FT	7–3	$ 512,044	23.5%	$120,330	$ 632,274
Staff nurse: PT	7–3	49,920	14.3	7,139	57,059
Staff nurse: FT	3–11	464,464	23.5	109,149	573,613
Staff nurse: PT	3–11	25,168	14.3	3,599	28,767
Staff nurse: FT	11–7	241,230	23.5	56,676	297,849
Staff nurse: PT	11–7	0	14.3	0	0
LPN: full-time	7–3	158,704	23.5	37,295	195,999
LPN: part-time	7–3	0	14.3	0	0
LPN: full-time	3–11	92,664	23.5	21,776	114,440
LPN: part-time	3–11	16,016	14.3	2,290	18,306
LPN: full-time	11–7	45,089	23.5	10,596	55,685
LPN: part-time	11–7	16,744	14.3	2,394	19,138
Aide: full-time	7–3	16,640	23.5	3,910	20,550
Aide: part-time	7–3	13,312	14.3	1,904	15,216
Aide: full-time	3–11	18,304	23.5	4,301	22,605
Aide: part-time	3–11	14,643	14.3	2,094	16,737
Aide: full-time	11–7	0	23.5	0	0
Aide: part-time	11–7	17,222	14.3	2,463	19,685
Subtotal		$1,702,108		$385,917	$2,088,025
Total		$1,954,620		$440,205	$2,394,826

about various additional costs that are incurred every year but not included or accounted for in the budget. Such hidden costs can result in a failure to meet the budget. However, the failure is not the result of poor control of operations but rather poor planning. To avoid such problems it is essential that managers understand how their staff uses its time and whether any factors are not adequately accounted for in the existing budget formulation.

※ EXPENSE BUDGET: OTHER-THAN-PERSONNEL SERVICES

The personnel budget is often by far the largest part of the operating budget for a nursing unit or department or a home health agency. However, a complete budget also requires inclusion of a budget for expenses for other-than-personnel services (OTPS). The nurse manager should exercise care in this portion of the budget, even if it is substantially smaller than the personnel budget. Miscalculations made in this element of the budget may lead to a need to cut back costs during the year. Often such cutbacks can only be made in the area of personnel. Thus an underestimated budget for clinical supplies may negatively affect a nursing unit's ability to provide high-quality care.

The nonpersonnel portion of the operating budget, the OTPS budget, includes a wide variety of items, such as clinical supplies, office supplies, minor equipment (noncapital budget items), seminars, books, and a variety of *overhead* items. Overhead is indirect costs charged to the unit or department from other departments. Some overhead is at least partly controllable by the unit, such as the cost of laundry. The more laundry used by a department, the higher the overhead charge for laundry. Other elements of overhead are completely outside the unit manager's control, such as administrative salary or building depreciation charges.

OTPS expenses may be for either fixed or variable items. Clinical supplies, for example, are variable. Their cost should be determined based on the expected number and mix of patients. Publications for the nursing department are a fixed cost. Assuming that publications (such as management journals or newsletters) are ordered by the organization only for the use of managers, the number of patients would have no effect on that cost. Managers must determine a budgeted amount for publications on a somewhat more subjective basis.

Table 12–11 provides a budget worksheet for OTPS costs. This worksheet is generally a summary of detailed supporting schedules providing calculations for each of the lines in the worksheet. The worksheet provides information on actual costs incurred to date, the budget for the current year, a projection of total costs for the current year, and the proposed budget for the coming year.

The projection for the current year can be done in one of two ways. The simpler approach is to divide the current year-to-date actual result by the number of months it covers to get an average monthly amount. That amount could then be multiplied by 12 to get an annual projection. A more accurate approach would be to assess whether the remaining months of the year are likely to be busier or slower than the year has averaged up to the current time. The projected annual totals could be estimated after adjusting for expected activity levels. These two approaches are primarily useful for variable costs.

※ TABLE 12–11. *Costs for Other-Than-Personnel Services (OTPS)*

	Year-to-Date Actual	Current Year Budget	Current Year Projection	Proposed Budget
Direct Unit Expenses				
Med/surg supplies	$126,533	$187,546	$191,249	$216,237
Office supplies	8,348	12,493	13,021	15,027
Noncapital equipment	14,325	17,094	17,000	18,255
Seminars	23,450	28,000	27,655	30,000
Publications	1,788	2,000	2,000	2,100
Other	7,351	10,000	10,000	10,500
Total direct unit OTPS	$181,795	$257,133	$260,925	$292,119
Overhead Expenses				
Administration	$ 28,345	$ 42,517	$ 43,394	$ 45,234
Depreciation—buildings	34,592	51,888	51,888	51,888
Depreciation—equipment	18,492	27,738	27,738	29,956
Laundry	13,295	21,340	22,431	24,390
Pharmacy	8,391	12,309	13,125	14,150
Laboratory	11,090	14,398	15,232	16,342
Duplication	3,113	4,310	4,100	4,100
Communications	14,321	19,430	19,834	21,079
Other	8,310	12,321	12,500	12,857
Total overhead OTPS	$139,949	$206,251	$210,242	$207,139
Total OTPS	$321,744	$463,384	$471,167	$499,258

For fixed costs, the manager must determine the typical expenditure patterns. If these costs are incurred reasonably evenly throughout the year, the average monthly approach is adequate. If all seminars and meetings take place during certain months of the year, then a specific calculation of remaining seminars will need to be made to project the current year total. Similarly, if publications and equipment are all purchased near the beginning of the year (to have their benefit throughout the year) or near the end of the year (after the manager has a feeling for whether spending cuts will be needed near year-end), then the manager will have to take those factors into account in making the current year projection.

Developing an accurate current year projection is worth a reasonable effort because it is an important starting point in planning the OTPS costs for the coming year. Much of that cost is based on an increase or decrease as compared with current-year spending. If the level of photocopying stays the same from year to year, this year's actual duplication costs serve as a primary guide to developing next year's budget.

Costs for the coming year can be developed based on sophisticated forecasting techniques (see Chapter 18), which rely on historical and current information as well as the manager's knowledge and intuition. A simpler, although possibly less accurate, approach is to project next year's budgeted cost as being the current-year cost increased by a percentage for inflation.

In some instances the manager will be able to prepare a budget based on specific circumstances. If turnover is expected to be unusually high because of planned retirements or maternity leave, a higher budget for training new staff may be necessary. The specific number of individuals who will need such training can be estimated and a budget developed. That number may not bear much relation to costs incurred currently or in the recent past. Rather, the costs will relate primarily to the number of new staff. As Graf points out:

> The key to budgeting nonsalary expenses . . . is to identify the most reasonable predictor . . . and to make expense projections based on that predictor. In some cases, more than one predictor may be needed. For example, assume that the delivery room's disposable linen account includes linen packs for . . . deliveries and . . . scrub clothes packs for fathers attending deliveries. The predictor for the linen packs is logically the number of deliveries. . . . The predictor for the scrub clothes packs, however, may be the attendance at prepared childbirth classes.[10]

The predictor approach will be quite useful for some OTPS accounts, but noncapital equipment typically requires a more direct approach. During the current year managers should accumulate lists of noncapital equipment needed for the unit. Any such items that cannot be accommodated during the current year within the existing budget would be explicitly included in the operating budget for the coming year. In addition, at budget preparation time the manager should consider and specify equipment needs. Therefore this category is less likely to be just a repeat of the prior year adjusted for patient volume or inflation, in contrast to a category such as medical/surgical supplies.

⨳ REVENUE BUDGET

Nursing is critical to the revenues of the organization. Without a nursing staff providing services, it is unlikely that hospitals, nursing homes, home care agencies, or a number of other kinds of health care organizations would be able to provide care and earn revenues. However, the association of revenues with nurses has been uneven. Some nurse managers have always had revenue responsibility; a few

---

[10] Ibid., p. 196.

examples include the OR, outpatient surgery, and clinics managed by nurses. In other cases, nursing has little if any revenue responsibility.

Even in cases where nursing does not have to calculate revenue for the budget or control revenue results, it is important for nurse managers to learn about the key determinants of revenue in their organization. The revenue base is critical to the organization's survival and its ability to provide resources to the various departments.

In recent years revenue has become more and more a direct concern for nurse managers. Patient classification systems have substantially increased the feasibility of variable billing for nursing services. Rather than simply including nursing as a part of the per diem charge, it is possible to charge patients for nursing each day at different amounts based on their classification for that day (see the discussion of variable billing in Chapter 8). Although home health agencies have always billed for nursing services, hospitals have only recently started to bill directly for nursing care, and nurse managers are becoming more involved in the revenue aspects of the budget.

Calculation of Budgeted Revenue

Gross patient revenue is the number of units of service times the price per unit. As discussed in Chapter 6, there are a variety of reasons for the net revenue received being less than gross patient revenues. Those reasons include contractual allowances, bad debts, and indigent care. Generally, nurse managers do not have to calculate reductions from gross revenues.

On the other hand, the units of service that are useful for estimating the expense portion of the budget are not necessarily appropriate for the revenue part of the budget. For example, the OR may calculate its expense budget by considering the number of each type of procedure it expects to have, with differing staffing and supplies costs for different types of procedures. However, patients are generally charged based on minutes or hours of operations. Therefore the OR would have to estimate both the total numbers of hours of operations (to get a revenue budget) and the total number of each type of procedure (to develop an expense budget).

In health care organizations, departments do not generally set prices. The prices the organization charges are set by the finance department based on a large number of factors, including government reimbursement regulations, prices of competitors, and a need to earn enough revenues in total to cover all costs and allow for desired expansions and improvements, if possible.

For example, the federal government sets the rates for Medicare hospital inpatients under the DRG system. Those rates cover the entire stay of the patient, and they are not broken out separately by unit or department. Similarly, state governments generally set rates for Medicaid patients. Health care organizations must estimate the amount that they expect to receive from those patients for whom they cannot set the price, such as Medicare and Medicaid patients. They then set prices for the remaining patients high enough to bring in remaining revenues needed by the organization to carry out its mission.

Even when revenues are per patient, such as DRG revenues, many health care organizations do have prices for the various services provided by many departments. Different services provided by a department will have different prices. In preparing a revenue budget it is necessary to get a price list from the finance office and apply it individually to each different type of patient. For example, there is likely to be a different standard charge for different types of outpatient surgery. Also, different payers often pay different amounts for the same procedure. A managed care organization may have negotiated a lower rate for surgery for its patients than the rate for self-pay patients. Once the revenue for each type of service is determined, the revenue for all the different services can be summed to arrive at total budgeted department revenue.

Variable Billing

The use of patient classification systems not only provides information for calculating staffing needs and personnel costs more accurately but also provides the ability to charge directly for nursing services. The main constraint most health care organizations face with respect to charging for nursing services (as opposed to lumping them in with per diem costs) is that there is no ready way to determine the different nursing costs the organization incurs for different patients. Patient classification systems eliminate that problem.

When patients are charged for various types of health care services, there is generally an attempt to charge patients for the resources they consumed. If a patient does not have an operation, there is no surgery charge. A patient who has a more expensive operation than another is charged a higher amount. Patients are charged for the number and type of x-rays, lab tests, and drugs they consume. As long as patients consume different amounts of a resource and those differences can be measured, then patients can reasonably be charged for the resources they consume. If those requirements are not met, costs are frequently lumped together in a catchall category such as the per diem charge.

It is clear that different patients consume different amounts of nursing care. Historically, however, there was not a reasonable method available to determine the differing nursing resources consumed by different patients. To track nursing resources consumed would have required extensive data-collection efforts at an extremely high cost.

Patient classification systems provide a solution to this problem. It is not necessary to measure the actual nursing costs of each individual patient. Instead, a special study establishes the average relative consumption of nursing resources by patients in each classification level. Suppose that a hospital's patient classification system indicates that level 2 patients consume 4.7 hours of care on average and level 4 patients consume three times as much care. A charging system can be established with patients being charged three times as much for each day that they are classed as level 4 as they are charged for each day that they are classed as level 2.

A number of hospitals have started to budget and charge for revenue based on variable billing tied to patient classification. The process is not complicated. Suppose that the hospital established nursing rates, based on an examination of nursing department costs, of $150 for a patient day at level 1, $250 for a patient day at level 2, $500 for level 3, $700 for level 4, and $1,100 for level 5, for a typical medical/surgical unit. Assuming the same mix of patients used in the example earlier in this chapter, budgeted revenue could be calculated as in Table 12–12.

Home health agencies charge different amounts for visits by different providers. Other health care organizations also charge for nursing services if they can determine varying nursing consumption by different patients.

※ BUDGET SUBMISSION, NEGOTIATION, AND APPROVAL

The three elements of the operating budget—personnel services expenses, other-than-personnel services, and revenues—must be compiled into a coherent total document for submission. The budget may not be accepted as submitted, in which case a period of negotiation and budget revision will take place. Finally the budget is approved.

The submitted budget should include an overview page that summarizes the revenues and expenses of the unit or department. In some cases, only expenses are calculated at the unit or department level, and revenues are not part of the operating budget process. In addition to the budget's overview or summary page there should be detailed schedules that support the requested amounts. Each number from the

※ TABLE 12–12. *Variable Billing Revenue Calculation*

Patient Classification	Number of Patient Days	×	Charge per 24-hour Period	=	Budgeted Revenue
1	1,100		$ 150		$ 165,000
2	3,000		250		750,000
3	2,600		500		1,300,000
4	1,400		700		980,000
5	900		1,100		990,000
Total	9,000				$4,185,000

summary page should be easily traceable to its supporting documentation through titles on the supporting schedules and/or by a series of references.

The supporting schedules should contain not only numerical calculations, like those in Tables 12–3 through 12–12, but also narrative support. The narrative defines the unit of service used for the budget, the sources of projections for the coming year, and explanations of why the requested amounts are needed. It should also discuss the ramifications of denying the full requested amounts.

Negotiation of the budget usually follows its submission. Because health care organizations' resources are limited, requests for funds are often in excess of the amount available. The subsequent reductions in the budget requests should be done in a way that best allows the organization to accomplish its goals and objectives. The budget negotiation process was discussed in Chapter 11.

Once the negotiation and revision process are completed, the budget can be approved by top management and the board. If they do not approve the submitted budget, it must be further revised until it is approved. The manager must then implement the approved budget.

※ IMPLEMENTING THE APPROVED BUDGET

The development of the operating budget and its ultimate approval are in many ways just the beginning of the budget management process. The manager must convert the approved resources into a working document that can guide specific staffing decisions throughout the year.

The manager must address a number of specific problems. First, a staffing schedule must be developed to allow the number of positions approved to be used to fill the daily staffing need. Recall that in the example there was a need for 30.5 shifts per day on average (including fixed staff [see Table 12–5]) and a total of fifty-nine staff positions to fill those shifts. It is necessary to determine when those fifty-nine individuals will be working.

That is a complicated task. Not only must there be coverage seven days per week, but holiday and vacation coverage must also be planned. Further, there must be flexibility to deal with sick leave, which does not occur on a planned basis. If turnover is expected, the manager must also be able to deal with low productivity of new workers during their orientation period.

An additional complicating factor is the seasonal nature of many health care organizations. There are busy periods and slow periods. Adequate staff must be available to work the busier periods; that requires maintaining a lower staffing level during slower periods. Sometimes that problem can be somewhat offset by using float pools, which allow for "borrowing" nurses from other units during busy periods and "loaning" nurses to other units during slow periods. That, however, requires a commitment on the part of the nursing department and the nursing staff to cross training.

Finally, a key element of the implementation process is control. An attempt must be made to keep as close to the approved plan as possible. Control aspects of budgeting are discussed in the next chapter.

⁂ IMPLICATIONS FOR NURSE MANAGERS

The operating budget often consumes more of a nurse manager's time than any other aspect of financial management; for that reason it is worthy of special attention. The three aspects of operating budgets are revenues, personnel expenses, and other-than-personnel expenses.

Revenue is becoming more important to nurse managers. For many years health care organizations received revenues as a reimbursement for costs. Governments and large third-party payers such as Blue Cross based the amount paid to health care organizations directly on the costs those organizations incurred. Recent years have seen a movement away from cost reimbursement. As a result, revenues must be managed to a greater extent. Over time, this will likely lead to more nursing involvement in the area of organizational revenues. At a minimum, nurse managers should prepare operating budgets with an understanding of the implications of the budgets for revenue.

Some proposed changes in operating budgets will lead to changes in revenues, and other changes will not. It is vital for nurse managers to consider whether a proposed change has an impact on both costs and revenues or solely on costs. Cutting costs may seem to promote organizational efficiency, but one must consider whether the expense reduction will affect the organization's revenues.

For example, suppose that hours per patient day of care were decreased to reduce costs. This might lead to a longer length of stay. The extra days would be costly in themselves. Furthermore, if the hospital had high occupancy, the increased length of stay would reduce the number of possible admissions. That would have a direct negative impact on revenues.

Increasing expenses may seem to jeopardize the organization's finances, but once again the short-run and long-run impact on revenues must be considered. Spending money to increase quality of care, for example, may improve the organization's reputation, leading ultimately to more patients and more revenues. Spending money to provide more nursing care hours per day may shorten average length of stay, allowing for more patients and therefore more revenues.

In placing a growing focus on revenues, the nurse manager must not reduce the effort spent on budgeting unit or departmental expenses. Nursing departments have the largest budget in many health care organizations. The amounts spent by nursing can have a dramatic impact on the organization. A 5% change, either up or down, in the costs of the nursing department will affect the organization by a greater total dollar amount than a 5% change in any other area. As a result, nurses have an obligation equal to that of other managers throughout the organization to carefully consider the resources needed by their units or departments to provide patient care.

The largest element of nursing operating budgets usually is labor. Personnel costs dominate, largely because the clinical care provided by the nurse is essential to the process of providing health care services. To account for labor costs as carefully as is warranted requires a lengthy and complicated budgeting process. A work-load budget must be developed specifying care hours needed. The work-load estimate must be as accurate as possible, adjusting for patient mix whenever possible. Care hours are converted to FTEs and positions. FTEs and positions are converted to dollar costs.

The process as described in this chapter is laborious for the manager. However, it is essential. Two critical things are at stake in the proper preparation of the personnel budget for nursing. One is the ability of the organization to survive; the other is the ability of the organization to provide patients with high-quality care.

Budgets not prepared with the greatest measure of care may lead to wasted resources. Overstaffing on one shift or one unit is a mistake that may lead to understaffing elsewhere due to inadequate total resources. The budgeting process attempts to allocate the organization's scarce resources to the areas where they are most needed to achieve the organization's objectives. Any resources allocated to a unit where they are not essential represent a failure to allocate those resources to parts of the organization where patients had a greater need for them.

The goal of budgeting is neither to maximize nor minimize a budget. It is important for managers to overcome the adversarial impulse that naturally arises in the budgeting process. The goal of budgeting is to develop a plan that places the organization's available resources in the appropriate places where the sum total accomplishment of the organization goal's will be the greatest.

KEY CONCEPTS

Workload budget Budget that indicates the amount of work performed by a unit or department, measured in terms of units of service. This information is used to prepare expense budgets.

Activity report Measures key statistics concerning current activity. It centers on the number of units of service and the relative proportion of the organization's capacity being used.

Average daily census (ADC) Number of patients cared for per day on average over a period of time.

Average length of stay (ALOS) Average number of days that each patient is in a hospital or nursing home.

Adjusted units of service Whenever possible, budgeting should be based on expected workload units of service adjusted for the specific mix of patients expected.

Care hours calculation Determination of the average required care hours per patient per twenty-four hours for each classification level and the total required care hours for all patients.

Expense budget: personnel services Budget for all personnel under the manager's direction.

Variable staff Staff needed to provide the required number of care hours, calculated as follows:

1. Determine the number of paid hours per FTE.
2. Determine the percentage of productive hours to total paid hours.
3. Multiply the number of paid hours per FTE by the percentage of productive hours to find the number of productive hours per FTE.
4. Divide required care hours by productive hours per FTE to find the required number of FTEs.
5. Divide the required care hours by the number of days per year that the unit has patients to find care hours per day. Divide that result by hours per shift to find the number of person shifts needed per working day.
6. Assign staff by employee type and among required shifts per day.

Fixed staff In addition to the staff calculated above are employees who do not vary with patient volume.

Establishing positions Daily staff requirements can be met by a variety of full-time and part-time positions that add up to the required number of FTEs. The breakdown between full-time and part-time is at the manager's discretion.

Calculating labor cost Each position's hours must be converted to a dollar basis considering straight-time salary, overtime rate, differentials, raises, and fringe benefit costs for each employee type.

Expense budget: other-than-personnel services Budget for all expenses for other-than-personnel services, including both direct unit or department expenses and indirect overhead expenses.

Revenue budget Plan for the unit's or department's revenues for the budget year. Variable billing is leading to an increased role of revenues in nursing budgets.

Budget submission Revenue and expense portions of the budget must be summarized and submitted for review together with detailed supporting calculations and narrative justification. Budget revisions may be required as the result of a series of negotiations over the submitted budget.

Budget implementation Managers must address a number of issues in implementing an approved budget, including development of a staffing plan that provides coverage for staff weekends, holidays, vacations, and sick leave as well as busy and slow periods.

SUGGESTED READINGS

Bender, A.D., "Budget Model Can Aid Group Practice Planning," *Healthcare Financial Management*, December 1991, pp. 50–59.

Cavouras, C.A., and J. McKinley, "Variable Budgeting for Staffing Analysis and Evaluation," *Nursing Management*, Vol. 28, No. 5, May 1997, pp. 34–36, 39.

Corley, M.C., and B.E. Satterwhite, "Forecasting Ambulatory Clinic Workload to Facilitate Budgeting," *Nursing Economic$*, Vol. 11, No. 2, March-April 1993, pp. 77–81, 114.

Douglas, D.A., and J. Mayewske, "Census Variation Staffing," *Nursing Management*, Vol. 27, No. 2, February 1996, pp. 32–33, 36.

Dreisbach, A.M., "A Structured Approach to Expert Financial Management: A Financial Development Plan for Nurse Managers," *Nursing Economic$*, Vol. 12, No. 3, May-June 1994, pp. 131–139.

Esmond, T.H., *Budgeting for Effective Hospital Resource Management*, American Hospital Association, Chicago, Ill., 1990.

Finkler, S.A., *Budgeting Concepts for Nurse Managers*, 3rd edition, W.B. Saunders Company, Philadelphia, Penn., forthcoming 2000.

Finkler, Steven A., and David R. Ward, *Cost Accounting for Health Care Organizations: Concepts and Applications*, 2nd edition, Aspen Publishers, Gaithersburg, Md., 1999.

Hernandez, C.A., and L.L. O'Brien-Pallas, "Validity and Reliability of Nursing Workload Measurement Systems: Review of Validity and Reliability Theory," *Canadian Journal of Nursing Administration*, Vol. 9, No. 3, September-October 1996, pp. 32–50.

Johns, V., "Capturing the Activity Factor: Impact on Volume," *Nursing Management*, Vol. 24, No. 12, December 1993, pp. 26–29.

Leftridge, D.W., and C.W. Lydford, "Decentralizing an Overtime Budget," *Nursing Management*, Vol. 24, No. 8, August 1993, pp. 52–53.

McLean, Robert A., *Financial Management in Health Care Organizations*, Delmar, Albany, N.Y., 1996.

Moss, M.T., and S. Shelver, "Practical Budgeting for the Operating Room Administrator," *Nursing Economic$*, Vol. 11, No. 1, January-February 1993, pp. 7–13.

Samuels, David I., *The Healthcare Financial Management and Budgeting Toolkit*, Richard D. Irwin, Burr Ridge, Ill., December 1997.

Sengin, K.K., and A.M. Dreisbach, "Managing with Precision: A Budgetary Decision Support Model," *Journal of Nursing Administration*, Vol. 25, No. 2, February 1995, pp. 33–44.

Shelver, S.R., and M.T. Moss, "Operating Room Budget Factors: A Pocket Guide to OR Finance," *Nursing Economic$*, Vol. 12, No. 3, May-June 1994, pp. 146–152.

Swansburg, Russell C., "Budgeting and Financial Management for Nurse Managers," *Jones & Bartlett Publishers*, Sudbury, Mass., March 1997.

Ward, William J., Jr., *Health Care Budgeting and Financial Management for Non-Financial Managers: A New England Healthcare Assembly Book*, Auburn House Publishers, Westport, Conn., January 1994.

CHAPTER

13

Controlling Operating Results

CHAPTER GOALS

The goals of this chapter are to:

- Introduce the concept of management control systems
- Explain the role of employee motivation in control
- Explore alternative incentive systems, including their strengths and weaknesses
- Consider the negative implications of unrealistic expectations
- Discuss the role of communication in the control process
- Clarify the importance of interim evaluation
- Define variance analysis and explain the reasons for doing variance analysis
- Discuss traditional variance analysis
- Outline some possible causes of variances
- Explain flexible budgeting
- Introduce flexible budget variance analysis notation
- Define volume, quantity, and price variances
- Provide variance analysis tools and examples
- Provide insight into the problems encountered when variance information is aggregated
- Introduce the concept of exception reports and explain their benefits
- Discuss revenue variances

⁂ INTRODUCTION

Organizations exercise control over operations through the use of a *management control system.* Such a system is a complete set of policies and procedures designed to keep operations going according to plan. Furthermore, a management control system detects any variations from plan and provides managers with information needed to take corrective actions when necessary.

The focus of health care management control systems is on *responsibility accounting.* Responsibility accounting is the assignment of the responsibility for keeping to the plan and carrying out the elements of the management control system. Such responsibility is generally assigned to managers of cost centers. This chapter discusses a variety of elements of the management control system, with special emphasis on a system for motivating managers and staff and on variance analysis techniques.

⁂ THE BUDGET AS A TOOL FOR MOTIVATION

The budgeting process primarily concerns individuals, not numbers. If the employees of an organization do not work to make the organization succeed, the numbers constituting a budget will have little relevance. Motivation of staff and managers cannot be overemphasized. If *people* are not motivated to carry out the budget, it is likely to fail. That is why budgets arbitrarily imposed from above without fair consideration of input from those expected to carry them out tend to do so poorly. It is why managers feel such a sense of frustration when they are denied the needed authority to go along with their responsibility. It is why budget flexibility is needed in the face of changing realities. Motivation is the critical underlying key to budget success.

Control is complicated by the fact that individuals act in their own self-interest. The primary goal of the nursing staff may be to help patients. However, they will have other goals as well. It is the basic nature of individuals for their own personal goals to be different from the goals of the organization they work for (Fig. 13–1). This does not mean that human nature is bad but only that there is such a thing as human nature and one is foolish to refuse to recognize it.

For example, other things being equal, most employees of a hospital would prefer a salary substantially larger than they are receiving. There is nothing particularly wrong in their wanting more money. In fact, ambition is probably a desirable trait in staff. Most nurse managers would like more staff to carry out their existing functions. However, all organizations must make choices concerning how to spend their limited resources.

Health care organizations will not provide employees with 100% raises because they lack the revenues to pay for those raises. While the nursing staff is not wrong to desire the raises, the organization is not wrong to deny them.

Thus the fact must be faced that even where morale is generally excellent and is

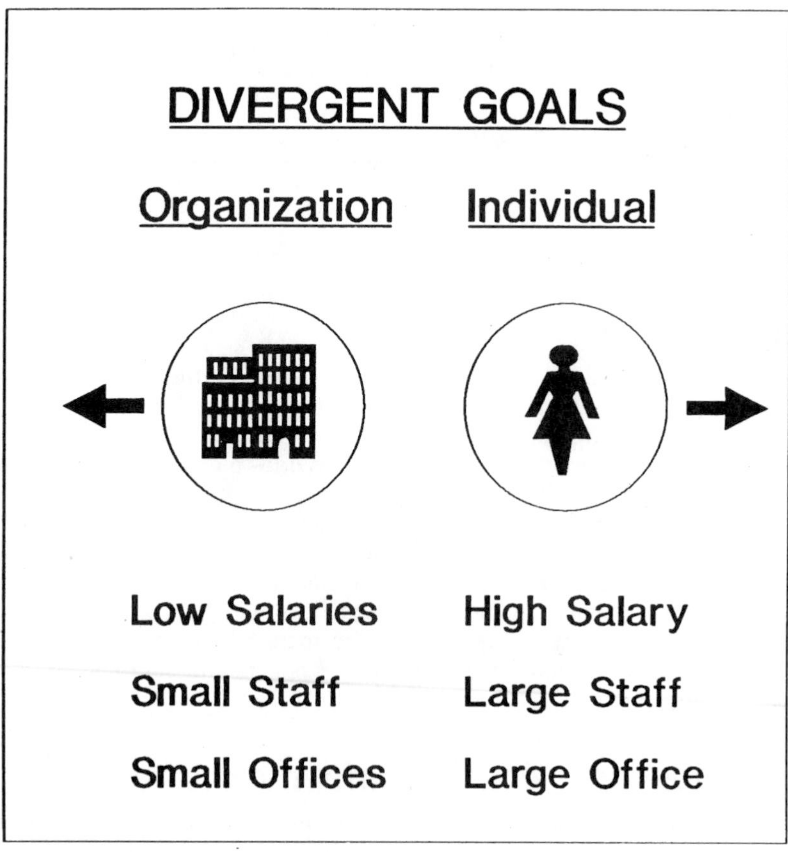

FIGURE 13–1. Divergent goals.

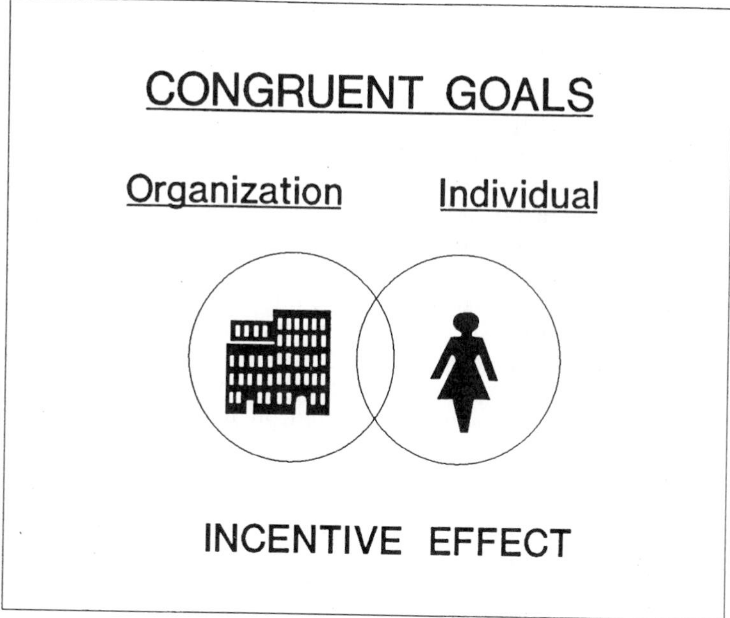

FIGURE 13–2. Congruent goals.

not considered a problem, an underlying tension will naturally exist. Even though the employees may want to achieve the mission of the organization in providing care, their personal desires will be for things the organization will choose not to provide. This is referred to as *goal divergence.*

The organization must bring together the interests of the individual and its own interests so that they can work together. In the budgeting process there must be some motivation for the people involved to want to control costs. Bringing the individuals' and organization's wants and desires together is referred to as *goal congruence* (Fig. 13–2). To be sure that the human beings will in fact want to control organizational costs, managers need to make sure that it is somehow in their direct best interests for costs to be controlled. Organizations generally achieve such congruence by setting up a system of incentives that make employees want to work toward the best interests of the organization.

※ MOTIVATION AND INCENTIVES

Although nurses are motivated by factors other than money, it would be foolish to ignore the potential of monetary rewards to influence behavior. As health care organizations search for the proper mix of incentives that will motivate managers and staff to control costs, financial incentives are frequently employed. The most basic financial incentives are the ability to retain a job and to get a good raise.

Another motivating tool is a bonus system. Since managers have many desires that relate to spending more money (e.g., larger offices, fancier furniture, larger staffs), formalized approaches need to be developed that will provide incentives to spend less money. For example, one can tell a nurse manager that last year the manager's department spent $2 million and that next year its budget is $2,080,000 (a 4% increase). However, for any amount that the department spends below $2,080,000, the manager and the staff can keep 10% of the savings. If spending is below the budgeted $2,080,000, the nurses benefit and the organization benefits. In this case goal congruence is likely to be achieved.

Many health care organizations have added bonus systems. These have both positives and negatives. The positives relate primarily to the strong motivation employees have to reduce costs. The negatives relate to the potential detriment to quality of patient care and to the potential negative effect on employee morale.

When an incentive is given to accomplish one end, sometimes the responses to that incentive are unexpected. Bonus systems may give a nurse manager an incentive to provide less staff nurse time per patient day. Health care organizations must be concerned about the impact their incentives will have on the quality of patient care. A strong internal quality assurance program is essential.

Further, bonuses are not necessarily the solution to all motivational problems. If everyone gets a bonus, no one feels that individual actions have much impact. As long as everyone else holds costs in check, all individuals may feel they do not have to work particularly hard to reap the benefits of the bonus. On the other hand, bonuses given only to some employees may create jealousy and discontent. This may create a competitive environment in a situation in which teamwork is needed to provide high-quality care.

There are incentive alternatives to bonuses. For example, one underused managerial tool is a letter from supervisor to subordinate. All individuals responsible for controlling costs should be explicitly evaluated with respect to how well they do in fact control costs. That evaluation should be communicated in writing. This approach, which is both the carrot and the stick, costs little to implement but can have a dramatic impact.

Telling managers that they did a good job and that their boss knows that they did a good job can be an effective way to get the manager to try to do a good job the next year. In the real world praise is cheap and in many cases effective. On the other hand, criticism, especially in writing, can have a stinging effect that managers and staff will work hard to avoid in the future.

⁂ MOTIVATION AND UNREALISTIC EXPECTATIONS

While motivational devices can work wonders at getting an organization's staff to work hard for the organization and its goals, they can also backfire and have negative results. This occurs primarily when expectations are placed at unreasonably high levels.

A target that requires hard work and stretching but is achievable can be a useful motivating tool. If the target is reached, there might be a bonus, or there should be at least some formal recognition of the achievement, such as a letter. At a minimum, the worker will have the self-satisfaction of having worked hard and reached the target.

But all those positive outcomes can occur only if the target is reachable. Some health care organizations have adopted the philosophy that if a high target makes people work hard, a higher target will make them work harder. This may not be the case. If targets are placed out of reach, this will probably *not* result in people reaching to their utmost limits to come as close to the target as possible.

It may seem as if the organization is shortchanging itself whenever someone achieves a target. The manager may think, "We set the target too low. Perhaps if the target were higher, this person would have achieved the higher target. Since the target we set was achieved, we haven't yet realized all of their potential." There are risks associated with that logic.

If people fail to meet a target because they are not competent or because they do not work very hard, the signal of failure sent is warranted. In fact, repeated failure may be grounds for replacement of that individual in that job. But if a manager is both competent and hard working, failure is not a message that should be sent. Even though it is desirable to encourage the individual to achieve even more, the signal of failure will be discouraging. When people work extremely hard and fail, they often question why they bothered to work so hard. If hard work results in failure to achieve the target, then why not ease off. Managers must be extremely judicious to ensure that all goals assigned are reasonable.

※ COMMUNICATION AND CONTROL

Communication is an essential part of a management control system. Communication should be an ongoing process. When a manager has a once-a-year meeting with the staff concerning the budget, it is quickly forgotten. To reinforce that meeting, a short weekly or monthly meeting should be held to discuss the budget. It is adequate to discuss just one or several items, such as bandage tape, diapers, chest tubes, disposable gloves, or sponges, at each meeting. It does not even have to be a separate meeting; it can be two minutes of any regularly scheduled meeting. The key is to make the staff aware of specific, definite, attainable goals that they can work toward. Further, by mentioning the budget often, awareness is created, and it becomes second nature to conserve the organization's resources.

If the manager does not mention the budget until after a month of excessive use, a strong admonition at that time will tend to create budget antagonism rather than cost control. When a nurse manager routinely conveys specific, measurable goals, cost control can become a routine part of the way nurses function.

※ USING BUDGETS FOR INTERIM EVALUATION

Interim evaluations are of particular importance in controlling operational results. If the manager simply prepares a budget, tells everyone what it is, and then puts it in a drawer until it is needed to help prepare next year's budget, an important element of motivation and control is lost. The budget has not been used to evaluate how well the unit, staff, and manager are doing and where improvements are possible. The role of evaluation should be primarily to focus on learning from past results to improve future outcomes.

Each month there should be comparisons between what was expected and what has been accomplished. First, this will allow the manager to give feedback to the staff nurses and to the manager's supervisor as to whether the budget's goals are being attained. Telling the staff the unit's goals without giving timely reports on whether they are being attained will weaken their motivation. Second, these monthly evaluations help to bring any unanticipated results to the manager's attention. Then the manager may be able to adjust staffing or take other corrective actions so that the budget will be met in future months.

Monthly information also allows a manager to provide early notice to a superior if a problem outside the manager's control exists. If the problem is controllable elsewhere in the organization (e.g., by the purchasing department), appropriate action can be taken. In evaluating any individual in an organization, one primary rule must be followed: *Responsibility should equal control.* If managers are held responsible for things they have no control over, the organization will reward and punish the wrong individuals. The result is invariably demoralization of managers and staff. Using budgets for control can help locate the cause of inefficiency and help prevent waste. In addition, in the hands of a skilled manager, budgeting can also help establish a defense for not meeting the budget (if there are valid reasons for spending in excess of budget, such as increases in noncontrollable costs).

We now turn our attention to the topic of variance analysis, one of the most widely used tools for interim evaluation.

※ VARIANCE ANALYSIS

Variance analysis is the aspect of budgeting in which actual results are compared with budgeted expectations. The difference between the actual results and the planned results represents a *variance,* or the amount by which the results *vary* from the budget. Variances are calculated for three principal reasons. One is to aid in preparing the budget for the coming year. By understanding why results were not as expected, the budget process can be improved and be made more accurate in future planning. The second reason is to aid in controlling results throughout the current year. By understanding why variances are occurring, actions can be taken to eliminate some of the unfavorable variances over the coming months. The third reason for variance analysis is to evaluate the performance of units or departments and their managers.

For variance reports to be an effective tool, managers must be able to understand the causes of the variances. This requires investigation of the variances. Such investigation in turn requires the knowledge, judgment, and experience of nurse managers. Variances can be calculated by financial managers. However, those finance personnel do not have the specific knowledge to explain why the variances are occurring. Without such explanation the reports are not useful managerial aids.

Causes of Variances

It is important to be aware of the fact that variance analysis is only a tool to point the manager in the direction to begin investigation. Variances can highlight an actual cost in excess of budget but cannot indicate whether it resulted from improvements in quality of care or from longer coffee breaks. The nurse manager must investigate and make the final determination of what caused a variance.

Variances may be caused by factors internal or external to the organization. Some common internal causes of variances include shifts in quality of care provided; changes in technology, in the efficiency of the nurses, and in organization policy; or simply incorrect standards. External causes of variances commonly include price changes for supplies, volume changes in workload, and unexpected shifts in the availability of staff.

Justification of Variances

Variance reports are given by finance to nurse managers for *justification*. The word justification, which is often used, is unduly confrontational. It focuses attention on the evaluation role of variance analysis instead of on the planning and control roles. The goal of the investigation process is to arrive at an explanation of why the variances arose. In the majority of cases, the variance report is being used to understand what is happening and to control future results to the extent possible. The focus should not be on a defensive justification of what was spent.

If variances arose as a result of inefficiency (e.g., long coffee breaks), then the process of providing cost-effective care is out of control. By discovering that inefficiency, actions can be taken to eliminate it and to bring the process back under control. In that case, future costs will be lower because of the investigation of the variance. The improvement comes, however, not from placing blame on those who failed to control past results but from using the information to improve control of future results.

※ TRADITIONAL VARIANCE ANALYSIS

At the end of a given time period, the organization compares its actual results with the budget. Suppose that the organization does this monthly. Several weeks after each month ends, the accountants gather all the cost information and report the actual totals for the month.

The simplest approach is to then compare the total costs that the entire organization has incurred with the budgeted costs for the entire organization. For example, suppose that the Wagner Hospital had a total budget for the month of

March of $4,800,000. The actual costs were $5,200,000. Wagner spent $400,000 more than it had budgeted. The difference between the amount budgeted and the amount actually incurred is the total hospital variance. This variance is referred to as an *unfavorable variance* because the organization spent more than had been budgeted. Accountants use the term *favorable variance* to indicate spending less than expected.

Assuming that the Wagner Hospital begins its fiscal year on January 1, its variance could appear in a format somewhat like the following:

This Month		
Actual: $ 5,200,000	Budget: $ 4,800,000	Variance: $400,000 U
Year-to-Date		
Actual: $15,150,000	Budget: $14,876,000	Variance: $274,000 U

In future examples the *year-to-date* information will be dispensed with for simplicity. The focus will be on the current month under review. In health organizations, nurse managers are generally provided with information for the year-to-date as well as the current month. The capital U following the variance refers to the fact that the variance is unfavorable. If the variance were favorable, it would be followed by a capital F.[1]

Why has Wagner had a $400,000 unfavorable variance for the month of March? If variance analysis is to be used to evaluate results, it is necessary to be able to determine not simply that the organization was $400,000 over budget but why. Given this simple total for the entire organization, the chief executive officer (CEO) has no idea of what caused the variance. The CEO does not even know which managers to ask about the variance, since all that is known is a total for the entire organization.

To use budgets for control, it must be possible to assign responsibility for variances to individual managers. Those managers can investigate the causes of the variances and attempt to eliminate the variances in the future. The key is that it must be possible to hold individual managers accountable for the variance. This leads to the necessity of determining variances by unit and department.

Unit and Department Variances

The overall Wagner variance of $400,000 is an aggregation of variances from a number of departments. Focus on the results for the nursing department.

THE WAGNER HOSPITAL
Department of Nursing Services
March Variance Report

Actual	Budget	Variance
$2,400,000	$2,200,000	$200,000 U

Apparently, half the variance for the Wagner Hospital for March occurred in the nursing services area. Now there is more information than there was previously. Previously it was known that there was an excess expenditure of $400,000, but it was not known how that excess came about. Now it is known that half of it occurred in the nursing area. The chief nurse executive (CNE) can be asked to explain why the $200,000 variance occurred.

---

[1]An alternative presentation to using U and F would be to use a negative number for an unfavorable variance and a positive number for a favorable variance. Alternatively, parentheses are placed around unfavorable variances, and no parentheses around favorable ones. Exercise caution in interpreting variance notation. Any systematic approach can be used to indicate favorable *vs* unfavorable variances. It would not be wrong to use parentheses or negative numbers for favorable variances and no parentheses or positive numbers for unfavorable variances, as long as the use is consistent throughout the organization.

Unfortunately, at this point the CNE has not been given much to go on. The CNE simply knows that $200,000 was spent that was not budgeted. Most hospitals would take this total cost for the nursing department and break it down into the various nursing units. Each nursing unit that has a nurse manager who is responsible for running that unit should have both a budget for the unit and a variance report that shows the unit's performance in comparison with the budget.

The variance for a particular nursing unit might appear as follows:

THE WAGNER HOSPITAL
Department of Nursing Services
Med/Surg 6th Floor West
March Variance Report

Actual	Budget	Variance
$120,000	$110,000	$10,000 U

Line-item Variances

Even when the total nursing department variance has been divided among the various nursing units, more information is still needed as a guide. Is the variance the result of unexpectedly high costs for nursing salaries? Does it relate to usage of supplies? To have any real chance to control costs, there must be variance information for individual line items within a unit or department. For example:

THE WAGNER HOSPITAL
Department of Nursing Services
Med/Surg 6th Floor West
March Variance Report

	Actual	Budget	Variance
Salary	$108,000	$100,000	$ 8,000 U
Supplies	12,000	10,000	2,000 U
Total	$120,000	$110,000	$10,000 U

This obviously is greatly simplified. There should be line items for each line in the unit's budget.

Understanding Variances

The objective of variance analysis is to determine why the variances arose. Nothing can be done with respect to the goal of controlling costs until the nurse manager knows where the unit or department is deviating from the plan and why.

Once the variance for each line item for each unit has been calculated, there must be a determination of whether to investigate the variance. It must be kept in mind that budgets are "guesstimates" of the future. They cannot be expected to come out exactly on target. Small variances can generally be ignored. Hopefully, over the course of a year the small unfavorable variances will be balanced out by small favorable variances. One of the most difficult aspects of variance analysis is determining when a variance is large enough to warrant investigation. Should a manager investigate $5, $50, $100, or $1,000 variances? How big a variance is too big to tolerate without investigation?

Unfortunately, there is no set answer. The solution favored by these authors is as follows: When managers look at a variance, they should assume that it will occur in the same amount month after month until the end of the year. For instance, suppose that a $500 unfavorable variance was found for January for nurses' aides salaries. If that variance occurred every month, it would total $6,000 for the year. If $6,000 is an unreasonably high variance, investigate the $500 January variance as soon as possible. Managers should also investigate variances that appear to be growing from month to month.

The key to controlling variances is to be timely, to correct behavior if necessary, and to use the information from variances to adjust patient charges promptly. If variances are not investigated promptly after each month's variance report is received, the budget will serve only as a planning tool and not a tool to help the organization control its operation. Information about last month's performance should be used to improve the performance for the remaining months of the year.

In some cases it will be found that the variances are simply out of the unit or manager's control. A shortage of a key raw material may drive the price of supplies up. If there appears to be a protracted change that is outside the control of the manager and will result in continuing unfavorable variances, it is important to bring this to the attention of the organization's rate-setting personnel. The sooner this is known and the rates charged are corrected upward, the better it is for the financial stability of the organization. However, rates are frequently negotiated for a year or more at a time. Therefore managers may need to focus more on decreasing costs than on assuming that rates can be increased.

Traditional variance analysis requires that the nurse manager proceed to use the unit line-item variance information to attempt to discover the underlying causes of the variances. Consider the $8,000 variance for salaries. Why was $8,000 more than budgeted spent on salaries? At this point we really do not know what caused the variance. Expenditure for staff in excess of the budgeted amount could have a number of possible causes. Without more information, corrective action cannot be taken.

One potential cause of the $8,000 salary variance is that the unit manager did not do a very good job in controlling the usage of staff. As a result, more hours of nursing care per patient were paid for than had been expected. Another possibility is that the patients were sicker than anticipated, and the higher average acuity level caused more nursing hours to be used per patient. Another possible cause is that the hourly rate for nurses increased. Still another possible cause of the variance is that there were more patients, and the additional patients consumed more nursing hours.

The most serious problem of traditional variance analysis is that it compares the predicted cost for a predicted number of patients with the actual cost for the actual patient volume. Unless the actual workload is exactly as predicted, there is very little chance that a unit will achieve exactly the budgeted expectations, because some costs are variable. Such costs will rise or fall if volume is greater or less than the budgeted level.

Many health care organizations are starting to use a more sophisticated variance approach based on a flexible budget. The main goal of that approach is to allow for changed expectations as the number of patients changes.

※ FLEXIBLE BUDGET VARIANCE ANALYSIS

Flexible budgeting is a system that requires more work than traditional variance analysis but can provide nurse managers with substantially more information. The key concept of flexible budgeting is that the amount of resources consumed varies with the volume of patients. Suppose that the following was the variance report for nursing department salaries:

THE WAGNER HOSPITAL
Department of Nursing Services
March Variance Report

	Actual	Budget	Variance
Salary	$1,000,000	$1,000,000	$0

It looks as if the department came in right on budget. Suppose, however, that the budget of $1 million for nursing salaries was based on an assumption of 25,000 patient days, but there actually were only 20,000 patient days. The department should have spent less than $1 million if any of the salary costs are variable. The original budget ignores that fact. The flexible budget is a restatement of the budget based on the volume actually attained. The flexible budget shows what a line item should have cost, given the volume level that actually occurred.

The flexible budget is prepared after the fact. The actual volume must be known to prepare the flexible budget for that volume.[2] Keep in mind that because some costs are fixed and some are variable, total costs do not change in direct proportion with volume. One would normally expect that a 10% increase in patient days would be accompanied by less than a 10% increase in costs, since only some costs are variable and increase as census does. On the other hand, a 10% reduction in workload would only be expected to be accompanied by a less than 10% reduction in cost because the fixed costs would not decline.

Use of the flexible budget technique allows the variance for any line item to be subdivided to get additional information. The variance is divided into three pieces: *volume variance, price variance,* and *quantity variance.*

The Volume Variance

The *volume variance* is defined as the amount of variance caused simply by the fact that patient volume has changed. For example, if the budget calls for 25,000 patient days but actually there were 30,000 patient days, it would be expected that it would be necessary to spend more. The additional cost of the resources needed for an extra 5,000 patient days constitutes a volume variance. Volume variances are generally outside the control of the nurse manager. Note that unfavorable volume variances are often accompanied by higher than budgeted revenue.

Many hospitals have adopted use of this aspect of flexible budgeting. Unit managers are asked to explain the differences between the actual amounts spent and the amounts that should be spent according to the flexible budget. Thus the noncontrollable volume variance is excluded from the variance that the manager is expected to justify or explain. While this is a major step in the direction of making variance analysis more relevant and useful, it does not yield all the potential benefits of flexible budget variance analysis.

The Price or Rate Variance

The *price* or *rate variance* is the portion of the total variance caused by spending more or less per unit for some resource than had been anticipated. For example, if the average wage rate for nurses is more per hour than had been expected, it would give rise to a rate variance. When the variance is used to measure labor resources, it is generally called a *rate variance* because the average hourly rate has varied from expectations. When considering the price of supplies, such as the cost per package of sutures, it is called a *price variance* because the purchase price has varied. The terms "price" and "rate" are often used interchangeably in practice.

The price or rate variance may or may not be under the control of the nurse manager. If the purchasing department predicts all prices used for supplies and then winds up paying a higher price than predicted, it should be possible to measure the price variance so that the responsibility can be placed with the purchasing

---

[2]As part of the budget preparation process, some organizations prospectively prepare flexible budgets. This provides the organization with a sense of what costs are likely to be at differing levels of workload.

department. If the nursing department bears the responsibility for price variances on supplies, the purchasing department will have no incentive to try to find the best prices. On the other hand, if the nurse manager hires temporary nurses directly from the agency, the responsibility for the rate variance may lie with the nurse manager. Were overqualified people hired? Was an attempt made to seek out an agency that would give the best rate? The manager who can exercise some control over the outcome should be the manager held accountable for the outcome.

The Quantity or Use Variance

The third general type of variance under the flexible budgeting scheme is the *quantity* or *use variance*. This is the portion of the overall variance for a particular line item that results from using more of a resource than was expected for a given work load. For example, if more supplies were used per patient day than expected, that would give rise to a quantity variance, because the quantity of supplies used per patient day exceeded expectations.

This variance is also frequently referred to as a *use variance* because it focuses on how much of the resource has been used. For example, if half a roll of bandage tape was used per patient day and the expected usage was only a quarter roll, there would be a use variance. The terms "quantity" and "use" are often used interchangeably.

THE MECHANICS OF FLEXIBLE BUDGET VARIANCE ANALYSIS

The first step in flexible budgeting is to establish the flexible budget for the actual patient volume. Given the actual cost for a particular line item and the original budgeted amount, it must be determined what that line item should have cost given the actual patient volume.

For example, consider the supplies budgeted for and used by the Med/Surg 6th Floor West nursing unit at the Wagner Hospital in March:

THE WAGNER HOSPITAL
Department of Nursing Services
Med/Surg 6th Floor West
March Variance Report

	Actual	Budget	Variance
Supplies	$12,000	$10,000	$2,000 U

The actual consumption was $12,000. The budgeted consumption was $10,000. Suppose that the budget assumed that there would be 500 patient days for this unit for March, but there actually turned out to be 600 patient days.[3] Assuming that the consumption of supplies would normally be expected to vary in direct proportion to patient days, the planned consumption was apparently $20 per patient day (the $10,000 supplies budget divided by the 500 expected patient days).

For 600 patient days at $20 per patient day, $12,000 would have been budgeted for supplies. This is the flexible budget. It is the amount the department would have expected to spend had the actual number of patient days been known. Notice that in this case the flexible budget and the actual amount spent are identical:

[3]It is assumed in this example that the average patient classification or acuity is unchanged. If average acuity is different from the expected level, it is logical that resource consumption in terms of nursing requirements will also differ from the budgeted amount. Acuity can be built into variance analysis through the flexible budget model. The portion of the variance resulting from changes in acuity can be separated and specified. See the reprinted article on this topic in the Appendix at the end of this chapter for further discussion of variance due to patient acuity.

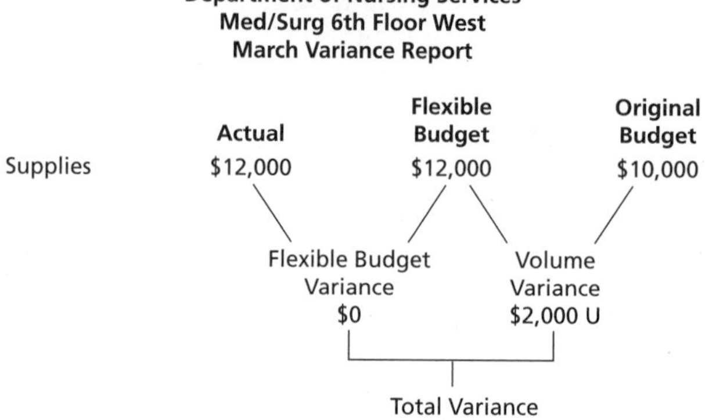

The difference between the original budget and the actual amount spent is the total variance. That is still $2,000 unfavorable. The difference between the original budget and the new flexible budget is the volume variance. In this case the difference is $2,000 U. Note that this volume variance is considered unfavorable because the flexible budget requires more spending than was expected. The increased number of patient days may represent more patients and more revenues. That may be favorable for the organization, but the accountant always refers to cost in excess of the original budget as an unfavorable variance. Unfavorable variances are not necessarily bad.

The difference between the flexible budget and the actual amount spent can be referred to as a flexible budget variance. Here the flexible budget variance is zero. The entire variance in supplies has been explained by the fact that there was a different volume of patients than had been anticipated.

What about the nursing salaries for the unit? Recall the variance report for nursing salaries:

THE WAGNER HOSPITAL
Department of Nursing Services
Med/Surg 6th Floor West
March Variance Report

	Actual	Budget	Variance
Salary	$108,000	$100,000	$8,000 U

To keep the discussion relatively simple, assume that nursing salary costs should vary in direct proportion to the number of patient days. In other words, assume that nursing salary costs are variable.[4]

Nursing salaries had been budgeted at $100,000, with an expectation of 500 patient days. That is a cost of $200 per patient day. Assuming nursing salary costs are

[4]This may assume more flexibility of nurse staffing than most organizations have. Hospitals may have some flexibility to transfer nurses from one shift to another or from a unit with a temporarily low occupancy to one with a higher occupancy, or per diem agency nurses can be used. In some cases, however, such flexibility may be quite limited. This is particularly so at unionized hospitals with strong work rules. Nurse staffing tends to be variable only if there is substantial change in patient volume. Flexible budget variance analysis can still be used. However, the process is more complicated. See Steven A. Finkler, *Budgeting Concepts for Nurse Managers*, 2nd edition, W.B. Saunders, Philadelphia, Penn., 1992, pp. 289–291, for the mechanics and an example. Bear in mind, however, that only significant variances require investigation. And significant variances are generally not the result of a minor shift in the number of patient days. Over major shifts in volume, staffing is likely to be reasonably variable.

variable, had it been known that there would be 600 patient days, $120,000 would have been budgeted. The variance report can be restated as follows:

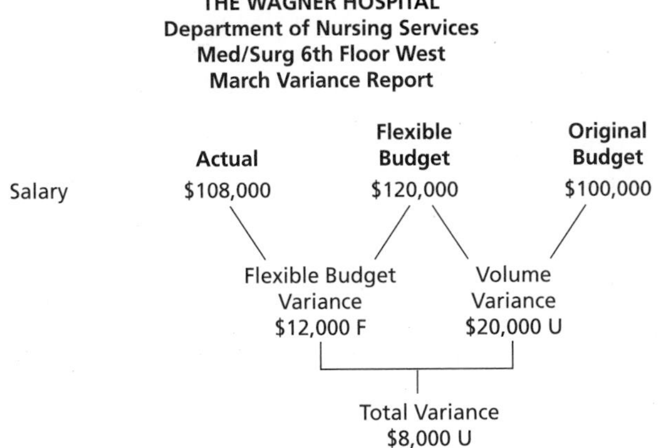

Subtracting the original budget from the flexible budget, the volume variance is found to be $20,000 U. When the flexible budget is subtracted from the actual cost, it turns out that the flexible budget variance is $12,000 F. Note that the volume variance is unfavorable because the extra patients require more spending. However, the actual amount spent was less than the flexible budget.

If the volume and flexible budget variances for salaries are combined, there is an unfavorable total variance of $8,000. (Note that since one of the variances is favorable and one is unfavorable, the smaller one must be subtracted from the larger one to get a combined total variance. The total variance will have the same label [i.e., favorable or unfavorable] as the larger of the two variances. Hence, $20,000 U – $12,000 F = $8,000 U.)

At this point in the analysis, there is not yet sufficient information to determine the causes of the flexible budget variance. Suppose that the CNE of the organization had come to the unit manager in the middle of April and complained about a total lack of cost control on the unit. The unit had a $2,000 unfavorable supplies variance and an $8,000 unfavorable salary variance. Based on traditional variance analysis (without using a flexible budget), there would be no way the unit manager could determine the cause of the problem.

Certainly the unit manager is aware of increased patient volume and would argue that extra patient days were a major factor. But how major? By using a flexible budget, it is possible to find out exactly what dollar impact the extra patient days should have had. In the example, flexible budgeting has shown that the entire variance in supplies is attributable to the extra patient days. The volume variance for supplies was $2,000 U, the same as the amount of the total supply variance. Furthermore, the volume variance was $20,000 U for salaries. The department manager should have expected to spend $20,000 more on nursing salaries than was in the original budget, given the 100 extra patient days. In fact, only $8,000 was spent above the original salary budget. Rather than being blamed for having gone over budget, the manager can now show that given the actual number of patient days, the unit actually spent $12,000 less than should have been expected!

Flexible Budget Notation

The next step in the process is to try to determine what caused the flexible budget variance. To do that it is necessary to formalize the flexible budgeting process by introducing some notation. The letter A will be used to refer to an actual amount, and the letter B to a budgeted amount. The letter P will stand for a price or rate, and the letter Q for a quantity. The letter i will be used to stand for an input, and the letter o for an output.

Inputs are the resources used to generate outputs. If one is considering how much was spent on nursing salaries, the input is nursing time. If one is considering the cost of bandage tape, the input is rolls of bandage tape. *Outputs* are a measure of what is being produced. Since improved health cannot readily be measured, proxies are used to measure how much output is produced. Frequently used output measures include patients, patient days, visits, treatments, and procedures.

The notation is combined to form six key variables. Pi stands for the *price of the input,* such as $1 per roll of bandage tape or $25 per hour for nursing salary. Qo stands for the total *quantity of output.* Qi stands for the *quantity of input* needed to produce one unit of output. The definitions of the notation can be formalized as follows:

- BPi: *b*udgeted *p*rice per unit of *i*nput
- BQi: *b*udgeted *q*uantity of *i*nput for each unit of output
- BQo: *b*udgeted *q*uantity of *o*utput
- APi: *a*ctual *p*rice paid per unit of *i*nput
- AQi: *a*ctual *q*uantity of *i*nput for each unit of output produced
- AQo: *a*ctual *q*uantity of *o*utput

The notation can best be understood in an example.

An Example of Volume, Price, and Quantity Variances

Suppose that Wagner Hospital had the following line item in its variance report for a nursing unit for the prior month:

	Actual	Budget	Variance
Nursing labor	$34,038	$28,800	$5,238 U

The unit manager wants to find out what caused the variance, so the following information is gathered:

- BPi: $24.00 per hour budgeted nursing rate
- BQi: 3.0 hours of budgeted nursing time per patient day
- BQo: 400 budgeted patient days
- APi: $24.40 actual average nursing rate per hour
- AQi: 3.1 hours of actual nursing time per patient day
- AQo: 450 actual patient days

Before proceeding to use these data, consider what is involved in obtaining the information. Information is only worthwhile if it is more valuable than the cost to collect it. All three budgeted items are already known. It would not have been possible to prepare an operating budget without a forecast of patient days, the average rate for nurses, and the budgeted hours per patient day (or the total budgeted nursing hours, which can be divided by the expected patient days to get the budgeted nursing hours per patient day). What about the actual information? The actual number of patient days is readily available. The actual wage rate and the amount of actual paid nursing time is available from the payroll department. Given the actual nursing time and the actual number of patient days, one can divide to get the nursing time per patient day. Therefore, all the data needed for flexible budget variance analysis are readily available.

The first step in utilizing these data is calculating the original budget in terms of the notation. The original budget is simply the expected cost per patient day multiplied by the expected number of patient days. In this case the expectation is that nurses will be paid $24.00 per hour; the department will pay for an average of 3.0 hours per patient day. Therefore, the expected cost is $72 per patient day. For the month, 400 patient days are expected, so the budget is $28,800 ($24.00 × 3.0 hours × 400 patient days). In terms of the notation, this can be shown as follows:

Original Budget
BQi × BPi × BQo
3.0 × $24.00 × 400
$28,800

That is, BQi, the budgeted quantity of input per patient day, is 3.0 hours; BPi, the budgeted price per hour of nursing time, is $24.00; and BQo, the budgeted quantity of patient days, is 400. If these three numbers are multiplied together, the result is the originally budgeted amount for nursing labor.

The next step is to find the flexible budget. Keep in mind that the flexible budget is the amount one would have expected to spend if the actual number of patient days had been known in advance. Therefore, leave the BQi at the budgeted 3.0 hours per patient day and the BPi at the budgeted $24.00 per hour. The only change is from a BQo of 400 patient days to a new AQo of 450 patient days. The flexible budget can then be calculated as follows:

Flexible Budget
BQi × BPi × AQo
3.0 × $24.00 × 450
$32,400

Note that the difference between the original budget and the flexible budget is caused by a difference in the number of patient days. Other than that, the calculations are the same. The originally budgeted amount of $28,800 can be compared with the flexible budget amount of $32,400 to determine the volume variance of $3,600 U. Since patient days are higher than expected, cost is higher than expected. This gives rise to an unfavorable variance. The comparison between the original budget and the flexible budget can be shown as follows:

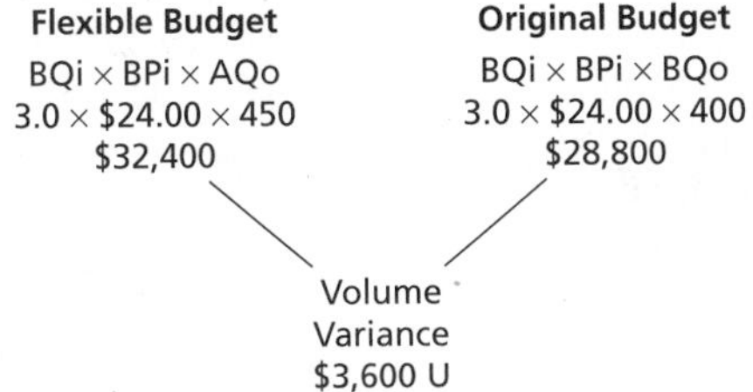

At this point the flexible budget can be compared to the actual results to find the flexible budget variance. First, restate the actual costs in terms of the notation:

Actual
AQi × APi × AQo
3.1 × $24.40 × 450
$34,038

Note that for the actual cost, the actual paid time per patient day, the actual price paid per hour, and the actual number of patient days are used. If desired, the flexible budget can be compared with the actual results to determine a *flexible budget variance:*

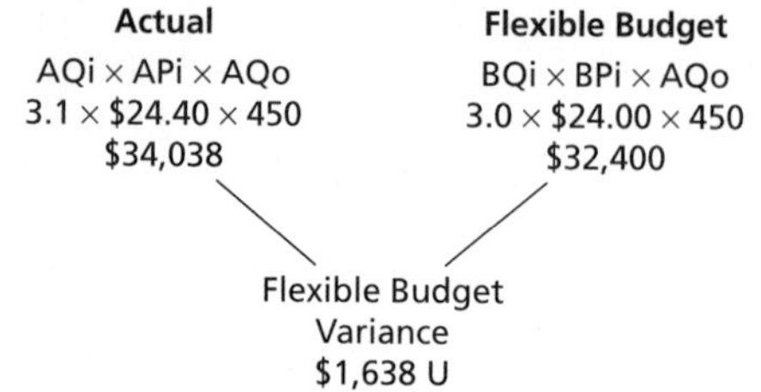

The flexible budget variance is $1,638 U. Since the total variance is simply being broken into its component parts, it should be possible to combine the volume variance and the flexible budget variance and come out with the total variance. The difference between the original budget and the actual result is $5,238 (i.e., $34,038 – $28,800). Consider all the information available so far in notation form:

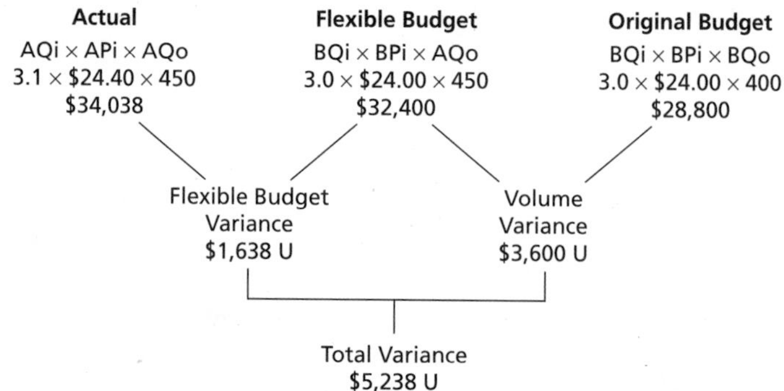

As can be seen, the total variance still is $5,238, but it has now been separated into a flexible budget variance and a volume variance. If the $1,638 U flexible budget variance is added to the $3,600 U volume variance, the result is the $5,238 total variance. The flexible budget variance is of greater concern to the nurse manager than is the volume variance. The volume variance is usually outside the nurse manager's control. The flexible budget variance is caused by the difference between the budgeted and actual price per hour for nursing services and by differences in the amount of nursing time per patient day. If possible, more should be found out about what makes up this variance.

To find out this extra information, it is necessary to derive something called a *subcategory*. This subcategory is simply a device to allow for separation of the flexible budget variance into two pieces: the price variance and the quantity variance. The subcategory is defined as the actual quantity of input per unit of output, multiplied by the budgeted price of the input, times the actual output level. In terms of the notation the subcategory can be calculated as follows:

Subcategory
AQi × BPi × AQo
3.1 × $24.00 × 450
$33,480

If the subcategory calculation is compared with the actual costs, the price variance can be determined:

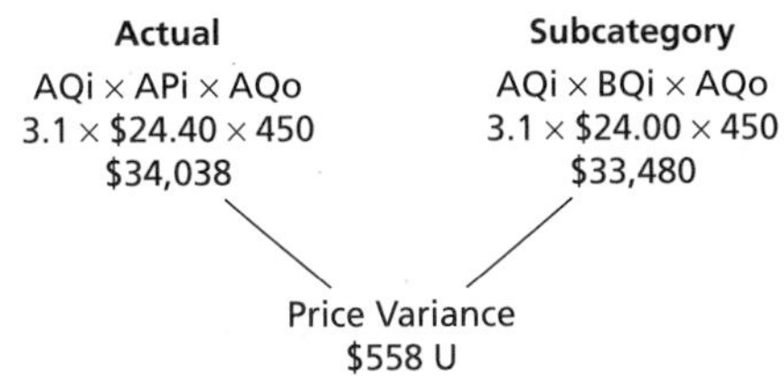

The only difference between the actual and the subcategory is in the hourly rate (Pi). The price variance of $558 U results from the fact that on average $24.40 was paid per hour for nursing time instead of the budgeted $24.00. It is possible that this occurs because of poor scheduling, which results in unnecessary overtime. Perhaps it is the result of a larger raise for nursing personnel than the nurse manager had been told to put into the budget. Perhaps the extra patient volume resulted in extra overtime or the addition of high-priced per diem agency nurses. All these possibilities should be investigated by the nurse manager.

What effect will added patient load have on the quantity of nursing time per patient? The quantity variance addresses that question. That variance is calculated by comparing the difference between the subcategory and the flexible budget. The only difference between those two numbers is a result of the nursing time (Qi) per patient.

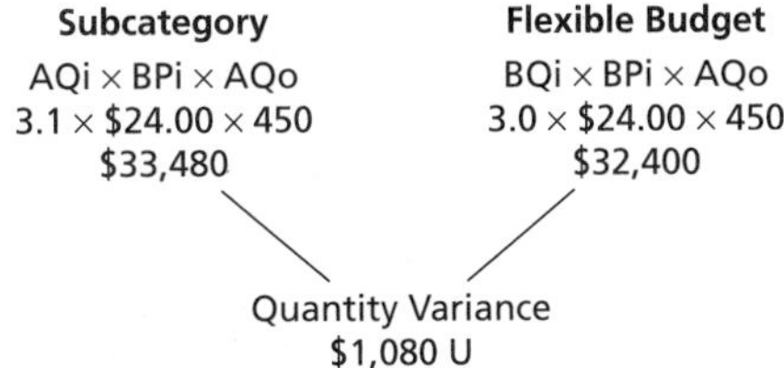

The quantity variance of $1,080 U can be explained in a number of ways. It is possible that because of the substantial increase in patient days over expectations, many part-time nurses were hired. These nurses were unfamiliar with the institution and therefore were not as efficient as the regular nurses. Another possibility is that the population was sicker than anticipated and required more care. An approach to measuring the part of the variance due to patient acuity is discussed in the article reprinted in the Appendix at the end of this chapter. Of course, there is also the possibility that supervision was lax and that time was simply being wasted. Again, variance information can only point out the direction; the manager must make the final determination regarding why the variance occurred and how to prevent it in the future.

To use flexible budgeting, one should have an idea of how the pieces fit together. Review the price and quantity variances, looking at how together they comprise the flexible budget variance:

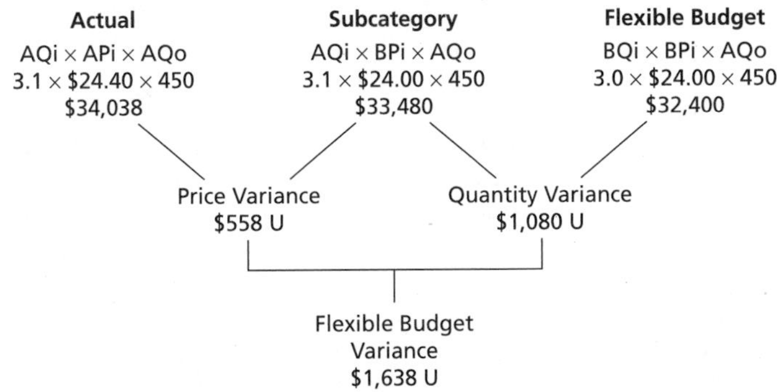

Notice that adding the price variance of $558 U and the quantity variance of $1,080 U results in the flexible budget variance. Recall that the flexible budget variance and volume variance add up to the total variance. Figure 13–3 shows that the three individual variances—price, quantity, and volume—add up to the total variance for the line item.

Recall that without flexible budgets the total variance for the line item would be the only piece of information available for analysis. There was an unfavorable variance of $5,238. Using Figure 13–3, it is possible to determine at the outset that of this total variance, $3,600 was caused by the increase in patient days. It is now also known that $558 of the variance was caused by having paid a higher average rate to the nurses than was anticipated and that $1,080 of the variance was caused by a longer average amount of nursing time per patient day than had been anticipated. Why these specific variances occurred is not known, but there is a much better focus on where the problem areas are.

A generic model for flexible budget variances is presented in Figure 13–4. In looking at this model, several things should be kept in mind. First of all, recall that basically all the necessary data are generally readily available. Second, these variances can be calculated on a computer.[5]

It sometimes is not obvious whether a variance is favorable or unfavorable. Looking at Figure 13–4, an easy rule of thumb is that as one moves from the right side toward the left, larger numbers on the left indicate unfavorable variance. For example, if the flexible budget amount is larger than the originally budgeted amount, the volume variance is unfavorable. If the subcategory is greater than the flexible budget, the quantity variance is unfavorable. This is true because as one moves from the original budget toward the left, movement is toward the actual result. If the actual result is larger than the original budget, more was spent than budgeted. The result is an unfavorable variance. Given the way this model is set up, this also holds true for each of the individual variances making up the total variance.

DETERMINATION OF THE CAUSES OF VARIANCES

What the nurse manager will not get from this analysis is the ultimate explanation of causes of the variances. The nurse manager will still have to investigate to find out *why* these variances have occurred. The analysis provides significant new information by pointing a finger in a specific direction instead of waving a hand in a vague direction.

For instance, if twice as many surgical supplies were used per patient day as expected, the nurse manager knows exactly what to investigate. The analysis does not tell why there was a variance, but it does tell where. Rather than simply saying that the operating room is over budget, it is known that the line item for surgical supplies is over budget. Furthermore, rather than simply noting that too much was spent for surgical supplies, it has been determined that the problem was not caused because there were extra procedures. Nor was it caused because the price of surgical supplies went up. It is specifically known that the problem lay in using more surgical supplies per procedure than had been budgeted. Managers must take over at this point and investigate why this occurred. Why were more surgical supplies used per procedure than expected? Was it sloppy use? Clear-cut waste? Was it pilferage? Was there a change in patient mix? Was there a major disaster that did not increase the number of procedures considerably but did bring in patients requiring a great amount of surgical supplies? Is the budget wrong and it is not really possible to get by with the budgeted amount of surgical supplies per procedure? Ultimately the nurse manager must find out the actual underlying cause of the variance.

---

[5]For more details on computerization of variances, see Steven A. Finkler, "Using Computers to Improve Variance Analysis," *Journal of Nursing Administration,* September 1991, reprinted in the Appendix at the end of Chapter 17.

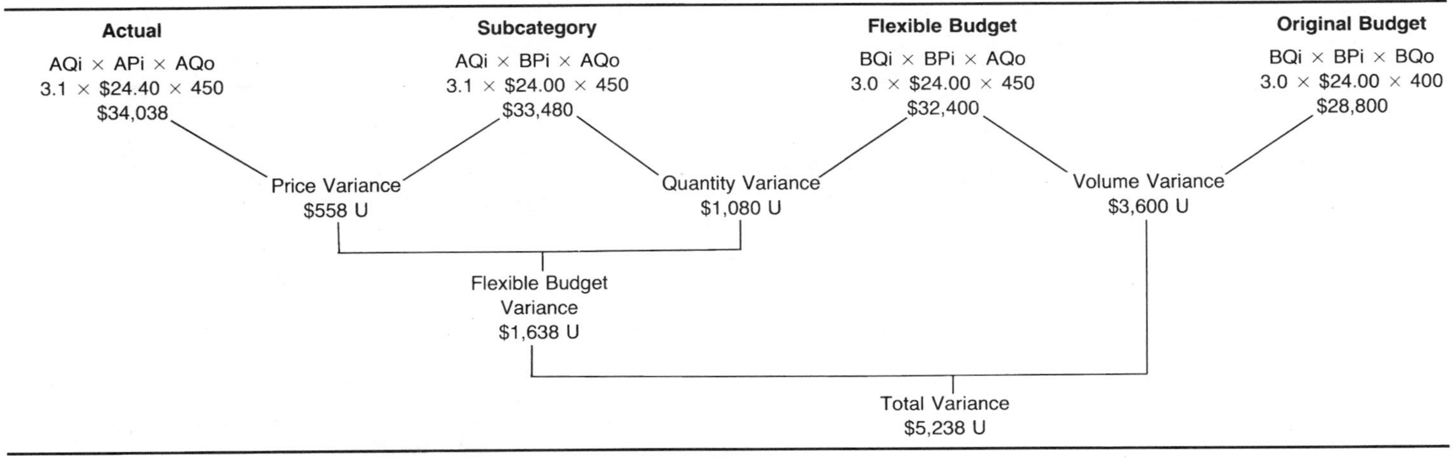

FIGURE 13–3. Price, quantity, and volume variances for 6th Floor West.

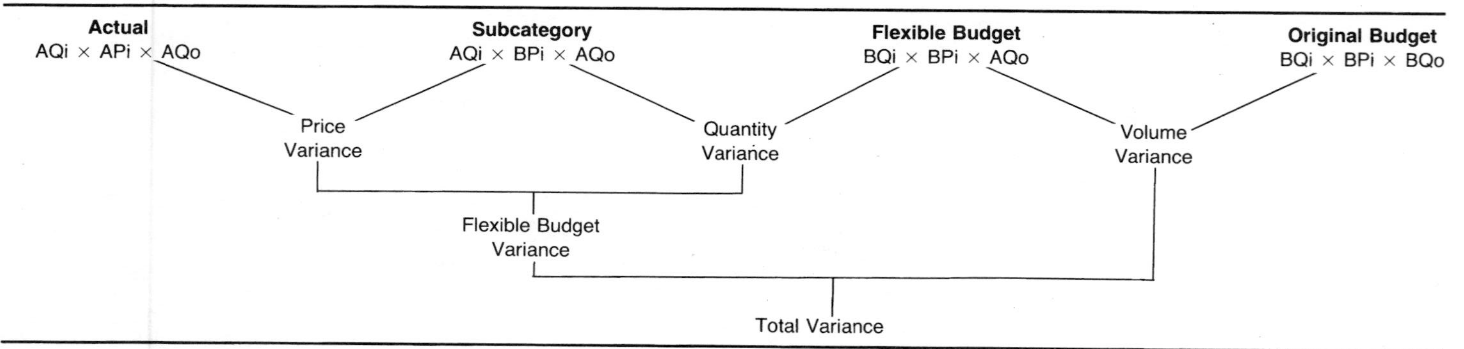

FIGURE 13–4. Price, quantity, and volume variances for a generic model.

※ AGGREGATION PROBLEMS

One problem that requires caution on the part of nurse managers is caused by the aggregation of information. When variances are combined, there is a tendency to lose information. Some of the favorable and unfavorable variances may offset each other. A summary report for a number of departments may appear to have little if any variance either in total or for a particular line item, such as salaries. However, one department might be well over budget and another well under budget. Both departments would warrant investigation.

The problem is not just at the interdepartmental level. The nursing department may appear to have little variance. However, two nursing units may have offsetting variances. Or it is possible that each nursing unit may appear to have little variance. However, within a nursing unit one line item may be offsetting another. For example, underspending in salaries could hide overspending in supplies.

Traditional variance analysis is adequate to disclose the types of aggregation problems discussed so far, if carefully used. By looking at each department and each unit individually and each line item rather than a summary for the department or unit, many aggregation problems are prevented. However, traditional variance analysis will not disclose a volume variance that offsets either a price or quantity variance. For example, if the number of patients is below budget and staffing is unchanged from the budget, there will be a favorable volume variance and an unfavorable quantity variance. The staff salary line might well show no variance in total. The nursing unit might well show no variance in total.

In this case the nurse manager of the unit is losing critical information. The volume variance is a strong signal. When volume is down, organizational revenues are probably down as well. The organization has a need to constrain costs. When staffing is unchanged even though there are fewer patients, costs may be excessive compared with available revenues. However, unless flexible budget variance analysis is used to disclose the quantity and volume variances, the manager will lack this information. As a result, the manager may not be able to move as quickly and decisively as the situation warrants.

※ EXCEPTION REPORTING

Aggregation problems create substantial difficulty. The only way to be sure that one variance is not being offset by another variance is by examining every single price, quantity, and volume variance of every single line item of every single unit of every single cost center of the organization. This creates a potentially unmanageable burden. Should the CEO of a hospital have to examine every individual variance for the entire organization? Should the CNE have to examine every individual variance for all units of the nursing department? The time required would be enormous. A solution to this problem is the use of *exception reports.*

Assuming a computer prepares all the variances for each cost element, it is a simple process for the computer to prepare a list for the CEO of only those individual variances that exceed a certain limit. This is called an exception report. It lists only the variances that are large. How large depends on the desire of the individual CEO. When tight, centralized control is desired, smaller variances are of interest. For example, while some CEOs might be interested only in monthly or year-to-date variances greater than 20% of the budget or $50,000, a CEO running a more centralized operation might be interested in variances greater than 10% or $10,000.

This does not mean that variances less than $10,000 must go unnoticed. Department heads, such as the CNE, would get a more detailed report for their departments, perhaps 5% or $1,000. Continuing the process, nurse managers would receive detailed exception reports for the variances in units under their supervision. Ultimately, the nurse manager who has direct control over a unit would want to review all variances for that unit. In all cases, if a nurse manager thinks a particular variance indicates a problem that is likely to grow worse in future months, the higher levels of nursing administration should be alerted to the problem rather than waiting until the variance is great enough to appear on the CNE's exception report.

※ REVENUE VARIANCES

The nurse manager's primary variance analysis effort is focused on expenses. This is predominantly because managers of health care organizations have a greater degree of control over expenses than they do over revenues. However, the information that can be yielded from revenue variance analysis is also important. For example, changes in revenue that result from changes in patient volume may be outside the control of the organization and its managers. Such changes, however, may require management actions or reactions to protect the organization's financial position.

Revenue variance methodology follows the same pattern as expense methodology. There is a traditional variance that tends to focus on the total revenue expected and actually achieved for a unit or department. There is also a flexible budget methodology that helps to identify the various underlying causes of variances. The total revenue variance for a unit, department, or organization can be broken down into a volume variance, a mix variance, and a price variance.

Consider an outpatient surgery department that has budgeted revenues of $1 million for the month just ended. Actual revenues were $850,000. Traditional variance analysis identifies a $150,000 unfavorable revenue variance. What caused the $150,000 shortfall?

The first step for flexible budget revenue variance analysis is to identify the revenue per patient. Unlike costs, which may be fixed or variable, revenues are all variable. Therefore the total $1 million budget could be divided by the number of patients budgeted to get an average revenue per patient. This allows calculation of a volume variance. Suppose that 800 patients were expected for the month. In that case the average revenue per patient was expected to be $1,250 (i.e., the $1 million total revenue ÷ 800 patients = $1,250 of revenue per patient) (Figure 13–5).

If there were actually only 750 patients, a flexible budget for revenue of $937,500 (i.e., 750 patients × $1,250 price) would be calculated. The revenue flexible budget indicates the amount of revenue that would have been budgeted if the number of patients had been forecast exactly correctly. The difference between the original budget for 800 patients and the flexible budget for 750 actual patients is an unfavorable volume variance of $62,500. Less revenue than expected is considered unfavorable.

The next calculation concerns the mix of patients. Not all patients would be expected to be charged $1,250. That figure represents an average. Assume that half the patients were expected to be type A patients charged $1,000 and half were expected to be type B patients charged $1,500. Any number of different types of patients with different prices is possible, but for this discussion we will limit it to just types A and B.

Suppose that of the 750 actual patients, 450 were type A and 300 were type B. Not only are there fewer patients than expected, but the mix of patients has changed as well. Less than half the patients are the more highly priced type B patients. Based on the actual number of patients and the actual mix, revenues would be expected to be $900,000 (i.e., 450 patients @ $1,000 + 300 patients @ $1,500). If we compare the flexible budget of $937,500 (the revenue expected for 750 patients) with this new "subcategory" value based on the actual mix, the difference is $37,500. This is the mix variance, which is unfavorable. The variance is unfavorable because there is a greater proportion of lower revenue patients.

This still leaves an unexplained variance of $50,000. This is a price variance. It is a result of charging a different price than expected. Although the outpatient surgery

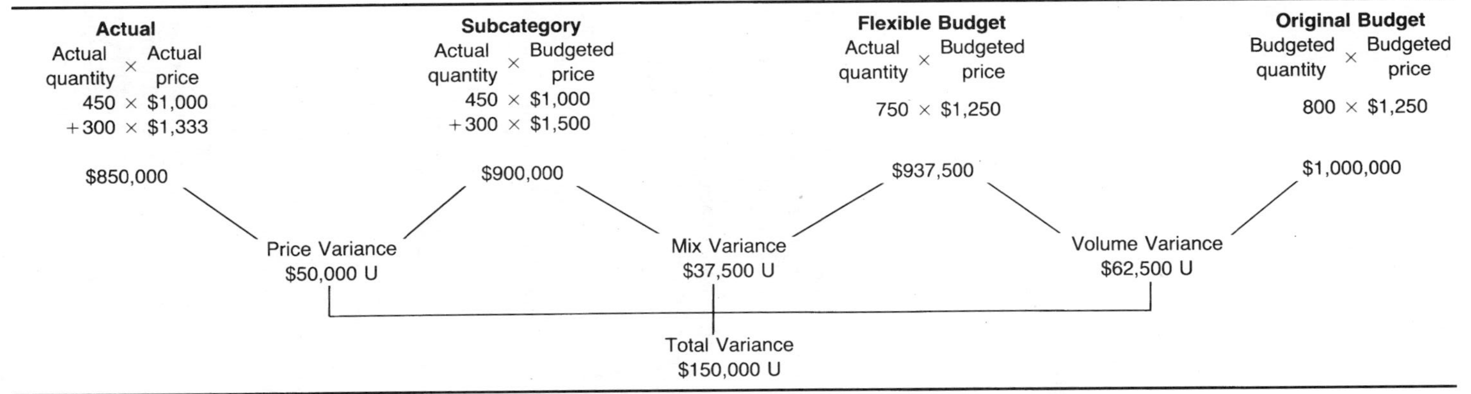

FIGURE 13–5. Revenue variances.

intended to charge $1,500 for type B patients, it is possible that because of government regulation or negotiated rates with insurance companies the average price for type B patients was only $1,333.33. In that case actual revenue would be $850,000 (i.e., 450 patients @ $1,000 + 300 patients @ $1,333.33). The $50,000 difference between the $900,000 from the mix calculation is an unfavorable price variance. It is unfavorable because the price was less than budgeted.

The calculations for these variances can be seen in Figure 13–5. Note that in each case the number of patients is multiplied by the price per patient. For the budget and flexible budget the total number of patients and the budgeted average price per patient are used. For the subcategory, the mix of patients is used, splitting the total into the number of actual patients of each type. For the subcategory the budgeted price for each type of patient is used. For the actual costs the actual number of each type of patient and the actual prices charged for each type of patient are used.

Often revenue variances are calculated based on the contribution margin rather than the revenue. (See Chapter 7 for a discussion of contribution margin.) Revenue places too great a focus on the total charge for different types of patients rather than on the profit implications of each type patient. A patient with very high revenue could have even greater expenses and cause losses. Another patient with only modest revenues could be quite profitable. Managers do not just need information about changes in revenues. They need to know whether the revenue changes are in profitable areas or unprofitable areas.

It is possible therefore to use the budgeted contribution margin rather than the revenue in all the calculations just discussed. There still would be a volume variance. Fewer patients would imply less overall contribution margin. There still would be a mix variance. However, whether the mix variance is favorable or unfavorable would depend on whether there is a greater or lesser proportion of the types of patients with higher contribution margins. The price variance would still depend on the actual price charged for each type of patient.

Whether variances are caused by changes in prices, the mix of patients, or the volume of patients is information that managers use in responding to increases or decreases in revenues. If the number of patients is falling, steps should be taken to try to find out why and to make sure that there are corresponding reductions in organizational expenses. If the mix of patients is changing, it may be necessary to shift resources within the organization. If prices differed from budget, an effort must be made to understand why and the overall implications for the organization's finances.

IMPLICATIONS FOR NURSE MANAGERS

Controlling the results of operations is as important as developing a feasible plan. Organizations use management control systems to ensure that every attempt is made to carry out the organization's plans.

Budgets can help control costs if they are used to motivate all managers and staff members. This requires communication of specific, measurable goals on a regular, frequent basis. Such a process will improve results as individuals make a self-motivated effort to achieve specified, attainable goals.

One must try to understand what incentives are needed to cause individuals to work toward the overall well-being of the organization. When a health care organization asks nurses to accomplish something, it is necessary to be concerned with why they would want to do it. Perhaps they will do it to benefit patient care. But that motive provides little incentive for cost control. Perhaps they will control costs out of loyalty to the organization. Perhaps they will control costs out of fear of losing their jobs. Perhaps they will control costs in hopes of earning a promotion.

Getting an understanding of what people will want to do and what they will not want to do is important. And once managers know what they will not want to do, they should carefully attempt to develop some clear motivational device that will give them an incentive to do what the organization needs to have accomplished. The key issue to remember is that organizations do not control costs; people do.

The difference between the budget and what actually occurs is called a variance. Comparison of actual results with budgeted expectations and analysis of the resulting variances should generally be done monthly. This enables midstream corrections that will improve year-end results. It also provides information for preparing the coming year's budget and for evaluating the performance of units, departments, and managers.

Most health care organizations prepare variance reports by comparing the information in the original budget with the actual results. There are several problems with this type of comparison. First, it does not tell as much about the cause of the variance as one would like to know; for instance, traditional variance analysis does not indicate whether a variance is caused by more resource use per patient or by higher prices for resources used. Second, traditional variance analysis ignores the fact that resource consumption is expected to vary with patient volume. Part of the variance will just be the result of changes in patient volume rather than being related to efficiency.

This has caused many health care organizations to start using a method called flexible budgeting. Flexible budgeting establishes an after-the-fact budget, that is, what it would have been expected to cost had the actual patient volume been known in advance. Using flexible budgets, it is possible to break a unit's or department's line-item variances down into components caused by (1) changes in prices or salary rates from those expected; (2) changes in the amount of input used per unit of patient volume or output, such as the amount of nursing time per patient day; and (3) changes in the patient volume itself.

Efficient management requires investigation and evaluation of variances on a timely basis, followed by actions to correct variances whenever possible. Managerial expertise and judgment are needed to investigate and evaluate the variances. Flexible budget variance analysis can make the manager's job easier by segregating the variance into its component parts. This allows the manager to spend more time understanding and explaining why the variance occurred instead of trying to isolate the portion of the variance attributable to patient volume changes, the portion attributable to resource usage per patient, and the portion attributable to the prices of the various resources consumed.

In considering variances the nurse manager should attempt to put finances in perspective. The financial health and survival of the institution are essential. However, the quality of patient care provided is also critical. Performance should be measured using more than one set of criteria. Meeting the budget is one measure of performance. Quality of care, patient satisfaction, nurse satisfaction, and innovation are a few of the other outcomes that nurse managers are trying to achieve. There should be a balance between evaluation of financial performance and evaluation of performance in nonfinancial areas.

This chapter has provided tools that can be used to identify the underlying causes of variances. Often this will allow the manager to explain a "poor" report. In some cases performance can be improved by using variance reports to learn where expenses are out of control. In other cases, spending over budget may mean that a trade-off was made. Some other objectives may have been achieved at the expense of financial goals. Which are more important? Each institution and its managers must make that decision in each specific case. Sometimes finances will be paramount. Sometimes they will not. If a nurse manager can meet the budget but fails to meet quality-of-care needs or can meet quality-of-care needs but fails to meet the budget, which choice is correct? Whichever choice is made, managers should be prepared to justify why they thought it was the right choice.

Although expense variances often require great attention, managers should also consider whether revenue variances are creating situations that require management intervention.

KEY CONCEPTS

Management control system Organizations exercise control over operations through the use of a complete set of policies and procedures called a management control system.

Responsibility accounting System of assigning responsibility for keeping to the organization's plan and carrying out the elements of the management control system. Responsibility is generally assigned to managers of cost centers.

Motivation The role of motivation of staff and managers in controlling operating results cannot be overemphasized. If people are not motivated to carry out the budget, it is not likely to be achieved. A variety of incentives, such as bonuses, can be used to help motivate staff and managers. If targets are set unrealistically high, the negative motivational implications are likely to offset any hoped-for benefits.

Communication Both the budget and actual results compared with the budget must be communicated throughout the organization. This is an essential element of control, and should be an ongoing process.

Responsibility should equal control If managers are held responsible for things they have no control over, the organization will reward and punish the wrong individuals. The result is invariably demoralization of managers and staff.

Interim evaluations These are of particular importance in controlling operational results. Each month there should be comparisons between what was expected and what has been accomplished.

Variance analysis Aspect of budgeting in which actual results are compared with budgeted expectations. Variances are used to improve future planning, allow for corrective actions to better control results in coming periods, and evaluate the performance of units or departments and their managers.

Traditional variance analysis Compares the budget with actual results for the most recent month and year to date for each line item in each cost center.

Flexible budget variance analysis Expands upon traditional variance analysis by dividing the total variance into price, quantity, and volume variances.

Price or rate variance Part of the total difference between the budget and actual that results from a higher or lower hourly rate or purchase price than budgeted.

Quantity or use variance Part of the total difference between the budget and actual that results from the use of more or less resources per patient than budgeted.

Volume variance Part of the total difference between the budget and actual that results from a different volume of patients than budgeted.

Aggregation of variances Managers should be careful to avoid failing to identify variances, because favorable variances and unfavorable variances offset each other when added together. Exception reports can be used to identify critical variances.

Revenue variances Can be calculated using either revenue or contribution margin to identify volume, mix, and price variances.

SUGGESTED READINGS

Bautista, C.L., "Meeting the Challenge of Cost Containment: A Case Study Using Variance Analysis," *Hospital Cost Management and Accounting,* Vol. 6, No. 2, 1994, pp. 1–8.

Cooper, J.C., and J.D. Suver, "Variance Analysis Refines Overhead Cost Control," *Healthcare Financial Management,* Vol. 46, No. 2, 1992, pp. 40, 42, 46.

Dove, H.G., and T. Forthman, "Helping Financial Analysts Communicate Variance Analysis," *Healthcare Financial Management,* Vol. 49, No. 4, 1995, pp. 52–54.

Feltau, Anne, "Budget Variance Analysis and Justification," *Nursing Management,* Vol. 23, No. 2, February 1992, pp. 40–41.

Finkler, Steven A., *Budgeting Concepts for Nurse Managers,* 3rd edition, W.B. Saunders, Philadelphia, Penn., forthcoming 2000.

Finkler, Steven A., "Control Aspects of Financial Variance Analysis," in *Health Services Management: Readings and Commentary,* Anthony R. Kovner and Duncan Neuhauser, eds., Health Administration Press, Ann Arbor, Mich., 1990, pp. 149–166.

Finker, Steven A., "Using Computers to Improve Variance Analysis," *Journal of Nursing Administration,* Vol. 21, No. 9, September 1991, pp. 9–15.

Finkler, Steven A., "Variance Analysis, Part I, Extending Flexible Budget Variance Analysis to Acuity," *Journal of Nursing Administration,* Vol. 21, No. 7/8, 1991, pp. 19–25.

Finkler, Steven A., "Variance Analysis, Part II, The Use of Computers," *Journal of Nursing Administration,* Vol. 21, No. 9, 1991, pp. 9–15.

Finkler, Steven A., "Flexible Budgeting Allows for Better Management of Resources as Needs Change," *Hospital Cost Management and Accounting,* Vol. 8, No. 3, 1996, pp. 1–5.

Horngren, C.T., G. Foster, and S.M. Datar, *Cost Accounting: A Managerial Emphasis,* 9th edition, Prentice Hall, Upper Saddle River, N.J., 1996.

Maitland, D., "Flexible Budgeting and Variance Analysis: Why Leave Staff Nurses in the Dark?" *Hospital Cost Management and Accounting,* Vol. 5, No. 9, December 1993, pp. 1–8.

Swansburg, Russell C., *Budgeting and Financial Management for Nurse Managers,* Jones & Bartlett Publishers, Sudbury, Mass., March 1997.

Voss, G.B., A. van Ooij, L.J. Brans-Brabant, and P.G. Limpens, "Cost-Variance Analysis by DRGs: A Technique for Clinical Budget Analysis," *Health Policy,* Vol. 39, No. 2, February 1997, pp. 153–166.

Wilburn, Debbie, "Budget Response to Volume Variability," *Nursing Management,* Vol. 23, No. 2, February 1992, pp. 42–45.

Variance Analysis

Part I, Extending Flexible Budget Variance Analysis to Acuity

Steven A. Finkler, PhD, CPA

The author reviews the concepts of flexible budget variance analysis, including the price, quantity, and volume variances generated by that technique. He also introduces the concept of acuity variance and provides direction on how such a variance measure can be calculated. Part II in this two-part series on variance analysis will look at how personal computers can be useful in the variance analysis process.

Recent years have seen a growing sophistication in the use of variance analysis by nursing departments. As cost containment has become more and more important to healthcare organizations, nurses have been among the leaders in pushing for techniques that can aid managers in controlling costs. Improved variance analysis—in particular, flexible budget variance analysis—is being adopted by an ever larger number of healthcare organizations.

Flexible budget variance analysis is based on the notion that budgets are prepared with a specific fixed volume of work in mind. When actual workload differs from budgeted expectations (which is more often than not the case), costs should be expected to change as well. That fact should be recognized in the variance analysis process. Flexible budget variance analysis explicitly recognizes this.

As healthcare organizations start taking workload *volume* into account in their variance analysis process, they should take the next major step in variance analysis. That step concerns the introduction of a technique for measuring the extent to which variances are caused by average patient *acuity* levels that differ from budgeted expectations. Over the last decade, hospital lengths of stay have been decreasing, but average patient acuity has been rising. If the increase in patient acuity exceeds a nursing department's anticipations, the results are invariably understaffing or overspending. However, mechanical processes are available that can calculate the portion of a variance that is attributable to unexpected changes in acuity.

In this article, the concepts of flexible budget variance analysis, including the price, quantity, and volume variances generated by that technique, are reviewed. The concept of an *acuity variance* is also introduced, and direction on how such a variance measure can be calculated is provided. Part II in this two-part series on variance analysis will look at how personal computers can be useful in the variance analysis process.

Flexible Budget Variance Analysis

Variance is the difference between a budgeted value and an actual result. Most healthcare organizations have been using variance analysis for a number of years. Until recently, however, that analysis tended to be rather unsophisticated. Actual results for each line-item of a department or unit budget were compared with budgeted amounts for the month and year to date. Differences between the actual result and the budget value were investigated to the extent possible.

There are several limitations to such information. The first and most critical problem is that the budget is based on an anticipated workload volume, whereas the actual costs incurred are based on the actual workload encountered. Given the information contained in this basic type of variance report, there is no easy way to calculate how much of the variance is due to the change in workload and how much to other factors.

Steven A. Finkler, PhD, CPA, Professor of Health Administration, Accounting, and Financial Management, Robert F. Wagner Graduate School of Public Service, New York University, New York.

Reprinted from *Journal of Nursing Administration,* Vol. 21, No. 7/8, July/August 1991, pp. 19–25.

A flexible budget is a revised budget prepared after each month is over, estimating the cost that should have been incurred for the actual workload encountered. Use of such an ex-post budget allows the manager to determine the extent to which variances are simply a result of increased or decreased workload. Because the workload is rarely controllable by the manager, it is possible to focus the investigation on the remaining portion of the variances.

Increased volume is often associated with increased revenues for the organization.

It should be noted that a flexible budget calculation is only appropriate for costs that are basically variable. For example, a 20% increase in patients on a unit would produce a 20% increase in supplies used. If the increase had been anticipated in advance, it is also likely that there would have been an increased level of staffing. On the other hand, the salary of head nurses and other nursing administrators is likely to be fixed. Costs that would not vary at all with changes in patient volume or acuity are not appropriate for flexible budget calculations.

Variance Components

The flexible budget approach allows any line-item for a variable cost to be divided into the portion caused by a change in the workload, called a *volume variance,* and a portion due to other causes. This latter portion, in turn, can be subdivided into a *quantity variance* and a *price variance.* The process involves taking the variance for a line-item for any unit or department, and subdividing it into several pieces or components. These individual pieces make it easier to track down the underlying causes of the line-item variances.

The volume variance is the change in resource consumption attributable to a change in workload volume. That volume might be measured in units such as patient days, admissions, hours of operating room time, emergency room treatments, or home care visits. In most cases, nursing has relatively little control over the volume of workload. If hospital occupancy levels rise from 80 to 85% nursing is expected to handle the increased number of patients. From a management standpoint, it makes excellent sense to separate out the volume variance because of the fact that the number of patients is usually not controllable. Further, increased volume is often associated with increased revenues for the organization. It makes little sense for the organization to discourage departments from handling increased volume. By holding a unit or department's spending to the level in its original budget, even if volume (and revenues) have increased, one merely encourages the unit or department to set up roadblocks to future patient increases.

The quantity variance is the change in resource consumption attributable to a change in the amount of resources used for each unit of output. For example, if paid nursing hours per patient day rise, that would give rise to a quantity variance. Quantity variances can arise as a result of a number of different causes. Unexpectedly high sick leave may result in more paid hours for the same number of patients, and therefore a higher nursing cost per patient. Changes in staff efficiency (e.g., longer lunch hours on the negative side or greater staff effort on the positive side) may lead to increased or decreased nursing cost per patient. A quantity variance also occurs if the workload changes and there is no staffing adjustment (upward or downward) made in response to the changing workload.

The price variance is the change in resource consumption attributable to a change in the price of inputs. For example, payment of a higher average hourly pay rate would create a price variance. Price variances may be under the control of nurse managers (e.g., poor staffing leading to unnecessary overtime premiums), or may be beyond their control (poor estimates by the purchasing department for the unit cost of supplies).

The Acuity Variance

If we total the volume, price, and quantity variances, we arrive at the total variance for the particular line-item under investigation. It is possible, however, to subdivide the quantity variance even further. Part of the quantity variance may result from a change in patient acuity levels from those anticipated.

Although acuity may change systematically as average length of stay declines over time, it is also a random element. In any given month or year, average acuity for a unit may be unexpectedly high or low, depending on the specific mix of patients in the unit during that time period. Such fluctuations in acuity are clearly beyond the control of the nurse manager, but he or she may have to respond with changes in staffing.

Flexible budget variance analysis can allow the quantity variance to be split between the portion caused by a difference between actual and anticipated acuity levels, and the portion caused by other factors. Before the advent of patient classification systems, measurement of an acuity variance was not possible. For hospitals that actively use patient classification systems, such measurement is now feasible.

Calculating Variances

To subdivide the variance for any line-item into volume, quantity, acuity, and price variances, a number of pieces of information are needed. First, it is necessary to know the budgeted workload level, the budgeted price of the resources used, and the budgeted amount of resources used. For example, consider the line-item cost of staff RNs in a medical/surgical hospital unit. The unit's workload would be measured in terms of budgeted patient days. The price would be the budgeted average hourly rate for staff RNs on the unit. And the amount of resource used would be the total budgeted staff RN hours for the unit. Note that this automatically takes acuity into account in the variance analysis because the total budgeted labor hours are the hours allowed for the budgeted number of patient days at the expected acuity level.

Ideally, the advantages of more sophisticated analysis should not be offset by the disadvantage of high cost to obtain additional data. All of the information needed so far is readily available from the data used to compile the budget. Flexible budget variance analysis also requires the same three pieces of data for the actual outcome. That is, it is necessary to accumulate information on the actual number of patient days, actual average salary rate, and actual number of paid labor hours. To calculate the acuity variance in addition to the price, quantity, and volume variances, it will also be necessary to know the actual number of patient days at each patient classification level.

The first three pieces of information should be relatively easy to obtain. Hospitals already generally keep track of the actual number of patient days by unit, the actual salary rates paid to staff, and the actual total number of paid hours for staff by unit. However, calculation of the acuity variance would require that patient classification information be collected on an ongoing basis. Each nursing department must make its own decision regarding whether the use of such information for variance analysis combined with its other potential uses, such as for improved staffing, make such data collection worthwhile. The information needed for flexible budget variance analysis, including development of an acuity variance is summarized in Table 1, which also includes hypothetical data for use in an example.

The original budget consists of the average price for the resource in question (e.g., staff RNs) multiplied by the budgeted amount of resource. Using the data from Table 1, the original budgeted amount is $100,000 ($20/hour multiplied by 5,000 staff hours). In contrast, the actual cost would be the actual average price paid for the resource multiplied by the actual amount of the resource used. The actual cost is $136,500 ($21/hour multiplied by 6,500 staff hours). Traditional variance analysis would compare the budget with the actual and note that the unit spent $36,500 more than its budget ($100,000 budget vs. $136,500 actual). However, it would not indicate anything about the source of that $36,500 variance.

A flexible budget should be calculated to reflect changes in workload from original expectations. The flexible budget is a computation of the amount that would have been budgeted, had the true workload level been known. The flexible budget consists of the budgeted amount of re-

TABLE 1. *Data Needed for Flexible Budget Variance Analysis*

Budgeted workload	1,000 patient days
Budgeted price of resource	$20 per hour
Budgeted amount of resource	5,000 hours
Actual workload	1,150 patient days
Actual price of resource	$21 per hour
Actual amount of resource used	6,500 hours
Actual acuity levels	200 at Level 1
	450 at Level 2
	300 at Level 3
	150 at Level 4
	50 at Level 5

source per unit of workload, multiplied by the budgeted price of the resource, multiplied by the actual workload level. In this case, the budgeted amount of resource is 5 hours per patient day (the budgeted total resource of 5,000 hours divided by the budgeted 1,000 patient days). Five hours per patient day, at $20 per hour, for 1,150 actual patient days yields a flexible budget value of $115,000 (5 × 20 × 1,150). Comparing the $115,000 flexible budget with the $100,000 original budget yields a difference of $15,000, which is an unfavorable volume variance. This would indicate that of the total $36,500 variance for the line-item, a portion equal to $15,000, is directly attributable to the fact that there were more patient days than expected. This portion of the variance would generally be considered beyond the control of the nurse manager.

In flexible budgeting, a calculation must be made to determine how much of a line-item variance results from changes in prices of the resources used. To make this calculation, the actual amount spent ($136,500 in this example) is compared with the amount that would have been spent had the actual price of the resource been as budgeted. In other words, using the actual amount of resources used but the budgeted price, how much would have been spent? In this case (Table 1), there are 6,500 actual staff RN hours. The budgeted price is $20. The product of those two number is $130,000. However, the actual cost for the nursing unit is $136,500 (6,500 hours × $21). The difference between the actual cost of $136,500 and the $130,000 cost using the budgeted price is $6,500. That is the price variance. It represents the portion of the total $36,500 variance attributable to the higher-than-expected hourly rate. Given the increased number of patient days, the use of either overtime or agency nurses might well be expected to drive up the average hourly wage, so this unfavorable price variance of $6,500 is not particularly surprising. However, it is large enough that it would probably warrant investigation to find its specific cause or causes.

The volume variance of $15,000 and the price variance of $6,500, combine to explain $21,500 of the total variance. However, the total variance for the line-item was $36,500. There is still $15,000 of variance that has not been explained. This is the quantity variance. It is caused by paying for more resource per unit of workload than expected. It is not attributable to more patients, but rather to the amount used per patient. Without patient classification information, the nurse manager would have to investigate the $15,000 quantity variance and try to ascertain its causes.

Calculation of the price, quantity, and volume variances is summarized in Figure 1. This figure includes the actual amount spent at the extreme left, and the original budget at the extreme right. In between are two other headings. The flexible budget, as previously noted, represents the amount that would have been budgeted for the actual workload of patient days had that workload level been known in advance. This does not reflect acuity-adjusted workload, but rather looks only at changes in patient-day volume. The value that is compared with the actual results to determine the price variance is referred to as the Budgeted Cost of Actual Resources Used. When this is compared with the flexible budget, the result is the quantity variance.

If patient acuity information is available, the quantity variance can be divided into the portion due to acuity and that due to other factors. This will require inserting a value in between Budgeted Cost of Actual Resources and the Flexible Budget in Figure 1. The new value will be called an Acuity Category. The difference between the Acuity Category and the Flexible Budget is the acuity variance. The difference between the Budgeted Cost of Actual Resources and the Acuity Category is a new quantity variance. The new quantity variance will be the same as the old quantity variance, except that it will exclude the portion of the variance due to changes in acuity. The key to this calculation is the ability to determine the number of paid nursing care hours that would have been budgeted had the actual acuity been known. For example, suppose that the hypothetical patient classification system in place calls for the following paid nursing care hours per patient day:

Patient Classification Level	Paid Nursing Care Hours
1	3.5
2	5.0
3	6.2
4	7.8
5	9.0

In the example being used (Table 1), the actual patient days at each level can be combined with the above chart to generate the hours of nursing care that would have been budgeted, had the

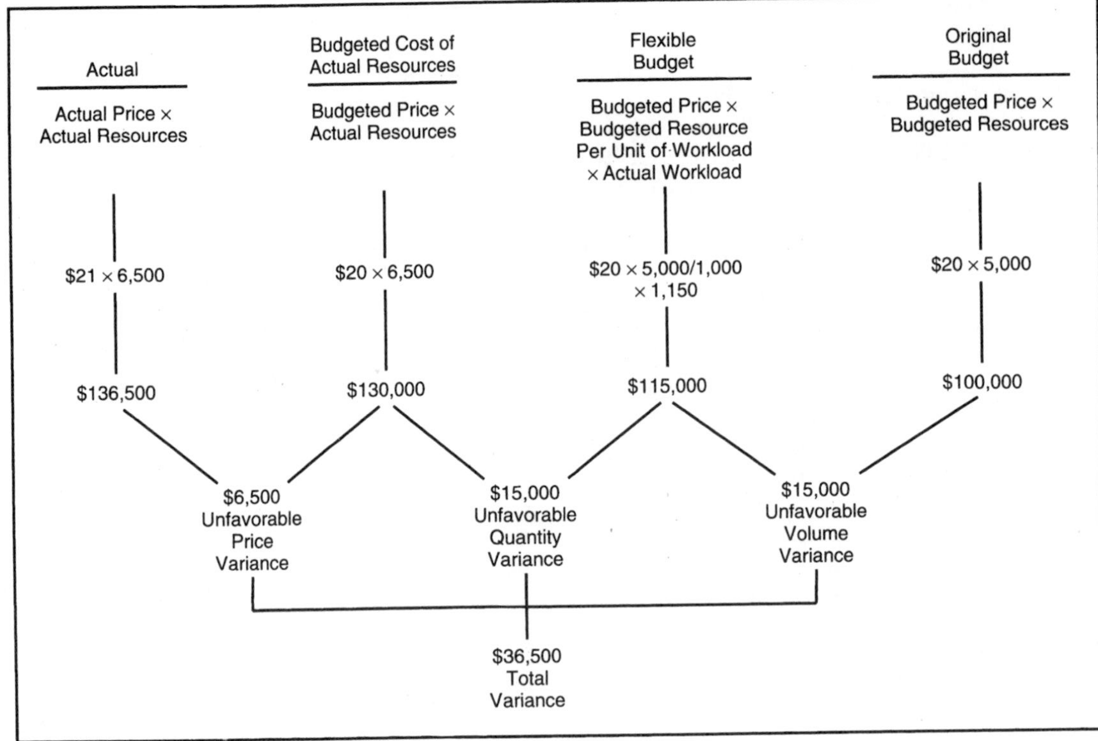

Figure 1. Calculation of price, quantity, and volume variances.

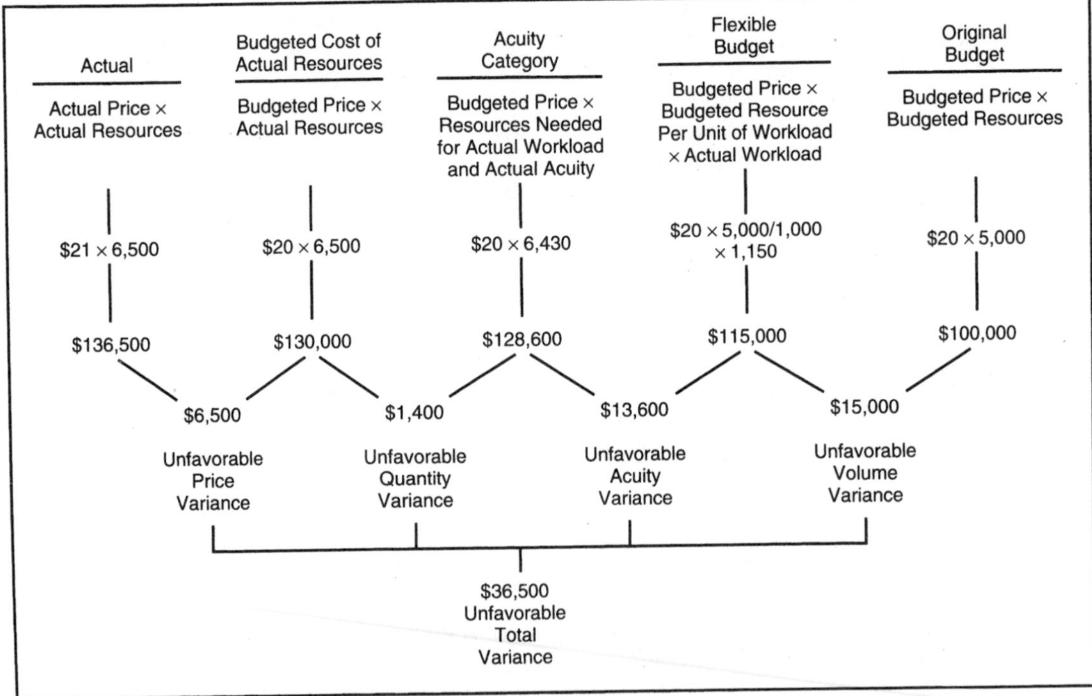

Figure 2. Calculation of price, quantity, volume, and acuity variances.

actual acuity level been known in advance. Essentially, the volume variance accounts for the fact that there were more or fewer patient days than expected. Similarly, the acuity variance will account for the fact that actual acuity differs from the level expected. The flexible budget asks the question, "how much should have been budgeted for the actual number of patients?," whereas the new Acuity Category (Fig. 2) asks, "how much should have been budgeted for the actual number of patients at the actual level of acuity?" Combining the patient classification scheme shown above with the data from Table 1, the number of nursing care hours that would have been budgeted, had the actual volume of patients and actual acuity levels been known, can be calculated as shown in Table 2.

Given that there would have been 6,430 budgeted nursing hours (Table 2) for the actual number of patient days and actual acuity, the acuity category can be calculated by multiplying the budgeted price of the resource, $20, by the 6,430 hours. The result is $128,600. When this is compared with the flexible budget value of $115,000 (Fig. 2), the difference is $13,600. That is the acuity variance. It is the result of actual acuity being higher than expected. When the $128,600 is compared with the Budgeted Cost for Actual Resources value of $130,000, the difference is $1,400. That is the new quantity variance. It represents the fact that more money was spent per patient, even after accounting for acuity. It could be caused by a wide variety of factors, and it could be investigated if the amount were considered large enough to warrant such an investigation.

It is important to note that although all variances in this example were "unfavorable," that does not mean that they were necessarily bad for the organization. Unfavorable simply means spent more than expected. If the extra patient days reflected more patients, revenue may have increased. Furthermore, if the increased acuity reflects a more complex mix of patients, the revenue per patient may be higher as well. Therefore, the unfavorable volume and acuity variances are not necessarily bad. A rule of thumb for determining whether a variance is favorable or unfavorable is that, moving from right to left in Figures 1 and 2, if the number on the left is larger, it indicates an unfavorable variance. However, managers must use thought, rather than rules of thumb, to determine if an unfavorable variance is good or bad.

Caveat

It is important to note one caveat regarding the development of the acuity variance. Budget line-items for nursing units and departments separate out each individual type of worker. Therefore it is appealing to determine the acuity variance for each line-item. However, patient classification systems do not usually isolate the amount of nursing care hours needed by class of care giver. When one calculates the number of nursing care hours needed for the actual acuity, it may be difficult to make that calculation for each separate type of employee. Therefore it may be necessary to aggregate some information in order to be able to calculate an acuity variance.

This is a less than ideal situation. Over time, patient classification systems may develop into more specific tools, looking at RNs, LPNs, and nurse's aides separately. In the meantime, however, the problem does create a complication for calculating acuity variances. Price, quantity, and volume variances are not affected by this problem.

※ **TABLE 2.** *Calculation of Required Paid Nursing Hours for Actual Number of Patient Days at Actual Acuity Levels*

Patient Classification	Nursing Hours Per Patient Day		No. of Patient Days		Required Nursing Hours
Level					
1	3.5	×	200	=	700
2	5.0	×	450	=	2,250
3	6.2	×	300	=	1,860
4	7.8	×	150	=	1,170
5	9.0	×	50	=	450
Total			1,150		6,430

Conclusion

At a minimum, nurse managers should be receiving variance reports that in some way allow for the impact of changes in the workload volume. As the number of patients increases, nurses should not have to explain that more patients consume more resources. Some type of volume variance measure is a necessity. The introduction of price and quantity variance calculations can also be a great aid. They can help nurse managers focus their variance investigations in specific areas.

The introduction of an acuity variance is somewhat more complicated. For organizations that have patient classification systems in place and in use, however, it represents an opportunity to move into the cutting edge of healthcare management in the area of variance analysis. Although adoption of flexible budget variance analysis methodology requires some effort, once used on an ongoing basis, it can continue to pay dividends in the form of improved explanations of variance causes and reduced variance investigation effort by all nurse managers, month after month and years into the future.

In Part II of this series on variance analysis, there will be a discussion of how the variances discussed in this article can be generated within a nursing department by the use of a microcomputer and a spreadsheet software program. The upcoming article will also discuss the use of a variety of types of graphs to aid in the process of variance analysis and justification.

Suggested Readings

Alward RR. Patient classification systems: the ideal vs. reality. J Nurs Admin 1983;13(2):14–9.

Curtin L. Integrating acuity: the frugal road to safe care [Editorial]. Nurs Manage 1985;16(9):7–8.

Finkler SA. Budgeting concepts for nurse managers. 2nd ed. Philadelphia: WB Saunders, 1991.

Francisco PD. Flexible budgeting and variance analysis. Nurs Manage 1989;20(11):40–5.

Nagaprasann B. Patient classification systems: strategies for the 1990's. Nurs Manage 1988;19(3):105–106, 108, 112.

Robbins WA, Jacobs FA. Cost variances in health care: when should managers investigate. J Nurs Admin 1985; 15(9):36–40.

Spitzer R, Poate W. Effective budgeting variance reporting. In: Spitzer R, ed. Nursing productivity: the hospital's key to survival and profit. Chicago, 5-N Publishers, 1986:21–5.

Wellever A. Variance analysis: a tool for cost control. J Nurs Admin 1982;12(7/8):23–6.

CHAPTER

14

Performance Budgeting

CHAPTER GOALS

The goals of this chapter are to:

- Introduce the concept of performance budgeting
- Identify weaknesses in traditional measures of performance
- Create an awareness of the importance of focusing on goals and measuring the accomplishment of goals
- Outline the specific technical steps in performance budgeting
- Identify potential measures for use by nursing in performance budgets

※ INTRODUCTION

The extreme financial pressure faced by health care organizations in recent years has resulted in substantial budget cuts. Managers are having to find ways to make do with less. A major concern in this environment is that the quality of patient care is likely to suffer. There is a growing call for evaluation of the outcomes of health care organizations. Budgeting can help managers by focusing to a greater extent on the results that departments and organizations achieve. This process, called performance or outcomes budgeting, is the topic of this chapter.

Performance budgeting is a technique that evaluates the activities of a cost center in terms of what the center accomplishes, as well as the costs of that accomplishment. It is an approach to budgeting specifically designed to evaluate the multiple outcomes of cost centers rather than a single budgeted output, such as the number of home care visits. Performance budgeting provides a mechanism for gaining a better understanding of the relationships between financial resources and the level and quality of results.

Traditionally, budgets focused primarily on the resources used by a department or cost center. There is detailed information on the number of nurses working in a unit and their pay rate. Supplies, educational seminars, and publications are all carefully considered. However, all of these are inputs. They are the resources the unit needs to achieve its objectives. Unfortunately, there has been little focus on objectives. What are the goals of the unit? What is it trying to achieve? Cost centers often define their goals only in the simplest terms, such as the number of visits, patient days, or procedures. Performance budgeting shifts the focus from the resources the unit plans to use to the various things it is trying to accomplish.

The first step in performance budgeting is to define the objectives or areas of accomplishment for the unit or department. These are called performance areas. Some examples of performance areas are quality of care, nursing satisfaction, patient satisfaction, productivity, and innovation. The second step is to identify the operating budget costs for the cost center being evaluated. In a nursing unit these costs include items such as the salary for the unit nurse manager, salaries for clinical staff, education costs, and supplies. The third step is to determine what percentage of available resources should be used for each performance area. The fourth step is to assign the budgeted costs for the center to the individual performance areas on the basis of those percentages. The fifth and final step is to choose measures of performance for each performance area and to determine the cost per unit of work load based on those measures.

WHEN IS PERFORMANCE BUDGETING APPROPRIATE?

In any organization that has multiple goals and objectives, performance budgeting may be useful. Performance budgeting allows the organization to define the various elements of performance that are important. It can then assess managers and departments based on their accomplishments in terms of those elements. Each department can have its own set of performance or outcomes criteria. Most existing budget measures focus on simple criteria, such as the number of patient days. Such measures are incapable of getting at issues such as quality of care per patient day or cost per unit of quality of care.

When nursing budgets are cut or inadequately increased for changes in patient acuity, wage rate increases, or other factors, there is often an expectation by top management that at least the same amount of work will be performed. Often this is an unreasonable and unrealistic expectation. While it is true that the number of patients or patient days may be cared for with a smaller budget, the amount of care given may not be the same. Performance levels and outcomes are likely to deteriorate. Unfortunately, rarely is there a linkage between the budget or amount spent and the amount of care provided, other than one simplistic measure such as the number of patient days.

If a nursing unit can care for 10,000 patient days in a year with a budget of $2,000,000, what happens if the budget is slashed to $1,750,000? If the unit still provides 10,000 patient days of care, traditional budgeting makes it appear that costs are down and output is unchanged. In reality, it is highly unlikely that outcomes are unchanged. Quality of patient care is likely to have declined along a number of dimensions. However, a traditional operating budget, focusing on the number of patient days, is unlikely to capture any of the changes that have occurred. A performance budget can help measure those changes.

THE PERFORMANCE BUDGETING TECHNIQUE

Determining Key Performance Areas

Nurse managers attempt to achieve a number of different objectives. Nursing units attempt to provide high-quality care. They attempt to satisfy patient needs and desires. They attempt to control costs. If you do not define clearly the performance that you hope to achieve, you cannot measure your success. The key is to develop a set of performance areas for measurement.

In developing performance areas, one should consider a variety of questions, such as: What important goals should be measured? What elements of a unit's performance are within the control of the nurse manager, and what elements are not? How should the nurse manager most productively spend working time? How should the nursing staff most productively use their time? How can the performance of a nursing unit be evaluated?

In addressing these questions, it is necessary to categorize the major elements of the manager's and unit's job or function. For example, consider a nurse manager of a thirty-bed unit. Some effort should go toward assuring a high level of patient care. Some effort should go to staffing the unit, some to controlling unit expenses, some to improving productivity, some to improving patient and staff satisfaction, and some to innovation and long-range planning. These are some key performance areas for the manager and unit. There may well be other important outcome areas that are not listed here. Managers must establish performance areas based on their own unit or department's specific circumstances.

Technical Steps in Performance Budgeting

Identifying the performance areas for a cost center is the first step in performance budgeting. The second step is to identify the existing line item budget for the cost center being evaluated. In a nursing unit, this budget includes the cost of items such as the salary for the unit nurse manager, salaries for clinical staff, education costs, and supplies.

The next step is to define how much of the resources represented by each line item are to be devoted to each of the performance areas. This requires that the manager develop a resource allocation model. This process forces the manager to think about what elements of the job are really important, and how important they are.

If, for instance, patient satisfaction is very important to the organization, the manager must consider whether an adequate amount of time and effort is being devoted to achieving patient satisfaction. The resource allocation for the performance budget explicitly notes the specific portion of the nurse manager's time, staff time, and other resources that should be spent on assuring patient satisfaction.

It is up to the nurse manager to decide how to allocate resources among the various processes that are associated with the desired outcomes. How much of the resources should be focused on quality of care? How much on staffing? A percent of the total effort should be assigned to each of the performance areas. The manager's allocations will likely not be the same for management time, staff time, and other resources. Each resource is allocated based on differing needs. For example, unit nurse managers might allocate 5% of their own time, 35% of clinical staff time, and 90% of supplies to direct patient care. A chart or table should be developed that shows the performance areas and the percent of each line item cost being allocated to each performance area.

The allocation of resources to different performance areas should be based on explicit decisions related to organizational priorities. However, when a performance budget is first introduced, it is easier to make allocations based on historical information. This information can be gathered by having everyone keep a log of their time for several weeks, or based on each individual's best guess of how they use their time. Once the performance budget is developed, more information will be available to the manager, and explicit choices can be made to reallocate resources in a more useful manner.

Once the percent of each resource to be used to achieve each performance area has been decided, a calculation must be made to determine how much money has been budgeted for each performance area. This can be done by taking the percent of each line item allocated to each performance area and multiplying it by the total amount of money in the budget for that line item. For instance, if the nurse manager's salary is $50,000, and 10% of the manager's working time is spent on improving quality of care, then $5,000 is calculated ($50,000 × 10%) as being spent on quality. If the staff nurses for the unit earn $500,000 in total, and they spend 5% of their efforts on improving quality, there is another $25,000 ($500,000 × 5%) being allocated to quality improvement. The nurse manager can total all the costs for each performance element. In this case, a total of $30,000 has been budgeted for improving quality of care.

The final step is to choose measures of performance for each performance area, budget a specific numerical objective for each area, and determine the budgeted cost per unit of each objective based on those measures. For instance, suppose that the nurse manager chooses to measure improvement in quality of care based on the number of medication errors. Suppose further that the performance budget calls for reducing the number of medication errors on the unit by 30 instances. Since $30,000 has been allocated to improve quality, it can be said that $1,000 has been budgeted per medication error eliminated. The next year the same amount of money might need to be budgeted just to maintain the level of care.

The performance budget specifies an amount of an outcome to be accomplished. For example, it might budget a certain specific number of fewer medication errors. The performance budget also specifies the inputs to be devoted to achieve that outcome. A certain amount of nurse time is budgeted for accomplishing the reduction in medication errors. Thus goals are matched with resources needed for their accomplishment. The process of performance budgeting can be clarified with an example.

PERFORMANCE BUDGET EXAMPLE

The first step in developing a performance budget is to determine the performance areas that the nurse manager intends to use. The following is one possible set of performance areas:

- Patient care
- Quality of care improvement
- Staffing
- Cost control
- Increased productivity
- Improved patient satisfaction
- Improved staff satisfaction
- Innovation and long-range planning

The second step is to get the cost information for the unit from the operating budget. Converting operating budget information into a performance budget will give a clearer focus of how the unit spends the budgeted amount of money. The operating budget already gives information such as the number of full-time equivalents (FTEs) by skill level. However, those are inputs rather than outcomes. The performance budget will provide information about results rather than just inputs. Suppose, hypothetically, that the line item operating budget for a nursing unit is $1,000,000 for the coming year, as follows:

Nurse manager	$ 50,000
Clinical staff salaries	800,000
Education	20,000
Supplies	40,000
Overhead	90,000
Total	$1,000,000

The third step is to determine the percentage of operating budget resources allocated to performance areas. Allocation of the nurse manager's time to performance areas might be as follows[1]:

[1]This simplified example treats the nurse manager's time as if it were all directly under the manager's control. A more realistic calculation might set aside an amount of time, such as 20%, for administrative mandated activities.

Quality of care improvement	15%
Staffing	15%
Cost control	20%
Increasing productivity	20%
Improving patient satisfaction	10%
Improving staff satisfaction	5%
Innovation and long-range planning	15%
Total	100%

By developing the allocation to areas of performance, a plan is provided for how the nurse manager's time should be spent and what areas are deemed to be either the most important or the most in need of the manager's efforts.

There is no reason to believe that all resources within a department or unit should necessarily be allocated in the same fashion. The time allocation for clinical staff might be as follows:

Direct patient care	30%
Indirect patient care[2]	30%
Quality of care improvement	5%
Cost control	5%
Increasing productivity	2%
Improving patient satisfaction	5%
Other	23%
Total	100%

The allocation of time for direct patient care seems low, but this is misleading. Since this budget is based on total unit costs, it includes non–worked time for sick leave, vacation, and holidays. It also includes worked time off the unit, such as education days. These items might account for most of the 23% "other" time. Furthermore, a substantial portion of time spent in quality of care improvement and improved patient satisfaction may in fact be additional direct patient care time with a specific focus on those two goals. Therefore this allocation might imply that about half of the time of nurses on the unit is spent on direct patient care.

To develop a full performance budget for the unit, it also will be necessary to determine how education, supplies, and overhead resources relate to the performance of the unit. Suppose that a reasonable expectation for the role of education in a given year is as follows:

Quality of care improvement	20%
Cost control	20%
Increasing productivity	20%
Improving patient satisfaction	10%
Improving staff satisfaction	10%
Innovation and long-range planning	20%
Total	100%

Supplies used by a nursing unit are primarily clinical supplies for direct patient care and, to a much lesser extent, administrative forms and other administrative supplies. Suppose that a reasonable expectation for the use of supplies is as follows:

Staffing	2%
Cost control	2%
Direct patient care	90%
Indirect patient care	5%
Other	1%
Total	100%

[2]For example, supervising staff or interacting with physicians.

There is no uniquely correct way to allocate overhead, since much of it is assigned arbitrarily to a nursing unit. Ultimately, performance budget measures will be used to assess the cost of devoting resources to a particular activity, such as improving quality of care. Since overhead is not likely to vary based on how much effort the manager and clinical staff devote to improving quality of care on the unit, it is reasonable to assign the unit's overhead all to direct patient care. However, this is an arbitrary allocation, and alternative approaches are possible.

Direct patient care	100%

The above percentage allocations are summarized in Table 14–1. Every line item category within the original operating budget has a percentage assigned to the individual performance areas.

The original operating budget can now be assigned to performance areas, as seen in Table 14–2. This table takes the total cost for each line item in the operating budget and multiplies it by the percentages in Table 14–1 to determine the budgeted cost for each performance area for each line item. For example, Staff Salary is budgeted at a total of $800,000 (Table 14–2, Totals column). Of this amount, 5% is allocated to quality of care improvements (Table 14–1, Quality column, Staff Salary row). As a result, 5% of $800,000, or $40,000, is allocated to quality of care improvements (Table 14–2, Quality column, Staff Salary row).

The total budgeted cost of each of the performance areas can be assessed. It is expected that the nursing unit will spend $51,500 in total on quality improvement efforts (Table 14–2, Quality column, Totals row), $8,300 on staffing, $54,800 on cost control, and so on. In Table 14–2, compare the *bottom row,* which gives the total for each key performance area, with the *Totals column,* which gives the total by line item from the original operating budget. The original operating budget appears to be primarily a fixed budget over which the unit has little control. It shows only the amount to be spent on each input resource consumed. However, the bottom row shows that implicit choices are being made about the allocation of the operating budget resources to different priority areas. Each column in Table 14–2 tells the amount of money budgeted for each performance area. The manager does in fact have at least some ability to modify how these resources are spent. It could be decided that relatively greater efforts should be made in one particular area and less in another. Knowing that $51,500 is budgeted for quality, $47,000 for patient satisfaction, and $366,000 for direct patient care is much more valuable information than knowing that $800,000 is budgeted for staff salaries. The focus has shifted from inputs to performance.

Note, however, that a performance budget has still not been fully developed. The allocation of operating budget to performance areas (Table 14–2) is a valuable plan that provides an indication of whether the unit is planning to proceed in the most appropriate manner. It does not go far enough, however. It is not specific in terms of quantifying the goals for each performance area.

Table 14–3 presents the next step—the actual performance budget. In Table 14–3, the performance areas have been moved from the top row to the left side of the table. For each area, the difficult task of choosing a performance measure and quantifying the budgeted level for each performance area must be addressed.

Health care organizations try to produce improved health. Since this cannot be measured directly in most cases, proxies such as the number of patient days of care are used. Performance budgets add additional proxies to assess the accomplishment of the organization's goals. In Table 14–3 it is seen that a budget can be developed that gives information about such items as the budgeted cost to attain a reduction in patient care planning errors. In this example, the budgeted cost is $5,150 for each 1% drop in the rate of failure to comply with patient care plan procedures (Table 14–3, Average Cost column, Quality Improvement row). The next section addresses the issue of developing proxies for performance measurement.

※ **TABLE 14–1.** *Summary of Percentage Allocation to Performance Areas*

	Performance Areas										
Cost Item	**Quality**	**Staffing**	**Cost Control**	**Productivity**	**Patient Satisfaction**	**Staff Satisfaction**	**Innovation and Planning**	**Direct Care**	**Indirect Care**	**Other**	**Totals**
Nurse manager	15%	15%	20%	20%	10%	5%	15%	0%	0%	0%	100%
Staff salary	5%	0%	5%	2%	5%	0%	0%	30%	30%	23%	100%
Education	20%	0%	20%	20%	10%	10%	20%	0%	0%	0%	100%
Supplies	0%	2%	2%	0%	0%	0%	0%	90%	5%	1%	100%
Overhead	0%	0%	0%	0%	0%	0%	0%	100%	0%	0%	100%

※ **TABLE 14–2.** *Allocation of Operating Budget to Performance Areas*

		Performance Areas									
Cost Item	**Totals**	**Quality**	**Staffing**	**Cost Control**	**Productivity**	**Patient Satisfaction**	**Staff Satisfaction**	**Innovation and Planning**	**Direct Care**	**Indirect Care**	**Other**
Nurse manager	$ 50,000	$ 7,500	$7,500	$10,000	$10,000	$ 5,000	$2,500	$ 7,500	$ 0	$ 0	$ 0
Staff salary	800,000	40,000	0	40,000	16,000	40,000	0	0	240,000	240,000	184,000
Education	20,000	4,000	0	4,000	4,000	2,000	2,000	4,000	0	0	0
Supplies	40,000	0	800	800	0	0	0	0	36,000	2,000	400
Overhead	90,000	0	0	0	0	0	0	0	90,000	0	0
Totals	$1,000,000	$51,500	$8,300	$54,800	$30,000	$47,000	$4,500	$11,500	$366,000	$242,000	$184,400

※ **TABLE 14–3.** *Performance Budget*

Performance Areas	Activity	Description of Output Measure	Amount of Output Budgeted	Total Cost of Activity	Average Cost
Quality improvement	Patient care planning	Patient care plan compliance	10% Reduction in failure rate	$ 51,500	$5,150 Per percent drop in failure rate
Staffing	Daily staff calculations	Number of daily calculations	365 Daily calculations	8,300	$22.74 Per daily calculation
		Reduction in paid hours per patient day	0.2 Hour paid per patient day		$4,150/.01 Hour reduction
Cost control	Reduce cost	Reduction in cost per patient day	$8 Per patient day	54,800	$6,850/$ Reduction
Increased productivity	Revise procedures Work more efficiently	Reduction in total unit cost per direct care hour	$3 Reduction per direct care hour	30,000	$10,000/$ Reduction
Increase patient satisfaction	Respond to needs	Complaints	10% Reduction in complaints	47,000	$4,700/1% Reduction in complaints
Increase staff satisfaction	Respond to needs	Turnover	25% Reduction in staff turnover	4,500	$180/1% Reduction in turnover
Innovation and planning	Planning sessions	Number of meetings	12 Meetings	11,500	$958.33 Per meeting
Direct care	Direct patient care	Hours of care	10,000 Hours	366,000	$36.66 Per direct care hour
Indirect care	Patient charting	Number of patient days	7,300 Patient days	242,000	$33.15 Per patient day
Other				184,400	
Total				$1,000,000	

⨳ DEVELOPING PERFORMANCE AREA MEASURES

To be able to create a performance budget that will be as useful as possible, there must be specific ways to measure accomplishments in each performance area. Some of the measures developed for the different performance areas will appear to be crude proxies at best. However, patient days is itself a crude proxy for the process of providing health care, which in turn is a proxy for improved health. Yet patient days is a very useful measure. Over time, performance budgeting will improve as better proxies are suggested and incorporated into the technique. What are some potential output measures for evaluating the results of a nursing unit? Each of the performance areas likely has some associated key activities that can be budgeted and measured.[3]

It will take a fair amount of thought to come up with a good set of performance areas and measures of performance. For example, are patient complaints an appropriate measure of patient satisfaction with the nursing unit? If the patients complain about nurses, is it because the quality of care or attention to patients is not what it should be, or simply that the patients are reflecting their general mood related to their illness. However, *increases* in the rate of complaints may well be a meaningful performance measurement.

Quality of Care

The quality of care measure will be addressed first, since quality always presents a particular measurement challenge. Earlier, the use of medication variances was suggested as one possible measure for the change in quality of care. Another possible approach is to focus on the patient care plan as a quality indicator. If staff are not skillfully developing patient care plans, ultimately patient care may suffer. Therefore it is possible to measure the quality of nursing by how well plans are developed. Measurement can be based on the *percent* reduction in the number of incomplete care plans or it can be based on the *number* of incomplete care plans. Many nursing units already measure the quality of their patient care planning. However, with performance budgeting, not only is the quality measured, but the measurement is also associated with the expected cost of improving compliance.

In the first row of Table 14–3, it can be seen that Quality Improvement is one performance area being budgeted for. The measure used for this performance area will be the percent reduction in incomplete patient care plans. A 10% reduction is budgeted. As Table 14–2 showed, $51,500 is devoted to this area of the budget. Therefore it is expected that each percent reduction in incomplete plans will cost $5,150. This represents the total $51,500 to be spent in this area divided by the volume of output expected, in this case, $51,500 divided by a 10% reduction equals $5,150 per percent.

This approach recognizes that improvements in performance cost money. It is insufficient to simply dictate that a nursing unit improve its patient care planning without providing additional resources to accomplish this end. Can this unit lower its failure rate even more? Yes, it probably can. However, the performance budget provides explicit information that improved patient care planning requires more attention from the nursing staff. Such additional attention requires real additional resources in terms of increased staffing. If additional staffing is not provided, the only way to improve patient care planning is to devote a greater percent of the staff's efforts to compliance in this area (unless productivity can be increased). However, this will mean devoting less time to other areas.

It is possible that a unit is satisfied with its patient care plans. The nurse manager

---

[3]The measures described are a mix of both process and outcome measures. They also overlap to some extent. Eventually, performance budgeting may be refined to a point where such problems can be overcome.

of the unit does not believe that it is worth a substantial effort to improve its patient care planning. However, even maintaining a given level of quality requires staff attention. Thus the performance budget might show a goal of no change in the number of incomplete plans. An explicit portion of the performance budget would still be allocated to the quality area, to achieve that steady state.

What happens if the overall budget for the nursing unit is cut? The performance budget allows determination of areas in which resources should be cut. If a choice is made to cut resources in an area that affects quality, it would not be surprising to detect later that the number of incomplete patient care plans is increasing. The performance budget would show how the cuts to the unit are expected to affect the various performance areas. Budget cuts must explicitly be assigned to the performance areas to be cut. Rather than expecting no impact of budget cuts, explicit choices are made, and the unit can demonstrate what outcomes are likely to deteriorate as a result of the budget cut.

Staffing

A nursing unit manager must make many staffing decisions throughout the year, as well as manage vacations, holidays, sick leave, and busy and slow periods. In Table 14–3, it is assumed that daily calculations are made for staff adjustments. This requires some managerial time each and every day.

Calculations by the unit manager to adjust unit staffing could conceivably be made weekly, or just once a month. If staffing were only adjusted monthly, extra staff might be assigned all month long so that there would be adequate staff for busy days. Less frequent work on staffing would save managerial time, but would likely result in higher staffing costs. Monthly calculations would only require the unit to devote about $250 of management resources to staffing annually instead of the $8,300 annual cost when staffing is adjusted daily. However, the cost of extra nursing staff might offset the savings. The performance budget serves a useful function by making explicit the costs of daily calculations.

The performance budget can also show the benefits of daily calculations. Suppose that it is expected that by adjusting staffing daily, seven days a week, to the desired staffing level for the actual workload, it is possible to reduce the overall average paid hours per patient day for staff by 0.2 hour (twelve minutes) per patient day. Presumably, by monitoring staffing needs very closely, it is possible to avert unneeded overtime, excessive use of agency nurses, or periods of overstaffing. If the 0.2 hour per patient day reduction is achieved by calculating staffing daily, $8,300 of the departmental budget will be devoted to staffing calculations. However, if the nursing unit has an average census of twenty patients, there would be a savings, on average, of four paid nursing hours per day (20 patients × 0.2 hour per patient day), or 1,460 nursing hours per year. The cost of 1,460 nursing hours would far outweigh the $8,300 investment in daily calculations to adjust staffing.

For example, suppose that the average nurse wage on the unit is $30 per hour. The total wage savings is $43,800. A return on investment can be calculated by dividing the savings of $43,800 by the cost of $8,300, or 5.28. In other words, $5.28 is saved for every dollar spent by doing staffing adjustments daily.

Cost Control

The purpose of cost control is to reduce or restrain increases in the organization's costs. For health care providers paid under a prospective payment system, such as capitation on diagnosis related groups (DRGs), reduced costs per patient directly improve the organization's financial health. The performance measure for cost control in Table 14–3 focuses on a reduction in the cost per patient day. The activity, reduce cost, really represents a goal rather than a description of specifically how the nurses in the unit are to go about accomplishing the goal. However, the budget shows a clear commitment in this area: $54,800 is allocated specifically to accomplishing this end. Referring to Table 14–2, it is possible to see how much of the cost control effort is expected to come from the nurse manager's time, how much from the staff, how much from formal education, and so forth. In this example, each staff nurse is expected to spend 5% of the time, or about two hours per week, specifically focusing on cost reduction. This could mean eight hours at a continuing education program once per month. It does not necessarily mean that each week each nurse will spend two hours on cost control.

In Table 14–3, it can be seen that the performance budget calls for a cost reduction per patient day of $8. The cost of the efforts in this area are budgeted to be $54,800. Most of this comes from requiring the staff to make a specific effort to find ways to contain costs. When the $54,800 budgeted cost for cost control is compared with the budgeted cost reduction of $8 per patient day, for each dollar saved in cost per patient day it will cost the unit $6,850.[4] That seems rather high. Perhaps the unit is spending more on this activity than it is worth. In some cases the performance budget may make explicit the fact that the unit is spending more to accomplish some end than it is worth.

However, care must be exercised in interpreting the performance budget. If $6,850 is spent to save a dollar per patient day, there must be a consideration of how many patient days there are likely to be. If the unit's average census is twenty, there will be 7,300 patient days during the year (20 patients per day × 365 days in a year), and the savings at $1 per patient day would be $7,300, or slightly more than the $6,850 cost. If the census is twenty-eight, the savings would be substantial. If the census is fourteen, the efforts to save money are costing more than they are saving.

Cost control is a general goal. While the cost per patient day is a rough proxy intended to measure success with respect to that goal, it may be that the cost control efforts are also saving money by getting patients discharged sooner. The shorter length of stay decreases overall costs. To determine the true payback for cost control efforts, it would be necessary to combine the savings from the reduced cost per patient day with the savings from the shorter length of stay. The same $54,800 effort for cost control will be working toward both of those ends. For this reason, although it is more complicated, it is often worth using several different measures of performance to more completely assess the unit and its accomplishments. This is discussed below, in the Multiple Measures section of this chapter.

Increased Productivity

The desired productivity outcome is for the unit to accomplish more with the same or less resources. Procedures may need to be revised to help the staff accomplish this. While it is difficult to specify exactly how this can be accomplished, it is not difficult to establish how to measure success. Assume that the organization is concerned about the cost of direct hours of care per patient day. If the total budgeted cost for the department is divided by the total direct patient care hours, a cost per direct care hour can be determined. It will probably be necessary to do occasional special studies to measure, on average, how many direct patient care hours are being provided.

Performance can then be assessed by the reduction in the overall unit cost per direct patient care hour. Such a reduction would indicate either a reduction in total costs or an increase in direct care hours. This approach has a big advantage over simply looking at the cost per patient day. If the cost per patient day declines, this could mean that patients are getting less care during each day. With this measure, cost of care is directly linked to the number of hours of direct care.

---

[4]Typically we find the cost per unit, such as the cost per percent reduction in turnover, or the cost per percent reduction in incomplete patient care plans. This is similar to finding the cost per patient day or the cost per discharge.

Patient and Staff Satisfaction

The key approach to satisfaction is to be responsive to the needs of individuals. Some hospitals use a formal instrument for collecting data on patient satisfaction. That would be a good tool to use for performance budgeting. However, even if the organization is not that sophisticated or is unwilling to spend the money on data collection that a formal instrument requires, performance budgeting can still be useful. One simply needs to be a bit more creative in establishing the measurement proxies.

For example, to measure patient satisfaction the number of complaints could be counted. It may be true that some complaints are unreasonable or are about things that are not controllable. Many dissatisfied patients may not complain. However, some reduction in the number of complaints may be a way to go about measuring improvement in patient satisfaction. As with other areas, it must be determined how much improved patient satisfaction it is hoped can be generated and whether the cost of the improvement is acceptable relative to the expected level of improvement.

Staff satisfaction might also be measured in terms of complaints. However, turnover rates might be a better indicator. If the hypothetical numbers in the example were correct, then taking actions to increase staff satisfaction that require $4,500 of total cost would be worthwhile, since it would cost only $180 for each 1% reduction in staff turnover on the unit. This is a small cost compared with the cost of recruiting and orienting new staff.

Innovation and Planning

Sometimes it is difficult to measure performance. Innovative activity is one example. Proxies for performance in this area tend to be particularly weak. On the other hand, one of the most important things that a manager can do is to be innovative and to foster innovation. By making innovative activity explicitly a part of the performance budget, the necessity of devoting energies to this area can be recognized even if the proxies available to measure performance are weak.

One measure of innovative activity and accomplishment is the number of procedure changes introduced based on recently published research. Another is the number of meetings related to change. The fact that meetings are taking place is probably an indicator that activity is going on in this area. Are the meetings themselves the end goal? No. Do more meetings necessarily mean that more is being accomplished? No. They do, however, provide some sense of the degree of innovative activity.

It is also beneficial to see how expensive meetings are (see Table 14–3). When managers and staff are aware of the cost per meeting, there is likely to be more serious work done, in less time, with fewer meetings.

Although meetings are used in Table 14–3, it is clearly a measure of process rather than of actual innovation. The number of useful innovative ideas generated might be a better measure. And certainly some formal system of rewards should be developed to give employees an incentive to generate innovative ideas.

Direct Care

The measure suggested for performance evaluation in this area is the direct care cost per direct care hour. Lowering the cost per direct care hour can be achieved either by increasing the number of hours produced for the same cost or by lowering the costs for a given number of direct care hours. This is not the total unit cost per direct care hour. Rather, it considers the total cost for only the hours of direct care provided, divided by the hours of direct care. This will generate information on the cost per hour of the direct care. If this cost can be lowered, it often implies that less overtime or fewer agency nurses are being used. Another common way to achieve this goal is to substitute less skilled caregivers (e.g., unlicensed assistive personnel) for RNs or to substitute less expensive RNs for more experienced, expensive RNs. Although these approaches may decrease costs, they may also adversely affect patient outcomes.

Indirect Care

Indirect care is more difficult to measure than direct care because it comprises a wide variety of activities, such as charting and communication with physicians. One approach is to measure the cost per patient day for these indirect activities. Reducing the cost per patient day for indirect activities is likely to indicate improved efficiency, unless the quality of the activities deteriorates. However, if there is a series of quality performance measures, such as patient care planning, adverse patient events, and other checks on quality, such deterioration would probably not go unnoticed.

Other

Some activities do not lend themselves to quantification and analysis. It is preferable to reduce the portion of the budget used for "other" purposes by as much as possible. However, to the extent that it exists, there is no simple way to measure performance with respect to the use of resources devoted to these activities.

This discussion is not meant to be comprehensive. Rather, it presents some examples of how specific measures can be associated with various performance areas. It is necessary for the nurse manager to closely manage staff to ensure that they follow the performance budget as closely as possible. If staff are included in the process of preparing performance budgets, they are more likely to strive to achieve the budgeted targets. One indication of the success of the performance budget approach is the extent to which the unit achieves its performance budget goals.

⁜ MULTIPLE MEASURES

In most of the above cases, one measurement was used for each of the various performance areas. This is not always an optimal approach. For example, the percent of patient care plans that are incomplete is not the only measure of quality available to nursing units. Adverse events such as medication errors or the number of patient falls could also be measured. As performance budgets become more sophisticated, it would not be unreasonable for the $51,500 allocated for quality to be subdivided. Perhaps half of the quality efforts will be related to patient care plans, one quarter to reducing patient falls, and one quarter to reducing the number of medication variances. In that case, the $51,500 in the performance budget would be subdivided into $25,750 for patient care plans, $12,875 for reducing patient falls, and $12,875 for reducing medication variances. The budgeted cost per fall prevented and the budgeted cost per medication variance avoided could be calculated in the same way as the budgeted cost for reducing failures to comply with patient care plan procedures was calculated earlier.

This multiple measure approach is clearly superior to use of one measure for each performance area. Since it is likely that the nurse manager will be trying to improve quality in many areas, assigning all $51,500 to one area is likely an overstatement of the cost per unit of performance in that area. It also ignores other important activities. Some quality improvement activities such as providing research-based care may improve several areas of quality, while other approaches such as a staff development program on decreasing medication errors may be specific to one area.

Suppose that the quality outcome area is subdivided and it is determined that ten medication variances can be eliminated by focusing some specific attention in that area. Suppose further that it would cost $12,875 to do this. The cost per medication variance eliminated would be $1,287.50. Is this too much to spend on this problem? Perhaps it is so low that even more should be spent to try to eliminate additional medication variances. The key is that this approach allows the manager to quantify the financial impact of many activities that are done now without any specific cost-effectiveness measurement. With this method it is possible to assess whether the results in a given area warrant the resource investment in that area.

In some cases, rather than allocating the cost to several different areas, it simply makes sense to aggregate the benefits yielded by the unit's efforts. For example, in the case of cost control, there may be efforts to reduce the cost per direct care hour, reduce supply costs, and also reduce the average length of stay. In real-life situations, it is probably hard to determine how much staff effort goes to reduced length of stay and how much effort to reduced direct hours per day. One solution is to calculate the benefits from both shorter length of stay and reduced direct hours per patient day and combine them. Thus the total benefits can be compared with the total costs.

※ IMPLICATIONS FOR NURSE MANAGERS

There is a wealth of information to be gained from performance budgeting. It is a tool that is likely to improve both the planning and control processes in hospitals substantially. Performance budgeting represents a proactive approach to management. This approach follows a basic concept of budgeting: managers prepare a *plan*, and attempt to manage according to that plan.

The starting point in performance budgeting is to determine the key performance areas. Next the operating budget is used to determine resources available. There is no conflict between the operating budget and the performance budget. They should work together. The operating budget focuses primarily on input resources. How much is going to be spent on RNs, how much on aides, and how much on supplies? The performance budget focuses on both processes and outcomes. How much is being budgeted to improve quality, how much to provide direct patient care, how much to innovate?

As health care organizations move forward in managerial sophistication, they must move beyond the focus on inputs and begin to focus on performance. Financial pressure to be more efficient can easily lead to deterioration in the quality of care provided. However, cuts in resources do not have to affect performance in a random or arbitrary manner. Performance budgeting can show where resources are being used. Movement toward a measurement focus on the cost of the goals of the nursing unit can allow the manager to make choices and to allocate scarce resources wisely among alternative possible uses.

Performance budgeting is time-consuming and challenging. In some cases, the allocation of money to goal achievement will be inexact or arbitrary. However, it has tremendous potential value in health care organizations. Performance budgets can allow for an indication of the level of quality of care expected in a planned budget. They can *explicitly* show quality decreases that are likely if budgets are cut without corresponding reduction in patient days. It is likely that as part of the evolution in budgeting, this is an approach that will gain ever wider use.

KEY CONCEPTS ※

Performance budgeting Technique that evaluates the activities of a cost center in terms of what the center accomplishes and the costs of that accomplishment. It is an approach to budgeting specifically designed to evaluate the performance of cost centers in terms of a variety of goals rather than a single budgeted output, such as home care visits.

Performance areas Objectives or areas of accomplishment for the unit or department.

Determining key performance areas In developing performance areas, a variety of questions should be considered, such as:

What are the important goals?
What elements of a unit's performance are within the control of the nurse manager, and what elements are not?
How should nurse managers most productively spend their time?
How should the nursing staff most productively use their time?
How can the performance of a nursing unit be measured?

Technical steps in performance budgeting

Identify key performance areas.
Identify line item budget costs for the cost center.
Define how much of the resources represented by each line item are to be devoted to each of the performance areas.
Calculate the dollars budgeted for each performance area. This can be done by taking the percent of each line item allocated to each performance area and multiplying it by the total amount of money in the traditional operating budget for that line item.
Choose measures of performance for each performance area, budget a specific numerical objective for each area, and determine the budgeted cost per unit of each objective based on those measures.

Multiple measures Selection of more than one basis for measurement of performance in each performance area.

SUGGESTED READINGS

Blustein, Jan, Karla Hanson, and Steven Shea, "Preventable Hospitalizations and Socioeconomic Status," *Health Affairs,* Vol. 17, No. 2, March/April 1998, pp. 177–189.
Bushardt, Stephen, and Aubrey R. Fowler, "Outcomes Evaluation Alternatives," *Journal of Nursing Administration,* Vol. 18, No. 10, October 1988, pp. 40–44.
Cobb, Martha Davis, "Evaluating Medication Errors," *Journal of Nursing Administration,* Vol. 16, No. 4, April 1986, pp. 41–44.
Donnelly, L.J., H. Jaffe, and D. Yarbrough, "Organization Management Systems Decrease Nursing Costs," *Nursing Management,* Vol. 20, No. 7, July 1989, pp. 20–21.
Finkler, Steven A., *Budgeting Concepts for Nurse Managers,* 2nd edition, Aspen Publishers, Gaithersburg, Md., 1992.
Fosbinder, Donna, and Helen Vos, "Setting Standards and Evaluating Nursing Performance with a Single Tool," *Journal of Nursing Administration,* Vol. 19, No. 10, October 1989, pp. 23–30.
Hatry, Harry P., James R. Fountain, Jr., Jonathan M. Sullivan, and Lorraine Kremer, eds., *Service Efforts and Accomplishments Reporting: Its Time Has Come,* GASB Research Report Series, Governmental Accounting Standards Board, Norwalk, Conn., 1989 through 1993.
Herzlinger, Regina E., and Denise Nitterhouse, *Financial Accounting and Managerial Control for Nonprofit Organizations,* South-Western Publishing, Cincinnati, Ohio, 1994.
Hill, Barbara A., Ruth Johnson, and Betty Garrett, "Reducing the Incidence of Falls in High Risk Patients," *Journal of Nursing Administration,* Vol. 18, No. 7 and 8, July/August 1988, pp. 24–28.
Lee, Robert D., Jr., and Ronald W. Johnson, *Public Budgeting Systems,* 6th edition, Aspen Publishers, Gaithersburg, Md., 1998.
Mann, Linda M., Cynthia F. Barton, Micaela T. Presti, and Jane E. Hirsch, "Peer Review in Performance Appraisal," *Nursing Administration Quarterly,* Vol. 14, No. 4, Summer 1990, pp. 9–14.
Saywell, Robert M., Jr., John R. Woods, J. Thomas Benson, and Margaret M. Pike, "Comparative Costs of a Cooperative Care Program Versus Hospital Inpatient Care for Gynecology Patients," *Journal of Nursing Administration,* Vol. 19, No. 3, March 1989, pp. 29–36.
Young, Sue W., Linda M. Daehn, and Christine M. Busch, "Managing Nursing Staff Productivity through Reallocation of Nursing Resources," *Nursing Administration Quarterly,* Vol. 14, No. 3, Spring 1990, pp. 24–30.

PART

V

MANAGING FINANCIAL RESOURCES

All managers of health care organizations manage resources. Determining which personnel and other resources to use and how to use them is a managerial function. A subset within the realm of organizational resources is represented by financial resources. To the same extent that clinical resources must be carefully used, financial resources must be managed efficiently.

Decisions concerning where and how to get financial resources—the source of financial resources—is one element of the management of financial resources. Some resources in for-profit organizations come from investments owners make in the organization. In not-for-profit organizations a common source of financial resources is charitable donations. Profits are a potential source of financial resources for all types of health care organizations. In the late part of the twentieth century it was common for health care organizations to borrow money to finance their operations.

Once the organization has financial resources, it must manage them efficiently. Decisions must be made concerning how much cash to have on hand. Management techniques must ensure that cash is received as promptly as possible. Managers must ensure that cash is available when needed for purposes such as employee payrolls or interest payments. This requirement to have control over the inflow and outflow of cash necessitates management of other assets and liabilities that directly affect cash. As a result, receivables, inventories, marketable securities, payables, and leases fall under the heading of management of financial resources.

While some managers perceive the management of financial resources as the strict domain of financial managers, that is not the case. For example, a financial manager can do little to control inventory levels. The nurse manager is in a much better position to make determinations regarding necessary inventory levels and to enforce policies established to prevent unnecessary stockpiling of inventory. Therefore the nurse manager and financial managers must work together in the management of financial resources to arrive at an optimal outcome for the organization.

Additionally, nurse managers should be aware of even those aspects of the management of financial resources that do not bear directly on their day-to-day activities. The decisions to borrow money or invest it have a direct bearing on the success of the organization and on the decisions it makes concerning the allocation of resources to various cost centers. Therefore it is beneficial for the nurse manager to be aware of the factors involved in the management of financial resources.

This part of the book is divided into two chapters. Chapter 15 focuses directly on the management of the short-term financial resources of the organization. Chapter 16 is concerned with the long-term financing of health care organizations.

Short-term financial resources appear in the current asset and current liability sections of the balance sheet. Such resources generally provide or require cash within a relatively short period, usually less than a year. These short-term resources and short-term sources of resources are referred to as the organization's working capital.

Long-term financing relates to the alternatives the organization has for acquiring financial resources that will not have to be repaid within less than one year. To be able to acquire capital assets—buildings and equipment—the organization must know that it can acquire money that does not have to be repaid in a short time. The choices it makes regarding such long-term financing can have dramatic effects on the ability of the organization to provide health care services and to compete in the health care marketplace. ※

CHAPTER

15

Short-Term Financial Resources

CHAPTER GOALS

The goals of this chapter are to:

- Define working capital and working capital management
- Describe the role of cash in the organization
- Explain techniques for cash management
- Distinguish between cash flows, and revenues and expenses
- Describe the cash budgeting process
- Provide a description of the elements of accounts receivable management
- Discuss factors related to efficient inventory management
- Define trade credit terms related to accounts payable
- Discuss elements of working capital management for other current liabilities

※ INTRODUCTION

Working capital is the organization's current assets and current liabilities. *Net working capital* is the current assets less the current liabilities. The term *working capital management* refers to management of the current assets and current liabilities of the organization. (A basic discussion of current assets and current liabilities is provided in Chapter 5.)

Working capital is sometimes referred to as "cash register money." When one opens a store for business, there must be some money in the cash register to make change for the first customer who makes a purchase. Additionally, some customers may charge their purchases. In those cases, the store will not receive any cash immediately, but it still must pay its suppliers for the items it has acquired for sale, and it also has to pay its employees. There must be adequate cash for the store to use during the lag time from when it must pay for its resources until it receives cash from its customers.

The cash resources of an organization are of concern to all its managers. Why should a nurse manager be concerned with issues such as cash flow and inventory levels? All organizations have limited resources. If intensive care unit nurses stockpile IV fluids, the organization will pay out more cash now for inventory than is otherwise necessary. This in turn could mean that medical/surgical nurses will be told that there is no cash available to buy needed supplies. Nurses sometimes cope with this situation by stockpiling whenever they get a chance so they will have the supplies when they need them. This creates a vicious cycle. Since all nurses try to keep high levels of inventory to protect their patients, the overall inventories are maintained at too high a level. This means that money has been spent on inventory rather than deposited in a bank and earning interest. The lost interest means that there is less total money available for purchases of supplies. A cooperative working relationship is needed throughout the organization to allow inventory levels to be maintained at adequate levels and money to be available for purchases when needed without unduly wasting resources by keeping high inventory levels.

One can envision a working capital cycle (Fig. 15–1) in which cash is used to buy inventory items such as clinical supplies. Then patients are treated, consuming inventory items and using employees' services. Then the organization bills patients and waits to collect payment. Finally cash is received, and the cycle starts again.

Working capital management is the role of the manager in ensuring that there is adequate cash on hand to meet the organization's needs and minimizing the cost of those resources. To do this, the manager must carefully control cash inflows and outflows. To be efficient, cash must not lie idle, so there should not be too much cash on hand. Cash not immediately needed should be invested, earning a return for the organization. Similarly, excess inventory should not be kept by the organization. The money spent to pay for inventory that is not needed can be used by the organization for some other purpose. Receivables from customers should be collected promptly so that the organization will have that cash available for its use.

By the same token, current liabilities must be managed carefully. The organization desires to have sufficient cash to pay its obligations when they are due. However, if the organization pays its bills before they are due, it will lose the interest it could have earned if it had invested its cash for a little longer rather than paying the obligation.

This chapter focuses on the management of all elements of working capital. The discussion begins with current assets. Then we will turn our attention to issues related to current liabilities.

※ CURRENT ASSETS

A number of current assets require careful management. The most essential financial resource is cash. Cash is what organizations must have to pay obligations as they come due. Cash is generally defined as both currency and balances available in bank accounts for withdrawal upon demand (e.g., checking accounts). Marketable securities provide managers with an outlet to invest idle resources while maintaining access to the resources when needed. In most health care organizations managers also focus a great deal of attention on accounts receivable. Such receivables often constitute the largest single element of working capital. Inventories also receive a great amount of attention because historically managers have had difficulty in managing them.

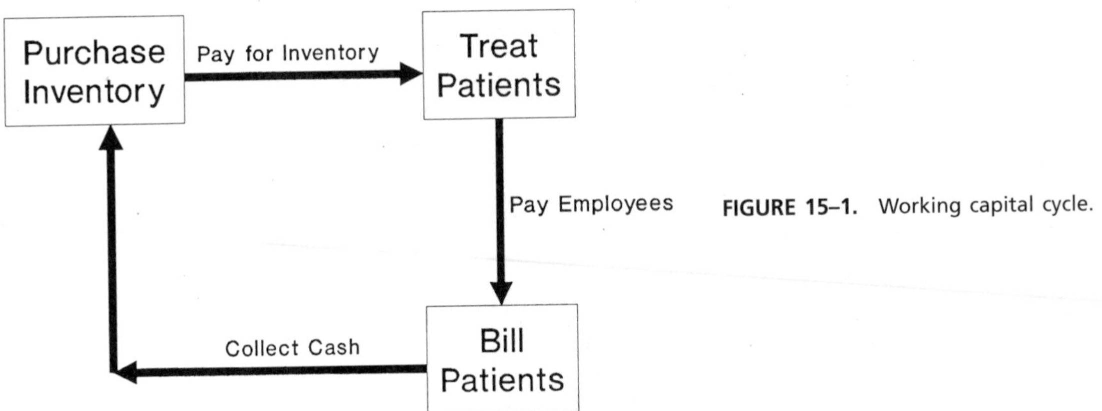

FIGURE 15–1. Working capital cycle.

Cash and Marketable Securities

Organizations have cash requirements for three main purposes:

- Transactions
- Safety
- Investments

Cash must be available for transactions, that is, the day-in and day-out normal operating expenses of the organization such as staff payroll and supplies. A health care organization cannot wait to receive patient payments before paying many of the organization's obligations; cash is needed for that purpose.

Safety is the second reason for holding cash. Managers are unable to anticipate all the organization's needs. Emergencies may require immediate, unexpected cash outlays. In some situations, managers may anticipate the likelihood of the event but not know when it is likely to occur. In other cases, the event may be totally unanticipated. Experience has proved that it is wise for the organization to have immediate access to cash just in case an unexpected need arises.

The third purpose for holding cash is to have cash available if a desirable investment opportunity arises. Such an opportunity may be the possibility of earning an attractive profit, or it may relate to the possibility of providing services to the community.

Given these reasons to hold cash, managers might desire to keep large amounts available, just to be safe. However, that is not necessarily an optimal approach. Cash does not generate a return for the organization. Often it sits in a non-interest-bearing checking account. Even if it is kept in a savings account, the rate of return is likely to be minimal. If the organization wants to maximize the benefits from all its resources, it must minimize the extent to which it has unproductive assets.

Therefore there is a conflict in cash management. The more cash on hand, the safer the organization, but the lower its return on invested money. The less cash the organization chooses to keep on hand, the better its financial profits, but the higher the risk. There is less protection against unexpected cash needs. Managers must walk a tightrope, attempting to determine a reasonable cash balance and keeping neither too much nor too little.

In a well-run organization, cash is actively managed. An initial projection is made regarding the timing of cash receipts from philanthropy, patients, the government, and insurance companies. A projection of the organization's required payments must also be prepared. The cash excess or shortfall is calculated for each period of time.

If a shortfall is anticipated, it may be possible to go to a bank and arrange for a line of credit to be available at the time cash is projected to be needed. Before doing that, however, other approaches should be considered. Can the financial managers take actions to process patient billings more quickly so that payments will be received sooner? Will the extra cost of speedier invoicing be offset by the interest saved by borrowing less money from the bank? What if payments to the organization's suppliers are delayed by thirty days to avoid borrowing money? How angry will that make the organization's suppliers?

If a cash surplus is forecast, it can be invested to earn interest, used to repay loans, or used to provide more health care services. Financial managers must ensure that the organization always has enough cash to meet obligations, but they should also be careful to ensure that the organization is not missing opportunities to provide additional health services because it is keeping too much cash in the bank. Either too little or too much cash leaves the organization in a less than optimal situation.

Short-term Cash Investment

Cash should rarely if ever be kept in non-interest-bearing accounts. In fact, even after checks are written, it is possible to invest the money in the interim period until the check is cashed. That period is called the *float*. Many banks have arrangements that allow money to be automatically transferred into a checking account as checks are presented for payment. Until that point the money can remain in an interest-bearing account.

Managers should make great efforts to ensure that cash is deposited into interest-bearing accounts as quickly as possible and withdrawn only when actually needed. All organizations should have specific policies that result in cash and check receipts being processed and deposited promptly.

Interest-bearing bank accounts pay relatively low rates of interest. Many alternatives are available for health care managers to invest cash at a higher rate of return. In most cases, however, this requires reducing the organization's ability to get immediate access to the cash. Short-term investments include treasury bills, certificates of deposit (CDs), and *repurchase agreements*. Treasury bills are issued for thirteen weeks, twenty-six weeks, or fifty-two weeks. However, they are traded actively, making it easy to convert them into cash when necessary. CDs generally tie up the organization's money for at least a month. However, they often pay interest rates higher than treasury bills. Repurchase agreements are flexible bank-related financial instruments. They can be for periods as short as one day. However, their interest rates are generally lower than those of treasury bills.

It is also possible for health care organizations to invest in other types of marketable securities such as corporate stocks and bonds. However, managers must exercise care in making such investments, since they are subject to market-rate fluctuations; that is, their value might fall while they are invested. While that reduction in value may be recovered if the securities are held for a period of time, the organization may well suffer a loss if it must liquidate the investment to get the cash. In general, risk and return represent a trade-off in investments. To earn a higher return on invested money, one must be willing to take a greater risk with the initial principal investment.

Cash Flow vs *Revenue and Expense*

Cash management concentrates on the inflows and outflows of cash. This is in contrast to the operating budget focus on revenues and expenses. Operating budgets consider overall profitability, but they do not consider when payments are made. Therefore the manager cannot use them to determine whether adequate cash will be available at any given point in time for the organization's needs.

At times cash management may cause the organization to make decisions that directly affect nurse managers and that seem to make no sense. For example, consider a request by nursing to buy bedside computers for nursing units at a total cost of $200,000. The computers are expected to have a useful lifetime of ten years and will improve the quality of documentation. This will result in improved care and will decrease overtime required for charting by $40,000 per year. The $400,000 of reduced overtime over the ten-year period is enough to make the initial investment of $200,000 financially sensible. Yet the financial officers may say that the organization cannot afford the computers. How can that decision make any sense?

Even though the computers would save more money than their cost, it is not clear that the organization can afford to purchase them. The entire price of $200,000 for the computers will have to be paid in cash this year, even though the overtime savings are expected to be only $40,000 this year. Where will the cash for the initial $200,000 purchase come from?

The potential for reduced costs or for increased profits does not by itself provide the cash needed to make the investment. It might be wise to lease the asset rather than pay all the cash up front. Maybe the organization can borrow the money from a bank. Perhaps it can raise the money through contributions. While the organization's managers should try to pursue various ways to get the cash for worthwhile investments—whether they are worthwhile because they are profitable or simply because they are good for patients—there is a responsibility to the well-being of the organization not to spend the money until it is first determined that there will be sufficient cash available to spend.

Financial officers must carefully consider the cash implications of the operating and capital budgets before they are approved. In effect, various departments submit their operating and capital budget requests. A *cash budget* is developed based on those requests. One reason that departmental budgets may be rejected is that the cash budget may show that the organization will simply run out of cash if it makes all the requested payments. If an organization finds itself without cash to meet its obligations, it may be forced into bankruptcy. Even if the organization is making a profit, without careful management it may run out of cash and get into financial difficulty.

Cash Budgets

As a result of the importance of cash balances, health care organizations generally prepare a cash budget for the entire coming year on a monthly basis. The format of cash budgets is fairly standard. Each month begins with a starting cash balance. The expected cash receipts for the month are added to this. These receipts may be broken down into categories such as inpatient, outpatient, other operating, and nonoperating or by payer (e.g., Medicare, Medicaid, Blue Cross, other insurers, self-pay patients, donations, and cafeteria sales). The starting cash balance is added to the total receipts to get a subtotal of available cash. Then expected cash payments are subtracted. Cash budgeting was introduced in Chapter 11.

Accurate cash budgeting requires managers to estimate how much cash will be received by type of payer. Different types of payers have different bad-debt rates and pay on different schedules. For example, Blue Cross might pay an organization more promptly than Medicare but less promptly than other private insurance companies. Payer-mix information, combined with knowledge about the lag time in payment by each type of payer, can be used to project cash receipts for each month.

For example, suppose that a health care organization had revenues of $500,000 for January and that the payer mix is as in Table 15–1. The payment lag times represent averages. Especially with respect to self-pay patients, there is likely to be a mix of faster and slower paying patients. Assuming that there are no bad debts, when will the $500,000 in revenue from January be received in cash? (See Table 15–2.) The payers with a one-month lag will pay in February, those with a two-month lag in March, those with a three-month lag in April, and those with a four-month lag in May. For example, a total of $225,000 from January revenues would be collected in April because in this example both Medicare and self-pay patients pay with a three-month lag.

If the expected cash balance for any month exceeds the minimum desired balance, the excess can be invested. This is true even if a surplus one month is followed by an expected shortfall the next. It may pay to invest the extra cash in a very short-term investment, such as a money market fund. In that way, the excess cash from one month can earn some interest and still be available to meet the shortage the next month. Borrowing can thus be avoided or minimized.

※ **TABLE 15–1.** *Payment Lag by Payer*

Payer	Percentage of Patients	Payment Lag Time
Medicare	30	3 months
Medicaid	20	4 months
HMOs	25	2 months
Other insurer	10	1 month
Self-pay	15	3 months

※ TABLE 15–2. *Timing of Cash Receipt of January Revenues*

Payer	Percentage of Patients		Total Revenue		Revenue Share	Month Collected
Medicare	30	×	$500,000	=	$150,000	April
Medicaid	20	×	500,000	=	100,000	May
HMOs	25	×	500,000	=	125,000	March
Other insurers	10	×	500,000	=	50,000	February
Self-pay	15	×	500,000	=	75,000	April

Maintaining Security over Cash

Of all the assets the organization has, cash requires the greatest care to ensure that it is not misappropriated. Systems must be put into place that have checks and balances. Individuals who handle cash should be different from those who reconcile cash receipts. Controls should exist for both cash receipts and cash disbursements.

Disbursements are often easier to protect. Whenever possible, payments should be made by check. Large checks should require two signatures. All checks should be numbered. All checks should require an authorization by someone other than the one involved in drawing the checks.

Cash receipts should be handled by individuals who are bonded, reliable, and take vacations. Bonding is an insurance procedure that protects the organization from cash theft by the insured individual. Reliable personnel are essential. The organization must have trustworthy individuals working in the cash area. Even with trustworthy individuals, it is a good practice to require individuals to take vacations. Knowing that someone else will be handling the function makes individuals less likely to do anything inappropriate that might be discovered in their absence.

Accounts Receivable

When an organization's customers do not pay for goods or services at the time they are provided, they are said to be buying the services "on account." An account is set up by both the buyer and seller to keep track of the amount owed. Providers of the service expect to ultimately receive payment, so they call the money owed them an *account receivable*. Buyers will ultimately pay the amount owed, so they have an *account payable*.

Management of accounts receivable focuses on speed, accuracy, and communication. Managers must try to minimize the time between provision of care and ultimate receipt of payment. Accounts receivable earn no return for the organization. The sooner cash is collected, the sooner the organization can use that cash for its operations or invest it. Also, efforts to collect cash quickly tend to reduce bad debts. For accounts to be collected on a timely basis, all documentation must be accurate and complete. Also, there should be great efforts to keep the lines of communication open between the organization and the payers.

The process of managing accounts receivable should start before a patient is admitted to a health care institution. Preadmission data collection is one of the most important activities an organization can undertake to ensure efficient collection of its accounts. Another essential feature is the establishment of credit policies. Who is the organization willing to treat, and under what circumstances? During a patient's course of treatment, there should be ongoing data collection. When a patient is discharged, there should be a review to ensure comprehensive inclusion of charges, and a bill should be issued. Receivables management does not stop at this point. Receivables should be monitored while outstanding, using an aging schedule. If necessary, the organization should use a collection agency to collect delinquent accounts. When cash does arrive, there should be specific procedures to safeguard it until its ultimate deposit in the bank. These elements are discussed below.

Preadmission Data Collection

The process of managing accounts receivable should start before a patient is admitted to a health care institution. Many organizations have a conference with the patient to determine the sources of payment for the patient's care. Patients may have Medicare, Medicaid, or other insurance coverage. If that is the case, all pertinent information should be recorded so that upon discharge a bill can be expeditiously processed. All forms should be completed, signatures obtained, and insurance companies called to verify coverage and obtain all necessary preadmission approvals. Many managed care organizations deny coverage if the patient was admitted without pre-notification to the company.

In some cases it may be determined that the patient is eligible for Medicaid but has not enrolled. Many health care organizations have specific policies regarding helping patients enroll for Medicaid. In fact, some hospitals actually have state Medicaid employees working in the hospital to enroll patients. Enrolling an eligible patient often represents the difference between a substantial payment for the care provided to that patient and receiving little payment, if any at all.

If the patient has no insurance coverage, financial planning for payment can take place at the preadmission conference. In some cases this will mean establishing a payment schedule so that patients can pay what they can afford over an extended period. In some cases it will be determined that patients have no capacity to pay, and they will be classified as indigent for medical purposes. In that case their care will be considered charity care. Some states provide financial assistance to health care organizations to reimburse some part of the charity care provided. However, careful documentation is required so that a claim can be properly filed. It is now common for patient bills to be sent electronically, decreasing the time from billing to payment.

Credit Policies

Some medical care is true emergency care, and standards in the United States require that such care be provided regardless of the patient's ability to pay. This certainly is justified on moral and ethical grounds. Other care, however, is elective. Health care providers have a greater ethical and legal latitude in deciding what nonemergency care to provide to whom. At the opposite extreme from emergency care are procedures such as cosmetic surgery. Few would blame a health care organization that refused to provide cosmetic rhinoplasty to an indigent patient.

Health care organizations must establish clear rules that guide their decisions on whether to offer credit to patients. These rules must reflect both the financial and the medical condition of the patient. There should be a clear policy on when patients are treated regardless of their ability to pay, and when they are not. Some organizations are more permissive than others for a variety of reasons. For example, one organization may have a better financial position than another and be better able to afford to provide charity care. Other organizations may have a mission to provide care to those patients who cannot pay.

To carry out the organization's credit policy, preadmission data collection is essential. In addition to providing the information needed for prompt, accurate billing, it provides information the organization needs to make its decisions on when to provide care. While it is distasteful to have to deny any care to anyone, it is a reality of the existing health care system. Organizations have credit policies to protect the organization so it can remain in business and continue to provide essential care to all.

Ongoing Data Collection

During a patient's course of treatment, there should be continuous collection of data. The organization must track the services that the patient is consuming so that they may properly be included in the patient's bill.

If data collection is postponed until discharge or shortly thereafter, there is the risk that some charges will be overlooked. The number of patient days, x-rays, and laboratory tests must all be accumulated on an ongoing basis.

Nursing has always had a responsibility to participate in this ongoing data collection in a number of ways. Inventory items used are recorded on the patient chart. Charge slips for various procedures are also often placed in the chart by the nursing staff. While it may seem cumbersome to have to place a charge slip for a catheter on the patient's chart, without that step the patient will not be billed for that item. In that case the organization will lose that money and have fewer resources available for the provision of patient care. Even with the growing trend of charging negotiated rates to managed care organizations, this remains important. Often the negotiated rate is a percent discount from full rates. Collecting 70% of the charge is better than collecting 0%. Also, it is easier to negotiate rates if management has a good knowledge of what resources patients consume.

This role is likely to grow in the future as variable billing for nursing services becomes more widely used. Specifically, to charge for nursing services it is necessary to have information on the patient's consumption of nursing resources. This is generally obtained from the patient classification system. While all acute care hospitals have such systems, they do not all actively use them. To charge patients for nursing, information on their daily classification level must be accumulated on an ongoing basis.

Discharge Review and Billing

At discharge, a number of activities must take place in short order. The original patient payment information must be reviewed to ensure that it is complete. Something as minor as a missing zip code in the patient address could lead to a payment delay of several months or more.

The diagnosis of the patient must be firmly and clearly established at discharge. Medicare DRG payments for inpatients rely on the DRG assignment. That assignment in turn relies on a number of factors recorded in the medical report, such as principal and secondary diagnoses, surgical procedures, and age. If any of those elements is missing, a DRG cannot properly be assigned, and payment will be delayed. Once a patient bill is "kicked out" of the system, a payment delay of at least several months is the rule rather than the exception.

When the record has been reviewed and found to be complete with respect to both payer information and clinical information, a bill should be promptly issued. Many large payers now accept electronic billing rather than requiring paper bills. Some payers require electronic submission of bills. This information may even be electronically transmitted, eliminating the entire time that a bill would normally be in transit.

Even a savings of two or three days can have a significant impact. For any one bill it does not seem to matter if there are a few delays. However, when all bills are considered, the impact of prompt billing is significant. For example, suppose that a large hospital issues $200 million in patient billings each year. Also assume that the hospital has outstanding loans from banks at 10% interest rate. If electronic processing of bills directly to payers means that each bill is collected three days sooner than it otherwise would be, the interest savings would be over $164,000 a year! ($200 million × 10% ÷ 365 = $54,800 interest per day. $54,800 × 3 days is approximately $164,000 per year.)

Electronic processing is only one element. Consider a hospital that processes laboratory charges only once a month. Bills for patients discharged in January could not be issued until laboratory charges are processed for January. That might not be completed until February 5. Then all the laboratory charges would have to be posted to the individual patient accounts. That might take another week. It is conceivable that in a totally manual system, it might well be February 15 until any bills are issued for patients discharged anytime in January. On average, it would be a month after discharge until a patient bill was issued.

Delaying billing by a month delays receipt of cash by a month. In a hospital with $200 million in charges, such a delay could cost over $1.5 million per year. It should be no surprise that most health care organizations have automated data entry and billing systems. Every day earlier that bills can be issued saves a significant amount of money.

Aging of Receivables

Once bills have been issued, it is important for the organization to monitor receivables and to follow up on unpaid bills. This is true not only for self-pay patients, who are viewed as bad-debt risks, but also for the government and insurers. Often the large third-party payers will not pay a bill if they find any problem with it. The health care organization must be on top of receivables to ensure that any problems preventing specific bills from being paid are resolved.

A tool used to keep track of potential accounts receivable problems is an *aging schedule*. An aging schedule shows how long a receivable has been outstanding since a bill was issued. For example, at the end of June a summary aging schedule might look like the example in Table 15–3.

The aging schedule allows managers to monitor outstanding receivables. In Table 15–3, we notice that only 53.4% of the receivables outstanding are outstanding for less than one month. Almost half the receivables are outstanding more than thirty days since the date the bills were issued. On the other hand, a relatively small 3% of outstanding receivables are more than ninety days old.

If large payers constitute a significant portion of the organization's revenue, the organization should attempt to arrange for periodic interim payments (PIP). In a PIP arrangement, the payer makes payments in advance of the receipt and processing of specific bills. For instance, in the example in Table 15–3 the hospital might find that every month it bills HMOs for about $700,000. Rather than wait for the billings, each month the HMOs might issue a payment of perhaps $500,000 for care to patients during the current month. The balance to be paid for each month's care would wait until the specific bills are received. This allows the health care organization to receive its revenues in cash sooner than would otherwise be the case. Unfortunately, in recent years payers, also under financial pressure, have been reluctant to make PIPs.

The over-ninety-day category in the aging schedule is a particular concern, even though it is a small part of the total. These accounts probably reflect problems encountered in processing the bills by third-party payers or inability or unwilling-

TABLE 15–3. *Sample Aging Schedule: June 30 Aging Report*

Payer	1–30 Days	31–60 Days	61–90 Days	>90 Days	Total
By Total Dollars					
Medicare	$ 802,054	$ 795,633	$402,330	$ 52,050	$2,052,067
Medicaid	325,020	342,943	85,346	28,345	781,654
HMOs	682,285	114,583	14,354	4,364	815,541
Other insurers	437,899	46,722	8,563	7,773	500,957
Self-pay	174,799	103,295	67,322	43,588	389,004
Total	$2,422,057	$1,403,131	$577,915	$136,120	$4,539,223
By Percent					
Medicare	17.7%	17.5%	8.9%	1.1%	45.2%
Medicaid	7.2	7.6	1.9	.6	17.2
HMOs	15.0	2.5	.3	.1	18.0
Other insurers	9.6	1.0	.2	.2	11.0
Self-pay	3.9	2.3	1.5	2.0	8.6
Total	53.4%	30.9%	12.7%	3.0%	100.0%

ness to pay by self-pay patients. The health care organization should have specific follow-up procedures, which should include sending monthly statements and making phone calls to determine why payment has not been made.

Some of this process can be avoided if indigent patients are clearly identified in advance. While the health care organization will want to pursue those individuals who can pay for the care they receive, it is a costly waste of effort to spend resources trying to collect payment from the truly indigent.

In some cases it is necessary to use a collection agency if other efforts have failed and it is believed that the patient can afford to make payments. This is a costly approach, since collection agencies retain as much as half of all amounts they are successful in collecting.

Cash Receipt and Lock Boxes

When cash arrives, there should be specific procedures to safeguard it. One common approach is to direct all payments to a *lock box*. This is generally a post office box that is emptied directly by the bank. The bank removes the payments and processes them directly to the organization's account. The paperwork associated with the payment is then forwarded to the organization.

There are two key advantages to this approach. First, since the bank empties the boxes at least once a day, the receipts are deposited to interest-bearing accounts immediately rather than sitting in a business office for several days or weeks until they are deposited. Second, there is substantially decreased risk that receipts will be lost or stolen. Maintaining security over cash resources is a key element of working capital management.

Inventory

The last major current asset category is inventory. This is the category that nurses are often directly involved with. Health care organizations tend to have a wide variety of inventory items, for example, clinical supplies, drugs, office supplies, food, and housekeeping supplies. The cost of inventory in health care organizations is generally much smaller than the amount of accounts receivable. Nevertheless, careful inventory management can result in significant savings. A general rule of thumb is that inventory levels should be kept as low as possible, consistent with patient needs. The less inventory on hand, the less money tied up in inventory.

The major problem health care organizations face with respect to inventory is the unpredictability of patient flow and patient needs. If the organization runs out of an item, it could mean the difference between life and death. However, that fact is sometimes used to justify excessive stockpiles of a wide variety of inventory items that do not have life-and-death implications. Management needs to develop a system that ensures that inventory is available when needed but also that it is used efficiently and that levels are kept as low as possible.

Inventory should be ordered and stored in a central area whenever possible. Although ready access to supplies justifies maintaining some items in a number of different areas, the amount in each area should be the bare minimum, with restocking from one central point. Otherwise, each area will have a large inventory, and resources will needlessly be tied up in inventory that may not be used for weeks or even months. This is an area that is sometimes difficult for staff nurses. Nurses do not like to run out of supplies. The nurse manager must balance the staff nurse needs for immediate access to supplies with the organization's needs to control inventory costs.

Perpetual Inventory

One approach that can be helpful is maintenance of a perpetual inventory of high-cost items. With a perpetual inventory each use of an item is recorded and a running balance maintained. This allows the organization to know how much it has of each item at any point in time. Reordering can take place when inventory falls below a certain level.

Generally less inventory is required when a perpetual system is used. There is less need to hold a large safety stock, since the manager always knows how much inventory is available. Reordering can take place whenever inventory of an item is low. Without a perpetual system it is necessary to take a physical count of inventory to determine how much is available. That is a costly, time-consuming process that is not frequently undertaken.

Perpetual inventory systems are costly and time-consuming as well. However, automated systems have reduced the cost of such perpetual systems substantially. Supermarkets, for example, use uniform price codes (bar codes) to automatically update their perpetual inventory records as each item is sold. If inventory is maintained on an automated perpetual system, managers have greater control over their stock and therefore can get by with less of each item.

Economic Order Quantity

Inventory not only entails a cash outlay when it is acquired, but also other costs related to inventory. It must be stored. That requires physical storage space. Over time inventory may become damaged or obsolete or its expiration date may pass. There are costs related to placing an order and having it shipped. There are potentially high costs of running out of an item. These many factors can be balanced using a method called the economic order quantity (EOQ).

EOQ is a quantitative technique that weighs all the pros and cons of ordering large amounts of inventory infrequently *vs* ordering small amounts more frequently. The result of an EOQ calculation is the optimal number of units that should be ordered each time an item is restocked and how frequently orders should be made. The EOQ technique is presented and explained in Chapter 17, along with other quantitative techniques of management.

⁂ CURRENT LIABILITIES

Management of current liabilities often receives less attention than current asset management, but it is also important. Careful planning and management of short-term obligations can save the organization significant amounts of money.

The typical current liabilities that most organizations have and that must be managed as part of working capital are accounts payable, payroll payable, notes payable, and taxes payable. Accounts payable represent amounts that are owed to suppliers. Payroll relates to obligations to employees. Notes payable represent short-term debt, usually loans from banks. Taxes payable include not only income taxes for proprietary organizations but also a variety of payroll taxes for all organizations.

The basic approach to management of current liabilities is deferral of payment and avoidance of borrowing to the extent possible. The longer the organization waits to make payments, the longer the cash will remain in the organization's interest-bearing accounts. This allows it to earn a return that can be used to provide more services. The less money the organization borrows and the later it borrows it, the less interest it must pay.

Accounts Payable

Accounts payable are often referred to as *trade credit.* Trade credit is generally free for a short time. After a purchase is made, the organization has several weeks or a month to pay the bill. After that time some suppliers charge interest; others do not. A more common practice than charging interest for late payments is to offer a discount for prompt payment.

Discount terms are often stated as 2/10 N/30. That means a 2% discount is given for payments received within ten days of the invoice date. Otherwise the full amount, referred to as the net (N) amount, is due thirty days from the invoice date. Sometimes only a 1% discount is offered, in which case it would be referred to as 1/10 N/30. Some vendors use terms based on the end of the month (EOM). For example, 2/10 EOM means that the buyer can take a 2% discount for payments made by ten days after the end of the month in which the invoice is issued. In general, trade credit is only offered to trustworthy buyers. In some cases, when the supplier has not had a long-term relationship with the buyer, goods will be sold cash on delivery (COD).

Does it pay to take the discount when it is offered? In most cases it clearly does make sense to take the discount. A formula can be used to determine the annual interest rate implicit in trade credit discounts:

$$\text{Implicit interest rate} = \frac{\text{Discount}}{\text{Discounted price}} \times \frac{\text{365 Days}}{\text{Days early}} \times 100\%$$

For example, suppose that your organization purchased $1,000 worth of goods and was offered terms of 2/10 N/30. A 2% discount on a $1,000 purchase is $20. This means that if the discount is taken, only $980 will have to be paid. If the discount is taken, payment is due on the tenth day rather than the thirtieth day. This means that payment is made twenty days earlier than would otherwise be the case.

$$\text{Implicit interest rate} = \frac{\$20}{\$980} \times \frac{\text{365 Days}}{\text{20 Days}} \times 100\% = 37.2\%$$

While the discount appears to be a very small percentage, on an annualized basis the rate is actually 37.2%! Effectively one can think of this as if the organization has an obligation of $980 due on the tenth day. If it waits an extra twenty days to make payment, the interest charge is $20. Twenty dollars of interest on a $980 loan for twenty days represents a 37% annual interest rate. Clearly, if the organization takes the discount, it is avoiding a high charge for deferring payment by a few weeks.

What if the organization does not have enough cash to take all discounts? In that case, it pays to incur short-term debt, that is, to borrow the money from the bank to pay the bill on the tenth day as long as the bank charges a rate less than 37%.

However, that assumes that the organization will in fact pay the bill on the due date if it does not take the discount. What if a hospital is in financial difficulty and is paying its bills after 150 days? That is an undesirable position to be in, as suppliers may stop making future sales. Nevertheless, it is not uncommon to find some health care organizations paying bills 90 days, 120 days, or even 150 days late. If a hospital would normally pay a bill after 150 days, then taking the discount on the tenth day means that payment is made 140 days sooner than it otherwise would be.

$$\text{Implicit interest rate} = \frac{\$20}{\$980} \times \frac{\text{365 Days}}{\text{140 Days}} \times 100\% = 5.3\%$$

In this situation the implicit interest rate is much lower. Any hospital paying after 150 days probably has a cash shortage. It is unlikely that this hospital could borrow from a bank for a rate as low as 5.3%. Therefore, in that situation it is not financially advantageous to take the discount. The decision to take or not take a discount is not automatic. It depends on both the amount of the discount and the implications for how much sooner payment must be made.

Payroll Payable

Payroll payables are generally very short. At the end of each payroll period, salaries and wages are paid and the obligation eliminated. This does not mean, however, that management has no ability to manage in this area.

First, there must be policy decisions regarding when and how often employees are paid. Paying some employees monthly instead of every two weeks effectively defers payment of half their salary by two weeks. Over the course of the year, that adds up to a significant amount of savings for the organization. Similar savings accrue from paying employees every two weeks instead of every week. Additionally, less frequent payments mean that there is less paperwork and other administrative costs.

Second, there is the issue of how long the delay is from the end of the payroll period until payment. If the payroll period ends on Friday and payroll is paid on the following Thursday, the organization has gained the use of the money for nearly an extra week.

On the other side of the ledger, one must give consideration to the organization's relationship with its employees. While it will require some time to process the amounts that are due to the employees and to print checks, a good relationship between employer and employees calls for payment of payroll as promptly as possible.

Short-term Debt

The most common type of short-term debt owed by health care organizations is *unsecured notes* payable to banks. Many health care organizations also borrow money from financing and factoring companies, using their accounts receivable as collateral. Additionally, some health care organizations issue commercial paper.

Unsecured notes are loans that do not have any collateral. *Collateral* is a specific asset pledged to the lender. If the borrower defaults on the loan, the lender can sell the collateral to recover its money. In the case of an unsecured note, if the organization fails to repay the money, the lender has no specific claim on an asset owned by the organization. Rather, it would be a general creditor and would share the assets of the organization with all the other general creditors. This makes lending money more risky and drives up the interest charged.

An alternative available to health care organizations is to put up accounts receivable as security or collateral for the loan. This is called *financing accounts receivable*. It is also possible to directly sell receivables. This is called *factoring*. The buyer of the receivables, called the factor or the factoring agent, takes on the risk that patients or third-party payers may not pay. Factoring tends to be an expensive alternative because of the risk that the factor takes. Financing is less expensive. The health care organization borrows money, and the receivables are simply backup security in case the organization fails to repay the loan. Since much of the receivables are due from the government, they are seen as reasonably good collateral. This may make borrowing with receivables as collateral less costly than an unsecured bank loan.

A last alternative is *commercial paper*. This is a form of borrowing in which the borrower issues a financial security that can be traded by the lender to someone else. This is an uncommon approach for any organization other than large, for-profit chains. Although the commercial paper is referred to as a security, it is generally unsecured.

In general, short-term debt bears a higher interest rate than long-term debt. This is because short-term debt is typically unsecured, while long-term debt is often secured by specific assets. Also, there are transactions costs related to the borrowing and repaying of loans. These costs are more substantial for short-term loans because they cannot be spread out over a long lifetime of a loan. Therefore, if an organization needs an amount of money for a long time, it usually borrows on a long-term basis. Long-term borrowing is discussed in Chapter 16. Short-term debt is generally used only for short-term needs.

Taxes Payable

Even not-for-profit organizations get involved with taxes. For the most part, these relate to FICA (Social Security taxes) and employee income tax withholding. FICA is paid by both the employee and the employer. The organization must withhold an amount for FICA from its employees and then must make payments to the government for both its share and the employees' share. The organization must also withhold a portion of each employee's wages and pay it to the government for the employee's income taxes. Generally, specific rules determine when these tax payments are due. Aside from not paying the taxes before they are due, there is relatively little management can do in this area.

※ IMPLICATIONS FOR NURSE MANAGERS

Nurse managers may question the importance of this chapter. Except for a minority of nurse managers, readers of this book are unlikely to be in charge of decisions concerning collection of accounts receivable and payment to suppliers. However, working capital management is important for all nurse managers.

It is important because managers do not just manage their cost centers; they manage a part of an organization, and they should understand the financial workings of the organization. It is important because in many instances the actions of nurse managers have an effect on working capital. And it is important because decisions made about working capital affect nurse managers and their cost centers or departments.

Nurse managers at one time were restricted primarily to clinical management. Over the last several decades their role has changed, and it continues to change. Nurse managers control the largest share of resources in most health care institutions. The financial management of the entire organization should be a concern of nurse managers. Inefficient use of working capital invariably has an impact on the resources available for patient care.

The impact nurse managers can have on working capital should not be understated. The most obvious area where nurses can have an impact is inventory management. Efficient control of inventory resources is one working capital ingredient. Another is payroll liabilities. Nurse managers, through their staffing decisions, do have an impact on that current liability. Decisions to purchase inventory and equipment come into play as well. The timing of such purchases should be made in light of their implications for working capital.

On the other hand, while delaying purchases of equipment until the equipment is actually needed makes sense, delaying it longer reduces quality of care. Understanding working capital management can help nurse managers understand why a financial manager would want to delay an acquisition as long as possible. That understanding should help the manager in a dialogue with financial management over the acquisition. Mutually beneficial solutions are more likely to be achieved when both parties understand the needs and concerns of their counterparts.

KEY CONCEPTS ※

Working capital Organization's current assets and current liabilities.

Working capital management Management of the current assets and current liabilities of the organization to ensure that there is adequate cash on hand to meet the organization's needs and to minimize the cost of short-term resources.

Cash requirements Cash is needed by organizations for three main purposes: transactions, safety, and investments.

Cash management Management of inflows and outflows of cash.

Cash budgets Starting cash balance, plus expected cash receipts, less expected cash payments.

Management of accounts receivable Minimization of the time between provision of care and receipt of payment. Accounts receivable earn no return for the organization. The sooner cash is collected, the sooner the organization can use that cash for its operations or else invest it.

Aging schedule Tool used to keep track of potential accounts receivable problems by showing how long each receivable has been outstanding since a bill was issued.

Inventory management Managers need to develop a system that ensures that inventory is available when needed, while keeping inventory levels as low as possible.

Management of current liabilities Process of deferring payment and avoiding borrowing to the extent possible. The longer the organization waits to pay, the longer the cash is in the organization's interest-bearing accounts, earning a return that can be used to provide more services. The less the organization borrows and the later it borrows, the less interest it must pay.

Trade credit Accounts payable. Often subject to credit terms such as 2/10 N/30. The implicit interest rate contained in such terms may be calculated as follows:

$$\text{Implicit interest rate} = \frac{\text{Discount}}{\text{Discounted price}} \times \frac{\text{365 Days}}{\text{Days earlier}} \times 100\%$$

Short-term debt Unsecured short-term loans.

SUGGESTED READINGS

Cleverley, William O., *Essentials of Health Care Finance,* Aspen Publishers, Gaithersburg, Md., February 1997.

Emery, Douglas, John D. Finnerty, and John D. Stowe, *Principles of Financial Management,* Prentice Hall, Upper Saddle River, N.J., 1998.

Finkler, Steven A., *Finance and Accounting for Nonfinancial Managers,* revised edition, Prentice Hall, Upper Saddle River, N.J., 1996.

Gapenski, Louis C., *Financial Analysis and Decision Making for Healthcare Organizations: A Guide for the Healthcare Professional,* Irwin Professional Publishers, Burr Ridge, Ill., January 1997.

Horngren, Charles T., Gary L. Sundem, and William O. Stratton, *Introduction to Management Accounting,* 10th edition, Prentice Hall, Upper Saddle River, N.J., 1996.

Keown, Arthur J., J. William Petty, David F. Scott, and John D. Martin, *Foundations of Finance,* 2nd edition, Prentice Hall, Upper Saddle River, N.J., 1998.

McLean, Robert A., *Financial Management in Health Care Organizations,* Delmar, Albany, N.Y., 1996.

Neumann, Bruce R., Jan P. Clement, and Jean C. Cooper, *Financial Management: Concepts and Applications for Health Care Organizations,* Kendall/Hunt Publishing, Dubuque, Iowa, May 1997.

Rosenblatt N.W., and D.G. Silverman, "Cost-Effective use of Operating Room Supplies Based on the Database of Recovered Unused Materials," *Journal of Clinical Anesthesiology,* Vol. 6, No. 5, September–October 1994, pp. 400–404.

Suver, James D., Bruce R. Neumann, and Keith E. Boles, *Management Accounting for Healthcare Organizations,* 3rd edition, Pluribus Press, Westchester, Ill., 1992.

Zelman, William N., Michael J. McCue, and Alan R. Milikan, *Financial Management of Health Care Organizations: An Introduction to Fundamental Tools, Concepts, and Applications,* Blackwell Publishers, New York, N.Y., January 1998.

CHAPTER

16

Long-Term Financial Resources

CHAPTER GOALS

The goals of this chapter are to:

- Describe the sources of long-term financing for health care organizations
- Explain the relative merits of equity financing *vs* debt financing
- Distinguish among the different equity sources of financing
- Consider the changing roles of equity sources of financing
- Explain the types of debt financing and the trade-offs for each type
- Introduce bond ratings and bond insurance
- Explain what bond refinancing is and why it takes place
- Explain the purpose of and methods used for feasibility studies
- Consider the future of long-term financing for health care organizations

※ INTRODUCTION

Chapter 15 covered a number of sources of short-term financing for health care organizations. We now turn to sources of long-term financing. Long-term financing represents sources of money that the organization can use for longer than a year. In many cases these sources are critical to the existence of the organization.

Most, if not all, buildings and equipment are financed on a long-term basis. It would probably be impossible to find a lender willing to make a ninety-day or six-month loan to acquire a building. It is unreasonable to expect that enough profits could be earned within a short period to repay the entire cost of a building. It is more likely that at the *maturity*, or due date, of the loan a new loan would be required to get the money to pay off the old loan. If a new loan cannot be obtained, the organization would likely have to default on its old loan. The lender would consider the risk of not being repaid too high.

As a result, long-term assets are generally acquired with money that the organization knows it can keep and use for a long time. The two principal sources of long-term money are debt and equity. Debt represents borrowed money. Interest must be paid during the period of the loan, and the original amount borrowed must be repaid. Equity represents ownership. In some cases equity represents money that outsiders have given the organization in exchange for owning it and having a claim on its profits. In other cases equity represents money that the organization itself owns.

⁜ EQUITY SOURCES OF FINANCING

The four principal sources of equity financing for health care organizations are philanthropy, corporate stock issuance, government grants, and retained earnings.

The main advantage of equity financing is that there is no legal requirement to make annual payments. This is in contrast to debt, which generally calls for at least annual payments of interest. Even if a health care organization has a bad year, it is legally required to make interest payments on its debt. If it does not have enough cash to make those interest payments, it might have to go out of business. That risk is not associated with equity sources of financing.

If a for-profit health care organization has a bad year, it can skip dividend payments to its stockholders. The usual form of stock, called *common stock,* has no requirements that dividends of any amount be paid, even if the organization is making a profit. A special form of stock called *preferred stock* requires a specific dividend each year, but in hard economic times payments can be delayed.

Other forms of equity such as retained earnings and philanthropic funds do not have required payments of any type. This freedom from interest payments relates to a concept called *leverage.* The greater the extent to which an organization uses debt financing, as opposed to equity, the more highly leveraged it is said to be. The benefit of leverage is that high leverage implies a low amount of required equity investment. The detriment of leverage is that it creates risk because of the need to make interest payments.

Philanthropy

Philanthropy represents gifts to the organization. These gifts may be small, or they may come in the form of multimillion dollar endowments. There may be costs related to generating the gifts, but once received they do not require interest or dividend payments, and the amount of the gift need never be repaid to someone outside the health care organization. Philanthropy has been a declining percentage of long-term financing for health care organizations.

The decline in philanthropy is probably caused by a number of factors, most of which are outside the control of any specific health care organization. These include changes in the tax rates, the introduction of Medicare and Medicaid, the proliferation of for-profit health care organizations, increased competition from non-health-care charities, cuts in federal support of social welfare, and the rising costs of generating philanthropic donations. Additionally, the existence of other sources for financing has made health care managers less aggressive in pursuing philanthropy.

Tax changes in the 1980s made it less advantageous to donate money to charitable organizations. Prior to that time many philanthropists were in a 70% federal income tax bracket. A donation of $1 resulted in a 70¢ tax savings. Considering the tax implications, it cost a person in that bracket only 30¢ to make a $1 contribution. With state income taxes added on, the effect was even more extreme. With the current lower maximum tax rates, each dollar contributed costs the donor more on an after-tax basis. For example, a gift of $1 million in 1980 might have cost a rich benefactor only $250,000 after considering the savings in federal and state taxes. That same contribution now might cost $650,000 after considering the tax savings.

Prior to the introduction of Medicare and Medicaid, many philanthropists believed that they had a mission to help provide for the health care of the poor and aged. With the government role that was created by Medicare and Medicaid, many philanthropists no longer believe that the same degree of need still exists. While it is true that many people are still uninsured or underinsured, the mere existence of a major role for the government in payment for health care possibly has made many people believe that the need for charity has disappeared from the health care industry.

At one time hospitals were viewed as community benefit organizations whose mission was to serve the people in the community. In many cases, especially in large cities, this is no longer true. Thus people in the community do not have the same sense of responsibility to the hospital.

This is probably reinforced by the fact that health care organizations view themselves more and more as businesses rather than charities. While running health care organizations in a financially sound, businesslike manner does not eliminate their charitable mission, it does change the way people perceive the industry. The proliferation of for-profit health care organizations tends to make the entire industry appear more like a business. And many people believe that the last place they would donate money is to a business.

At the same time that health care organizations were losing some of their allure as a charity, there has been tremendous growth in the non–health care not-for-profit sector. More charities are competing for dollars, and they are learning how to do it better. This increased volume of charities and improved fund-raising skills has occurred at the same time as a government cutback in social services. During the 1980s the federal government pushed more of its social welfare function back to localities. The result was numerous cuts. Many charitable organizations stepped in to try to restore some services. That created an additional, highly visible outlet for philanthropic giving.

Another problem with philanthropy for health care organizations has been the rising cost of generating philanthropic donations. As competition for philanthropy has grown, organizations have had to develop more sophisticated and more expensive approaches to generating gifts. Expensive advertising campaigns join the more traditional dinners as a way to raise money. Full-time personnel must be hired to work at the task of "development" (i.e., gift generation).

Most, if not all, of the above factors contributing to the decreasing role of philanthropy cannot be greatly influenced by managers of an organization. Nevertheless, many not-for-profit health care organizations have dropped the ball with respect to raising philanthropic funds. Not only have philanthropists started to view health care as a business, many health care managers have as well. There is a need to distinguish between running the organization in a businesslike manner and being a for-profit corporation.

Many health care managers believe that among Medicare, Medicaid, Blue Cross, private insurers, Health Maintenance Organizations (HMOs), and other payers, there should be enough revenue to run a health care business. The error in that perception is that in the case of not-for-profit organizations health care is not a business. The mission is not centered on making money but on providing service to the community. Not-for-profit organizations inherently undertake some activities at a loss because of their mission. One way to offset those losses is to earn high profits on other services. Most health care organizations try to accomplish that. However, another way to offset those losses is to actively solicit donations from a wide variety of sources, including past patients and community leaders.

Realistically, however, while efforts to receive donations should continue and perhaps even be stepped up, philanthropy can no longer be viewed as the major source for long-term financing. The costs of the health care industry have grown too high. New buildings are so expensive that in most cases their cost has gone beyond the reach of the best philanthropic efforts.

Corporate Stock Issuance

A major growth area in health care financing during the 1980s and 1990s was the issuance of corporate stock. In direct contrast with philanthropy, this approach says that health care can in fact be a business. Individuals can give money to health care organizations in exchange for stock. The stock makes the individuals the owners of the business. As the business earns profits, it distributes part of them to the owners in the form of dividends. The owners can sell the stock to someone else as a way of getting back their original investment, perhaps with a profit. The new owner of the stock can then receive the future dividends from the business's profits.

The issuance of stock has slowed considerably in the health care industry. Oxford Health Plans, an HMO, saw its stock plunge from over $80 per share to under $20 during 1997 because of poor financial results. Large for-profit hospital chains also found difficult financial conditions and saw their stock prices plunge. The for-profit sector is still growing and still seen as potentially profitable. Apparently, however, the rapid growth of the health care for-profit sector, which saw it take over approximately one third of all acute care hospital beds in less than two decades, is over. Nevertheless, many new health care organizations are still getting their start using stock issuance to get much of their initial financial resources.

Stock issuance is only available to for-profit organizations. It is unlikely that health care organizations will generally switch to being for-profit simply to access this form of financing. Such a step would likely have wide ramifications for the organization. On the other hand, organizations that are already for-profit must decide how much equity financing of this form they want. It is possible to issue enough stock to raise all the necessary long-term financing for an organization. However, that may not be an optimal strategy.

When stock is issued, a major benefit to the owners who invest money in the business is the dividend flow. Dividends are a distribution of profits. They are paid after taxes have been calculated on profits. Interest, on the other hand, is a tax-deductible expense. By issuing some stock and some debt, some of the payments for financing become tax deductible, therefore lowering the taxes paid to the government. That is one reason that most for-profit organizations have a mixture of stock and debt.

Government Grants

Government grants were a common financing mechanism at one time, especially for hospitals. Hill-Burton funds were available in the 1950s for the construction of new hospital buildings. In recent years, however, there has been a growing reluctance by the government to create more capacity in the health care system. Studies have demonstrated that increased capacity tends to create higher levels of utilization. Further, there is an excess of capacity for health care services in many areas of the country. As a result, government grants are no longer a significant source of financing for health care organizations. They are available, however, for programs such as the development of primary care clinics.

Retained Earnings

The last significant source of equity financing is retained earnings. Each year that a health care organization makes a profit, that profit is either paid to owners in the form of a dividend or else retained in the organization. Money retained can be used for short-term operations or to finance long-term assets.

Retaining earnings is a critical factor in the long-term survival of health care organizations. To stay viable, it is necessary to replace plant and equipment as they physically deteriorate or become technologically obsolete. In addition, organizations must add new services and technology to remain current as health care changes. The combination of inflation plus technological change plus expanding community needs often drives the cost of replacement buildings and equipment well above the cost of the original items. It would not be surprising for an old hospital building that cost $50 million to build sixty years ago to be replaced now for $250 million. If profits have been earned, retained, and invested, the organization will have some of the money needed for the new facility.

Even on a less grand scale, retained earnings are essential. Suppose that a hospital wishes to buy a patient monitor for $25,000. If it goes to a bank to borrow the money, the bank will want the hospital to make a down payment of probably 20% or more. The reason for this is discussed later under Mortgages and Long-term Notes. If there is adequate philanthropy or cash from stock issuances, the hospital will be able to buy the equipment. If not, it is likely that it will only be able to acquire the equipment if it has enough money for the down payment available from earnings that have been retained and have not yet been used for another purpose. Retained earnings represent a source of equity financing that is of growing importance to health care organizations.

※ DEBT SOURCES OF FINANCING

Relatively few health care organizations are entirely free from debt. The need to raise large amounts of long-term financing causes many, if not most, health care organizations to borrow money. There are a number of different approaches to borrowing. Depending on the specific circumstances for which money is needed, at times some approaches will be superior, while at other times other approaches will be more suitable.

The major forms of long-term debt are mortgages, long-term notes, leases, and bonds. Mortgages and long-term notes generally represent money that a bank lends to the organization. However, it is possible to have a mortgage or note with a nonbank. For instance, some equipment manufacturers will lend the buyer money to acquire equipment. Leases are arrangements to rent equipment or facilities under a contract. Bonds are formal borrowing arrangements in which the debt is transferrable. The issuer of the bonds receives money and owes the buyer. The buyer in turn can sell the bond to another party, to whom the issuer is then obligated.

Mortgages and Long-term Notes

Mortgages and long-term notes are referred to as *conventional debt.* A long-term note is a loan. It is sometimes secured by collateral, and sometimes is unsecured. If secured, the collateral is often in the form of financial securities rather than physical property. The obligation to repay the loan is generally evidenced by a formal legal document, called a note, that is signed by the borrower. When a note is secured by a specific piece of physical property such as a building, piece of equipment, or land, it is referred to as a mortgage. If the borrower fails to repay a mortgage, the lender can foreclose on the property, sell it, and pay the borrower only the amount realized from the sale that exceeds the outstanding loan balance.

Mortgages and long-term notes are common, can be issued with little delay, and require relatively little paperwork and involvement of lawyers. They tend to be more expensive than bonds but less expensive than leasing.

Mortgages are often used to finance a specific acquisition. Usually lenders require that the borrower make a down payment of anywhere from 20% to 50% of the purchase price of the asset. This protects the lender in case there is a payment default and the asset cannot be sold for its full original cost. Mortgages generally call for monthly payments of a constant amount. The payments consist of interest on the balance of the loan that was outstanding during the previous month, plus a repayment of a portion of the original loan. Over time the amount of interest in each payment declines and the amount of loan repayment in each payment rises. At the end of the term of the mortgage, the loan has been fully repaid. In contrast, notes generally call for monthly payments of interest only. At the maturity date of the loan, the full amount of the original loan is repaid.

For example, suppose that an HMO wanted to purchase equipment for a new group practice office. The total cost of the equipment needed is $500,000. The HMO plans to invest $100,000 of its own funds and borrow $400,000. Suppose that if it borrowed on an unsecured long-term note, the interest rate would be 14%. If it took

※ **TABLE 16–1.** *Payment Schedule for a Long-term Note*

Year	Loan Balance Start of Year	Interest Payment	Loan Repayment	Total Payment	Loan Balance End of Year
1	$400,000	$56,000	$ 0	$ 56,000	$400,000
2	400,000	56,000	0	56,000	400,000
3	400,000	56,000	0	56,000	400,000
4	400,000	56,000	0	56,000	400,000
5	400,000	56,000	0	56,000	400,000
6	400,000	56,000	0	56,000	400,000
7	400,000	56,000	0	56,000	400,000
8	400,000	56,000	0	56,000	400,000
9	400,000	56,000	0	56,000	400,000
10	400,000	56,000	400,000	456,000	0
				$960,000	

a mortgage, using the equipment as collateral, the interest rate would be 12%. The collateral lessens the lender's risk, so a lower interest rate is available. Assume for this example that payments are only made once a year. What are the annual payments under the two alternatives?

The long-term note has annual payments of $56,000, as seen in Table 16–1. This is 14% of $400,000. The loan balance of $400,000 remains constant over the 10-year life of the loan. At the end of the loan there is an interest payment, plus a payment for the full $400,000.

The annual mortgage payments on a $400,000 loan are $70,794.[1] Note that this is a higher amount than the annual $56,000 payment on the long-term note, even though the interest rate on the mortgage is only 12% and the rate on the note is 14%. This is because the mortgage payments include not only interest but also repayment of a portion of the original loan (see Table 16–2).

Note that in the early years most of each payment is interest. However, because there is some repayment of the original loan, each year a smaller amount is owed. Since less money is owed, there is less interest. The annual payments are a constant amount. If the amount of interest decreases each year, the amount of the annual payment available for paying off the loan increases. Thus, in the later years most of each payment is loan repayment rather than interest. By the end of 10 years the loan is fully paid off.

Note that in total the mortgage payments came to $707,940, and the note payments came to $960,000. The reason for this is that there is more interest on the note. This is partially because of the higher interest rate and partly because for the note the full $400,000 is owed during the entire ten years, while the mortgage obligation declined over the ten years.

Leases

Leases are rental agreements evidenced by a contract referred to as a *lease*. The *lessee* rents a building or equipment from the *lessor*. Unless otherwise agreed, at the expiration of a lease the lessor continues to own the property. It is possible, however, to design the lease to transfer the property to the lessee at the end of its term. It is

[1]The $70,794 constant annual payment is exactly the amount of money that is needed to provide for a 12% interest payment on the outstanding balance of the loan, plus repayment of the loan so that there is no remaining balance at the end of ten years. That number can be calculated using the time-value-of-money techniques discussed in the appendix to Chapter 11. In this case the number of compounding periods is 10, the interest rate is 12%, the present value of the loan is $400,000, and the annual payment is being sought.

※ TABLE 16–2. *Payment Schedule for a Mortgage*

Year	Loan Balance Start of Year	Interest Payment	Loan Repayment	Total Payment	Loan Balance End of Year
	(A)	(B)	(C)	(D)	(E)
1	$400,000	$48,000	$22,794	$ 70,794	$377,206
2	377,206	45,265	25,529	70,794	351,677
3	351,677	42,201	28,592	70,794	323,084
4	323,085	38,770	32,023	70,794	291,060
5	291,062	34,927	35,866	70,794	255,195
6	255,195	30,623	40,170	70,794	215,025
7	215,025	25,803	44,991	70,794	170,034
8	170,034	20,404	50,390	70,794	119,645
9	119,645	14,357	56,436	70,794	63,209
10	63,209	7,585	63,209	70,794	0
				$707,940	

(A) Loan balance at the start of the year is the original loan balance in the first year. In subsequent years it is the ending balance from column E for the previous year.
(B) 12% interest rate multiplied by loan balance in column A.
(C) = (D) – (B).
(D) = Annual payment calculated using time-value-of-money techniques. See Chapter 11 appendix.
(E) = (A) – (C).

also possible to design the lease to give the lessee the option to purchase the property at the end of the lease for a specified price. Leases usually call for equal payments payable at the beginning of each month.

Lease payments generally have three components, although the lessee is only told the total monthly payment. The first component pays for part of the cost of the property being leased. This is equivalent to the principal portion of a mortgage payment. The second component is an interest charge equivalent to the interest portion of a mortgage payment. The last component is profit for the lessor.

In many ways leases are simply an alternative to mortgages. In both cases the organization wishes to have the use of an asset, but it does not have the cash to go out and buy the asset. It needs to use cash from someone else, either the mortgage lender or the lessor. Leases in effect obligate the lessee to make monthly lease payments for a number of years into the future in the same way that the user of the equipment would be obligated to make monthly mortgage payments had the property been purchased with a mortgage. It is because of the long-term obligation to make payments on a lease that accountants treat long-term noncancelable leases as long-term debt.

Other things being equal, leases are more costly than mortgages. In either case the user of the property must ultimately pay the cost of the property. In either case the user of the property must pay interest for the use of the money needed to buy the property. That interest includes a profit for the lender. In the case of a lease, however, the lessor has generally borrowed the money to buy the property. Suppose that the lessor borrows from a bank to finance the asset purchase. The bank and its depositors must receive interest, and the lessor must also earn a profit. This extra party to the transaction, the lessor, adds the need for additional profits and therefore creates additional costs to the lessee. The bank and its depositors *and* the lessor earn a profit. With a mortgage, only the bank and its depositors need earn a profit.

Then why would one lease rather than buying a property and taking a mortgage? For one thing, leases do not require a down payment. If the organization does not have the 20% to 50% of the asset cost needed for a down payment, then the lease may be viewed as advantageous even if it is more expensive. Another advantage of leasing is that the leasing company may be better able to sell the used property than the user of the property.

Consider a home health agency that provides cars to its nursing staff for making home visits. At the end of three or four years the agency may wish to replace the cars. The agency probably cannot get a high value for the cars when it sells them because it is not an expert in the used car market. On the other hand, if the cars are leased, the leasing company can probably sell the cars for a reasonable price because it is an expert. By sharing the extra amount received on the ultimate sale with the lessee, the lease may become attractive.

Another potential advantage of leasing is that in some leases the lessee can call for the equipment to be replaced if it becomes obsolete. This removes some risk that health care organizations take when they buy equipment. On the other hand, the leasing company will probably charge a higher monthly amount to pay it for taking that risk.

The total rate being charged to cover interest and profits on a lease can usually be estimated using the time-value-of-money techniques. Suppose that a nursing home is considering buying some equipment for $200,000 or leasing it for $5,000 per month for five years. If it purchases the equipment, there will be an immediate down payment of $50,000, plus monthly mortgage payments based on a 12% interest rate, for five years. If it leases the equipment, it will have sixty monthly payments of $5,000. If the number of months equals sixty, the payment each month is $5,000, and the present value of the equipment is $200,000, then the annual interest rate on the lease is approximately 18%.[2] This is substantially higher than the bank rate of 12%. On the other hand, the nursing home would need only $5,000 at the start for the first month, as opposed to $50,000 for a down payment.

Bonds

Bonds are formal certificates of indebtedness. The certificate indicates a promise to pay interest, usually semiannually, and the face value of the bond at a specified maturity date. Bonds are financial obligations that can be traded from one party to another. For example, Mr. Smith can lend money to the health care organization (i.e., he can buy a bond) in exchange for a promise that interest plus the original loan will be repaid. That promise is evidenced by the bond certificate. In turn Mr. Smith can sell the bond certificate to someone else, and the borrower will then owe the money to the new owner of the bond instead of to Mr. Smith. Bonds are issued by the borrower. Sometimes it is said that the borrower sells the bonds or floats a bond.

Bonds are an advantageous way of obtaining debt for several reasons. First, the borrower obtains the money directly from the ultimate lender. Second, bonds tend to disperse risk.

In the case of a bank loan, the borrower gets money from a bank, which in turn gets money from depositors. The depositors must make a profit and the bank must make a profit. With a bond, the money is borrowed directly from individuals, who might otherwise put their money in a bank. By eliminating the middleman bank, the depositors can be paid more than the bank would pay them, and the borrower can pay less than would be paid to a bank. Both the borrower and the ultimate lender are better off if they can eliminate the bank's role.

The second major advantage is that there is dispersal of risk. If a bank were to lend $100 million for a hospital expansion, it would take on a tremendous amount of risk. If the hospital were to default, the bank would be faced with a huge potential loss. Bonds, however, are often divided into hundreds or thousands or even hundreds of thousands of relatively small loans. For a $100 million total debt, each

---

[2]Using the methods from the appendix to Chapter 11, i = ?% per month, N = 60 months, the present value is $200,000, and the monthly payments = $5,000. Note that with a lease, payments are made in advance of each period rather than at the end of each period.

lender may lend as little as $5,000. Thus no one single person or organization takes on the full risk of one organization's defaulting on a loan.

With mutual funds, investors may effectively disperse their risk even further. An individual could invest $5,000 in a mutual fund that has combined the investments of thousands of individuals to buy hundreds of different bonds. Thus an individual's risk from any one hospital's defaulting might be several hundred dollars or less. By lowering risk, the borrower lowers the interest rate that must be paid to adequately reimburse the lender for the risks taken.

Bonds are also advantageous because they do not require down payments for projects, and they may have extremely long maturity periods. Forty-year bonds are not uncommon. These factors can be very important to a health care organization borrowing money to construct a new building. The organization can have the full depreciation period of the building to accumulate the money needed to pay for its construction.

Usually bonds pay interest *semiannually*. Every six months a payment is made based on a stated interest rate and the face value of the bond. Bonds are generally issued in denominations of $5,000 and multiples of $5,000, such as $10,000, $25,000, and $100,000. The total amount issued by the borrower is generally large, often over $100 million. At the due date or maturity of the bond the original face amount must be repaid.

Although bond interest is paid at the stated rate and the face value is repaid at maturity, the bonds may actually be issued for a greater or lesser amount than the face value. That is because interest rates fluctuate in the financial marketplace. Bond certificates may be printed indicating a promise to pay a 10% interest rate. If the issuer finds that market conditions have changed and no one is willing to lend money unless it is possible to earn a 10.1% return on the money, then a discount will have to be offered to get anyone to buy the bonds.

Thus on a $10,000, 20-year, 10% bond paying interest semiannually, the issuer might accept payment of $9,915. In exchange for the $9,915, the borrower will make payments of $500 twice a year for twenty years (i.e., the $10,000 face multiplied by 10% a year, divided by two payments per year), plus a payment of $10,000 at the end of twenty years. The borrower received $9,915 but repays $10,000. This converts the 10% stated interest rate to the 10.1% market interest rate.

If interest rates fall, the bond will be issued at a premium. If interest rates in the marketplace are only 9.8% and this bond offers 10% based on a face value of $10,000, investors will be willing to pay more than $10,000 to get the bond.

A number of decisions must be made before bonds are issued. These decisions can have a dramatic impact on the interest rate that must be paid on the outstanding bond obligations. Bonds may be issued in either taxable or tax-free form. The issuer can request to have the bond rated. The issuer can also purchase insurance that guarantees the payments of bond interest and principal. Another decision concerns whether to make interest payments or let the interest accrue and pay both the interest and face value at the maturity date. That is called a zero-coupon bond. After bonds have been issued, another question that sometimes arises is whether the bonds should be refinanced. These issues are discussed below.

Taxable vs *Tax-free Bonds*

A taxable bond is one on which the lender of the money (also called the buyer of the bond) must pay income tax on the interest received. Under certain conditions it is possible to offer bonds free of federal income tax and free of state and local income taxes in the state or locality issued. The advantage of a tax-free bond is that people are willing to lend money in exchange for a lower interest rate if they can avoid paying taxes.

Suppose that a hospital wanted to borrow money and found that with a taxable bond it would have to pay 12% interest. However, there are a number of potential lenders from the state where the hospital is located. Many of these lenders are in a combined federal and state income tax bracket of 33%. That means that they will have to pay one third of any interest received in taxes. If they could earn the interest free of taxes, it would save a lot of money. In fact, if the hospital paid just two thirds as much interest, or 8% interest on a tax-free bond, the lenders would still have just as much money after taxes!

In fact, not all lenders are necessarily in such a high tax bracket. Also, some lenders may be from another state, which will tax the bond interest. As a result, it is likely that the hospital can issue the bond for a rate somewhere between 8% and 12%. If the bond is issued at 10%, that can still mean a savings of millions of dollars per year to the hospital.

One key to this savings is the ability to borrow money directly from individuals. Note in Figure 16–1 that individuals (households) lend about 40% of the money organizations receive from tax-exempt bonds, but they lend only about 7% of the money received by for-profit corporations or foreign borrowers.

To issue a tax-free bond, however, requires compliance with a number of federal

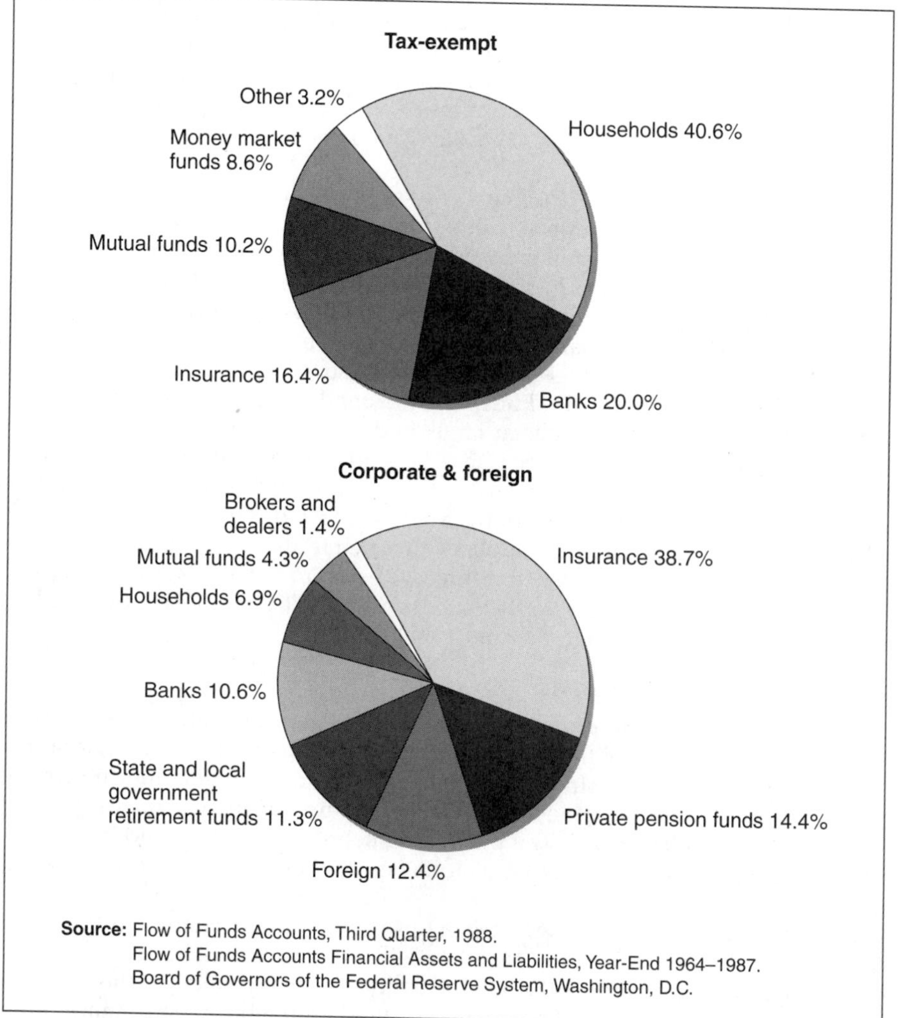

Source: Flow of Funds Accounts, Third Quarter, 1988.
Flow of Funds Accounts Financial Assets and Liabilities, Year-End 1964–1987.
Board of Governors of the Federal Reserve System, Washington, D.C.

FIGURE 16–1. Holders of tax-exempt, corporate, and foreign debt. (Reprinted from John Aderholdt and Pardue, Charles, "A Guide to Taxable Debt Financing Alternatives," *Healthcare Financial Management,* July 1989, p. 60, with permission of Healthcare Financial Management Association.)

and state regulations. Generally, a health care organization itself cannot issue a tax-free security. That is a privilege reserved for governmental bodies. For that reason, tax-free bonds are usually referred to as *municipal* bonds. In most states there are governmental bond-issuing authorities. They act as a link allowing not-for-profit health care organizations to issue tax-free securities. However, they usually assume no liability for repayment.

Given the possibility of avoiding taxes, why would taxable bonds ever be issued? There are several reasons. First of all, for-profit organizations are generally not given access to the tax-free market. Second, laws govern the total amount of bonds that can be issued on a tax-free basis. If that ceiling has been exceeded, only a taxable bond offering may be possible. The most common reason for issuing taxable bonds, however, is because it is possible to have lower expenses related to the issuance of the bond.

A number of costs are related to the issuance of bonds. Legal fees are one type of cost; placement fees are another. Bonds tend to require a great deal of sophisticated legal work to properly protect all parties. There is legal counsel for the issuer, counsel for the investors, and counsel for the investment firm that finds the buyers. Additionally, substantial amounts of money are paid to the investment firm, called the *underwriter* of the bond. The underwriter is generally an investment banking company that places the bonds with investors. A health care organization does not typically have direct access to the thousands of potential investors necessary to issue a bond successfully. Investment bankers have that large client base and are expert at finding buyers for bonds.

Despite the high legal and placement costs, it is worthwhile to issue bonds. Even a 1% savings in the interest rate as compared with conventional debt would save $1 million per year on a $100 million bond flotation. To borrow that much money for forty years, issuance costs of $2 or $3 million may be considered reasonable.

However, for a smaller bond such as $5 to $20 million or a shorter term bond such as ten years or less, the issuance costs may be too much. Taxable bonds do not require that the organization go through nearly so great a legal and regulatory process as tax-exempt bonds do. Further, if the bond is issued to a small group of investors rather than to the public at large, both legal and placement costs can be reduced even further. In such a case it may be worthwhile to pay the higher interest rate on a taxable bond. Consider that a 2% interest difference on a $7 million, three-year bond would amount to only about $400,000. If the costs of a tax-exempt issuance always exceeded a million dollars, the taxable approach would make sense. Why not just borrow $7 million for three years from a bank? The bank would probably charge a higher interest rate than even a taxable bond. Recall that the bank represents an extra middleman that must make a profit.

Bond Ratings and Insurance

A primary reason for issuing bonds rather than using conventional debt is to get a lower interest rate. One of the most important determinants of interest rates is risk. If investors perceive an investment to be risky, they require a higher return than they otherwise would. The way they get a higher return on money they lend is by charging a higher interest rate. The purpose of bond ratings and bond insurance is to lower perceived or actual risk levels to lower the interest rate that must be paid on a bond.

Two dominant bond-rating agencies in this country are Standard and Poor's and Moody's Investor Services. For a fee, they will evaluate the issuer of a bond and assign a rating to the quality of the bond. Quality is a measurement of the likelihood that the borrower will make all payments required by the bond. The highest rating is triple A, indicated by AAA or Aaa. The ratings then decline to double A, single A, triple B, double B, single B, and down into the C and D range. Anything below single B is considered a risky, speculative investment.

Triple A bond ratings are reserved for only the safest investments. Extremely few, if any, health care organizations can merit a triple A rating on the basis of their financial condition. Even double A ratings tend to be reserved for the most elite of health care organizations. Ratings of single A and below are common in health care. The specific rating assigned to an organization's bonds will have a significant bearing on the interest rate it must pay.

There is no requirement that an organization have its bonds rated. The organization can avoid paying a fee to the rating agency and simply issue "nonrated" bonds. The fee for rating a bond is high, since the bond rater must continue to follow the organization's financial condition over the life of the bond so that it can change its rating if the financial circumstances of the organization change. Failure to have a bond rated is not an indication that the bonds are a safe or unsafe investment. It may simply mean that the bond offering is too small to warrant the expense of a rating. However, many investors are reluctant to invest in such bonds.

Another alternative to rating is bond insurance. The premium for bond insurance is even more costly than obtaining a rating. The borrower pays a company to insure its obligations under the bond. Two major insurers of tax-free bonds are the American Municipal Bond Assurance Company (AMBAC) and the Municipal Bond Insurance Association (MBIA). Both organizations undertake a study of the financial situation of the bond issuer to assure themselves that the chance of default is extremely low. If they are satisfied, they issue the insurance.

Both Standard and Poor's and Moody's currently give an automatic rating of triple A to any bonds that are insured. We say currently because substantial defaults could affect the financial status of the insurer, in which case the ratings of the bonds could be lowered. The benefit of obtaining a triple A rating in terms of interest rates is so great that it often makes insurance a worthwhile investment for the bond issuer, if the organization's financial condition is sufficient to allow it to obtain the insurance.

Zero-coupon Bonds

Typical bonds pay interest semiannually. Another type of bond, called a *zero-coupon* bond or simply a "zero," does not make periodic interest payments. Instead, the interest is calculated every six months and is added onto the outstanding loan balance. At the maturity date the payment consists of the original loan plus all the accrued interest. Note that every six months the accumulated obligation grows, and in future periods interest accrues on prior interest as well as on the original principal amount. In other words, since interest is not paid out every six months, compound interest applies to all amounts owed the lender.

Zero coupon bonds are issued at deep discounts, and the interest is built into the face value of the bond. For example, a $10,000, 10%, twenty-year-maturity, zero-coupon bond might be issued for $1,420. The $10,000 payment at maturity would cover both the original $1,420 loan and also the interest from the entire life of the loan.

Zeroes have a great advantage in that they do not require any payments of interest until the maturity date. At the same time, there is also an increased risk. Lenders generally receive at least interest over the life of a loan. If they have to wait until the very end of a loan before they receive any payment at all, they are likely to demand a higher rate of interest to compensate them for that increased risk.

Zero-coupon bonds get their name from an era when bond certificates had a coupon attached for each interest payment. The lender would clip a coupon every six months and present it for payment. At that time bonds were often issued in bearer form. When a bond was sold by one party to another, the borrower was not informed. Whoever presented the coupons for payment was assumed to be the owner. For reasons of safety (to avoid loss or theft) and for tax purposes (to avoid people not paying taxes on taxable bonds), bonds are no longer issued in bearer form. They are all *registered.* The borrower maintains a record of the owner of the bond. The interest payments are automatically made without presentation of a coupon. Zero-coupon bonds were so called because they had no coupons attached, since there were no periodic interest payments.

Debt Refinancing

From time to time organizations review their bond obligations and consider whether it would be advantageous to *refinance* the debt. Generally, refinancing means that the organization pays off outstanding debt with high interest rates and substitutes new debt with a lower interest rate.

Interest rates in the financial markets tend to rise and fall with the economy. When there are recessions, interest rates fall. This is largely because there is not much business demand for money. When demand is low, the price of borrowed money (i.e., the interest rate) falls. When the economy is strong and there is a great demand for loans, the price rises.

Sometimes a health care organization borrows money despite relatively high interest rates because there is a pressing need for the assets that will be bought with the money. The economy's cycles take a long time. It might be five years, ten years, or even longer before interest rates decline. When the rates do decline, however, the organization must consider whether it pays to refinance the outstanding bonds.

Refinancing is not automatic for a number of reasons. First, there are all the costs related to a new bond issuance. These costs are high but make sense when spread over a long period. If the bonds are refinanced every five years, the issuance costs could overwhelm much, if not all, of the interest rate benefit. Second, when bonds are issued, assurances are given to the lenders (i.e., the buyers of the bonds) that they will earn the stated interest rate. Often a penalty is charged to the issuer of the bond for early repayment of the bonds. The borrower may have to pay not only the face value of the bonds but also an extra amount.

The amount of the penalty, if any, depends on the *call provisions* of the bond. Call provisions are the conditions in the bond agreement that specify the rights the borrower has to call in the bond early and pay it off. If the call provisions are easy on the borrower, the original interest rate will be high. If the call provisions make it difficult to call in and pay off the bond, the interest rate is somewhat lower. When the bond is first issued, a trade-off must be made as the call provisions are established.

So far, we have considered refinancing from the point of view of calling in and paying off an outstanding bond at its face value. A related element of refinancing is the purchase of the organization's own bonds on the open financial market. However, unlike the refinancing done when interest rates fall, purchase refinancing is likely to occur when interest rates rise. If interest rates climb, the market price of bonds drops. Why would anyone want a bond that pays 10% when new bonds pay 12% or 13%?

If interest rates have risen and bond prices have fallen and if the organization has some cash available, it can buy its own bonds at the market price. The advantage of this is that the price is less than the organization will have to pay if it waits for the maturity of the bond.

Frequently organizations establish a *sinking fund* when they have an outstanding bond liability. A sinking fund is a pool of money accumulated for a specific purpose. The purpose of a bond sinking fund is to accumulate money to eventually pay the bond face value at maturity.

If interest rates have risen and the bonds are selling below their face value, money from the sinking fund can be used to buy the bonds and retire them early. By retiring the bonds, the interest payments for those specific bonds purchased no longer have to be paid. And by buying them below face value, the organization saves the difference between the price paid and the face value that would eventually have had to be paid. On the other hand, the money is no longer in the sinking fund, earning interest at the relatively high current rate.

※ FEASIBILITY STUDIES

When large amounts of money are borrowed on a long-term basis, the lenders often require that the borrower undertake a feasibility study to demonstrate the organization's capacity to repay the loan. The organization will generally hire an outsider such as a certified public accounting firm to perform the study. Feasibility studies evaluate all the financial implications of the proposed investment. They show expected revenues and expenses over a long period, usually five to ten years.

A feasibility study will not only show the expected profitability of a particular investment or venture but will also project pro forma financial statements for the entire organization.[3] In addition, feasibility studies include ratio analysis showing the capacity of the organization to cover the interest charges and principal payments on its total debt, including the proposed borrowing.

One of the most telling elements of the feasibility study is the ratio that relates to interest coverage.[4] If the organization cannot make interest payments when due, it risks having to seek protection of the bankruptcy laws and possibly even closure. Therefore lenders are interested in how much cushion is anticipated for coverage of such payments.

Another element of feasibility studies that is considered fairly important relates to the attitude of the staff of the organization. If the majority of people in the organization believe in a project and are committed to its success, that does not guarantee success. But when the majority are opposed to a project, disinterested, or not committed to it, there is a strong likelihood of failure.

If a commissioned feasibility study raises serious questions about the success of an expansion or new venture, the organization should seriously consider the weaknesses that have been raised. Not only will there be a question about whether financing can be obtained, there is also the more important question concerning whether the organization is making a mistake in undertaking the project.

※ THE FUTURE OF HEALTH CARE FINANCING

To thrive an organization must be able to maintain its major facilities. Buildings must be modernized and eventually replaced. Equipment must be kept up-to-date. This all requires major capital investments, which in turn require cash resources.

The source of financing for health care has changed quite a bit over the last fifty years, and there is a likelihood that it will continue to change. Before the 1960s, philanthropy was a major source of cash for long-term investments by health care organizations. Then the government became the major supplier of cash resources. Most recently, long-term debt has become the single largest element for new construction.

However, the continued availability of debt is not assured. There are movements to eliminate tax-free bonds. That would severely hurt health care organizations, hospitals in particular. Even with the continued existence of tax-free bonds, there is cause for concern. The introduction of DRGs in 1983 had a dramatic effect on the health care bond market. Lending money to organizations in the health care industry has been a riskier investment since the shift of hospital Medicare payments from cost-based reimbursement to the DRG prospective payment system. The basic ability of the organization to issue bonds depends on its actual and perceived risk as an investment.

Approximately half of all hospital revenues come from Medicare and Medicaid patients. In the pre-DRG era the bond market perceived those revenues as nearly risk free. Certainly hospitals could count on receiving their annual stream of revenues

---

[3]Pro forma financial statements are discussed in the section on business plans in Chapter 20.

[4]A discussion of ratios is included in Chapter 6.

from the government. That allowed hospitals to incur large amounts of long-term debt at relatively favorable interest rates.

With the advent of DRGs, the guaranteed revenue base was affected. Payments were shifted to a fixed fee rather than cost reimbursement. Substantial losses might occur on Medicare patients. In fact, the number of hospital closures has increased dramatically since the introduction of DRGs.

To the bond market, that represents increased risk. The change not only increases the chances that hospitals will lose money on Medicare patients but also increases the likelihood of additional regulatory changes that might hurt all health care providers. Whether this is likely to close off a major source of financing for health care, or simply make it more expensive, cannot be determined at this time. However, the poor financial health of the health care industry makes it more likely that long-term debt will become less and less available. On the other hand, this is offset at least somewhat by the limited availability of federal guarantees for long-term debt of some health care organizations.

Where will the resources come from in the future? Some have suggested that corporations will have to get together to generate the monies needed. In effect that proposal is a return to philanthropy but at the corporate level, since individuals do not have the vast sums necessary for modern health care facility construction.

Another view of the future is that the government will take over the health care system, similar to the approaches of England and Canada. In that view the government will decide what facilities are needed and will build them using tax dollars.

Yet another view is that many health care organizations will go out of business, reducing excess capacity. The remaining organizations will be financially healthy and will continue to have access to the major debt markets.

We have no special insight regarding a solution. We do, however, clearly see a problem. Nationwide, and particularly in certain regions such as the Northeast, the severe financial distress of health care institutions such as hospitals and nursing homes has prevented some of them from replacing or even adequately maintaining their facilities. Given this state, there is clearly the potential for a health care financing crisis in the early part of the twenty-first century.

※ IMPLICATIONS FOR NURSE MANAGERS

The highest levels of nurse managers in any health care organization must be involved in the specific long-term financing decisions. Other nurse managers also have an important role in the financing process.

The decision to finance using conventional debt, tax-free bonds, or leasing will have a dramatic impact on the financial well-being of the institution. This decision should not be left solely to financial managers, because they may lack vision about the organization. They have greater financial expertise than nurse managers, but they may not have as good judgment about the clinical aspects of the organization.

This fact is evidenced by the interest that lenders, bond raters, and bond insurers all have in the attitude and thoughts of the staff of a health care institution. If the physicians are unhappy, they will not admit patients. If the nurses are unhappy, patients will not want to come to the institution. Financing should be done for investments that will make the organization as a whole work better. The nursing staff can provide critical input in this area.

It is important to bear in mind that major long-term financing such as a bond issuance is not an area of expertise of *anyone* in most health care organizations. Except for the larger academic medical centers, bond floatation may be something that occurs just once in the career of a chief executive officer, chief financial officer, or chief nurse executive. The input of all areas of the institution can help the organization make the correct decisions.

Some other types of long-term financing are more common. Mortgages and leases are used with great frequency. However, the choice of a mortgage or a lease is not strictly financial. Rather than having financial managers make such decisions on their own, nurse managers should provide input to the process. From a departmental or unit point of view, what are the advantages of a lease or the advantages of ownership as compared to a lease? Does the lessor provide some essential support service that is otherwise not readily available? Perhaps the equipment is subject to repeated breakdown. A lease arrangement may provide cheaper service than ownership plus a service contract.

Nurse managers should not assume that the financing of the organization is something outside their management sphere of activity or expertise. A participatory team attitude and approach between nursing and finance is more likely to result in financing decisions that will benefit the entire organization, including nursing services.

KEY CONCEPTS

Long-term financing Sources of money that the organization can use for longer than one year.

Debt Borrowed money. Interest is generally paid on the debt.

Equity Represents ownership sources of financing. In some case equity represents money that outsiders have given the organization in exchange for an ownership interest. In other cases equity represents money that the organization itself owns. The four principal sources of equity for health care organizations are philanthropy, corporate stock issuance, government grants, and retained earnings.

Philanthropy Gifts to the organization.

Stock issuance Sale of ownership interests in the organization; only available to for-profit organizations.

Government grants Direct payments to health care organizations, usually to finance construction.

Retained earnings Profits earned by the organization and retained in the organization to finance assets.

Long-term debt Represents borrowed sources of financing. This includes mortgages, long-term notes, leases, and bonds.

Mortgages and long-term notes Conventional loans to the organization. Notes are sometimes secured by collateral and sometimes are unsecured. A note secured by a specific piece of physical property such as a building, piece of equipment, or land is referred to as a mortgage.

Leases Rental agreements evidenced by a contract referred to as a lease. Considered long-term debt because they obligate the organization to making payments over a period of years.

Bonds Formal certificates of indebtedness. The certificate indicates a promise to pay interest, usually semiannually, and the face value of the bond at a future specified maturity date.

Call provisions Elements of the loan agreement between a bond issuer and a bond purchaser indicating the rights of the bond issuer to call in and pay off the bonds early and specifying penalties that must be paid if a bond is retired early.

Bond sinking fund Pool of money accumulated for the eventual repayment of the face value of outstanding bonds.

Feasibility study Analysis designed to determine the organization's capacity to repay a long-term loan.

SUGGESTED READINGS

Cleverley, William O., *Essentials of Health Care Finance,* Aspen Publishers, Gaithersburg, Md., February 1997.

Emery, Douglas, John D. Finnerty, and John D. Stowe, *Principles of Financial Management,* Prentice Hall, Upper Saddle River, NJ, 1998.

Finkler, Steven A., *Finance and Accounting for Nonfinancial Managers,* revised edition, Prentice Hall, Upper Saddle River, N.J., 1996.

Gapenski, Louis C., *Financial Analysis and Decision Making for Healthcare Organizations: A Guide for the Healthcare Professional,* Irwin Professional Publishers, Burr Ridge, Ill., January 1997.

Horngren, Charles T., Gary L. Sundem, and William O. Stratton, *Introduction to Management Accounting,* 10th edition, Prentice Hall, Upper Saddle River, N.J., 1996.

Keown, Arthur J., J. William Petty, David F. Scott, and John D. Martin, *Foundations of Finance,* 2nd edition, Prentice Hall, Upper Saddle River, N.J., 1998.

McLean, Robert A., *Financial Management in Health Care Organizations,* Delmar, Albany, N.Y., 1996.

Neumann, Bruce R., Jan P. Clement, and Jean C. Cooper, *Financial Management: Concepts and Applications for Health Care Organizations,* Kendall/Hunt Publishing, Dubuque, Iowa, May 1997.

Suver, James D., Bruce R. Neumann, and Keith E. Boles, *Management Accounting for Healthcare Organizations,* 3rd edition, Pluribus Press, Westchester, Ill., 1992.

Zelman, William N., Michael McCue, and Alan R. Milikan, *Financial Management of Health Care Organizations: An Introduction to Fundamental Tools, Concepts, and Applications,* Blackwell Publishers, Cambridge, Mass., January 1998.

PART

VI

ADDITIONAL MANAGEMENT TOOLS

※

Most nurse managers recognize the importance of financial management. To successfully manage finances the nurse manager must understand the underlying financial concepts. The preceding chapters describe these concepts. In addition to understanding the concepts, it is necessary to have sound financial information on which to base financial decisions. The first step in getting information is to know what to ask for.

Nurse managers generate some of the information they need themselves. Other information is readily available in health organizations; the nurse manager needs to ask for it. Still other information is available but not in a format that is useful for the nurse manager. Some information is not available and must be generated either by the nurse manager directly or by other departments in the organization.

The following chapters describe management tools that can be used both to generate information and to reconfigure it into a useful format. In addition, the kinds of information that are useful in making financial decisions are explored.

Chapter 17 relates the use of information systems and computers to financial management. The chapter begins with a description of computer hardware and software. The use of computers is reviewed. Major types of software for microcomputers are identified, and their use for forecasting, costing, personnel management, budgeting, and acuity systems is described. Finally, the future use of computers in financial decision making is assessed.

Chapter 18, Forecasting and Other Methods for Decision Making, focuses on quantitative and qualitative methods useful to nurse managers. The chapter begins with a discussion of probability, which forms the basis for many of the methods discussed later in the chapter. The use of specific techniques to predict future events, such as patient volume and staffing needs, is stressed. Finally, this chapter provides methods for inventory control and tracking a project.

Chapter 19 begins with a discussion of why marketing is important for nurse managers. The difference between marketing and advertising is clarified. Marketing concepts are then defined. The elements of a marketing plan and the role of these elements is discussed. ※

CHAPTER

17

The Use of Computers in Financial Management

CHAPTER GOALS

The goals of this chapter are to:

- Describe computer hardware and software
- Identify the use of computers for information management
- Describe the use of computers for financial management
- Discuss special purpose software, such as that used for forecasting, costing, personnel management, budgeting, and acuity systems
- Analyze the future use of computers in financial management
- Discuss the implications of computers for financial management for nurse managers

※ INTRODUCTION

The purpose of this chapter is to describe the use of computers in nursing financial management. Computers are tools to help the nurse manager summarize and organize information. Computers decide neither what information is provided nor the format in which it is displayed. Previous chapters identified the types of financial information the nurse manager needs to effectively manage a unit or an organization. This chapter focuses on how the computer can be used to collect and summarize that information.

※ COMPUTER HARDWARE AND SOFTWARE

Computers and their related pieces of equipment such as printers, monitors, and terminals are referred to as *hardware*. The instructions that tell computer equipment what to do are referred to as *software*.

Types of Computers

The three major types of computers are mainframes, minicomputers, and microcomputers. Mainframe computers are large (both physically and in computing capacity), fast, and expensive; microcomputers are small and inexpensive; minicomputers fall somewhere in between. Computers are made by a number of manufacturers such as IBM, Dell, Gateway, Compaq, Apple, and Unisys. Computer manufacturers make a large variety of models. Some manufacturers make only mainframes or microcomputers; others make all types of hardware. Within the category of microcomputers, for example, a company may make as many as fifty different models.

When health care organizations first used computers to manage financial information, they used mainframe computers. They either purchased or leased time on a mainframe. Sometimes they leased time on a mainframe and accessed the computer over telephone lines. Many hospitals and nursing homes contracted with a computer services company to provide both the time on the computer and the staff services to process financial information.

Some health care organizations purchased minicomputers, hired information systems staff, and processed their own financial information. In the 1980s, as the cost of microcomputers decreased and their processing speed increased, health care organizations began investing in them. Mainframe or minicomputers are still required and used by most large health care organizations to perform the major financial operations such as billing. Many clinical information systems operate using terminals linked to a mainframe computer. However, an increasing number of nurse managers are using microcomputers for managerial functions.

Telling Computers What to Do

Computers require software to operate. Software is a *program* or set of instructions for the computer. All computers must use a type of software called an operating system, the basic language used to give the computer instructions about what to process. When a computer is purchased, an operating system is purchased as well. Windows 98 is a widely used microcomputer operating system. However, the operating system only provides a starting point. Someone must program or write the instructions for the computer to follow for various specific applications. Initially, individuals (programmers) wrote specific sets of instructions for each computer and each application. It soon became clear that many organizations had common needs and that all could use the same set of basic programs. Since many people want to use a computer to calculate the arithmetic sum of a set of numbers, one person wrote a program (software) to calculate sums for his or her own organization. Proprietary companies wrote more sophisticated software using the operating system to perform complex operations. Other people can use the software (usually by purchasing it) to do sums. These programs are often called *software packages* or *packages*.

To understand the use of computers for financial management the nurse manager must know both the hardware and software capabilities available at the institution. Since hardware is often more expensive than software, once an organization owns hardware, it is less likely to purchase new equipment. Some commercially available software can operate on a variety of computers; other software will operate only on one model of computer. Some software packages are sold prepackaged, and little or no tailoring is needed; other software is designed (at much greater expense) to meet the specific needs of a particular organization.

⋇ USES OF COMPUTERS

The three principal uses of computers for nursing are for general information, clinical applications, and financial management.

General Information Management

Computers are tools to store and process information. In health care organizations, computers are used for various types of information, including keeping a calendar or telephone directory, word processing, and spreadsheets. When information is computerized, it is often called *electronic*. Over time the number of applications continues to grow.

Clinical Care

Computer uses for clinical care fall into two general areas. The first area is assessment of patients. This includes computers used in laboratories to measure blood levels, in radiology for magnetic resonance imaging (MRI), and for physical assessment measures such as blood pressure. Each of these applications requires both hardware and software.

The second clinical care area is storage and management of patient information. Often called the hospital information system or nursing information system, these computer systems store data such as patient demographics; admission, transfer, and discharge information; and documentation of nursing care provided.

While clinical information systems are not directly related to financial management, data produced by these systems can be used to make financial decisions. Clinical systems are used to directly link the use of services to the billing for them. Ultimately, financial management is based on the allocation of resources; clinical information systems offer the nurse manager data about the use of resources in the organization.

Clinical information systems that combine information from a variety of sources, such as laboratory, radiology, dietary, and nursing, are called *fully integrated* systems. In these systems the data are entered once and are accessible all over the organization (with the appropriate confidentiality precautions). These integrated systems improve the flow of information.

Financial Management

Computers can greatly aid nurse managers in the area of financial management information. The first step for the nurse manager is to decide what financial information is needed for management. This includes information the manager needs from others and information the manager must report to others. Earlier chapters of this book discuss various types of information needed for financial management, such as budget information and variance reports. An example of computerizing some aspects of variance analysis is provided in the article reprinted at the end of this chapter.

Later chapters also discuss financial information that can be generated by a computer, such as forecasting analyses. After identifying the needed information, the nurse manager should identify information currently available in the organization. Some information may already be routinely reported to managers (e.g., occupancy, average length of stay, payroll). Next the manager should identify information that is likely available but not systematically reported. After assessing whether the required information can be obtained in a useful format, the nurse manager must decide how best to collect and analyze unavailable data.

Computerizing everything is not always the best solution. Using a computer for data management has equipment and human costs. Adding to and retrieving information from a computer requires an ongoing human resource commitment. Without that commitment the benefits of computerizing may not be worth the cost. For example, setting up a computerized checkbook system requires that all entries be entered in timely fashion. If data are not entered on an ongoing systematic basis, the computerized system is no better than the paper record with missing entries.

The key to the use of computers is that they must accomplish one of two things. One is to electronically generate information that currently is generated manually, thus saving human effort. The other is to generate information that would not otherwise be available and whose value is greater than the cost of obtaining it.

Mainframes and Financial Management Information

Most hospitals and many other health care organizations have mainframe computers for patient billing and other aspects of organizational financial management. In many cases the chief nurse executive (CNE) was not involved in planning these systems. In almost all health care organizations the CNE receives periodic reports generated by the system, and in many organizations first-line nurse managers also receive regular reports. Often the format of these reports is designed by the financial or information systems departments and does not give the nurse manager the type of information needed. In some cases the information is provided months after appropriate decisions based on that information should have been made.

As a nurse manager you may want to know the average length of stay by Diagnosis Related Groups (DRG) for each unit for which you are responsible. Your hospital provides the CNE with the average length of stay by DRG hospital-wide. While that information as reported for the entire hospital is useful for overall hospital efforts to decrease length of stay, it may not assist you in identifying variation in length of stay by unit.

After assessing information needs, the first step is to learn what information is currently collected electronically. Many health organizations have information systems departments. Data may be collected by the information systems department or by the finance department, the nursing department, or other departments. Data collected by other departments may be useful to you. By understanding how finance, personnel, or information systems departments collect and organize data, you will be able to identify the data that you can request. Most health organization finance systems can prepare special reports on request. However, you should keep in mind that such requests are often time-consuming and expensive. If you will be requesting these data on a regular basis, you should communicate that.

Computers allow for storing, processing, and reporting huge amounts of information quickly. First, the nurse manager can easily become overloaded with computer-generated reports. Second, processing and reporting data is not costless. What may appear to be a simple request may take hours of programming by the information systems department.

Clear communication with the data processing department is essential to obtaining appropriate information. The first step is to carefully determine what information is needed. Next, that specific need must be clearly communicated to the correct department. The nurse manager should be sensitive to the fact that many demands are placed on the information systems department. There should be an exchange of information concerning how hard it will be to generate the data and how valuable the data will be. In some cases the cost of obtaining the data may exceed the benefit. Finally, the nurse manager should give a sufficient amount of time to generate the information. Undertaking this process of communication and consideration will make the nurse and information managers partners in meeting the needs of the organization.

Microcomputers and Financial Management Information

Many types of microcomputer software applications are useful for financial management. There are currently two standard microcomputer hardware systems, IBM and MacIntosh. *Clones,* equipment made by competitors and intended to function on a completely compatible basis, are available for both and are usually substantially cheaper. Although many software applications are available for IBMs and MacIntoshes, some are available for only one or the other. Information is not difficult to transfer between the two types of hardware, as conversion processes do exist.

Five major types of software are especially useful for financial management:

- Word processing
- Data base
- Spreadsheet
- Statistical packages
- E-mail and Internet

Both general purpose and application-specific programs are available for each of these. General purpose programs require that the person using the program set up many of the parameters.

Word processing software is used to prepare correspondence and reports. While not directly related to financial management, the presentation of budget justifications, business plans, and other proposals virtually requires that the nursing department have this capability. WordPerfect and Word are examples of commercially available software for word processing.[1]

It is strongly suggested that most people in the organization use the same word processing package. Because the use of computers developed gradually in most organizations, each department and even each person in a department initially may have selected and used different software. Unfortunately, although most software is *compatible,* in a way it is like asking a computer that understands French to read something in Spanish. Although there are ways to "translate" files, in some cases the translation is not very good, particularly formatting such as spacing and paragraphs. While staff initially may be resistant to learning a new program, in the long run having everyone use the same program will save hours of retyping.

Related to word processing programs are graphics programs that present information in pictorial form. Powerpoint, Corel Presentations, and Freelance Graphics are examples of such programs.[2] These programs can be used to produce slides and overhead transparencies. They are often referred to as presentation graphics programs. These programs can produce charts and graphs. Word processing programs now include the capability to produce graphics.

Data bases are compilations of related information systematically organized. The telephone directory is a data base of names, addresses, and telephone numbers, usually organized alphabetically by last name. Most nursing departments have numerous data bases. The nursing department and each nursing care unit likely have a data base of employees. The nursing department also maintains a data base of equipment inventory. These data bases may be handwritten, on 3×5 cards, or typed on paper. They also may be electronically stored for use on a computer.

Many data base software packages are available commercially. Access and dBase are examples of data base software programs.[3] The software may be designed for general applications and may be useful for a variety of tasks, or it may be designed for specific applications. General application programs tend to be more difficult to learn but are flexible and offer the advantage of integrating a variety of data bases.

Specific-application data bases such as those used for health records are often easier to learn to use but may limit the integration of data. Data bases allow one to store information in a systematic manner and then retrieve information according to criteria one chooses.

Once you have decided to use a computerized data base, choosing which software to use will depend on a variety of factors. The general rule is to use what everyone else in the organization is using unless there is a compelling reason not to. First, there will be people to help you use the program; second, your data bases will be compatible with theirs.

Because most nonelectronic data bases are organized in only one way (e.g., alphabetically, by date, by dollar amount), it is difficult to look for information by other than the organizing category. For example, if you received a garbled message that someone called you and his phone number was 348-8125, how would you determine who called? You might remember that this is the number of the supply salesperson who has been bothering you about buying new equipment. You could

---

[1]WordPerfect is a trademark of Corel; Word is a trademark of Microsoft.

[2]Powerpoint is a registered trademark of Microsoft Corporation; Corel Presentations is a trademark of Corel Corp., and Freelance Graphics is a trademark of Lotus Development Corp.

[3]dBase is a trademark of Borland International; Access is a trademark of Microsoft.

look through your phone book page by page and find out who the person is. You will likely just call the number and see who it was. With a computerized data base of phone numbers you can ask the computer to locate the name of the person with this phone number. The computer will look through your list of phone numbers and identify the name associated with that number. However, it is not always cost effective to computerize every data base you have.

Spreadsheets are large ledger sheets often used by accountants for financial calculations. A spreadsheet has columns and rows of cells. These cells contain text or numbers that can be manipulated. Electronic spreadsheets allow cells to contain formulas for mathematical manipulation. The formulas are decided by the person who develops the spreadsheet, and can contain any mathematical formula. The power of an electronic spreadsheet is the speed with which a whole series of numbers can be recalculated.

Spreadsheets are often used for budgeting. For example, Figure 12–6 in Chapter 12 shows a spreadsheet for the calculation of positions needed. As you probably know, the calculations can be tedious, particularly if someone changes one of the underlying assumptions and the entire budget must be recalculated. There are several commercially available spreadsheet packages. LOTUS 1-2-3 and Excel are examples.[4] As with data base programs, both general purpose and specific programs are available. The same general rules apply. It is often advisable to use what the rest of the organization uses and get a generic program unless there is a compelling reason not to.

Although spreadsheets can be used to perform statistical analyses, there is also specific statistical software used to perform such analyses. Statistics refers to both the way in which data are organized and analyzed and the data themselves. Nurse managers frequently perform statistical analyses and use the results from these analyses. They need to know the average number of sick days, the range of sick days, the average staff salary per category of worker, or the average overtime per unit per day. An example is an estimate of the average number of sick days per month for different categories of staff. One approach is to estimate based on memory. The usual approach is to count the sick days per category of worker, add up the days, and divide by the number of workers.

All statistical calculations can be done with pencil and paper. They can be done more quickly with a calculator, and often even more quickly with a spreadsheet or a statistical software program on a computer. It is not always more efficient to do tasks with a computer. For example, to calculate the average number of nurses who worked during a five-day period, it may be easier to use a calculator. Using a computer is more efficient for manipulating a large quantity of numbers, for performing complex analyses such as forecasting that are time-consuming to do by hand, and for repetitive tasks.

A variety of software programs are available for purchase. The most sophisticated programs were initially designed for use on mainframe computers and have been rewritten for microcomputers. SPSS – PC + (Statistical Package for the Social Sciences Personal Computer Version) is an example.[5] The versions for microcomputers do not include as many options as the mainframe versions, but they are more than adequate for most nursing departments and are now "user friendly." Additional statistical programs are available that were developed for microcomputers. Careful use of these programs is advised for those nurse managers who have not studied statistics.

Electronic communication has dramatically changed the way people communicate. Two examples of this are e-mail (electronic mail) and the Internet. Most large organizations have e-mail, and many individuals also have e-mail through a

---

[4]LOTUS 1-2-3 is a trademark of the LOTUS Development Corporation; Excel is a trademark of Microsoft.

[5]SPSS – PC + is a trademark of SPSS, Inc.

commercial account. E-mail allows the writer to send a "typed" message virtually immediately to someone else within and often outside of the organization. Advantages of e-mail over U.S. or interoffice mail (called "snail mail" by computer types) are its speed and low cost. In terms of speed, an e-mail message to almost anywhere in the world is received within minutes. Thus e-mail has the speed of a telephone at less than the cost of mailing a letter. Unlike a telephone call, there is a written record of the interaction, and the respondent does not have to provide an immediate answer. Using e-mail can eliminate the need for a secretary to type memos. Another advantage is that the same message can be sent to multiple recipients, and a message received can be forwarded to someone else. E-mail can also be used to send and receive files such as those produced using a spreadsheet. The recipient can then review the spreadsheet on his or her computer and print it out only if necessary. On the negative side, many people think that e-mail is impersonal, and in some cases the nurse-manager may not want a written record of the interaction.

The Internet is a complex system of electronic "sites" that can be used to obtain information or for a nurse manager to provide information to others. Most government agencies now have sites. For example, the New York State Education Department provides a site that contains the name and license number of all registered nurses in the state. This provides an inexpensive source of information about licensure status. The federal government's National Institutes of Health provides information on many health problems. A longer discussion about the Internet is beyond the scope of this book, but readers are urged to read the references at the end of this chapter.

Special Purpose Software

The previous section described the general types of software that can assist the nurse manager. The following section describes how these general purpose programs can be used for specific financial management activities, and discusses special applications programs.

Forecasting

Chapter 18 discusses forecasting in depth. Computers can be extremely useful in forecasting. Forecasting is used to predict the future. One of the best predictors of the future is the past. Obviously, the past is not a perfect predictor, and other factors must be taken into account. Statistical models can be used to predict the future based on past performance and assumptions about the future. Both spreadsheets and statistical software packages are useful for forecasting. Table 18–5 in Chapter 18 shows a computer printout of the estimated hours of nursing care needed for a nursing unit, based on historical hours.

Costing

Determining the cost of providing nursing care is discussed in Chapter 8. Goals are to determine the cost of providing care to a particular patient, to groups of similar patients, or to a group of patients on a particular unit. The more valid and reliable data collection is at the patient level, the more reliable and valid the aggregated data will be. Much of the literature on determining the cost of nursing care advocates using acuity systems. The section below on acuity discusses the use of computers for acuity measurement.

However, as discussed in Chapter 8, using acuity is not the only way to determine costs. Costs are really a dollar determination of resources used. How can computers be useful in determining resources used? In the nursing department the major resources consumed are personnel and supplies. Clinical information systems can provide an electronic data base of resources consumed. Each time a supply is used for a patient, it is noted in the electronic record and the appropriate cost is allocated. Each time the nurse notes that care is provided, that resource use can be captured by the computer and the appropriate costs determined. There are potential flaws in this system. It requires the nurse to note every care activity. Although noting activities on a computer may be easier than writing them, many nursing activities are not documented in either system.

The same activity provided for two different patients may require different amounts of time. This is obvious for something such as patient education, but it is also true for activities such as initiating a venous line. Depending on the use of the cost estimates, standard measures of resource use may be acceptable (see Chapter 8 discussion of standard costs). For example, Hospital A may assume that starting a line takes ten minutes, recognizing that there may be variation from patient to patient.

Some health care organizations use *bar coding*. Each patient's wristband contains a bar code. Each time the nurse begins care, and again when care is completed, the nurse uses a scanner to *scan* the patient's bar code. Data are then collected about real time spent providing care to patients. The scanner is also used to identify supplies that patients consume. Computers then use these data to tabulate resources used. However, nursing includes both the care giver and care integrator roles.[6] The care integrator role involves communication with other health providers and family members and is less easy to document with the scanner.

While using computers may decrease the time required to collect and analyze data to determine the cost of care, the expense is still not trivial. The nurse manager must make the decision about the level of detail that is necessary and the cost/benefit of collecting the data.

If the nurse manager does not believe it is cost effective to document the cost of care provided to each patient on every unit, the computer can still be useful for summarizing available cost data. The manager can use a spreadsheet program with existing data from payroll combined with data generated from unit variance reports and acuity numbers to estimate costs on various units.

Personnel Management

Personnel management requires the systematic organization of information about employees, such as staff skill levels, work preferences, health background, salary, work history, and other factors. A computerized data base is a helpful tool for organizing this material. In most health care organizations payroll is computerized. In most organizations with a personnel department distinct from the nursing department, it is likely that some personnel data are computerized, although that will vary from organization to organization.

From a financial management viewpoint the nurse manager needs to have information to most efficiently use these personnel resources. One main use of data bases is for staffing. The organizational structure of the organization will have an impact on the way data bases are set up. For example, a home health agency may want a data base of all RNs employed. This data base will include demographic information, health status, continuing education record, full- or part-time status, and preferred work hours. It is particularly useful to include special skills such as knowledge of foreign languages and expertise in parenteral fluid administration in the data base. The data base may also include vacation time used. If nurse managers need a nurse to work on the weekend, they can use this data base to identify a nurse in the appropriate geographic area who has the requisite skills and who is willing to work extra shifts.

Staffing is the major responsibility of the nurse manager. Special application

---

[6]McClure, M. L., and J. J. Nelson, "Trends in Hospital Nursing," in L. H. Aiken, ed., *Nursing in the 1980s: Crisis, Opportunities, Challenges*, J. B. Lippincott, Philadelphia, Penn., 1982, pp. 59–73.

programs are available for staffing. These programs are combinations of data bases and spreadsheets. Examples are ANSOS and RESQUE. Private computer consultants will also develop software programs to meet the needs of organizations. Data about available staff are stored in the data base. Staffing needs are identified by nurse managers, often using an acuity system.

Staffing rules are determined by the nurse manager. Rules can include: (1) no nurse can work more than seven consecutive days; (2) no nurse can work more than every other weekend; (3) each nurse must have at least two consecutive days off. Using the established rules, the computer provides staffing options. These programs can also incorporate individual preferences. For example, Nurse A prefers not to work Thursday evenings and requires Mondays off to attend school. For years nurse managers have been staffing units and taking staff preferences into account. The use of a computer greatly reduces the time needed to do this and can quickly adjust for changes in staff requirements. This frees the nurse manager to spend time on other elements of management.

The advantage of spreadsheets is the ability to quickly determine "what if" options. For example, "what if" the number of sick days increases or three more staff decide to go back to school and need to switch work days? The most sophisticated systems can provide staffing patterns based on acuity and patient need. While staffing is a general management function rather than a specific aspect of financial management, efficient use of available staff will likely improve the financial strength of the organization.

Budgeting

Chapter 12 discusses the budgeting process. Budgeting is often seen as one of the most painful parts of a nurse manager's responsibility, but computers can dramatically decrease the frustration and tedium of budget preparation. Budget preparation involves collection of historical data, estimates of future resources and needs, and proposed allocation of resources to meet those needs.

Using the computer for forecasting, costing, and personnel will give the nurse manager many of the data needed for successful budgeting. A spreadsheet is the most common computer application for budgeting. Commonly used software packages are LOTUS 1-2-3 and Excel. Exhibit 17–1 shows a simple spreadsheet for overtime hours. Overtime hours for each of five workers for five months are shown. Total overtime hours are shown in row 11. Assume the nurse manager realizes that overtime hours for Smith and Jones were erroneous. Instead of working three and two hours, respectively, in May, they each worked ten hours. Exhibit 17–2 shows the corrected spreadsheet. The nurse manager corrects only the hours for the individuals, and the spreadsheet automatically recalculates the total shown in cell

※ EXHIBIT 17–1. *Example of Spreadsheet*

	A	B	C	D	E	F	G	H	I	J	K
1			Nursing Hospital—4 South West: Overtime Hours								
2											
3			Jan.		Feb.		Mar.		Apr.		May
4											
5	Smith		28		30		16		12		3
6	Jones		25		25		14		8		2
7	Kovner		34		35		24		14		5
8	Finkler		15		28		20		10		2
9	Moga		40		35		18		13		2
10											
11	Totals:		142		153		92		57		14

※ EXHIBIT 17–2. *Revised Example of Spreadsheet*

	A	B	C	D	E	F	G	H	I	J	K
1			Nursing Hospital—4 South West: Overtime Hours								
2											
3			Jan.		Feb.		Mar.		Apr.		May
4											
5	Smith		28		30		16		12		10
6	Jones		25		25		14		8		10
7	Kovner		34		35		24		14		5
8	Finkler		15		28		20		10		2
9	Moga		40		35		18		13		2
10											
11	Totals:		142		153		92		57		29

K11. This same spreadsheet can be used to calculate "what if" scenarios. For example, if overtime increased to fifteen hours per worker, what would be the implications of total overtime? These are, of course, simple examples of the complicated calculations the computer can do automatically.

It is becoming increasingly common for health care organizations to use flexible budgeting (discussed in Chapter 13). Spreadsheets can be particularly useful in calculating, understanding, and justifying flexible budget variances (see, for example, the article reprinted at the end of this chapter). A series of multiplications is used to identify the actual cost, the budgeted cost of actual resources used, the acuity category, the flexible budget, and the original budget. Further calculations are required to determine the price, quantity, acuity, and volume variances. In some institutions these calculations are performed by the finance department. If these data are not available, the nursing department can create a spreadsheet template to do these calculations. Secretarial staff can type in the information, and nurse managers can benefit from sophisticated variance data.

Information can be presented in a variety of formats. The appendix at the end of this chapter provides a reprinted journal article that gives examples of ways to show the information contained in a variance report generated by LOTUS 1-2-3. Note that there are a number of cells with "xxx" or "err." The "xxx" represents data not yet available, and "err" represents where the program has been unable to carry out a calculation because the needed data have not been made available. Data can be presented in a variety of graphic formats. Figure 17–1*A* shows variances in the form of a bar graph, and Figure 17–1*B* shows the same information in the form of a pie chart. Figure 17–1*C* shows variance data for six months in line-graph form.

Acuity Systems

It is becoming more and more common for staffing to be based on actual patient care needs. This has led to a greatly increased focus on measurement of patient acuity.

Home health agencies base the amount of care provided (usually visits per week and total number of visits per episode of care) on the patient's need for care. This assessment of need is usually ordered by the physician, but in actuality it is determined by the nurse doing the initial assessment and on an ongoing basis by the nurse providing care. Increasingly, payers request more systematic determination of care required, often limit the number of visits that are paid for, and sometimes pay a set amount for an episode of care.

The Joint Commission on Accreditation of Healthcare Organizations (JCAHO) now requires that hospital staffing be based on patient needs. While hospitals have always done this, JCAHO now expects some evidence of systematic assessment of patient needs. Most hospitals use some type of acuity system to make this determination.

Numerous articles describe approaches to determining acuity, and many hospitals have developed their own system. The usual method is for nurses to rate the patient's needs periodically (usually once per day), to sum the scores for each

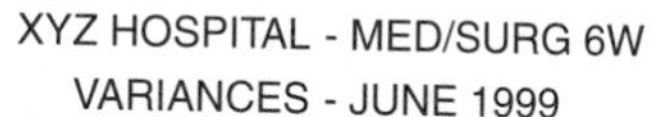

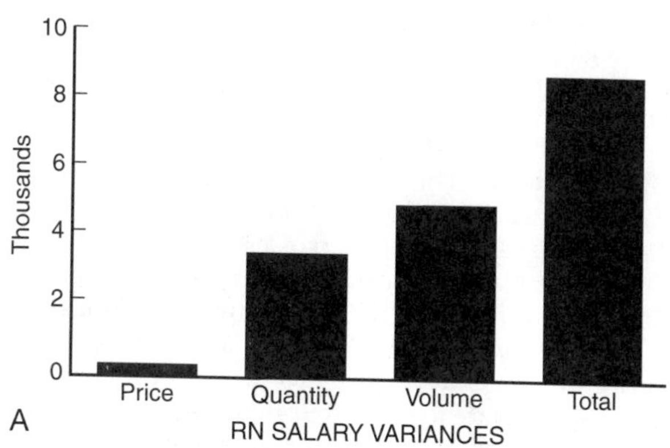

XYZ HOSPITAL - MED/SURG 6W
VARIANCES - JUNE 1999

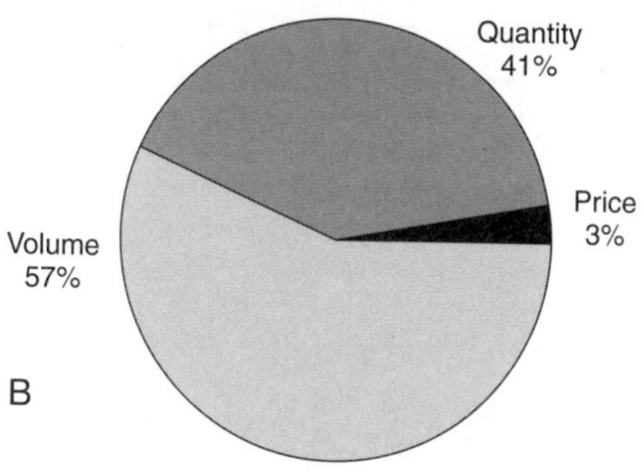

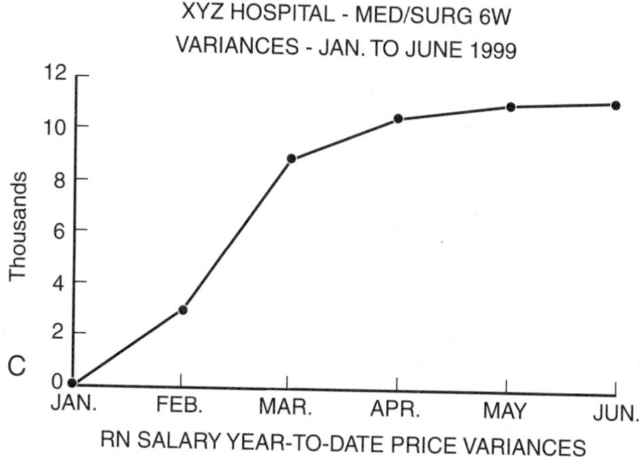

FIGURE 17–1. *A,* Bar graph of price, quantity, and volume variances for June. *B,* Pie graph of June price, quantity, and volume variances. *C,* Line graph for year-to-date price variances.

patient, and, based on a predetermined relationship for score to hours of care needed, determine the required staff for the next time period (often the next twenty-four hours). Usually the score sheets are sent to a centralized location for tabulation. The average acuity measures over time are also reviewed for long-range planning for staffing requirements.

The entire process can be computerized. In the most sophisticated model the nursing plan of care is entered into a clinical information system. Data from the plan of care are electronically transmitted into an acuity system, patient acuity is determined, and those data are analyzed to determine future staffing needs and aid in budgeting. This totally electronic system is beyond the resources of most health care organizations. Figure 17–2 depicts a staffing system integrated with the clinical information system. Information generated by nurses about patient needs determines appropriate staffing needs.

Most acuity systems require completion of a paper form on each patient to determine acuity. This form can be a *scansheet*. Scansheets are forms with preprinted markings, usually filled out with a number 2 pencil. These forms can then be read electronically by a computerized scanner and directly entered as data. Those data can then be analyzed by the computer and printed for review by the nurse manager. This process decreases data entry time by clerical staff and dramatically decreases transcription errors. Both Medicus and GRASP have the capability to provide this service to hospitals. Hospitals using other systems, including their own, can purchase software to do this. Scanners and customized forms can be purchased from National Computer Systems and other vendors.

For those hospitals that choose not to invest in a scanner, a spreadsheet program is useful to calculate staffing requirements based on acuity. The spreadsheet program

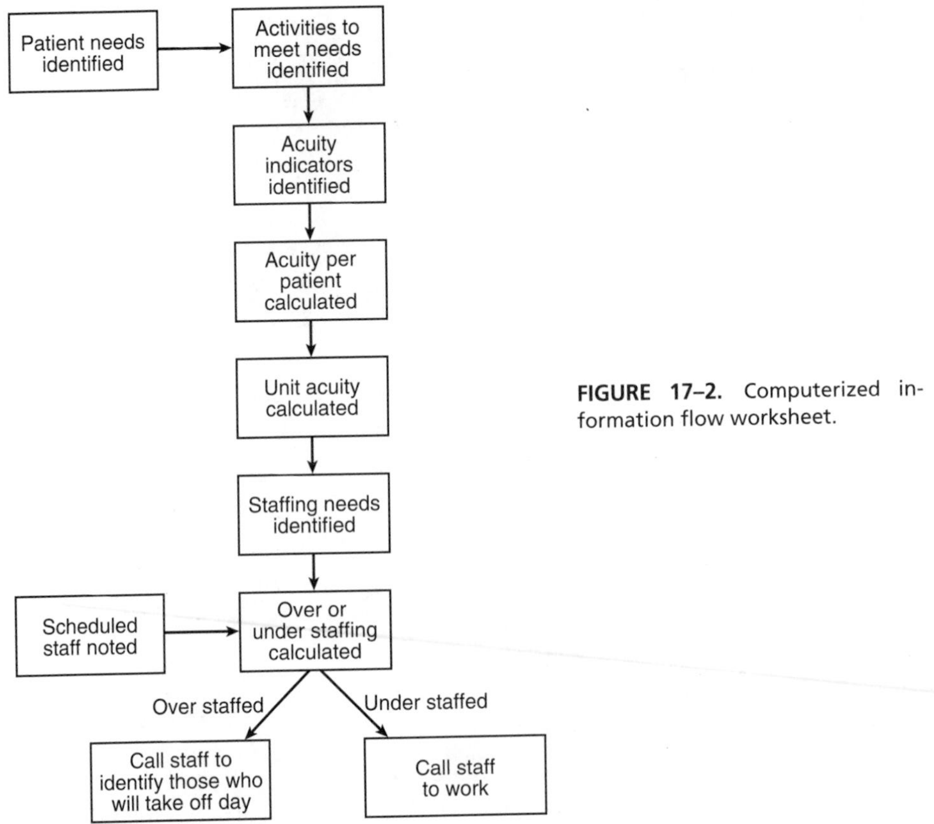

FIGURE 17–2. Computerized information flow worksheet.

can be set up to perform routine calculations. Data on the acuity status of each patient are entered manually, and the calculations of weighing and summing are performed by the computer.

⁜ THE FUTURE

The section on clinical information systems discusses the fully integrated system. In an ideal future vision, financial, personnel, and clinical systems are fully integrated. In the health care world of the future, as the nurse, physician, and other health care providers plan care for a patient, the providers required to provide care will be alerted. As the care is ordered and provided, data will be electronically stored and appropriate bills generated. Reports of care provided to patients will be identified, as well as care provided by various categories of workers and even individual workers. These data can then be summarized in a variety of formats so that the nurse manager can analyze the way care is provided for types of patients by type of nursing staff and by individual nurses across all settings.

Decision-support systems are available that can analyze or recommend solutions. Programs are available to simulate a health organization. The programs can be developed for a specific hospital, nursing home, or home health agency. The programs are similar to sophisticated spreadsheets in that they allow the user to present "what if" scenarios. After the work flow in the organization is analyzed a complex computer model is developed. Using this model the nurse manager can test on the computer a variety of organizational models and estimate the impact that changes will have on the other parts of the organization.

For example, what if the admitting department assumed the responsibility for orienting the patient to the hospital? What would the implications be in terms of paper flow, personnel, and costs? Obviously, the work level for admitting would increase. However, with the computer simulation this could be more exactly anticipated. The modeling approach can handle the impact of many concurrent changes simultaneously. What if admitting handled orientation, sent an admitting staff person with the patient to the unit, and each unit had its own food preparation area and small lab for routine tests, and transport workers used beepers and guaranteed less than a ten-minute response time?

When organizations explore changing the way care is provided, implications for the various departments are almost always considered. However, the implications of multiple simultaneous changes are more difficult to analyze. A computerized model can assist with the assessment of multiple simultaneous changes. The options are simulated on the computer without disrupting even one pilot unit prior to implementation.

⁜ IMPLICATIONS FOR NURSE MANAGERS

One of the most difficult decisions about using computers is determination of the set of activities that should be done by the manager and those activities that others (e.g., secretaries, clerks, nursing staff, finance) should do. We believe that all nurse managers should use computers. The skill level required can be reached by taking a one-semester college course in information systems or some combination of one-day workshops. Some managers have the capacity to be self-taught using the computer and a few books.

We also think the nurse manager should take a seminar in use of spreadsheets and data bases. These are essential management tools. We think that using computers and related software will greatly increase the nurse manager's ability in the area of financial management. That does not mean that the manager must learn or become proficient in all (or any) of the software used. Realizing the benefits of the software is the key; implementing the use of the software for many applications can be left to nonclinical personnel if the nurse manager prefers.

The level of skill required can be compared to the level of clinical knowledge required by a nurse manager. Managers must understand the concept of parenteral fluid administration. They must know what can be done to provide fluids and what can go wrong. Does that mean they must be proficient at working every new pump the organization uses? Probably not. Might there be times when the manager needs to set the dials? Maybe. The manager should know enough about the principles to be able to read and understand the manual or know where to get the help needed. Other managers want to know how to work every piece of equipment. They want to be able to "do the work themselves" that they expect their subordinates to do.

Computers are like that. The nursing office may provide staff to develop computer spreadsheet programs for unit budgets. Nurse managers may be expected to hand in changes and then wait for results. Sometimes the wait may be too long. The organization may have central staff to set up the spreadsheet shell (tailored model for the application, often referred to as a template) and even enter the numbers. Perhaps you don't need to do that. With enough knowledge of the program you can change the numbers and try different options. Finally you may want to do it all yourself.

Our experience is that it is useful to know the basics of how to use a few software programs. Although we have staff to assist us, our experience is that the day before a research grant budget is due, our colleagues want to use that same staff. We'd rather do it ourselves. However, neither of us is a software expert, and we rely on organizational experts to help us. We believe there should be a computer on every nurse manager's desk and that it should be used.

The nurse manager can use computers to assist in financial management. The manager can use the computer for data base management, financial simulations, e-mail, research over the Internet, and report generation. In addition to general programs for these uses, specialized programs are available for staffing and acuity.

KEY CONCEPTS

Hardware Computers and their related pieces of equipment such as printers, monitors, and terminals. The three major types of hardware are mainframes, minis, and microcomputers.

Program Set of instructions for the computer to do a task. Some programs are tailored for specific organizations. Other programs used to perform a specific task can be purchased "off the rack."

Software packages Computer programs. All computers use a type of software called an operating system, which is the basic language used to give the computer instructions. In addition, software is available to perform a variety of functions, such as word processing, budgeting, and statistical analyses.

Electronic data Computerized information.

Fully integrated Information system in which all the components are able to communicate with each other. In health care organizations these systems integrate clinical and financial information from a variety of sources, such as dietary, nursing, and radiology. The data are usually entered only once and are available all over the organization (with the appropriate confidentiality precautions).

Word processing Electronic production and storage of documents. Word processing software is used to prepare correspondence and reports. The presentation of budget justifications, business plans, and other proposals can be improved using word processing software.

Data base Compilation of related information systematically organized. Electronic or computerized data bases are used to organize information in the nursing department. Examples of data bases are an equipment inventory or personnel directory.

Spreadsheet Large ledger sheets often used by accountants for financial calculations. Spreadsheets have columns and rows of cells. The cells contain text or numbers that can be manipulated. Electronic spreadsheets contain formulas in some of the cells. When a number is changed in one cell, other cells are automatically recalculated according to the formulas.

Special purpose software Software used for a specific purpose, such as budgeting, statistics, or assessing acuity.

Statistical software Computer software used to perform statistical calculations.

Acuity systems Systems to assess how much care is required by patients. These systems are developed for a particular hospital or can be purchased. Special purpose software is available to determine acuity.

Scansheet Form with preprinted markings and markings added, usually with a number 2 pencil, which can be read by an optical scanner.

SUGGESTED READINGS

Acker, Francoise, "Computerization of Nursing Units and Formalization of Nurses' Work," *Sciences Sociales et Sante,* Vol. 13, No. 3, September 1995, pp. 69–92.

American Nurses Association, *Nursing Data Systems: The Emerging Framework,* American Nurses Publishing, Washington, D.C., 1996.

Ball, M., K. Hannah, S. Newbold, and J. Douglas, *Nursing Informatics: Where Caring and Technology Meet,* Springer-Verlag, New York, N.Y., 1995.

Benson, J.A., J.E. Michelman, and D. Radjenovic, "Using Information Technology Strategically in Home Care," *Home Healthcare Nursing,* Vol. 14, No. 12, December 1996, pp. 977–983.

Cavouras, C., and J. McKinley, "Variable Budgeting for Staffing: Analysis and Evaluation," *Nursing Management,* Vol. 28, No. 5, 1997, pp. 34–39.

Cleland, V.S., H.A. DeGroot, and L. Forsey, "Computer Simulations of the Differentiated Pay Structure Model," *Journal of Nursing Administration,* Vol. 23, No. 3, March 1993, pp. 53–59.

Dick, Richard S., and Elaine B. Steen, eds., *The Computer-Based Patient Record,* National Academy Press, Washington, D.C., 1991.

Dillon, Thomas W., Dorothea McDowell, Fatalloah Samilimian, and Denise Conkin, "Perceived Ease of Use and Usefulness of Bedside-Computer Systems," *Computers in Nursing,* May/June 1998, Vol. 16, No. 3, pp. 151–156.

Edwardson, S.R., and J. Pejsa, "A Computer Assisted Tutorial for Applications of Computer Spreadsheets in Nursing Financial Management," *Computers in Nursing,* Vol. 11, No. 4, July-August, 1993, pp. 169–175.

Hendrickson, G., C.T. Kovner, J.R. Knickman, and S.A. Finkler, "Implementation of a Variety of Computerized Nursing Information Systems in Seventeen New Jersey Hospitals, *Computers in Nursing,* Vol. 13, No. 3, pp. 96–102.

Jacobs, S.M., and S. Pelfrey, "Decision Support Systems: Using Computers to Help Manage," *Journal of Nursing Administration,* Vol. 25, No. 2, 1995, pp. 46–54.

Kahn, M.G., "Three Perspectives on Integrated Clinical Databases," *Academy of Medicine,* Vol. 72, No. 4, April 1997, pp. 281–286.

Karr, J., and R. Fisher, "A Patient Classification System for Ambulatory Care," *Nursing Management,* Vol. 28, No. 9, 1997, pp. 27–29.

Marr, P., E. Duthie, K. Glassman, et al., "Bedside Terminals and Quality of Nursing Documentation," *Computers in Nursing* Vol. 11, No. 4, July-August 1993, pp. 176–182.

McCormick, K.A., "Including Oncology Outcomes of Care in the Computer-Based Patient Record," *Oncology,* Vol. 9, No. 11, November 1995, pp. 161–167.

McCormick, K., "Nursing on the Electronic Highway," *Collegian,* Vol. 3, No. 4, October 1996, pp. 21–24.

Mills, M., C. Roman, and B. Heller, *Information Management in Nursing and Health Care,* Springhouse, New York, N.Y., 1995.

Moynihan, James J., and Marcia L. McLure, *EdI: A Guide to Electronic Data Interchange and Electronic Commerce Applications in the Healthcare Industry,* Irwin Professional Publishers, Burr Ridge, IL, October 1996.

Nicoll, L.H., and T. Oullette, *The Nurses' Guide to the Internet,* Lippincott-Raven, Philadelphia, Penn., 1996.

Redes, Sharon, and Margaret Lunney, "Validation by School Nurses of the Nursing Intervention Classification for Computer Software," *Computers in Nursing,* Vol. 15, No. 6, November-December 1997, pp. 333–338.

Richards, Julie, "Implementing a Computer System: Issues for Nurse Administrators," *Computers in Nursing,* Vol. 10, No. 1, January-February 1992, pp. 9–13.

Saba V., and K. McCormick, *Essentials for Computers for Nurses,* 2nd edition, McGraw-Hill, New York, N.Y., 1995.

Simpson, R.L., "CIOs and Trends in Health Care Computing," *Nurse Management,* Vol. 28, No. 9, September 1997, pp. 20–21.

Staggers, N., "Electronic Mail Tips and Tricks," *Computers in Nursing,* Vol. 14, No. 5, 1996, pp. 264–266.

Stoughton, L.L., "Electronic Communications: Email in the Emergency Department," *Journal of Emergency Nursing,* Vol. 22, No. 4, 1996, pp. 336–338.

Turley, J., "Toward a Model of Nursing Informatics," *Image: Journal of Nursing Scholarship,* Vol. 28, No. 4, 1996, pp. 309–313.

Waterworth L., and S. Abbatt, "Benefits of An Electronic Clinical Information System: An Intensive Care Nursing Perspective," *Intensive Critical Care Nursing,* Vol. 13, No. 5, October 1997, pp. 289–292.

Werley, Harriet H., Elizabeth C. Devine, Celia R. Zorn, et al., "The Nursing Minimum Data Set: Abstraction Tool for Standardized, Comparable, Essential Data," *American Journal of Public Health,* Vol. 81, No. 4, April 1991, pp. 421–426.

Wilson, D., and M. Neiswanger, "Information System Support of Changes in Health Care and Nursing Practice," *Holism Nursing and Informatics: Holistic Nursing Practice,* Vol. 11, No. 1, 1996, pp. 84–96.

Zielstorff, R., "Capturing and Using Clinical Outcome Data: Implications for Information Systems Design," *Journal of the Medical Informatics Association,* Vol. 2, No. 3, 1995, pp. 191–196.

Variance Analysis

Part II, The Use of Computers

Steven A. Finkler, PhD, CPA

This is the second in a two-part series on variance analysis. In the first article (*JONA*, July/August 1991), the author discussed flexible budgeting, including the calculation of price, quantity, volume, and acuity variances. In this second article, the author focuses on the use of computers by nurse managers to aid in the process of calculating, understanding, and justifying variances.

In recent years, there have been great strides in the degree of sophistication of variance analysis in healthcare organizations. This is the second in a two-part series on variance analysis. In the first article, flexible budgeting was discussed, including the calculation of price, quantity, volume, and acuity variances. Many healthcare organizations use some form of flexible budget variance analysis, but many do not. The focus of this second article is on the use of computers by nurse managers to aid in the process of calculating, understanding, and justifying variances.

Part I concluded that, at a minimum, nurse managers should be receiving variance reports that in some way allow for the impact of changes in the workload volume. As the number of patients increases, nurses should not have to waste their time explaining that more patients consume more resources. Therefore, some type of volume variance measure is a necessity. The calculation of price, quantity, and acuity variances can also be a great aid. Such variances can help nurse managers focus their variance investigation attention on the specific areas in which the variances arose.

The calculation of flexible budget variances is a straightforward matter with a personal computer (PC). Even if variance reports provided to nursing departments do not provide such information, nurses can readily calculate the variances on a PC. This article describes what is involved in computerizing flexible budget variance analysis. Furthermore, even in departments that receive flexible budget variance information from the finance or information systems departments, the *form* of the information is not always conducive to understanding the variances. This article also focuses on the development of graphs to aid nurses in understanding, investigating, explaining, and justifying variances.

Steven A. Finkler, PhD, CPA, Professor of Health Administration, Accounting, and Financial Management, Robert F. Wagner Graduate School of Public Service, New York University, New York City.

Use of an Electronic Spreadsheet

Basics

The basic role of an electronic spreadsheet is to make repetitive, quantitative calculations less laborious. The key to the value of electronic spreadsheets is that a model is developed that uses formulas based on relationships rather than specific numbers. For example, if employee benefits are calculated in an institution as 20% of salaries, and a department's salaries are expected to be $100,000, we could expect benefits to be $20,000.

In a spreadsheet model, however, we would simply indicate that benefits are 20% of salaries. If subsequent changes in forecasts lead us to believe that salaries are going to be only $90,000, the computer can automatically update the amount of benefits because it has been programmed with the 20% relationship between salaries and benefits. A long sequence of calculations, with each calculation being affected by the result of some earlier calculation, can be linked in the spreadsheet model. One change in a beginning assumption will set off a series of recalculations by the spreadsheet program, and hours or days of manual arithmetic can take place in seconds on the computer.

To make a spreadsheet a useful tool for any specific application, it cannot be used directly from the manufacturer. Someone must program

Reprinted from *Journal of Nursing Administration*, Vol. 21, No. 7/8, July/August 1991, pp. 19–25.

the specific relevant relationships. There is no need for nurse managers to perform the actual programming. It is quite feasible, as well as reasonable in cost, to employ a programmer to generate a specific model (or template). Once the template has been developed, the use of a spreadsheet is quite simple.

There are a large number of electronic spreadsheets for use on microcomputers. The examples used in this article are based on LOTUS 1-2-3 (Lotus Development Corp., Cambridge, Massachusetts), the most widely used spreadsheet program.

Spreadsheets and the Calculation of Variances

In Part I, flexible budget variances were calculated manually. The mathematics involved are not advanced. A series of multiplications are required to determine the actual cost, the budgeted cost of actual resources used, the acuity category, the flexible budget, and the original budget. Several subtractions are then required to determine the price, quantity, acuity, and volume variances.

For one unit, for one time, for one line item, the calculation of the variances is not unduly time-consuming or difficult. If we were to suppose, however, that a hospital had 30 different nursing units, each with a separate unit budget, it would be necessary to perform those calculations 30 times for each variable cost line item. Furthermore, we would have to perform the calculations every month in order to have the information we need to investigate variances on a timely basis. Devoting the time of 30 nurse managers on a regular basis to perform a series of repetitive mathematical tasks is not a good use of their time.

In some cases, finance or information systems will provide the variance information. If they do not, then the nursing department can have a simple spreadsheet template created, specifying the mathematical relationships in the variance calculations. The template can be used on a monthly basis by secretarial staff to generate a wealth of information promptly and efficiently for the nurse managers to use. Nursing departments can have the benefit of sophisticated variance information, relieve unit managers of numerous repetitive calculations, and in all likelihood increase accuracy as well by reducing arithmetic errors.

There are many different ways that the variance information can be reported once it has been calculated. For example, our printed report could appear as the one shown in Table 1. In this example, only one line item is shown. Typically, each unit would have a number of line items for their flexible budget variance report. Additionally, the report would include columns for an acuity variance if the institution has a patient classification system that collects the necessary data, as discussed in Part I. The report could also show more detailed information, month by month for each specific line item, if desired.

The exact form of the report is quite flexible once the variance information has been calculated. Each manager can design a reporting form to suit their needs. Therefore, the remainder of this article will not focus on the form and content of the report. Instead, it will consider some of the tasks that are required, who is capable of performing them, some of the types of graphs that can be generated for the purposes of analysis, and the types of analysis that can be done.

Table 1 represents the portion of a spreadsheet model that would be printed out each month. The remainder of the spreadsheet appears in Table 2. This section of the spreadsheet would be updated each month, but would not necessarily be printed unless specific detailed information were desired.*

Note that there are a number of cells in Table 2 with either a dash or the letters ERR. The dashes represent data that are not yet available. The ERRs indicate areas where the program has been unable to carry out a calculation because needed data have not been made available. As each month's information is entered into the computer, those error messages automatically are replaced with variance information. Once a template is designed, it is used to calculate all flexible budget variances for that unit month after month, year after year.

At the beginning of each year, a secretary could be assigned the task of inserting all budgeted data. This task can be performed by one secretary for all units, or individually unit by unit. In this example, all that is involved is typing in the values for budgeted patient days, budgeted rate, and budgeted RN hours, for each of the 12 months. A total of 36 numbers have to be typed. For each line item, there would be a budgeted rate and budgeted amount of resource. If ABC Hospital, Med/Surg Unit 4B, also wanted variance information for LPN labor and for nurse's aides, it also

* A computer disk with the example template is available from the author at the Robert F. Wagner Graduate School of Public Service, New York University, 738 Tisch Hall, 40 West 4th Street, New York, NY 10003.

※ TABLE 2. *Flexible Budget Variance Report*: June 1991 and Year-to-Date Variances*

This is Month Number_____ 6

	This Month						Year-to-Date					
			Variances						Variances			
	Budget	Actual	Price	Quantity	Volume	Total	Budget	Actual	Price	Quantity	Volume	Total
RN salaries	$90,000	$98,847	$247	$3,600	$5,000	$8,847	$652,000	$684,333	$11,333	$6,000	$15,000	$32,333

* ABC Hospital Med/Surg Unit 4 B Variance Report.

※ TABLE 2. *Remaining Portion of Computer Template*

	Jan	Feb	Mar	Apr	May	Jun	Jul	Aug	Sep	Oct	Nov	Dec
Workload measure												
Budgeted pt. days	1,200	1,230	1,140	1,050	1,000	900	900	850	950	1,000	1,050	1,100
Actual pt. days	1,180	1,200	1,200	1,100	1,040	950	—	—	—	—	—	—
RN salary information												
Budgeted rate	$20.00	$20.00	$20.00	$20.00	$20.00	$20.00	$21.00	$21.00	$21.00	$21.00	$21.00	$21.00
Budgeted RN hours	6,000	6,150	5,700	5,250	5,000	4,500	4,500	4,250	4,750	5,000	5,250	5,500
Actual rate	$20.00	$20.50	$21.00	$20.30	$20.10	$20.05	—	—	—	—	—	—
Actual RN hours	5,930	5,990	5,890	5,550	5,360	4,930	—	—	—	—	—	—
RN salary variances												
This month												
Price	$0	$2,995	$5,890	$1,665	$536	$247	ERR	ERR	ERR	ERR	ERR	ERR
Quantity	$600	($200)	($2,200)	$1,000	$3,200	$3,600	ERR	ERR	ERR	ERR	ERR	ERR
Volume	($2,000)	($3,000)	$6,000	$5,000	$4,000	$5,000	ERR	ERR	ERR	ERR	ERR	ERR
Total	($1,400)	($205)	$9,690	$7,665	$7,736	$8,847	ERR	ERR	ERR	ERR	ERR	ERR
Year-to-date												
Price	$0	$2,995	$8,885	$10,550	$11,086	$11,333	ERR	ERR	ERR	ERR	ERR	ERR
Quantity	$600	$400	($1,800)	($800)	$2,400	$6,000	ERR	ERR	ERR	ERR	ERR	ERR
Volume	($2,000)	($5,000)	$1,000	$6,000	$10,000	$15,000	ERR	ERR	ERR	ERR	ERR	ERR
Total	($1,400)	($1,605)	$8,085	$15,750	$23,486	$32,333	ERR	ERR	ERR	ERR	ERR	ERR
Budget this month	$120,000	$123,000	$114,000	$105,000	$100,000	$90,000	$94,500	$89,250	$99,750	$105,000	$110,250	$115,500
Actual this month	118,600	122,795	123,690	112,665	107,736	98,847	ERR	ERR	ERR	ERR	ERR	ERR
Budget year-to-date	120,000	243,000	357,000	462,000	562,000	652,000	746,500	835,750	935,500	1,040,500	1,150,750	1,266,250
Actual year-to-date	118,600	241,395	365,085	477,750	585,486	684,333	ERR	ERR	ERR	ERR	ERR	ERR

would be necessary to type in the budgeted average hourly rate for each of these types of employees, and the budgeted number of paid hours. It would not be necessary to type in the budgeted patient days, since the workload measure will remain constant for all line items for a given unit. It should not take a secretary much more than several days to enter the initial budget data for all 30 units at ABC hospital, for each line item for which flexible budget variance information is desired, for all 12 months.

Each month, the variances can be calculated by having the secretary enter the actual information for that month. For example, assume that the hospital's fiscal year begins in January. In July, the secretary is asked to prepare a June variance report. The secretary would start by entering 6 as the month number at the top of the template (Table 1). This monthly numerical indication is needed so that the computer program knows which set of data to show as being the variances for the current month and year-to-date. The variance numbers in Table 1 come from the June column in Table 2. However, it is not necessary to type those numbers. They are automatically transferred from the June column in Table 2 to Table 1, once the computer knows that it is Month 6.

The next step for the secretary each month is to enter the actual data for the month into the computer template. In this example, in the June column of Table 2, the secretary would type the actual values for patient days, rate, and hours: 950, $20.05, and 4,930, respectively. Once those three pieces of information are entered, the computer calculates the four variances for the month and the four variances for the year to date and transfers that information to the Table 1 portion of the template automatically. If the table also contained lines for variances for LPNs and nurse's aides, then the secretary also would have to enter actual average rates and hours for those types of employees. The Table 1 portion can then be printed out, providing a monthly flexible budget variance report. (The actual formulas used for the calculations are discussed in Part I.)

This monthly process of data entry and report production should take less than 2 days each month for one secretary for all 30 units. However, it is important to establish a system that generates the raw data (actual number of patients for each unit, etc.) each month for the secretary to input.

Different nursing units will use slightly different templates. Some units may use orderlies, while others may not. Some units may use the number of patient days as a measure of workload, while others may use emergency room treatments or hours of operations. Although the templates may vary somewhat from unit to unit, the process of entering information at the start of the year as well as each month will be basically the same for all units. If desired, a master template can be prepared, which takes the data from each of the unit templates and prepares a summary report for the nursing department as a whole.

Graphics

Once variance information has been generated and is available, it must be analyzed and investigated by nurse managers. The knowledge, judgment, and experience of the nurse manager is critical to understanding what is causing the variances. The use of flexible budget variance analysis is meant to be a time-saving aid to the nurse manager. Rather than just being faced with the total variance for any line item, the manager knows how much of the variance is due to more patients, how much to higher prices paid for a resource such as nursing labor, and how much to the amount of nursing labor per patient. This can simplify the variance investigation process substantially. Using graphics to display the variances is another step in providing the nurse manager with tools to improve variance analysis capability.

The advantage of graphs is that in many cases a visual display of relationships either highlights certain items that would otherwise go unnoted, or else makes it easier to spot certain relationships and key focal points. The discussion that follows highlights only a few of the possibilities. It should be noted that, once the spreadsheet model is constructed, LOTUS 1-2-3 or similar software can generate graphs based on a few additional instructions to the computer, with no additional input of data. All the graphs discussed below were generated from the data in Table 2. A standard set of graphs can be developed and built into the template. The same graphs can then be produced each month with automatically updated information.

One type of graph that is frequently used is a bar graph. Figure 1 is an example of a bar graph showing the price, quantity, volume, and total variances for RN salaries for the month of June 1991. This graph gives a very quick and vivid picture of the extent to which each type of variance is having

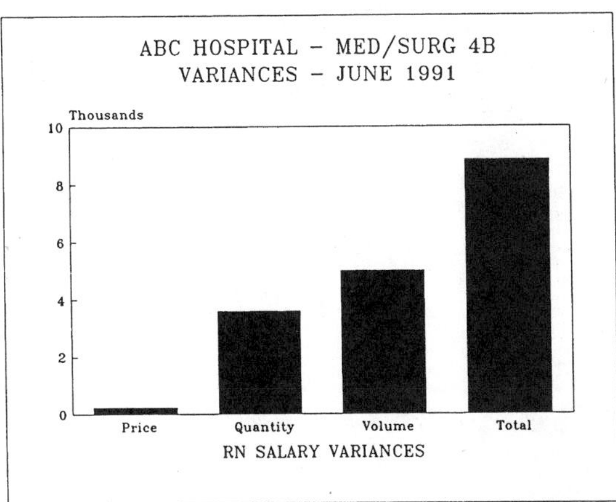

Figure 1. Bar graph of price, quantity, and volume variances for June.

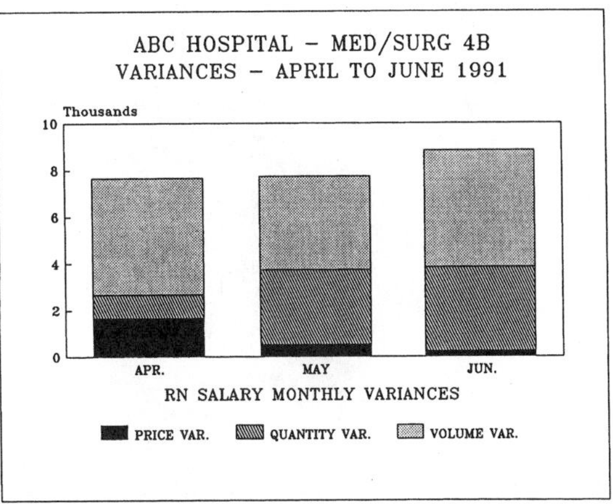

Figure 3. Stacked bar graph for April through June variances.

an impact on the total variance for this line item for this month. For example, Figure 1 emphasizes the importance of investigating the quantity and volume variances. Although the volume variance is not usually under the control of the nurse manager, if it becomes significant in amount she must try to understand it, because if it persists it will have considerable significance for future staffing decisions. Figure 2 provides somewhat more information at a glance by showing not only the price, quantity, volume, and total variance for June, but the variances for the 6-month year-to-date period as well.

An alternative to a simple bar graph is a stacked bar graph. In Figure 3, one can see the price, quantity, and volume variances all in one bar for each month. In this graph, the user quickly notes that the total variance has been rising despite the fall in price variance. The main change took place in the middle segment. The quantity variance increased substantially during the 3 months. Despite some advantages, stacked bar graphs can become quite confusing if any of the variances are negative numbers. The combination of a positive and negative variance in one bar makes interpretation of the graph quite difficult. Since variances can be either favorable or unfavorable, stacked bar graphs should be used for variances only with a great deal of caution.

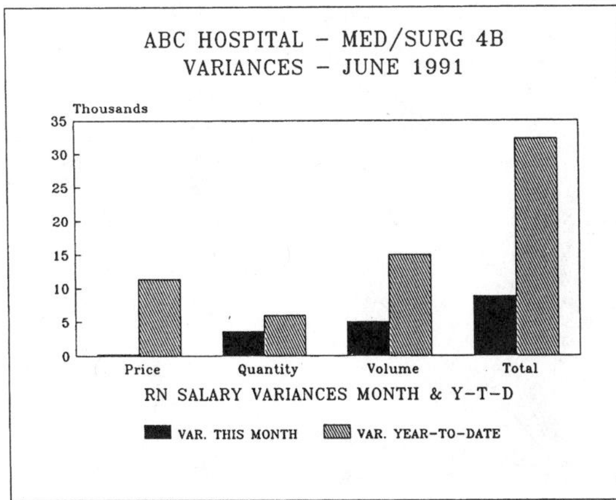

Figure 2. Bar graph with June and year-to-date variances.

Another way to look at information is from the perspective of the relative size of each variance compared with all variances—in proportions rather than specific dollar amounts. A pie graph (Figs. 4–5) provides a very easy and quick assessment of which variances are large in size relative to the other variances. In some instances, displaying this information in the "exploded pie" format of Figure 5 may be preferred, although the information content is the same in both graphs. In Figure 5, the quantity variance is highlighted by the explosion of that section away from the remainder of the pie. This helps to emphasize the size of the quantity variance, which is often viewed as being the one variance most directly under the manager's control. Figures 4 and 5 show the volume and quantity variances in June to be quite significant, and substantially less effort could be spent investigating the price variance. Pie graphs are somewhat limited as the amount of data to be pre-

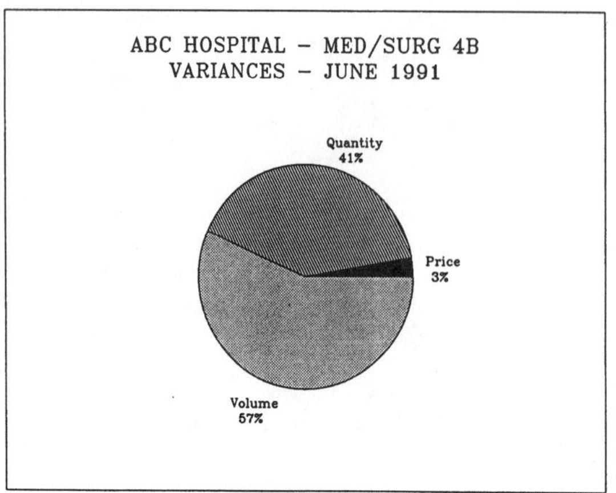

Figure 4. Pie graph of June price, quantity, and volume variances.

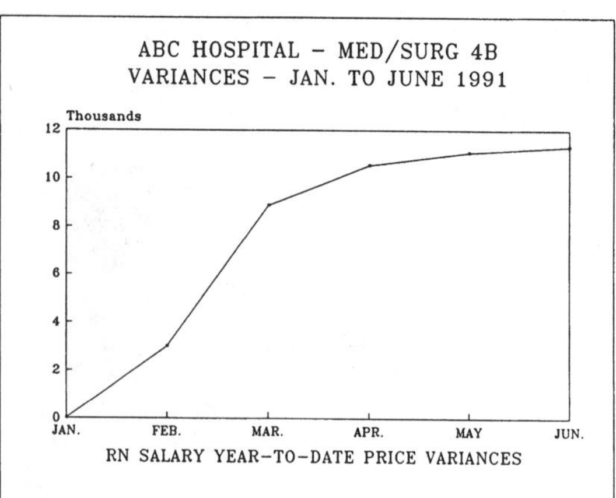

Figure 6. Line graph for year-to-date price variances.

sented increase. It would not be possible to show both the monthly values and the year-to-date values on one pie graph.

For information that reflects what is happening during a period of time, a line graph often is a helpful tool for evaluating possible problematic trends. However, even a potentially good format, such as a line graph, will not make our information useful unless we carefully decide on the appropriate information. For example, Figure 6 presents a line graph for year-to-date information on the price variance through June. Our first reaction to this graph may one of concern over the large and apparently growing variance. The year-to-date variance is substantial by the end of June. The monthly price variance information of Figure 7, however, should produce a different reaction. Although the price variance was a problem in the early months of the year, it does seem to have been brought substantially under control. The graph quickly informs the user that the price variance has been decreasing for a number of months and has now reached a quite modest level. Although this data could be obtained from the numbers in Table 2, in many cases it is hard to ferret information out of a table full of numbers; a selected graph (Fig. 7) quickly conveys what has been happening. Figure 8 shows monthly quantity variances. In contrast to the price variance, we quickly observe a problem. The quantity variance is modestly unfavorable in the first month (January) and then favorable for two months (February and March). In the last several months, however, there appears to be a serious unfavorable trend. This would warrant immediate attention.

When desired, more than one set of informa-

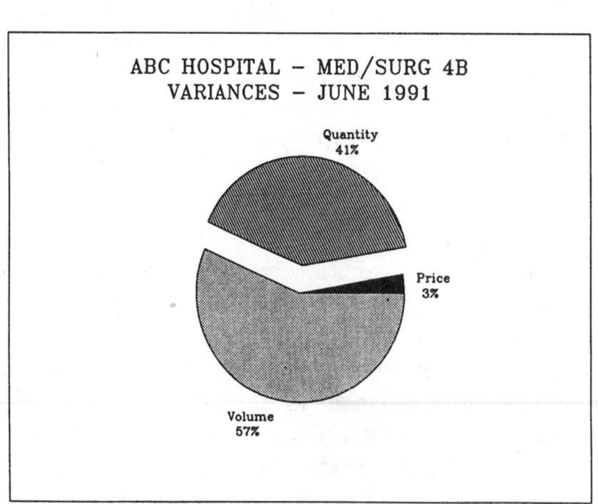

Figure 5. Pie graph with exploded section.

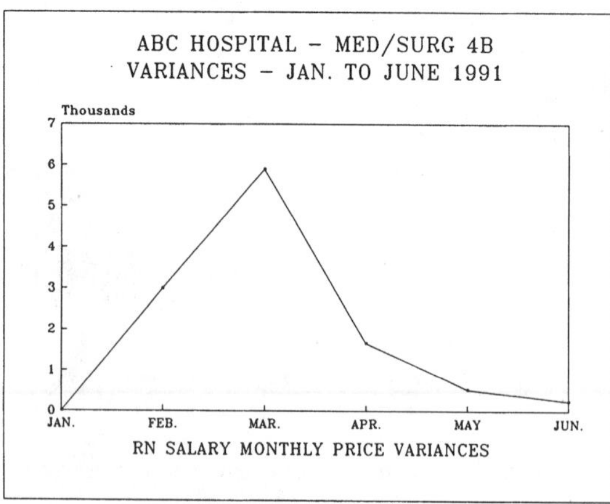

Figure 7. Line graph for monthly price variances.

tion can be shown on a time graph simultaneously. For example, Figure 9 shows monthly price, quantity, and volume variances. However, adding more items to a line graph may not always be desirable. In Figure 9, the price and volume lines intersect in March. Look at those two lines carefully. It is quite easy for the viewer's eye mistakenly to switch from one line to another at the intersection point. If that occurs, the use of the graph will be damaging because it will be conveying misinformation. In a case such as this, presenting the same information in three separate line graphs, or in a bar graph format, may be more informative.

Essentially, graphs do not present information that we don't already have in the form of numbers. After all, these graphs were derived directly from the information in Table 2. They can be very helpful, however, in spotting areas that need prompt attention and trends that may be early warning signals of oncoming problems.

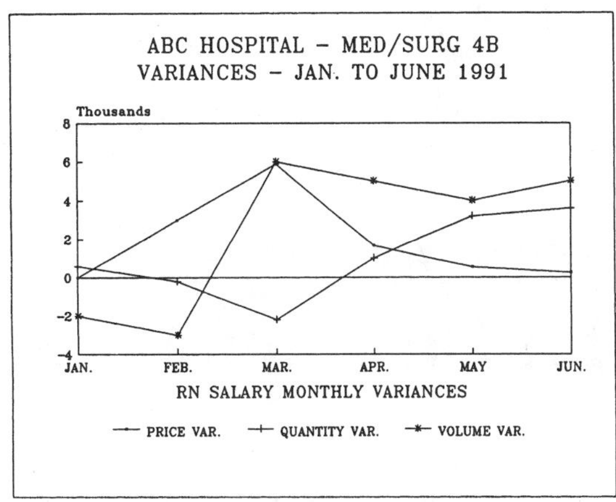

Figure 9. Line graph for monthly price, quantity, and volume variances.

Conclusion

Variance analysis is an area of growing attention as control of costs becomes more and more vital to the financial well-being of healthcare organizations. Adequate data for variance analysis often are not being generated by the organization's financial and information systems departments. Recent advances in terms of availability of reasonably priced PCs, however, has placed the ability to generate useful variance information within the reach of most nurse managers.

Calculations that would be an imposing task, if performed manually each month for each line item for each unit or department, can be processed by a spreadsheet program in rapid fashion. Some data will still have to be collected, but once the system is in place, the monthly effort involved in collecting actual information should be quite small for each unit. The data entry, computation, and generation of reports can be done by secretarial or other support staff and should not take an unreasonable amount of time.

In addition to yielding information on price, quantity, volume, and possibly acuity variances, as opposed to simply a total for each line item, it is also possible to use the computer to make the information much more usable through the generation of graphs. A variety of types of graphs, if thoughtfully considered, can generate supplements to variance reports, which should reduce the time needed to grasp the impact of the information and be an aid in both variance investigation and interpretation.

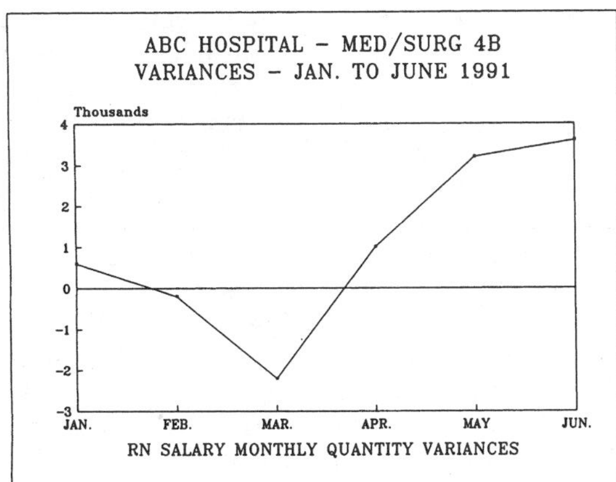

Figure 8. Line graph for monthly quantity variances.

Suggested Readings

Austin C. Information systems for health services administration. Ann Arbor, MI: Health Administration Press, 1988.

Finkler SA. Microcomputers in nursing administration: a software introduction and overview. J Nurs Adm 1985;15(4):18–23.

Hannah KJ, Ball MJ. Nursing and computers: past, present, and future. J Clin Comput 1984;12(6):179–84.

Spitzer R, Poate W. Effective budgeting variance reporting. In: Spitzer R, ed. Nursing productivity: the hospital's key to survival and profit. Chicago: 5-N Publications, 1986:21–25.

Tortora ML. Integrating computers into the nursing environment. Nurs Forum 1989;24(2):8–12.

CHAPTER

18

Forecasting and Other Methods for Decision Making

CHAPTER GOALS

The goals of this chapter are to:

- Describe quantitative methods useful for nurse managers in decision making
- Discuss probability theory
- Explain forecasting techniques used to predict resource use, patient volume, and income
- Discuss the reasons for forecasting
- Discuss the use of microcomputers for forecasting
- Explain the use of qualitative approaches to forecasting
- Explain the use of other quantitative methods such as linear programming and expected value for decision making
- Discuss quantitative methods of inventory control
- Describe the use of techniques for tracking projects

⁜ INTRODUCTION

Uncertainty exists when there is doubt about future events. The delivery of health care is uncertain. We do not know for certain who will need nursing care tomorrow. Yet the nurse manager must make decisions each day about the allocation of resources. Many of the resource allocation decisions are about what to do today. Others are decisions about expending resources in the near or distant future.

An example of a decision that must be made today occurs when two RNs call in sick. Should the manager replace one or both of them? Should the manager use agency nurses or try to find in-house overtime staff? The manager makes these decisions based on organizational policies, experience, and knowledge about what is currently happening on the unit. Decision making requires the exercise of managerial judgment. Many decisions must be made with less information than the nurse manager would like. Everything seems under control on the unit. There are four empty beds and no one waiting in the emergency room (ER) for admission. However, what if the unit gets three new admissions? Is that likely?

Nurse managers must also make decisions about resource allocations for the next year. What should the staffing pattern be? What will occupancy be? Which units will need new infusion pumps? These long-range decisions are often made with even less information than is available for daily decisions. Some information is available, however. Other chapters in this book suggest what information is needed to make financial decisions.

It should be remembered that the nurse manager, along with other key managers, decides organizational and program goals. These goals then form the basis for the decision-making process. The methods outlined in this chapter assume that the manager has decided what key decisions need to be made. For example, many of the methods described can be used to determine whether a decision will likely lead to increased profits. If the manager does not have increased profits as a goal, knowing how to maximize profits will not be very useful. As in many managerial issues, the first question is, "What is the question?" It is up to the manager to decide what question to ask. The focus of this chapter is the use of forecasting and other techniques to assist nurse managers in making judgments about the questions they have posed.

PROBABILITY THEORY: FOUNDATION FOR FORECASTING AND DECISION MAKING

Probability is the likelihood that an event will occur. Managers of health organizations depend on knowing the probability of events' occurring to plan for care. We know with complete certainty where the hospital ER is today. We are very certain it will still be there tomorrow. We know with less certainty that it will be there three years from now. We know with a great deal of certainty that at least one patient will come to the ER for care in the next twenty-four hours, but what is the likelihood that someone will come to the ER in the next hour? What is the likelihood that 100 people will come to the emergency room in the next hour? The answer to these questions is unknown, yet the probability of each possible answer to these questions can be based on information that is known.

Suppose we expect to have 100 maternity patients who will deliver babies. We know from our past records that it is highly likely that thirty patients will have cesarean sections and seventy patients will have normal vaginal deliveries. The type of delivery affects the unit's staffing needs. If a patient arrives at the unit, before we have any other information we know that the chance of a C-section is 30 out of 100. We could also say that if 1,000 patients arrive this year, the percentage of C-sections would be about 30 and the percentage of vaginal deliveries would be about 70.

Mathematically, if an event can happen in X ways and not happen in Y ways, the probability of its happening is $X/(X+Y)$. The possibility of its not happening is $Y/(X+Y)$. To determine probabilities it is necessary to specify events. Each patient either has a C-section or does not. These events are mutually exclusive and are the two possible events upon the arrival of a patient who will deliver a baby. If events are mutually exclusive, the sum of the probability of each event's occurring must equal 100%.

Two general rules apply to probability. One relates to the likely occurrence of one or another mutually exclusive event. The second is the likelihood that each of two mutually exclusive events will occur simultaneously or in succession. For example, what is the likelihood of rolling a 1 on a die on the first try or a 2 on the die on the second try? We know that the likelihood of rolling a 1 is $\frac{1}{6}$. We also know that the likelihood of rolling a 2 is also $\frac{1}{6}$. The likelihood that either of these events will occur is $\frac{1}{6} + \frac{1}{6}$, or $\frac{1}{3}$.

The likelihood of rolling a 1 is $\frac{1}{6}$, of rolling a 2 is $\frac{1}{6}$, of rolling a 3 is $\frac{1}{6}$, of rolling a 4 is $\frac{1}{6}$, of rolling a 5 is $\frac{1}{6}$, and of rolling a 6 is $\frac{1}{6}$. The sum of $\frac{1}{6} + \frac{1}{6} + \frac{1}{6} + \frac{1}{6} + \frac{1}{6} + \frac{1}{6}$ is 1. We know that if we roll a die, a 1, 2, 3, 4, 5, or 6 will result. Therefore the likelihood of one of these numbers' being rolled is the sum of each probability, or 1. The *additive probability rule* states that the likelihood of either one event or another event's occurring is the sum of the likelihood of each event's occurring.

The likelihood of two specific events' *both* occurring is much less. The likelihood of rolling a 1 on the first try and a 2 on the second try is $\frac{1}{6} \times \frac{1}{6}$, or $\frac{1}{36}$. The second rule of probability is the *multiplication rule;* the likelihood of two or more events is the product of each event.

Nurse managers implicitly use probability theory on a frequent basis. The nurse manager in the ER knows that there is a 90% probability that two people are in the ER waiting to be admitted. The nurse manager knows there is 100% probability that it will take the lab more than ten minutes to send someone up to draw blood. The nurse manager knows that one in four, or 25%, of the nurses who are asked to work an extra shift will say yes. These probability estimates, sometimes called "guesstimates," are based on previous experience of the nurse manager and the manager's colleagues.

The probability that events will occur in the future can be based on historical data. The following example shows how to estimate the probability of staff's calling in sick on a weekend day shift based on historical data. The nurse manager knows that for a three-month period there were thirteen weekends, each with two days, or a total of twenty-six day shifts ($13 \times 2 = 26$). There were five nurses scheduled for each of these shifts. Therefore a possible 130 nurse shifts were scheduled ($26 \times 5 = 130$). During this time ten nurses called in sick. There were sick calls for ten of the possible 130 shifts, or 8% of the time. Therefore the likelihood of a sick call on this unit on a weekend is about 8%, calculated as follows:

Day shifts scheduled = 13 weeks × 2 days = 26
Nurses scheduled per shift = 5
Total nurse shifts possible = 26 × 5 = 130
Actual number of sick calls for day shift = 10

Probability = Actual number of sick calls ÷ Total nurse shifts
P = 10 ÷ 130 = 8%

In future planning for staff the manager can assume that about 8% of weekend day shifts will require coverage for sick leave. This may not turn out to be exactly correct, but it provides the manager with a reasonable estimate.

In some cases the nurse manager does not have historical data on which to base probabilities and must estimate. For example, suppose the hospital now has twelve-hour shifts. Historical data for sick time are based on eight-hour shifts. The nurse manager believes that some nurses take a sick day because they are really tired and just need a day off. The manager thinks that nurses who have four days off per week will take fewer sick days than those who have two days off and therefore estimates the sick-time probability at less than 8%—perhaps 5% or 6%. Such an estimate is referred to as *subjective probability*. It relies not only on the scientific application of the laws of chance but also on the judgment of the manager. The need for nursing units to be managed by experienced and skilled nurses exists partly because of the frequency and importance of decisions based on the manager's subjective probability estimates.

The concepts of probability are used in the following sections that describe forecasting and other quantitative approaches to decision making.

⁜ QUANTITATIVE METHODS FOR FORECASTING

The preparation of budgets and other financial decision making requires a number of preliminary steps, including forecasting. A budget cannot be prepared without knowing the types of patients that the organization will likely be treating. A staffing plan to implement a new liver transplant unit cannot be developed without an estimate of the number of patients the unit will serve. And financial decisions cannot be made without knowledge of who the competition is and the actions competitors are likely to take. Similarly, a budget cannot be prepared without knowing information such as *how many* patients are likely to be treated or *how sick* they are likely to be. That is where forecasting comes in.

Forecasting techniques allow for prediction of how many patients or patient days the organization or a particular unit or department will treat. Forecasting allows prediction of how sick the patients will be. If a nurse manager were to attempt to prepare an operating budget without some prediction of these elements, there would be no way of determining how much staff is needed. Forecasting can help to estimate how many chest tubes the intensive care unit will need or how many heparin locks a medical/surgical unit will consume. This will enable the nurse manager to plan the supplies portion of the unit's budget.

Forecasting is a tool that helps in the preparation not only of the operating budget but also of other budgets. If trends in the demographics of the community can be forecast, it is possible to prepare better long-range and program budgets. If it is forecast that a growing portion of the patient population will be Medicare patients, it can be determined what impact that will have on how quickly the organization gets paid. That will help in preparation of the cash budget.

The range of items that can be forecast is unlimited. It is possible to predict patients, patient days, various supply items, the percentage of total operations performed by a specific doctor, and so on. Generally, forecasting focuses on items that the manager must respond to rather than items that can be controlled. For example, a nursing unit may forecast how sick the patients will be. It cannot control severity of illness, but its budget must be a plan that responds to how sick the patient population is expected to be.

Forecasting should be undertaken as an early step in the budget preparation and financial decision-making process. Virtually all managers forecast in some manner. Unsophisticated managers may forecast by simply using their best judgment or by assuming that the previous year's results will occur again the next year. It has been found that more formalized analysis of historical data can yield more accurate predictions than such less sophisticated approaches. These predictions in turn form a basis for many decisions in the planning process.

A formalized forecasting process can be divided into several steps. The first step is collection of historical data. The next step is graphing the data. The third step is analysis of the data to reveal trends or seasonal patterns. The fourth and final step is developing and using formulas to project the item being forecast into the future.

Before these steps are considered, one point must be stressed. When a forecast is made, it is just an estimate of the future based on probabilities. Sophisticated approaches to forecasting allow the projection to be an educated estimate, but it is still an estimate. Your intuitive hunch or gut feeling should not be ignored. The most sophisticated methods lack the feel for the organization that a manager develops over time. Never accept forecasts on the blind faith that if it is mathematical or computerized, it must be superior.

Quantitative forecasts are merely aids or supplements that managers should take into consideration along with a number of other factors, many of which often cannot be quantified and entered into formalized predictive models. The best forecasts result from neither naive guessing nor advanced mathematics, but from an integration of quantitative methods with the experience and judgment of managers.

Data Collection

The first step in formalized forecasting is collection of historical data. Consider several examples. A nurse manager who wishes to make the most basic of projections—workload—will first have to decide upon a workload measure, such as patients or patient days. Then it is necessary to determine what the workload was in the past so that it can be projected into the future. This is referred to as a *time-series* approach to forecasting. Historical changes over time are used to help anticipate the likely result in a coming time period.

The method discussed in this section is broadly applicable. To predict diaper usage in the maternity unit, data on the number of diapers used previously can be used. Once the number of diapers needed is predicted, it will probably be necessary to focus on the expected cost per box of diapers. If the purchasing department has a good degree of certainty about the price of diapers for next year (such as a purchase contract specifying price), this would be a pretty accurate approach. On the other hand, if it was desired to predict the total cost for diapers directly rather than focusing first on the expected number of diapers, it would be possible to gather information on what total amount was spent on diapers in the past and use that for a direct cost estimate.

In other words, it is possible to first forecast diaper usage and then calculate the projected cost or to forecast diaper cost directly. The preferred choice will depend partly on whether information about the number of diapers to be used in the coming period is considered valuable. Similarly, both the number of patient days and the patient severity of illness can be predicted. Then those data can be used to project the number of nursing hours needed, or historical information about the number of nursing hours consumed can be used to directly forecast nursing hours.

Appropriate Data Time Periods

There is often a tendency to try to make do with annual data. In fact, many operating budgets are annual budgets, specifying the total amounts to be spent on each line item for the coming year. However, when a manager is preparing an operating budget, it makes a lot of sense to use monthly rather than annual predictions of costs.

The easiest way to make monthly predictions is to take annual budget information and divide it by twelve. In many industries it would be possible to use such a simple approach; production in one month may be much the same as in any other month. In the health care sector, such an expectation is not reasonable. If for no other reason, the weather alone is likely to cause busy and slow periods. Winters are often busier for health care organizations than summers. Health care organizations must be prepared to have more staff available in busier periods. It is desirable to plan more vacations in slow periods and fewer during peak periods. Thus it is important to be concerned with month-to-month variations within each year as well as with the predictions for the year as a whole.

Furthermore, the number of days in a month will affect monthly costs. Many health care organizations, such as clinics, labs, or radiologists' offices, might only be open weekdays. Some months have as many as twenty-three weekdays, while other months have as few as twenty weekdays. A three-day difference on a twenty-day base represents a 15% difference. Clearly a difference that large would have a significant impact on the resources required for the month. Similarly, for a hospital it is quite likely that the number of weekdays will have an influence, since on certain days of the week admissions and discharges tend to be higher.

Monthly budgets are also important because they can be compared with actual results as they occur. If there is a difference (variance) between the plan and the actual results, the cause can be investigated, and perhaps a problem can be corrected immediately. Such variance analysis is the topic of Chapter 13. Without monthly subdivisions of the budget, it might be necessary to wait until the end of the year to find out if things are going according to plan. By then, of course, it will be too late to do anything about it for this year.

Thus it is important for most health care institutions to have costs broken down on a monthly basis and in a manner that is more sophisticated than dividing the year's expected cost or volume by twelve. Therefore the data collected should generally be historical *monthly* data. For each type of item to be forecast (patients, chest tubes, diapers, costs) twelve individual data points are needed per year, representing values for the item being forecast for each month.

How far back should the data go? One year seems convenient, and it provides twelve data points. However, one year's worth of data provides only one piece of information about January, not twelve. If this January was unusual (either very costly or unusually low in cost), that would not be readily apparent. It is likely that next year would be inaccurately predicted to be like this year. Therefore more than one year's data is needed.

The use of ten years of data is often suggested for forecasting, although that has weaknesses as well. It is possible that so much has changed over ten years that the data are no longer relevant. For that reason, it would seem that five years of data (or a total of sixty months) is a reasonable rule of thumb. If a nurse manager knows that things have not changed much on the unit in a long time, using more years of data will make the estimate a better predictor. If there have been drastic changes recently, five years might be too long. Judgment is needed. One of the most important things a manager does is exercise judgment. Throughout the budgeting process, as in other managerial functions, a manager can never escape from the fact that thoughtful judgment is vital to the process of effective management.

What Data Should Be Collected?

It is necessary to collect historical data on the items to be forecast. Too often managers stop at that point because those data are sufficient to make a forecast. However, those data points are not all the data that are really needed to make a *good* forecast.

Forecasting techniques mindlessly predict the future as an extension of the past, even though many things change over time. Whenever forecasting is done, the manager should question whether factors have changed that will make the future different from the past. Are things changing? For instance, are demographics shifting? When it is predicted that next January will be like the previous five Januarys, is the fact that last July there was a large influx of refugees into the community being ignored? Is a sudden shift in population caused by the closing of the town's auto plant being ignored? The forecasting formulas to be developed will not take these recent factors into consideration. Forecasting formulas are based solely on historical information. The manager should collect additional data to use as a judgmental adjustment to forecast results.

For example, availability of personnel can have a dramatic impact. For years many health care organizations suffered from a shortage of available nurses. The result was high overtime payments to staff nurses and high agency charges for per diem nurses. If there has been a noticeable increase in the number of nurses available, a manager should realize that the average hourly cost for nursing can be brought down by the elimination of much overtime and agency cost. A quantitative model for forecasting will not take that into account. Information about nurse availability must be collected, and the manager should give specific consideration to that information.

Note that a unit manager does not have to be a one-person information service. The personnel department can be asked about the outlook for hiring additional staff nurses. Administrators can be asked whether changes in third-party coverage are likely to have any impact. It is unreasonable to expect a home health agency's director of nursing to budget correctly for the coming year if the number of allowable Medicare-reimbursable visits has changed and he or she does not know about it. Most home health agency financial officers would quickly be aware of such a change. That information should promptly be communicated to the chief nursing officer. It is vital to open communication links with other managers throughout the organization to ensure receipt of necessary information that could help in the budget process.

Some changes will not be easy to get information about. For instance, there may be no central clearing person to provide an update on changing technology that will dramatically shift the demand for nursing personnel. Nevertheless, a unit manager must try to get that information and consider its likely impact on the unit. To some extent, nurse managers may have better information on changing technology than the organization's administrators. First of all, nurse managers have clinical knowledge superior to administration's. Second, nurse managers are likely to know what kinds of changes physicians in their clinical area are planning to implement.

It is also important for nurse managers to be aware of the organization's long-range plan, program budgets, and capital budgets. Many hospitals tend to guard budget data closely, with an "eyes only" attitude. Only people with an immediate need are allowed to see any budget other than their own. It is important that administrators begin to understand that managers do need to see any budget that even indirectly may affect their unit or department. For example, if a new service winds up consuming a significant amount of nursing time that had not been planned on, much of it will likely be at overtime rates or will result in overtime elsewhere in the hospital. Had the service been planned for, overtime premiums might have been avoided. If a manager is to be held responsible for that overtime, then the manager is entitled to have the information needed to anticipate demands on the unit and to plan for adequate staffing.

Graphing Historical Data

Having collected all the relevant data that might help predict the future, the next step is to lay out the historical data on a graph. In the forecasting approach discussed here, time is plotted on the horizontal axis. For instance, suppose that the unit manager wants to predict next year's total nursing hours starting with January 2001. Assume that it is currently October 2000 and that historical data from the past five years are going to be used. Data for October through December 2000 are not yet available. Therefore the horizontal axis begins with October 1995 and goes through September 2000 (Fig. 18–1).

The vertical axis provides information on the item to be forecast. This is nursing hours in Figure 18–1. The forecasting methods discussed later in this chapter allow a manager to predict workload estimates for the future, such as the number of patients and the number of patient days, the actual amounts of resource consumption (e.g., the number of nursing hours or the number of rolls of bandage tape), or to predict costs. Depending on the procedures of your specific institution, some of these forecasts may be made by the accounting department rather than by nurse managers.

If costs or some other financial measure expressed in dollars is being predicted

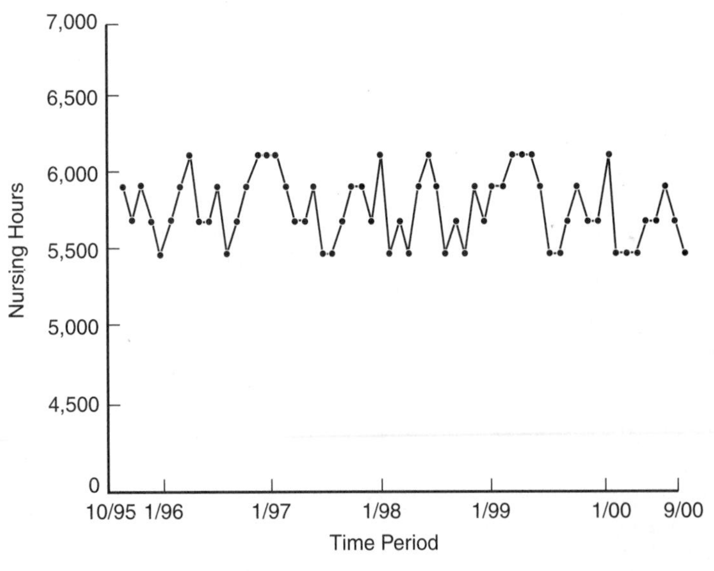

FIGURE 18–1. Basic graph for nursing hours forecast.

directly, the impact of inflation must be considered. If inflation is ignored as forecasting is done, the forecast becomes more complicated because it must predict not only a workload measure, such as the number of diapers for the coming year, but also the rate of inflation for the coming year. The problem of inflation and adjustments that can be made to allow for it are discussed in Chapter 7.

If a prediction is being made for next year's nursing hours (Fig. 18–1), the first point graphed is the number of nursing hours worked in October 1995. The next point is the number of nursing hours in November 1995, and so on. It is important to keep in mind that this forecasting approach is a time-series analysis; that is, the variable on the horizontal axis is always time. In time-series analysis, whether the manager is trying to predict workload, resources, or cost, the basic process is to look at how much of that item was used in the past and project that into the future. To make such predictions, the manager will need to be able to analyze the underlying cause of variations in the data that have been graphed.

Analysis of Graphed Data

Before any predictions can be made, it is necessary to assess the basic characteristics of the data that have been graphed. For instance, do the data exhibit *seasonality?* Is there a particular *trend?* Do variations from month to month and year to year appear to be simply random fluctuations? There may be patterns related to the passage of time that can be uncovered.

A visual inspection can usually give a good picture of the type of pattern that exists. Here it is important to focus on a reasonably long period, at least several years, as opposed to several months. By just looking at the past few months, it is possible to get a distorted impression of what is occurring. For instance, see Figure 18–2. (NOTE: These are not the same data as shown in Fig. 18–1.) It appears that the number of nursing hours has a definite downward trend, but this graph covers a period of only six months.

Figure 18–3 shows the pattern for the full year. Now the graph gives a totally different impression. The number of nursing hours has not been steadily decreasing over time. For the first half of the year it was decreasing, and for the second half it was increasing. The pattern observed is not likely to be indicative of a long-term decline. It is still not possible to tell, however, if some basic change has occurred that caused a downward trend to reverse or if the pattern is seasonal behavior. Next year will the number of nursing hours continue to rise, as it appears to be doing near the end of the year, or will it turn downward, as it did at the beginning of the graphed year? To answer that question it is vital that data for at least several years be graphed.

Now look at Figure 18–4, which covers a period of five years. A pattern of falling and then rising hours occurs each year. This is clearly a seasonal pattern rather than a trend. Each year the same pattern repeats itself.

When data for a sufficient number of years are graphed, the pattern that becomes apparent will generally fall into one of four categories: random fluctuations, trend, seasonality, and seasonality and trend together. Each of these patterns will be discussed.

Random Fluctuations

It would be quite surprising if a unit or department consumed exactly the same amount of any resource two months or two years in a row. One year the winter will be a little colder than another, and more people will get pneumonia. Another year prices will rise a little faster. One year some staff members will take more sick days than another. Yet these events are not likely to be trends—it does not get colder and colder year after year. Nor are they seasonal. They are just random, unpredictable events.

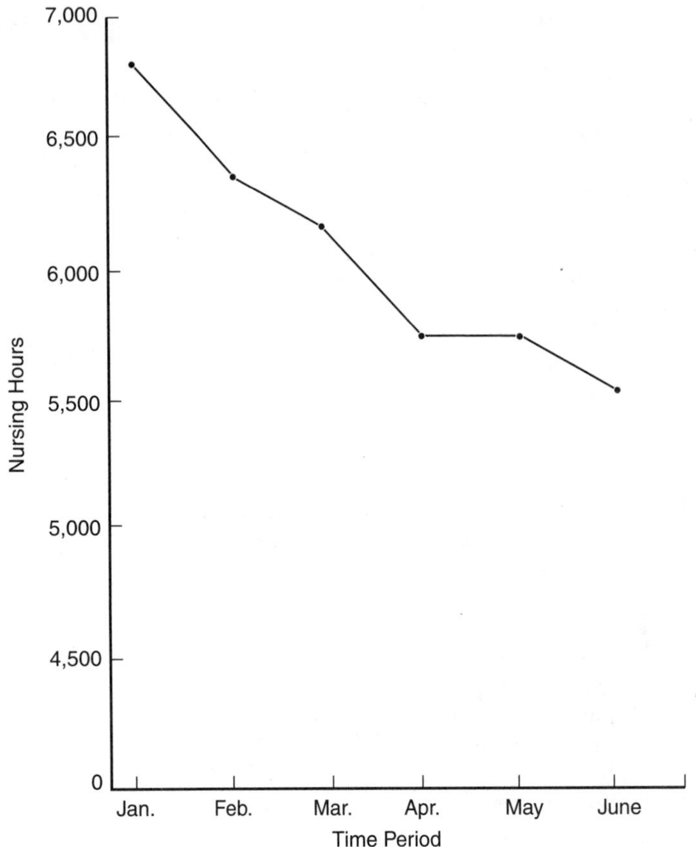

FIGURE 18–2. Six months' data for nursing hours.

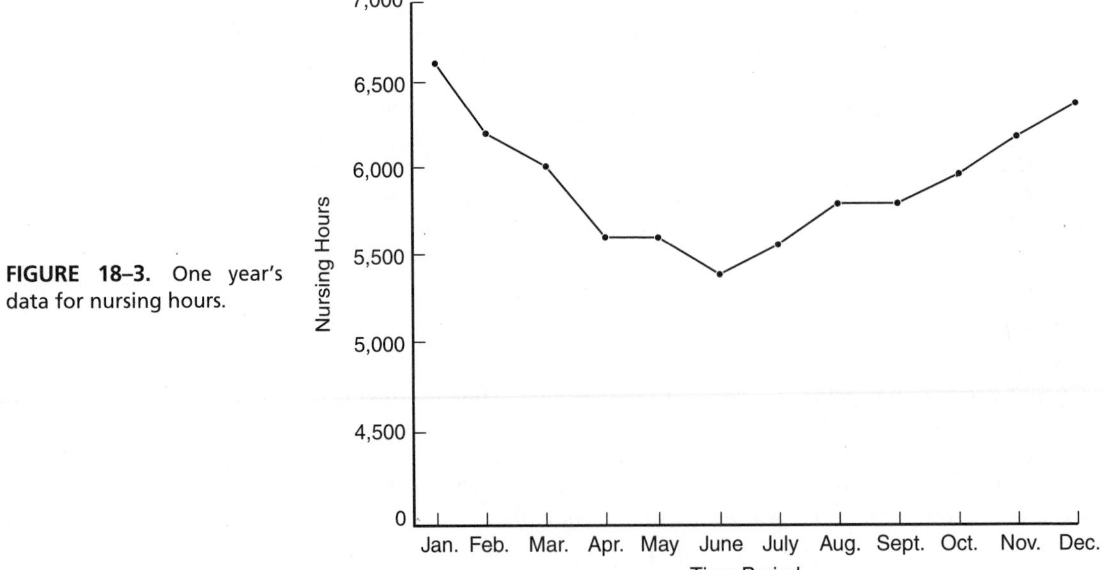

FIGURE 18–3. One year's data for nursing hours.

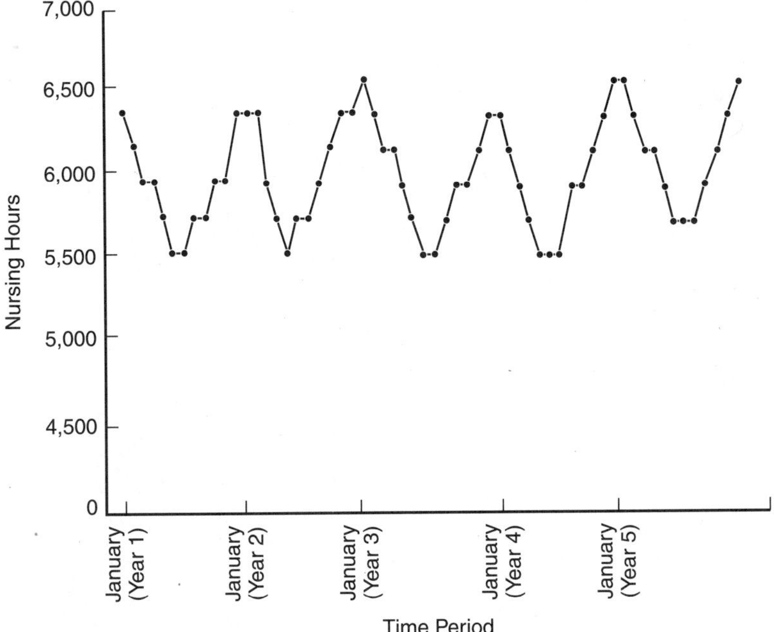

FIGURE 18–4. Five years' data for nursing hours forecast: seasonality.

A graph exhibiting random patterns only should look something like Figure 18–5. As can be seen, there is no clear upward or downward trend. You may also notice that each year there is no discernible seasonal pattern. The month of May is not usually particularly busy nor particularly slow. May is a low month in the first year and a high month in the next year, relative to the values for the other months in those years.

Seasonality

Seasonal patterns are sometimes visible to the eye, as was the case in Figure 18–4. In health care, one is especially likely to see seasonal patterns because of seasonal disease patterns and as a result of the weather. Winter months bring different ailments than summer months do. For hospitals and home health agencies, this will affect overall patient volume. On the other hand, nursing homes may be running at full occupancy all year round. Therefore the number of patient days at a nursing home might not show any seasonality, although the specific care needs of the patients in a nursing home are likely to vary with the different seasons of the year.

Seasonality may not always be easy to spot. Therefore, it might be a worthwhile exercise to examine certain months that are known as peak or slow periods. Suppose that January is compared with June for each of the last five years and it is found that January almost always has higher levels of the item being forecast than June does. In that case seasonality does exist, even if it is not readily apparent when the graph is visually inspected.

Trend

In Figure 18–6, note that although the graph has its ups and downs, there is a clear upward trend. Because nursing hours rather than dollars are being considered here, this is not caused by inflation. Rather, it is probably caused either by an increased number of patient days or by an increased amount of nursing time provided per patient day.

The underlying causes of observed patterns will not be determined in the

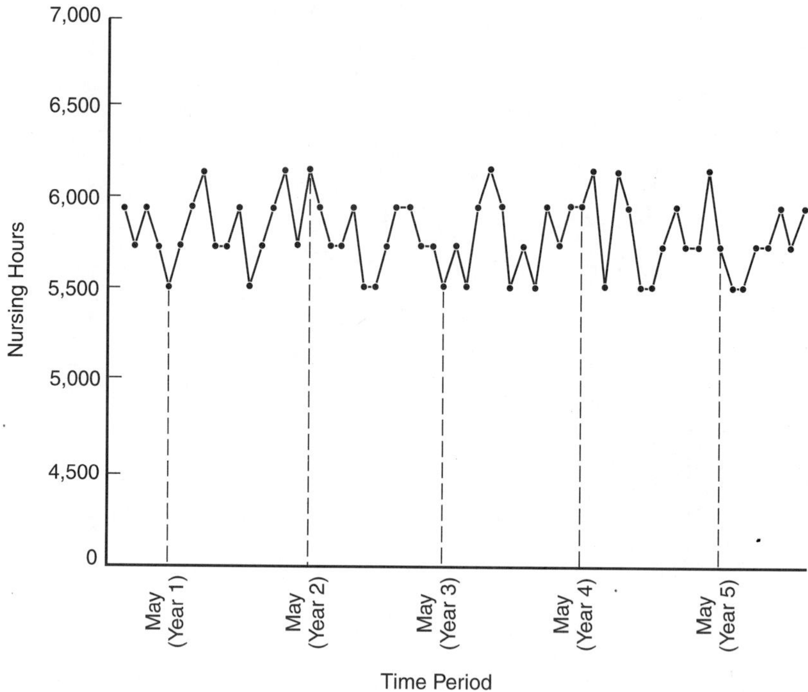

FIGURE 18–5. Five years' data for nursing hours forecast: random fluctuations.

forecasting process described here. The focus is strictly on projections of past items into the future. Whatever the cause, it appears that a definite trend exists. Unless there is information about expected patient days or a new policy regarding the relative ratio of nurses to patients, it would have to be assumed that this trend will continue. However, managers should try to understand the underlying causes of

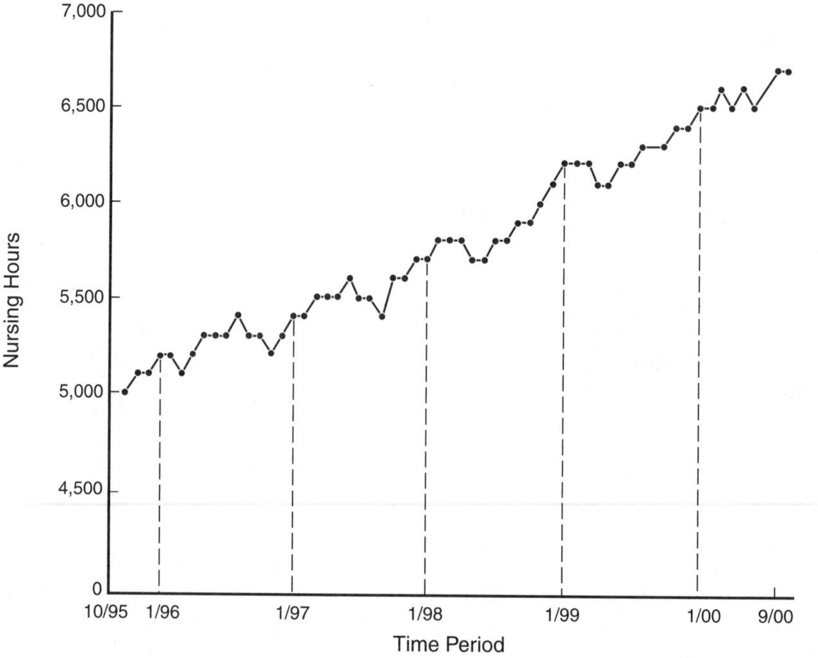

FIGURE 18–6. Five years' data for nursing hours forecast: trend.

patterns such as trends. This will better enable them to forecast correctly if something does change the underlying cause of the pattern.

Note further in Figure 18–6 that although the overall trend is upward, there is no discernible seasonal pattern. For example, January does not appear to be consistently high or low each year relative to the other months of those years.

Seasonality and Trend

It is common for health care organizations to experience at least some seasonality. At the same time, due to increasing patient volume or the effects of inflation, upward trends are common as well. Downward trends may also occur. It is not at all unusual therefore for the organization to experience both seasonal influences and trends at the same time. Figure 18–7 shows an example of a historical pattern exhibiting both seasonality and trend.

Often the trend is more obvious than the seasonality in patterns that contain both. In these cases, it becomes especially useful to make several comparisons to see if certain months are always higher or lower than other months. Valid forecasts require an awareness of seasonal patterns if they exist.

Forecasting Formulas

At this point historical data have been gathered and graphed, and there has been a visual inspection of the graphs for apparent trend or seasonal patterns. It is finally time to begin using the information to make forecasts for the coming year. The approach taken for forecasting depends to a great degree on whether seasonal patterns, trends, both, or neither are present.

An approach to forecasting each of these patterns is discussed below. First, however, it should be noted that the formulas assume limited use of computer technology in performing the forecasting function. Much of the tedium and difficulty of the forecasting process is avoided if a sophisticated computer forecasting program is used. Although the formulas discussed below are valuable in situations in which a computer approach is unavailable, a computer solution is preferred. It takes less

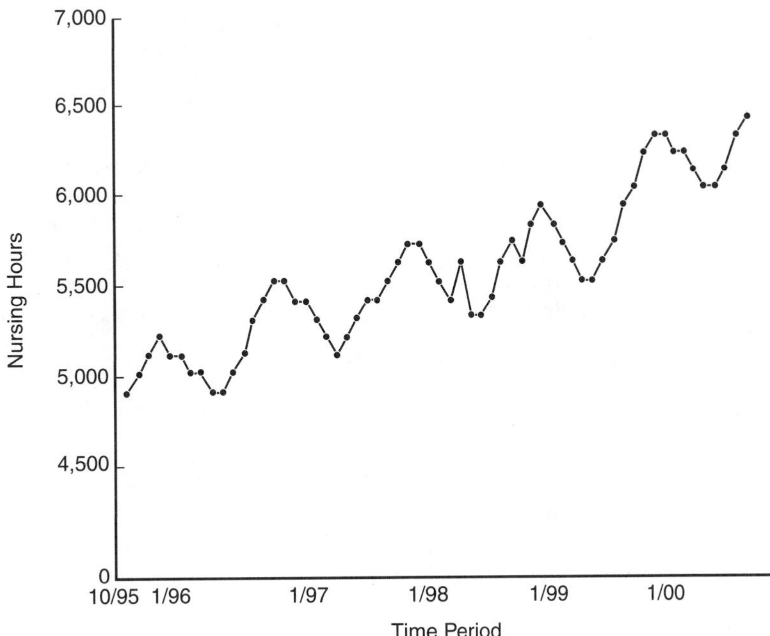

FIGURE 18–7. Five years' data for nursing hours forecast: seasonality with trend.

management time and can produce superior results. The costs of appropriate software are readily offset by the saved managerial time. A computer approach to forecasting is presented later in this chapter.

Random Fluctuations

The easiest forecasting occurs when there is no seasonal pattern or trend. For example, consider the budget for office supplies for the office of the chief nurse executive (CNE). The need for these supplies may not vary much over time or with the particular workload faced by the clinical nurses.

The most obvious approach in this case would be to simply add up the sixty monthly data points for the past five years and divide by sixty. That will give a monthly average. If every month is like every other month in terms of the item being forecast, this would be a reasonable approximation.

Caution must be exercised, however. Different months have different numbers of days. Even if there is no strong seasonal influence or trend, longer months may consume more of a resource. Months that have more weekdays may consume more of a resource. It may be necessary to adjust for factors such as days in a month or weekdays in a month. For example, if weekdays use much more of a resource than weekends, rather than dividing the total for the last sixty months by sixty, the total could be divided by the number of weekdays in the past sixty months. The result is a predicted value per weekday. That value can be multiplied by the specific number of weekdays in each month in the coming year to get the appropriate forecast for each month.

Seasonality

If seasonality exists in the item being forecast, it means that some months are typically low and other months are typically high. If all sixty months for the last five years are averaged together, the seasonality becomes lost in the broad average. An approach is needed that is more sensitive to fluctuations within each year. The most obvious approach is to add together the values for a given month for several years and divide to get an average for just that month. For example, the last five February values can be totaled and then divided by five. That provides a February average for the last five years that can be used as a prediction for next February.

This approach is not always acceptable. Suppose that seasonal variations do not repeat in the exact same month each year. For instance, suppose that February is usually the coldest month, causing patient days to peak because of many flu cases. Sometimes, however, January or March is colder. Because of this variation in seasonality from year to year, a better prediction may result from adding January plus February plus March for the last five years. Thus February is based on January, February, and March. This total is divided by fifteen to get a prediction of February for next year. Then March is estimated by adding February plus March plus April for each of the last five years and dividing by fifteen.

The key to this *moving-average* approach is to add up not only the month in question for the last five years but also the month preceding and the month following the month being predicted. This formula will often give a good prediction. However, there are also problems with this approach. Peaks and valleys in activity will be understated. For instance, what if January is typically the busiest month of the year, and both December and February are less busy? By averaging December and February with January, the slower December and February will cause the busier January to be understated in the forecast.

How can a nurse manager determine whether predictions will be improved by using calculations such as this? Should the manager simply take an average of five Februarys or use January, February, and March information for five years to predict next February? One good way to make that determination is to use historical data (excluding data from the most recent past year) to predict the results of the past year.

For instance, if 2000 has just ended, take data from 1995 through 1999 and use them to predict 2000. Since the actual results for 2000 are known, the prediction can immediately be compared with the actual results. This is a good way to test any formula to see if it is a reasonable predictor.

Keep in mind two things, however. First, no forecast can predict the future perfectly. The future is uncertain, and all the specific events that will occur can never be fully anticipated. Therefore the prediction should not be expected to match the actual results precisely. Second, the predictions or forecasts using formulas must be adjusted based on the manager's own knowledge about the future. The formulas just use information about the past. If managers have some information about the future that leads them to believe that the future will not follow the patterns of the past, that information must be used to adjust the predictions of the formulas. The role of an intelligent manager should never be relinquished to the mathematical precision of a formula.

When a formula is tested by seeing how well it can predict what actually happened last year, there should be a determination of whether the predictions based on the formula are closer to what actually happened than the predictions that would have been used in the absence of the formula. If so, then it is a useful tool. Otherwise, the formula should be either modified or discarded.

Trend

If a trend is observed, it is desirable to project that trend into the future. Trends are usually represented by a straight line. However, trends tend to have some random elements within them. If one were to draw a straight line, it would not generally go through each historical point. Some points would be above the line and some would be below the line. A manager could just eyeball the points on the graph and try to draw a line that is as close as possible to all the points and that extends into the future. However, such manual attempts are likely to be inaccurate.

If the line is drawn too high or too low, the estimates for the future will also be too high or too low. Even worse, if the slope of the line is too high or too low, the error will be magnified, as seen in Figure 18–8. In this figure the solid line represents

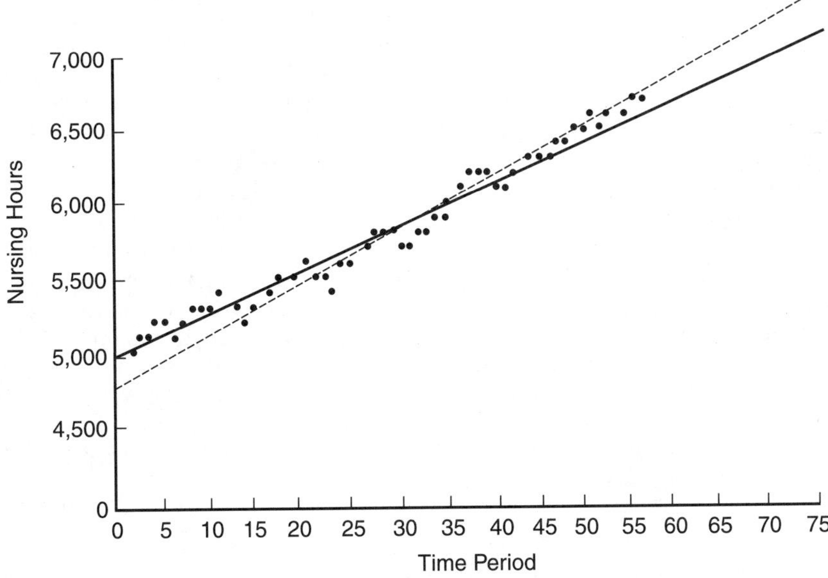

FIGURE 18–8. Nursing hours forecast for trend with no seasonality: judgmental *vs* regression results.

the best straight line that uses the known data to forecast the future. The dashed line represents a judgmental, eyeball estimate. Note that near the center of the graph, the two lines are relatively close. However, to the extreme right side of the graph, in the area of the forecast for the coming year, the two lines have diverged to the point that the number of nursing hours predicted differs a great deal, depending on which line is used.

One solution to this problem is to use a statistical technique called *regression analysis*. The goal of regression analysis is to find the unique straight line that comes closest to all the historical data points. Regression analysis can be readily performed by a nurse manager using many types of hand-held calculators or on a computer using statistical software packages such as the Statistical Package for Social Sciences (SPSS), spreadsheet packages such as LOTUS 1-2-3, or forecasting packages such as SmartForecasts for Windows.

Regression analysis is a technique that applies mathematical precision to a scatter diagram. The scatter diagram used in regression analysis is a graph that plots points of information. Each data point represents a dependent variable and one or more independent variables. The independent variable is sometimes referred to as the causal variable. It is responsible for causing variations in the dependent variable.

When making forecasts, time is considered an independent variable, and a second variable is considered a dependent variable. For example, the dependent variable could be the number of patients treated by the organization. As time passes, the organization may have more or fewer patients. The change in the number of patients over time may reflect a random pattern, seasonal effect, trend, or seasonality and trend. If a trend exists, regression analysis will generate a line that is a good predictor of the future.

Regression is a tool that can help managers to manage better. The major difficulty in using regression is simply a fear of the process (and this relates not only to nurse managers but to all managers). However, when using a computer program, regression analysis does not require the user to do extensive mathematical computation. The computer carries out all the calculations.[1]

Since regression analysis requires the manager to provide numerical values, months and years cannot be used by their names for the independent variable. An independent variable cannot be referred to as January 1995. Instead the month names can be replaced by assigned numerical values. The historical months used for the analysis can be identified as one through sixty instead of October 1995, November 1995, and so forth to September 2000. Table 18–1 presents the data. After feeding the information into a calculator or computer (e.g., in month 1 there were 5,000 nursing hours; in month 2 there were 5,100 nursing hours; and so on through month 60, with 6,700 nursing hours), the calculator or computer is instructed to "run" (compute) the regression. When the computation is complete, it is possible to determine how many nursing hours are expected in months 64 through 75, which represent the twelve months of next year. Note that months 61 through 63 have been intentionally skipped over. There are neither historical data points nor forecast points plotted for those three months. That is because those months represent the remaining months of the current year, for which data are not yet available. The goal is to develop predictions for the months in the coming year.

The results are shown in the scatter diagram in Figure 18–9. The regression results are plotted as a solid line for 2001 and are extended back from 2000 to 1995 with a dashed line. The specific predictions of nursing-hour requirements for 2001, by month, are as follows:

---

[1]Although regression is easy to perform with a computer, the user should have some familiarity with regression to interpret the regression results and their significance. See the discussion of regression in Chapter 7 or a statistics text.

January	6,772	May	6,884	September	6,995
February	6,800	June	6,911	October	7,023
March	6,828	July	6,939	November	7,051
April	6,856	August	6,967	December	7,079

Note in Figure 18–9 that the projections for the next year all fall on the trend line, even though in the past many points are not on the extended (dashed) trend line. Actual results over the coming year are not really expected to fall right on the line; however, in the absence of any other information, the points on the trend line are the best prediction that can be made for the actual uncertain outcome. To guess higher than the trend-line value would probably be too high; to guess lower than the trend-line value would probably be too low.

Seasonality and Trend

Seasonality together with trend poses a more complex problem; yet it is likely to be a common occurrence, so the reader should pay special attention to the approach discussed here. This example uses the data provided in Table 18–2. The first step is to use regression analysis to predict a trend line for the coming year. Once a set of results for the regression is plotted for each month in the coming year (January 2001 through December 2001) it should be noted that there is no seasonal appearance to

※ TABLE 18–1. *Nursing Hours—Historical Data for Trend with No Seasonality*

Data Point	Date		Nursing Hours	Data Point	Data		Nursing Hours
1	October	1995	5,000	31	April		5,800
2	November		5,100	32	May		5,700
3	December		5,100	33	June		5,700
4	January	1996	5,200	34	July		5,800
5	February		5,200	35	August		5,800
6	March		5,100	36	September		5,900
7	April		5,200	37	October		5,900
8	May		5,300	38	November		6,000
9	June		5,300	39	December		6,100
10	July		5,300	40	January	1999	6,200
11	August		5,400	41	February		6,200
12	September		5,300	42	March		6,200
13	October		5,300	43	April		6,100
14	November		5,200	44	May		6,100
15	December		5,300	45	June		6,200
16	January	1997	5,400	46	July		6,200
17	February		5,400	47	August		6,300
18	March		5,500	48	September		6,300
19	April		5,500	49	October		6,300
20	May		5,500	50	November		6,400
21	June		5,600	51	December		6,400
22	July		5,500	52	January	2000	6,500
23	August		5,500	53	February		6,500
24	September		5,400	54	March		6,600
25	October		5,600	55	April		6,500
26	November		5,600	56	May		6,600
27	December		5,700	57	June		6,500
28	January	1998	5,700	58	July		6,600
29	February		5,800	59	August		6,700
30	March		5,800	60	September		6,700

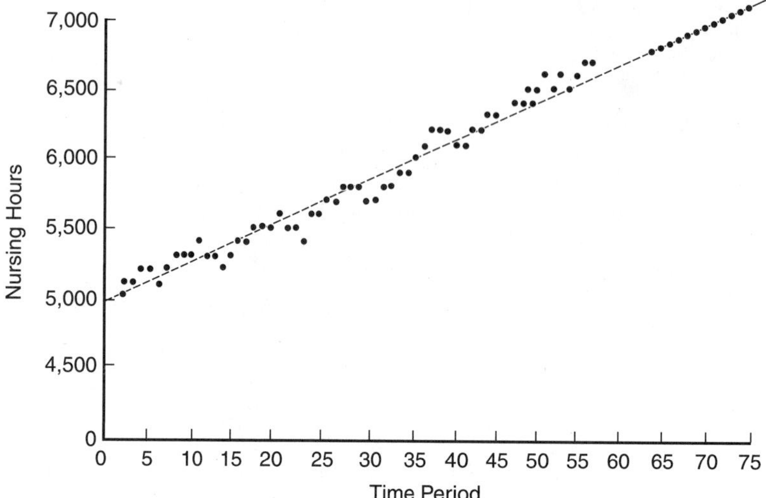

FIGURE 18–9. Nursing hours forecast for trend with no seasonality: regression results.

※ **TABLE 18–2.** *Nursing Hours—Historical Data for Trend with Seasonality*

Data Point	Date		Nursing Hours	Data Point	Date		Nursing Hours
1	October	1995	4,900	31	April		5,500
2	November		5,000	32	May		5,400
3	December		5,100	33	June		5,600
4	January	1996	5,200	34	July		5,300
5	February		5,100	35	August		5,300
6	March		5,100	36	September		5,400
7	April		5,000	37	October		5,600
8	May		5,000	38	November		5,700
9	June		4,900	39	December		5,600
10	July		4,900	40	January	1999	5,800
11	August		5,000	41	February		5,900
12	September		5,100	42	March		5,800
13	October		5,300	43	April		5,700
14	November		5,400	44	May		5,600
15	December		5,500	45	June		5,500
16	January	1997	5,500	46	July		5,500
17	February		5,400	47	August		5,600
18	March		5,400	48	September		5,700
19	April		5,300	49	October		5,900
20	May		5,200	50	November		6,000
21	June		5,100	51	December		6,200
22	July		5,200	52	January	2000	6,300
23	August		5,300	53	February		6,300
24	September		5,400	54	March		6,200
25	October		5,400	55	April		6,200
26	November		5,500	56	May		6,100
27	December		5,600	57	June		6,000
28	January	1998	5,700	58	July		6,000
29	February		5,700	59	August		6,100
30	March		5,600	60	September		6,300

the line predicting next year; it simply shows an upward trend (see Fig. 18–10 for 2001).

The next step is to extend the trend backward into the five years for which there are historical data. This is fairly straightforward, since it simply requires extending backward a straight line that has been already located for the coming year (see the dashed line on Fig. 18–11).

Once the line has been extended backward, the manager must calculate how much above or below the line the actual value was each month for the last five years. Those amounts must then be converted into a percentage. For example, in January 1996 (Fig. 18–11) there were 5,200 nursing hours, but the trend line was at a vertical height of 5,000. The actual value was 200 hours above the trend. Because it is a trend, however, it is necessary to convert it to a percentage. In this case, it is a positive 4%, because 5,200 is 4% above the trend-line point of 5,000.

Now simply revert to the seasonal approach. Add together the percentages that December, January, and February are over and under the trend line for the last five years and divide by fifteen. The result is a prediction of the percent above or below the trend line January will be next year. Find the point on the trend line next year for January and multiply it by the moving-average percent to find how much above or below the trend line the predicted point is. This process can be repeated for each month of the coming year. For example, Table 18–3 shows the actual number of nursing hours incurred and the extended trend-line information for December, January, and February for five years.

The trend-line prediction for January 2001 from Figure 18–11 is 6,204. This is before adjustment for seasonality. In the calculation shown in Table 18–3, it was determined that for January the moving-average percentage is a positive 3.2%. By adding 3.2% of 6,204 to the trend-line value of 6,204, the resulting prediction adjusted for seasonality is 6,403. That point has been plotted for January 2001 on Figure 18–11. Similarly, to get the 2001 forecast for the entire year, this process should be repeated on a moving-average basis for each month in turn.

Using Computers for Forecasting

The previous section on forecasting formulas demonstrates how complicated forecasting can become when historical data are influenced by both trend

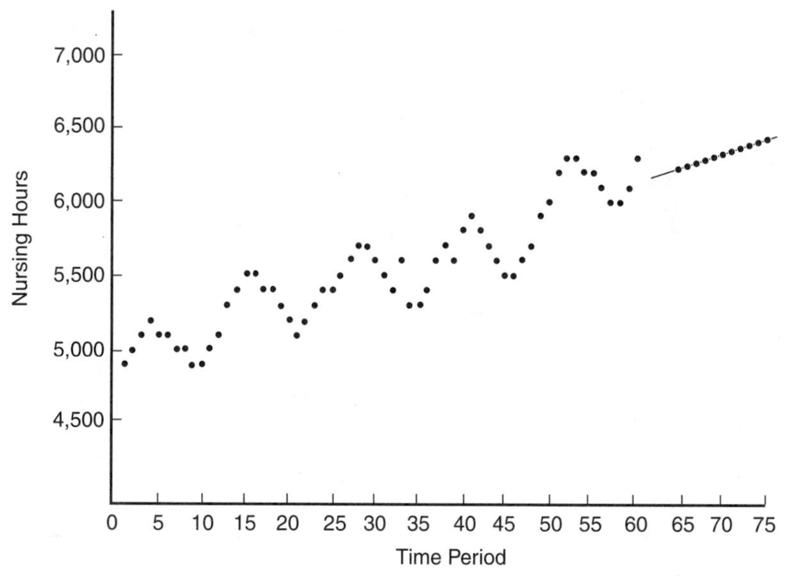

FIGURE 18–10. Nursing hours forecast for trend with seasonality: regression results.

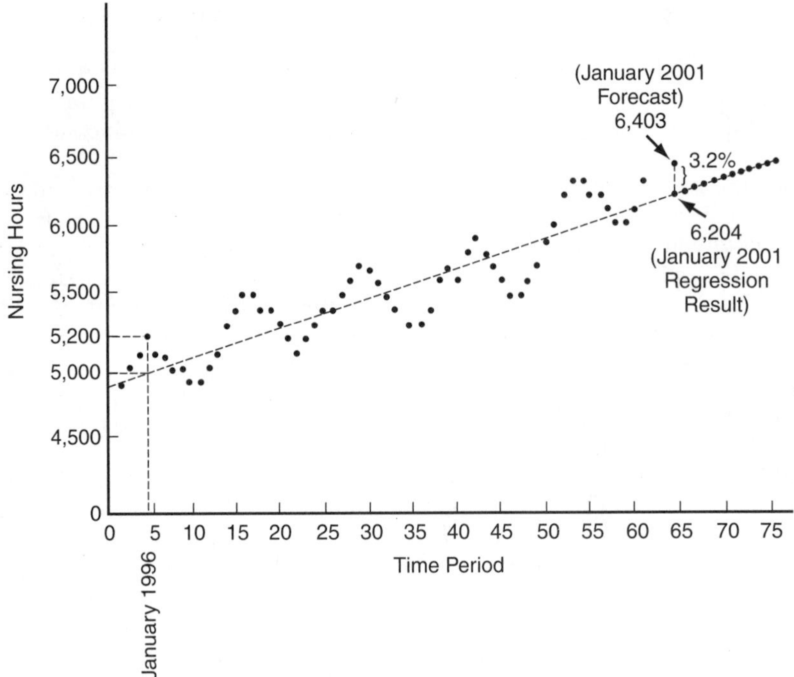

FIGURE 18–11. Nursing hours forecast for trend with seasonality: regression results extended back into historical data.

and seasonality. However, health care organizations frequently do have at least seasonality; both trend and seasonality are not uncommon. In recent years, nurse managers' ability to deal with such patterns has improved dramatically as a result of personal computers and specially designed computer software. These computer programs make the work of forecasting easier and the results more accurate.

※ TABLE 18–3. *Calculation of Moving Average Percent for January 2001*

Month		Actual	Trend Line	Difference	Difference as a Percentage of Trend Line
December	1995	5,100	4,980	120	2.4%
January	1996	5,200	5,000	200	4.0
February	1996	5,100	5,020	80	1.6
December	1996	5,500	5,221	279	5.3
January	1997	5,500	5,241	259	4.9
February	1997	5,400	5,261	139	2.6
December	1997	5,600	5,461	139	2.5
January	1998	5,700	5,482	218	4.0
February	1998	5,700	5,502	198	3.6
December	1998	5,600	5,702	(102)*	(1.8)*
January	1999	5,800	5,723	77	1.3
February	1999	5,900	5,743	157	2.7
December	1999	6,200	5,943	257	4.3
January	2000	6,300	5,963	337	5.7
February	2000	6,300	5,983	317	5.3
Total					48.4%
Divided by 15 =					3.2%

*Negative amounts.

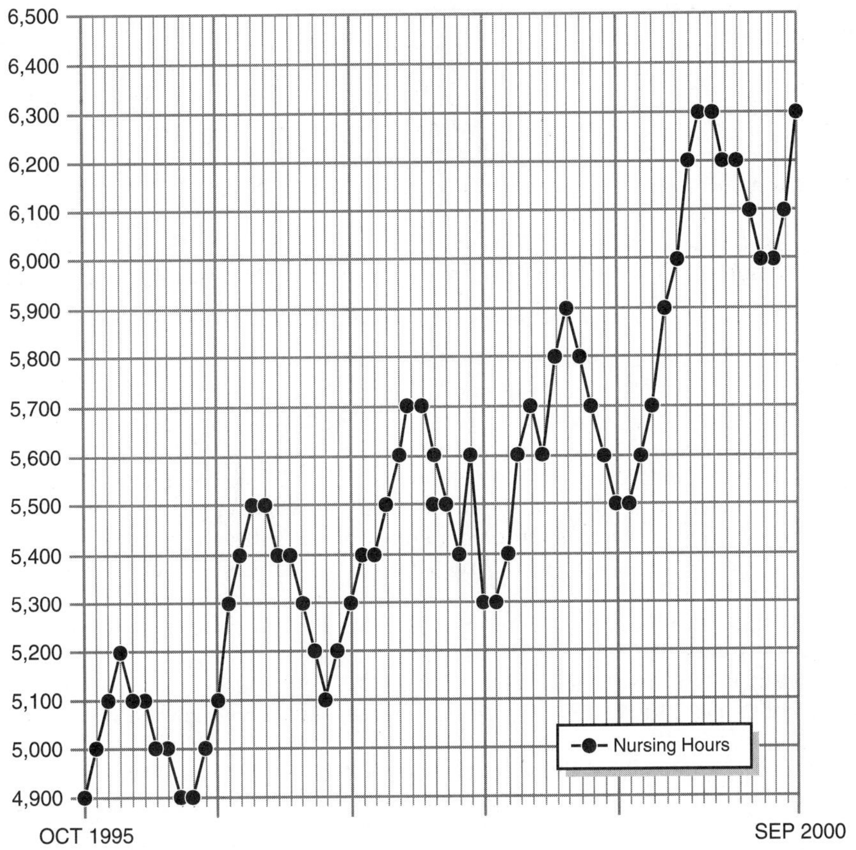

FIGURE 18–12. SmartForecasts II time plot graph of historical data.

A number of forecasting programs are available. This section discusses forecasting using one such program, SmartForecasts for Windows.[2] This program is an example of computer forecasting software that is not limited to linear forecasting. Regression analysis produces a straight-line forecast. When there is seasonality, certain months are always above the regression line and others are always below it. Software such as SmartForecasts for Windows can generate *curvilinear* (curved line) forecasts. That means that the forecast line generated will come closer to the historical points, and therefore its projections are likely to be closer to the results that will actually occur.

SmartForecasts provides a data entry format similar to an electronic spreadsheet (e.g., LOTUS 1-2-3 or Excel), with columns and rows. Each column represents a time period, and each row represents a variable to be forecast, such as patients or nursing hours.

Reconsider the forecast for the data from Table 18–2 using SmartForecasts for Windows. After the data are entered, one of the first steps is to print a time plot graph to get a visual sense of the data. Examination of the time plot in Figure 18–12

---

[2]SmartForecasts for Windows is a trademark of Smart Software, Inc., 4 Hill Road, Belmont, MA 02178; telephone (617) 489-2743. Version 4.16 was used for Exhibits 18–1 to 18–4, Figures 18–12 and 18–13, and Tables 18–4 and 18–5 in this chapter. This chapter does not attempt to demonstrate all the capabilities of this software. The software program is used simply as an example of the use of computer forecasting.

Permission has been obtained from the vendor for the use of these examples. The use of the examples in this chapter does not represent a formal endorsement of the product.

quickly alerts the user to the seasonal nature of the data; closer inspection reveals the upward trend.

A number of different forecasting models are available within the software program. SmartForecasts allows the user to forecast nursing hours using regression analysis. However, if regression analysis is used, given the seasonality observed in the time plot, the same problem will occur as existed in Figure 18–10, requiring the same manual adjustments shown in Figure 18–11 and Table 18–3.

The key advantage of this software and other programs like it is that it allows use of a curved line for forecasting. This should remove the necessity to adjust the trend line for seasonality. However, which forecasting approach should be used? Available methods include exponential smoothing, moving average, multiseries analysis, and so on.

Moving average approaches were used in the earlier section on forecasting formulas in this chapter. However, will that approach give the best result if other advanced statistical techniques are available? The best approach until one is very familiar with forecasting is to use automatic forecasting, which lets the computer choose the best approach. With the automatic approach the computer will calculate the forecast with a number of different methods to see which predicts best.

Figure 18–13 is the forecast graph generated by the software program. What does the graph consist of? The historical data points are connected by a solid line. The forecast during the historical (past) periods is dotted. Compare this dotted line with the regression line shown in Figure 18–11. During the first five years in Figure 18–11 the actual points are usually substantially above or below the regression line. Therefore it is reasonable to assume that as the line is used to project next year, each month's actual result is likely to be substantially above or below the forecast trend line.

Although the statistical theory is complex, effectively, the closer the forecast line comes to the actual results in the past, the more likely the forecast line is to come

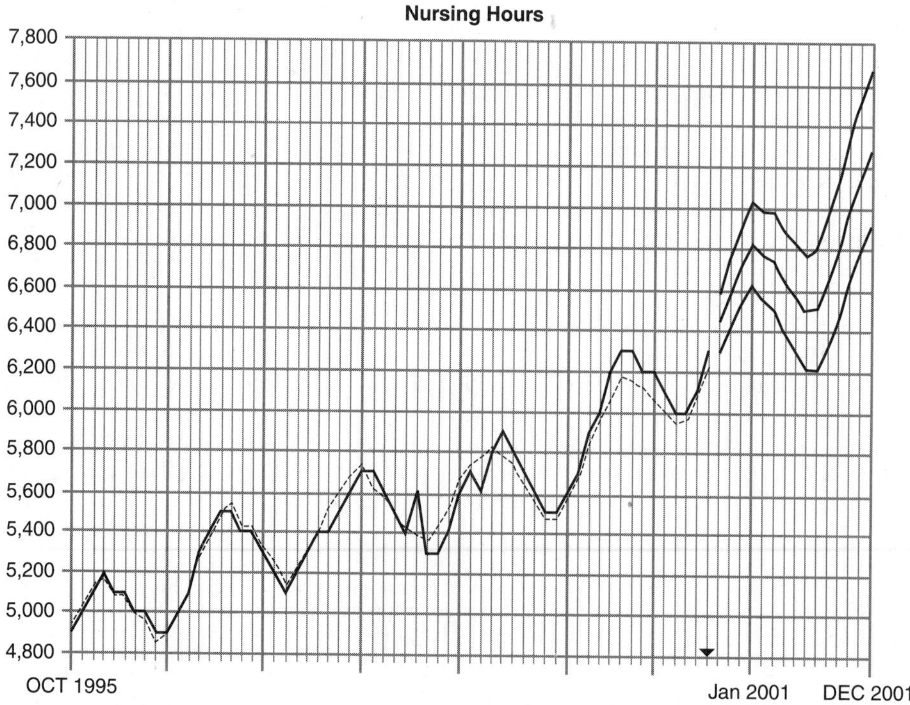

FIGURE 18–13. SmartForecasts II forecast of nursing hours.

※ **TABLE 18–4.** *Tournament Rankings for AUTOMATIC Forecasts of V1 Nursing Hours*

Rank	Method	% Worse than Winner
1	Winters' multiplicative, weights = 22%, 22%, 22%	(winner)
2	Winters' additive, weights = 20%, 20%, 20%	1.3
3	Double exponential smoothing, weight = 8%	57.2
4	Linear moving average of 12 periods	65.0
5	Simple moving average of 1 period	118.3
6	Single exponential smoothing, weight = 59%	118.9

close to the actual results in the future. When the computer performs forecasting automatically, it examines how close the forecast line is to the historical actual points for each of a series of different forecasting methods. The computer can be given a command to examine the relative accuracy of the different forecasting methods examined. Table 18–4 shows the results of the competition among forecasting methods for this example. The best technique is Winters' multiplicative method. Winters' is a curvilinear approach that works extremely well for seasonal data. The data points are only 1% to 3% farther away from the forecast line for the next best method, another form of Winters' forecasting. However, using alternatives to the Winters approaches generates much less accurate results.

In Figure 18–13 it is evident that the dotted forecast line for the first five years followed extremely closely the actual results. In some cases the solid and dotted lines are so close that they cannot be distinguished from each other. Therefore, the forecast line, when projected through 2001, is likely to give a fairly accurate estimate.

In the graph shown in Figure 18–13 there are solid lines above and below (bracketing) the forecast line projected into the future. These lines represent a margin-of-error interval. Forecasts can never be expected to be exactly correct. It is possible, however, to use statistics to get some idea of how large the difference might be between the forecast and the actual result. In this case, based on the statistical analysis there is a 90% likelihood that the actual result will fall somewhere between these solid lines. But graphs, while visually informative, are hard to read when it is time to write the actual forecast. Another computer command provides a numerical table of the forecast results. See Table 18–5 for the forecast results.

This table shows not only the forecast but also the margin of error or confidence interval above and below the forecast. If desired, that interval can easily be changed so that there is 95% or 99% confidence that the actual result will fall within the range of values between the lower limit and upper limit estimates. If the percentage is raised to a higher confidence level, the interval around the forecast line becomes wider. For example, for January 2001 the prediction is 6,821 nursing hours, and there is 90% confidence that the actual nursing hours will not be less than 6,622 nor more than 7,020. If a manager wants to be 99% confident that the actual results will not exceed the boundaries of the projection, the lower limit value becomes lower and the upper limit higher.

In practice it is rarely necessary to be so precise. While 95% or 99% confidence may be important for academic research studies, in practice, managers tend to have a greater degree of latitude. In fact, the SmartForecasts software program is preset by the manufacturer to give a 90% confidence. While it is simple for the user to change that confidence level, given the way the software is set up, one must question whether it is desirable. Essentially, a 90% confidence interval implies that nine times out of ten the actual result will fall within the bounds of the interval. That is an extremely good result for most managers' forecasts.

Compare the result from Winters' multiplicative method (Table 18–5, Fig. 18–13) with the earlier result obtained by the combined regression analysis–moving-

※ **TABLE 18–5.** *Forecasts of V1 NURSING HOURS Using Multiplicative WINTERS' METHOD*

	Approximate 90% Forecast Interval		
Time Period	**Lower Limit**	**FORECAST**	**Upper Limit**
OCT 2000	6,284	6,434	6,584
NOV 2000	6,405	6,572	6,740
DEC 2000	6,520	6,704	6,888
JAN 2001	6,622	6,821	7,020
FEB 2001	6,549	6,766	6,983
MAR 2001	6,502	6,737	6,973
APR 2001	6,391	6,641	6,891
MAY 2001	6,306	6,570	6,834
JUN 2001	6,210	6,493	6,775
JUL 2001	6,205	6,507	6,809
AUG 2001	6,311	6,633	6,956
SEP 2001	6,449	6,788	7,126
OCT 2001	6,634	6,996	7,358
NOV 2001	6,769	7,143	7,516
DEC 2001	6,897	7,282	7,666

average approach (see January 2001 in Fig. 18–11). As can be seen, the results differ. This is because the approach used earlier is less accurate than Winters' method. Earlier the January 2001 number of nursing hours was projected to be 6,403, while Winters' method predicts it to be approximately 6,821. In fact the earlier estimate is below the lower limit value of the 90% confidence interval. It is clear that using more sophisticated techniques can generate results that differ markedly from the manual approaches used before computer software was readily available. It is probable that the manual moving-average calculation will be more accurate than simply a judgmental guess. However, the computer-based Winters' solution is likely to be even more accurate.

It is also possible to refine Winters' method even further. The computer makes some general assumptions when it performs forecasts under the automatic approach. If Winters' method was immediately selected as the forecasting method instead of selecting automatic, some additional options would be provided to improve the forecast further. Specifically, the SmartForecasts software can be informed of the relative importance of the most recent level, trend, and seasonal factors. If the user knows that the trend is changing due to shifts in the underlying demographics of the community population, it is possible to give more weight to the most recent trend, as compared with the trend in the earlier years.

Not only can information be supplied to enable the computer to be more accurate, such as the relative importance of the recent trend, but it is also possible to modify the results of the computer analysis. Results can be adjusted directly on the forecast graph, or historical data points can be modified on the basis of some judgment or knowledge the user has that is not reflected in the historical information. This is especially helpful when there is an outlier data point. For example, suppose that a rare event caused data for one month to be atypical. That data point can cause the forecast to be thrown off substantially. A better forecast may be obtained by judgmentally adjusting that data point's value. Judgmental adjustments are also needed because computer-generated forecasts assume that factors that affected nursing hours remain the same in the future as they were in the past. That may not be the case.

Most managers initially use a forecasting program only to forecast one item at a time. However, as one becomes more adept at using computer-based forecasting, the program would probably be used to generate forecasts on a number of different variables. The user will also want to be able to save the data file to avoid having to reenter data each time an analysis is to be performed. The SmartForecasts program has its own data files, and the data can also be stored in a wide variety of formats for future use, including LOTUS 1-2-3 worksheet files, ASCII (generic) files, or DIF files. By the same token, data in another format such as LOTUS, ASCII, or DIF can be read into SmartForecasts.

SmartForecasts is one of a number of forecasting programs that can be used on a microcomputer. The most significant aspect of using sophisticated software programs is that they can generate a substantially improved result. The ability of the forecast line to curve in synchronization with the actual historical seasonal pattern decreases the required effort by the manager substantially, while enhancing the result.

※ QUALITATIVE METHODS FOR FORECASTING

The discussion in this chapter has assumed that reasonably reliable historical data are available. However, there will be many instances, especially in the case of new ventures, where a forecast will be needed for a budget even though there are no reliable historical data. Subjective estimates will be required. In such cases regression analysis or even computerized curvilinear forecasting will be inadequate to provide a solution. Two approaches commonly used to aid in making reasonable subjective forecasts are the Delphi and nominal group techniques.

In both approaches a team or panel must be selected who are likely to have reasoned insights with respect to the item being forecast. Although no one may have direct knowledge or experience, an attempt should be made to select a qualified group. Industrial experience has shown that by arriving at a consensus among a team of experts, subjective forecasts can be reasonably accurate.

Nominal Group Technique

The *nominal group technique* is one in which the group of individuals is brought together in a structured meeting. Members write down their forecasts. Then all the written forecasts are presented to the group by a group leader without discussion. Once all the forecasts have been revealed, the reasoning behind each one is discussed. After the discussions, each member again makes a forecast in writing. Through a repetitive process, eventually a group decision is made.

Obviously there are weaknesses to the nominal group technique. One problem concerns lack of information. If different forecasts are made based on different assumptions, it may be impossible to reach consensus. Another problem concerns politics and personalities. As members of the group defend their forecasts, extraneous issues having to do with whose idea it is may bias the group decision.

Delphi Technique

With the *Delphi technique* the group never meets. All forecasts are presented in writing to a group leader, who provides summaries to all group members. For those forecasts that differ substantially from the majority—either high or low—a request is made for the reasoning behind the forecast. That information is also shared with group members. Then a new round of forecasts is made. This process is repeated several times, and a decision is made based on the collective responses.

Delphi has several particular advantages. By eliminating a face-to-face meeting, confrontation is avoided. Decisions are based more on logic than on personality or position. The dissemination of the respondents' underlying reasoning allows erroneous facts or assumptions to be eliminated.

These two methods both make use of the fact that individual managers cannot be expected to think of everything. Different individuals, bringing different expertise and different points of view to bear on the same problem, can create an outcome superior to what any one of them could do individually. It is a cliche to say that two minds are better than one. Nevertheless, it is true that in many forecasting instances, the Delphi and nominal group approaches can substantially improve results.

※ OTHER DECISION-MAKING TOOLS

A number of other tools can aid managers in making decisions. In particular, the remainder of this chapter will focus on the following techniques:

- Expected value
- Linear programming
- Inventory control
- Gantt chart
- Critical path method and program evaluation and review technique (PERT)

Expected Value

One approach to making decisions in the uncertain world of health care is to estimate the probability that certain events will occur. An *expected value* is a weighted average using the probabilities as weights. For example, assume that the nurse manager of a home health agency is considering two possible approaches to providing nursing care to the elderly. On the basis of previous experience, reading the literature, and talking with managers of other similar agencies, the manager makes the predictions of cash receipts for care provided under each approach, as shown in Table 18–6. The expected value for each project in Table 18–6 is the weighted average of the possible cash flow outcomes. Each cash flow is weighted by its probability. Therefore the expected value of Project A, denoted as E(A), is as follows:

$$\begin{aligned} E(A) &= 0.3 \times 5{,}000 &&= \$1{,}500 \\ &+ 0.5 \times 8{,}000 &&= 4{,}000 \\ &+ \underline{0.2} \times 10{,}000 &&= \underline{2{,}000} \\ &\underline{\underline{1.0}} &&= \underline{\underline{\$7{,}500}} \end{aligned}$$

The expected value of Project B is:

$$\begin{aligned} E(B) &= 0.1 \times \$\ 3{,}000 &&= \$\ 300 \\ &+ 0.8 \times 6{,}000 &&= 4{,}800 \\ &+ \underline{0.1} \times 11{,}000 &&= \underline{1{,}100} \\ &\underline{\underline{1.0}} &&= \underline{\underline{\$6{,}200}} \end{aligned}$$

※ **TABLE 18–6.** *Projected Cash Receipts for Two Different Projects*

Project A		Project B	
Probability	**Cash Flow**	**Probability**	**Cash Flow**
.30	$ 5,000	.10	$ 3,000
.50	8,000	.80	6,000
.20	10,000	.10	11,000

Thus if the goal of the agency were to choose the option that maximized revenue, option A offers the greatest likelihood of achieving that goal. Such an option is probably desirable if it has no negative impact on quality.

When using the expected value approach, it is essential to bear in mind that the expected value provides information on the *average* outcome. Sometimes the results will be better; sometimes they will be worse. Over a large number of decisions they should average out to the expected value.

For the example above, Table 18–6 indicates that the possible outcomes for Project A are $5,000, $8,000, or $10,000. The expected value of the project is $7,500. However, $7,500 is not one of the possible outcomes. When we say that the expected value is $7,500, we recognize that we really expect the outcome to be $5,000 or $8,000 or $10,000. Sometimes the result might turn out to be the low $5,000, sometimes the high $10,000, and sometimes $8,000. Over time, however, we would expect the average cash flow from many projects with similar possible outcomes to be $7,500.

The nurse manager should also remember that expected value is based on the assumed probabilities. The manager should get the best estimate of the probabilities that the event will occur, but this information is not perfect. Often it is based on subjective estimates by managers. Even with the best information poor outcomes can occur. All decisions must be made on the basis of information available at the time the decision is made. As the probability data indicate, by choosing option A there is still a .30 chance that cash flow will be only $5,000. That may occur, but that does not mean that it was a poor decision. Even further, the actual result might be lower than $5,000. It is possible that an unanticipated event may cause actual results to be lower or higher than the manager even believed was probable. However, use of techniques such as expected value should still improve a manager's ability to assess information and make correct decisions.

Linear Programming

Linear programming (LP) is a technique to determine how best to allocate scarce resources to achieve a certain goal. It is based on solving simultaneous equations. Given that two or more resources are available, the linear programming model helps determine the best combination to achieve a desired goal. The goal is usually to maximize an outcome such as revenues or sales or minimize an outcome such as personnel costs. The equations developed for these models can be solved for a specific value either graphically or mathematically.

Efforts to achieve goals are often limited by a number of constraints. Most nurses do not want to work weekends or nights. Yet some nurses must work those shifts to maintain a desired level of quality. The nurse manager of the OR wants to increase the hours of OR time, yet most surgeons do not want to operate on Saturday. In complex organizations, balancing the various constraints in achieving goals is complicated.

Linear programming can assist the nurse manager in making complex decisions that are constrained by a variety of factors. The first step is to develop the objective function. This equation states the relationship between the objective and other organizational factors. Developing the objective is not so simple as it would appear. Is the objective of the nursing unit to maximize revenue, maximize patients served, maximize quality, minimize errors? One advantage of LP is that any objective can be tempered by constraints established by the manager. Therefore an objective could be to maximize profits but not let quality fall below 3 on a nursing quality scale.

For example, suppose that the OR has been told it should maximize its profits. The objective function would be

$$\text{Profits} = \text{Revenues} - \text{Expenses}$$

where revenues are the sum of revenues from all operations, and expenses are the costs of all operations. For simplicity, assume that there are three types of operation:

hernia, heart, and gallbladder surgery. The average price charged for a hernia operation is $1,000. The average price charged for heart surgery is $10,000. The average price for a gallbladder procedure is $5,000. At first glance, one would not think it would be complicated to determine which mix of operations would be most profitable. Clearly, devoting all OR space to heart surgery will yield the largest total revenue.

However, it will not necessarily yield the maximum profit. Suppose that heart surgery takes five hours, while gallbladder cases take only two hours on average, and hernias only one hour. One could do five gallbladder operations (total revenue $25,000) in the time it would take to do two heart operations (total revenue $20,000). Therefore, in preparing an analysis one would want to consider the length of each procedure as well as the revenue, assuming that the total hours of procedures is limited.

Thus we have an objective function: maximize profits. We also have a constraint: the total number of hours of operating room time available. We also have several existing conditions: total revenue is the sum of the revenue of each case; total cost is the sum of the cost of each case; hernia operations take one hour; gallbladder operations take two hours; heart operations take five hours.

It seems to be getting complicated, but we have only begun to establish all the conditions. Dr. Smith does hernia operations; Dr. Jones does gallbladder operations; Dr. Brown does heart procedures. Dr. Brown will only operate from 6 AM to 4 PM on Tuesdays through Fridays. Dr. Jones will operate anytime from 6 AM to 8 PM on Mondays through Saturdays. Dr. Smith will operate from 6 AM to 10 PM on any day except Tuesdays, when she has office hours until 1 PM in the afternoon. On Tuesdays she will operate from 2 PM to 10 PM. However, Dr. Smith will not perform surgery more than five days per week. Anytime that the surgeons cannot operate at this hospital, they will operate at the hospital across town. Therefore, if the patients cannot be done within the OR schedule, the revenue will be lost. The problem is growing in complexity.

The OR contains six suites. However, because of difficulties in recruiting nurses it has been determined that we will probably only staff one room for one shift on Sundays and two rooms for two shifts on Saturdays. On weekdays, three rooms will be staffed for one shift and three rooms for two shifts, if necessary. Nurses working on the second shift get a $3 per hour premium. The complexity grows.

Hernia operations, although low priced, are relatively simple and require only one nurse during the procedure. The nurse may be experienced ($27 per hour) or inexperienced ($20 per hour). Gallbladder operations require one nurse for the procedure, and the nurse may be experienced or inexperienced. Heart surgery requires two nurses, and they must both be experienced.

Note that not only is the problem growing in complexity, but the number of constraints is growing as well. Even if we wanted to provide only heart surgery, we probably could not because we would be constrained by both Dr. Brown's operating schedule and by the need for experienced nurses only for that procedure. The equations would have to include the possible supply of shifts by inexperienced nurses and the supply of shifts by experienced nurses.

How can all the various factors be simultaneously taken into account to ensure that the OR time is preferentially given to the correct surgeon to maximize the OR's profit? Linear programming establishes an approach that solves multiple equations simultaneously to arrive at the optimal result. Human beings are not nearly so adept at taking all the factors into account and balancing them to determine the actual profit-maximizing solution. Note that in the real world the OR might have hundreds of different types of procedures and dozens of nurses and surgeons to balance.

Computer programs are now available that perform linear programming. Therefore it is not necessary to be able to work out the mathematics (which involve inversion of a linear algebra matrix). The nurse manager needs to be able to specify the relationships and constraints. Using computer software, the manager can spend less effort on trying to solve the problem and more effort on trying to correctly specify the relationships. Only the unit's or department's manager usually has adequate knowledge about such relationships to accurately specify them.

Will the organization schedule staff in the manner LP deems is most profitable? Will it keep the number of ORs open the optimal number of shifts as determined by the mathematical solution? Will it create the specific patient mix that generates the most profit? Very possibly not. Hospitals and other health care organizations tend to be very political places to work. As discussed in Chapter 3, managers must learn to understand and take into account the various unofficial lines of authority. Sometimes it is better to give in a bit to a demanding surgeon than to fight that surgeon and possibly lose the surgeon and all the surgeon's patients.

The LP solution to each problem generates not only the optimal solution but also an ability to determine the cost of giving in to politics. The profits can be calculated at the optimal-mix solution. The profits can then be calculated at a solution that would appease either all the surgeons or perhaps just the most vocal surgeon. In either case, the manager can now determine how much profits would decline from the optimal because of the accommodations being made. A rational decision can then be made concerning whether it is worth the reduced profit in the short run to keep the surgeons happy.

For small sacrifices in profit, it probably pays to keep the surgeons happy. For large sacrifices in profit, the organization may want to find some other way to appease the surgeons (fancier office or title) rather than foregoing the extra profits. The key is that the manager who uses linear programming can easily determine how much profit it will cost the organization to keep the surgeons happy.

The LP model also has the capability to determine (automatically) the impact on the objective function of the relaxation in certain constraints. For example, how much extra profit would be earned if Dr. Smith were willing to start her surgery hours one hour earlier on Tuesdays? It may be that the optimal mix and scheduling of patients result in the nurses on Tuesdays being paid for a full shift, even though they have no surgical duties during one hour of the shift. If Dr. Smith performed one more hernia operation on each Tuesday, it would allow the unit to eliminate one Saturday shift a month. This would generate much more efficient use of staff, lowering the average cost per operation. Once the impact on profits of such a change is known, it can be determined how hard we should work to induce Dr. Smith to make that change.

The key to LP is that it helps managers obtain information to make improved decisions. Using LP, the nurse manager will be able to assimilate a huge amount of information and provide guidance to make decisions and achieve the organization's goal.

The following example is presented so the reader can understand how LP works. Suppose the goal of the nurse manager is to provide care at the lowest cost per patient. Most decisions have some inherent constraints. In this case the manager has determined that to maintain an adequate level of quality when the census is thirty, at least six staff must work on the day shift. The unit has a "partners" or "dyad" nursing model. Therefore, there must always be a number of RNs equal to or greater than the number of aides. RNs are paid $200 per shift, and aides are paid $80. What is the best combination of RNs and aides that will achieve the desired goal?

Objective Function: Minimize Average Cost per Patient

Minimum cost = [$200 × (Number of RNs) + $80 × (Number of aides)]
÷ Average patient census

Let R = number of RNs; A = number of aides.

Minimum cost = $(200R + 80A)/30$

The manager identified two constraints that can be mathematically depicted as:

1. The number of RNs *(R)* plus the number of aides *(A)* must be at least 6:

$$R + A \geq 6$$

2. The number of RNs must be at least equal to the number of aides:

$$R \geq A$$

Although the nurse manager's constraints indicate that the number of RNs must be equal to or greater than the number of aides, to simplify the calculation in this example assume that the number of RNs must equal the number of aides. In addition, to simplify the calculation assume that the number of aides plus the number of RNs must be equal to 6. Therefore we remove the greater than signs and have the following equations:

$$R + A = 6$$
$$R = A$$

Using algebra, these equations are solved simultaneously. The second equation states that $R = A$. In the first equation if we substitute A for R we get the following:

$$A + A = 6$$
$$2A = 6$$

By dividing both sides by 2 we get:

$$\frac{2A}{2} = \frac{6}{2}$$

$$A = 3$$

Thus if the unit is staffed with three RNs and three aides, costs are minimized. Minimum cost = [($200 × 3 RNs) + ($80 × 3 aides)]/30 = $28 per patient per shift.

We recognize that this trivial example is intuitive. In the more complex situations of the real world, all the known constraints would be depicted and the many equations would be solved simultaneously using a computer.

Inventory Control

Operations management is the area of management that analyzes the use of resources to produce the desired product. Most of this book focuses on nursing personnel as the major resource used in providing nursing care. Although nursing personnel are the costliest resource in providing nursing care, nurse managers are often also responsible for management of clinical and other supplies. In areas such as the OR, supplies are a major expense. On other nursing units and for outpatient programs, supply costs can be considerable. One aspect of the management of supplies is the appropriate use of supplies. Another aspect of management of supplies is *inventory management*. Inventory management refers to the appropriate ordering and storage of supplies. This section focuses on inventory management.

Horngren and Foster describe five categories of costs associated with supplies: (a) *cost of the product*, (b) *ordering costs*, (c) *carrying costs*, (d) *stockout costs*, and (e) *quality costs*.[3] Cost of the product, that is, what the organization must pay for the product, can be affected by quantity discounts and timing of payment. Ordering costs include those costs associated with the order, such as clerk time for preparation

[3] Horngren, Charles T., and George Foster, *Cost Accounting A Managerial Emphasis*, 7th edition, Prentice-Hall, Inc., Englewood Cliffs, N.J., 1990, p. 741.

of a purchase order. Carrying costs are often called *opportunity costs* or those costs of having money tied up in inventory rather than in a revenue-producing endeavor such as an interest-bearing bank account. Stockout costs are the costs incurred when the supply is not available but is needed. If this is a supply item that the nurse must have for patient care, often the supply must be purchased at a higher price from a local vendor. Finally, quality costs are those costs incurred to ensure that the product is of the required quality. This may include costs such as inspection or replacement or patient harm done by using a low-quality item.

Nurse managers are most often concerned with stockouts. Because many of the supplies used have a direct impact on the quality of patient care provided, nurse managers are particularly sensitive to this issue. In some cases supplies are not readily available from other sources. Patient care will suffer, or a patient may need to be transferred to another institution and revenues will be lost. Although the manager cannot predict with certainty what supplies will be needed, previous experience and expectations about future patient care needs can be used to estimate supply needs.

At the unit level the nurse manager is usually concerned with balancing the space required to store supplies with the goal of avoiding a stockout. The following example shows how to calculate the reorder point for catheter kits. Suppose that the nurse manager knows that the unit usually uses about 0.2 catheter kits per patient day.

Identify the average daily census on the unit = 25
Identify average catheter kits used per patient day = 0.2

Calculate daily usage = Census × Usage per patient day
= 25 × 0.2
= 5 kits needed per day

Identify safe level of supply on unit = 10
Identify lead time to order supplies = 2 days
Reorder point = (Lead time × Average daily use) + Safe level
= (2 × 5) + 10 = 20

Assuming that the census remains at about twenty-five, catheter kits should be reordered when there are twenty remaining.

This simple approach to determine inventory supplies, however, does not tell the manager how much to order. The amount ordered is based on a calculation that takes into account the carrying costs or the ordering costs.

Economic order quantity (EOQ) is an approach to determine the balance between ordering costs and carrying costs. The goal of inventory control is to minimize costs while not encountering a stockout. The manager estimates the optimal quantity of supplies to order and lead time necessary to place that order. For example, suppose that based on historical use the nurse manager on a medical/surgical unit knows that when the unit has twenty-five patients the staff uses 5,000 syringes per year. It takes two days from the time the request is made to the time the supplies reach the floor. Preparing a central supply request costs $5 of a clerk's time. The central accounting office has determined that the organization currently borrows money at a rate of 10% to pay some of its bills and that it costs the organization $.50 per unit for insurance, storage, and other carrying costs per year. This $.50 includes 10% interest on the average inventory level.

Table 18–7 shows an example of the calculations that can be used to estimate the balance between ordering costs and carrying costs. *A* is defined as the demand for the supply for the year. *E* is the size of each order. The average inventory on hand therefore is *E* ÷ 2. There is one purchase order for each order, so the total number of purchase orders per year will be *A* ÷ E. The cost of placing orders is the cost per

※ **TABLE 18–7.** *Economic Order Quantity for Purchase of Syringes*

A	Demand	5,000	5,000	5,000
E	Order size	50	316	5,000
E ÷ 2	Average inventory	25	158	2,500
A ÷ *E*	Number of purchase orders	100	16	1
P(A ÷ *E)*	Annual ordering costs @ $5.00	$ 500	$ 80	$ 5
S(E ÷ *2)*	Annual carrying costs @ $0.50	13	79	1,250
C	Total annual relevant cash	$ 513	$ 159	$1,255

purchase order *(P)* multiplied by the number of orders *(A* ÷ *E)*. The total cost of carrying inventory is the cost to carry one unit for one year *(S)* multiplied by the average inventory level *(E* ÷ 2). The total inventory costs, *C,* in addition to the purchase price of the units is the order cost $P \times (A \div E)$ plus the carrying costs $S \times (E \div 2)$. The nurse manager has estimated that the demand *(A)* for syringes is about 5,000 per year (or about fourteen per day). In the example shown, three possible order sizes *(E)* are identified: 50, 316, and 5,000.

The easiest approach might appear to be the third alternative: order once per year. In that case there would be just one order, at a cost of $5. However, the average inventory on hand would be 2,500 syringes. That would result in high carrying costs of $1,250. The total cost is $1,255. At the other extreme, an order of fifty syringes is sufficient stock for the unit. The costs to the organization of that alternative are $513.

Both the first and third alternatives are substantially more expensive than the EOQ, which is 316 (cost = $159). Ordering a little more than once per month (sixteen times per year) will minimize costs of inventory. The EOQ is calculated with the following formula:

$$EOQ = \sqrt{\frac{2AP}{S}}$$

$$= \sqrt{\frac{2 \times 5{,}000 \times \$5}{\$.50}}$$

$$= 316$$

This formula approach does not take into account that there are sometimes discounts for quantity. The manager should consider what discounts are available and calculate the higher carrying costs associated with larger orders to determine if it is worth taking the discount.

For example, suppose in this problem that there was a $250 discount in purchase price for five orders of 1,000 units each as opposed to sixteen smaller orders. To order 1,000 units at a time, there would be five orders at a cost of $5 each. Therefore the order cost would be $25. The carrying cost would be $S \times (E \div 2)$, or $.50 × (1,000 ÷ 2) = $250. The total costs would be $275. This is $116 higher than the EOQ cost of $159. If we can reduce the purchase cost of the inventory units by $250, the savings will more than offset the $116 increase in inventory management costs. Five orders per year instead of sixteen will be justified.

Even if the nurse manager is not responsible for inventory control, an appreciation of the costs incurred in inventory may make the manager and the staff more sensitive to the issues. It is common for nurse managers to stockpile supplies. Because nurses believe that they cannot provide care without certain supplies and because they have run out of supplies in the past, often extra supplies are hidden for future use. Organizations incur costs associated with inventory. The use of organizational resources can be optimized by efficient inventory control.

※ PLANNING AND TRACKING A PROJECT

Organizations often have the opportunity to pursue new ventures or programs. Careful analysis of the steps involved in the planning and implementation of such projects will lead to smoother implementation.

Successful implementation of a project requires the completion of many activities in a timely fashion. A variety of specific techniques can be used to aid in planning and implementation of a project. Examples of these approaches are the Gantt chart, PERT, and the critical path method. Each of these methods provides an approach for laying out the specific steps to be taken and when each activity must be accomplished. There are computer software programs that apply many of these approaches.

A major benefit of these techniques is that they force the manager to think through all the steps necessary to complete a project. To use them successfully the manager must outline the timing of the necessary steps. In addition they serve as a map of how the project is proceeding. In many cases certain steps must be completed before other steps can occur. If a necessary step is not completed, further work on the project cannot proceed. These methods highlight such "bottleneck" points.

For example, if a hospital plans to open a hospital-based home care agency, the nurse manager may be responsible for the successful implementation of the project. Planning for the project may include activities such as obtaining a certificate of need, hiring staff, renovating space, and developing a marketing strategy. Some of these steps cannot be completed until a prerequisite step is completed. Some may be done concurrently.

The initial step in using any of these techniques is to identify the activities that must be completed. Next the manager estimates the time required to complete the activity and finally the sequence of tasks in relation to other activities.

Gantt Chart

A *Gantt chart* depicts necessary activities or goals in a matrix format with the horizontal axis indicating the time frame and the vertical axis the activities in the project. Exhibit 18–1 shows a Gantt chart for implementation of a skin risk assessment program on two units of a hospital.

The vertical axis shows the activities that must be completed. The horizontal axis shows when the various activities will occur and the expected date of completion. For example, item 5 states "Collect baseline data." Collection of baseline data is expected to take two months. Prior to this period, the nursing staff will need to develop a consensus for a skin assessment protocol to use to collect baseline data. Item 5 will occur during April and May. However, item 6, "Implement education program on two units," will not occur until June, or after the baseline data are collected. Note that data analysis begins in October, even though some data are being collected during that month.

Critical Path Method and PERT

The *critical path method* is a diagram or model of the sequencing of events that must be completed for successful implementation of a project. The first step is to identify all activities that must be completed. The second step is to identify approximately how long it will take to complete the activities. With this information the work flow is diagramed. See Figure 18–14 for an example of a critical path to conduct a comprehensive zero-based budget review. Various methods of depicting an activity (often identified by a number) and the time required to complete the activity are noted. Those points that must be completed prior to the next step are identified and highlighted. In many projects only a few steps are critical. An activity may take a month to complete, but the time line may show several months to

※ **EXHIBIT 18–1.** *Example of GANTT Chart*

	2001											
Project Timeline	**JAN**	**FEB**	**MAR**	**APR**	**MAY**	**JUN**	**JUL**	**AUG**	**SEP**	**OCT**	**NOV**	**DEC**
1. Hire projector director	X											
2. Review literature	X											
3. Train data collectors	X	X										
4. Develop consensus on skin assessment			X									
5. Collect baseline data				X	X							
6. Implement eduation program on two units						X	X	X				
7. Collect post data									X	X		
8. Analyze data										X		
9. Prepare report for QA committee											X	
10. Place for further implementation or options												X

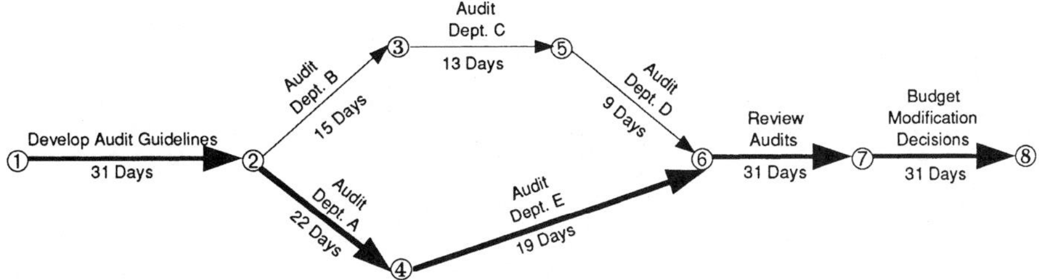

FIGURE 18–14. Critical path method. (Reprinted from *Hospital Cost Management and Accounting,* Vol. 3, No. 6, p. 3, with permission of Aspen Publishers, Inc., © 1991.)

complete the activity. However, some steps in a project are critical, and subsequent steps cannot be done until these steps are completed. These critical steps must be carefully monitored. The critical path is generally shown as a bold line on a diagram.

In Figure 18–14 the days needed to complete an activity are noted under the activity. It can be seen that developing audit guidelines will take thirty-one days. The top path shows that auditing departments B, C, and D will take fifteen, thirteen, and nine days, respectively, for a total of thirty-seven days. The bottom path indicates that auditing departments A and E will take twenty-two and nineteen days, respectively, for a total of forty-one days. This path is part of the critical path and is shown in bold. Activity 6, Review Audits, cannot be completed until this path is completed.

Steps 2-4-6 are critical because a delay of even one day in that path will delay the entire project by a day. By contrast, a delay in path 2-3-5-6 will not delay the project at all. Since this latter path takes thirty-seven days, as compared to forty-one days for the critical path, it has four days of slack. It is not worthwhile to push to shorten work in departments B, C, or D. However, any savings in time in the work in departments A and E could speed up the entire project.

PERT (program evaluation and review technique) is a more sophisticated version of the critical path method.[4] All activities are noted in a network format with events and activities identified. Time estimates are made for optimistic, likely, and pessimistic outcomes. Figure 18–15 shows a PERT chart for a simple project.

The development of a PERT network often begins at the end and works backward to identify those activities that must be completed. The project depicted must be completed in sixteen weeks. Three sets of activities must be completed. The numbers in triangles indicate the earliest week that an activity can start, and the squares indicate the latest week in which an activity can start and the project still be completed on time. The circles indicate the likely time frames. The activities on the top and bottom rows can be completed in four weeks (two weeks plus two weeks) and three weeks, respectively. The middle set of activities will take at least eleven weeks to complete, but twelve weeks are allowed. This path is shown in bold because the entire project cannot be completed until activities on this path are completed, and these activities must be done in sequence. Sophisticated tables may be prepared in addition to the graphic depiction outlining the slack time and the probabilities that events will occur.

For some projects it is necessary to complete the activities as quickly as possible. It may be possible to complete the project sooner, but that will require additional expenditures. For example, it may be possible to complete activity D in five weeks if extra resources are devoted to that activity. The project manager can estimate the time savings and related costs, and estimate whether these costs are justified. In the

[4]See, for example, Warner, D. M., D. C. Holloway, and K. L. Grazier, *Decision Making and Control for Health Administration,* 2nd edition, Health Administration Press, Ann Arbor, Mich., 1984, for a detailed description of PERT and other quantitative methods for decision making.

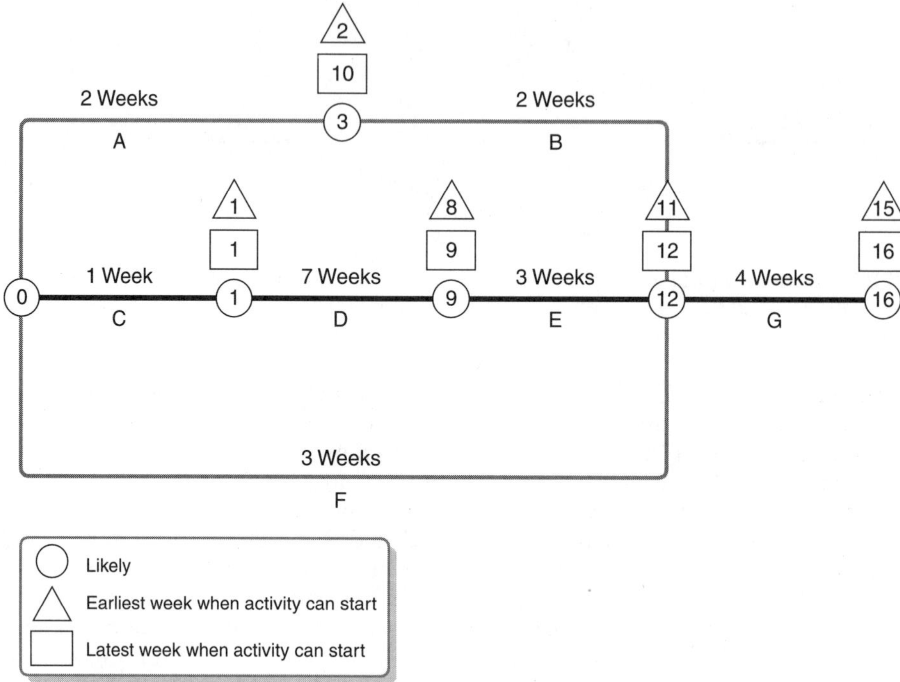

FIGURE 18–15. Example of program evaluation and review technique (PERT).

example above it is unlikely that the costs could be justified. However, the additional revenues generated by opening a new transplant unit two months earlier may justify incurring additional expenses to complete the project more quickly.

In all these methods the person responsible for each activity is usually identified. This identification then offers the manager in charge of the project an opportunity to hold someone accountable for the completion of the various components. That tends to create an environment in which there is increased likelihood of completion of the various phases of the project on a timely basis.

※ IMPLICATIONS FOR NURSE MANAGERS

Forecasting is an essential part of the budgeting process. Some items such as number of patients, length of stay, and acuity are essential ingredients of an operating budget. Preparation of an operating budget cannot begin without some prediction of the values for these variables. The same holds true for other types of budgets.

Most forecasting is based on the theories of probability. Probability, the likelihood that an event will occur, is usually based on historical data.

Managers have great flexibility in selecting the variables that they choose to forecast. They can forecast the number of patients, patient days, the quantity of a resource that will be consumed (e.g., the number of chest tubes needed or the number of nursing care hours), the amount that will be spent on supplies or personnel, or the acuity level of patients. Any variable for which historical data are available can be forecast using the methods presented.

The forecasting process consists of collecting data, graphing the data, analyzing the graphed data, and preparing prediction formulas. Care must be exercised regarding consideration of things that are changing and that will prevent the future from being like the past. For example, a change in federal regulations concerning types of treatments covered by Medicare might have a dramatic impact on volume.

While managers are aware of such changes, computerized formulas are unlikely to take discrete, recent changes into account. The human role in the forecasting process is critical to generating accurate forecasts.

Analysis of the graphed data helps a manager determine whether the item to be forecast has been exhibiting seasonal or trend behavior, both, or neither. Formulas can then be used to make predictions of the future.

It is important for managers not only to use common techniques of management but also to be prepared to be leaders in the development of new uses. The first decade of the twenty-first century will likely see a rapid increase in the use of computers by health care managers. The first wave of microcomputer use in the late 1970s and early 1980s saw widespread introduction of personal computers in positions where the same rote function was performed over and over. Computers clearly increase productivity by being faster at performing a calculation currently done many times. The next wave of computer use in the middle to late 1980s often represented a novelty. Computers were widely introduced, but in many cases they were used only as sophisticated typewriters (word processors).

Managers use personal computers to manage better—not just to do an existing calculation faster and not just to type nice-looking letters, but to manage better. Forecasting is one area where the results of a manager's efforts will be superior because the use of a computer can allow a greater degree of sophistication to be merged with the already existing judgment and experience of the manager.

Specific decision-making tools such as expected value, linear programming, and EOQ can be used by the nurse manager to make better decisions. In addition, approaches such as the Gantt chart and PERT can be used by the nurse manager to plan and manage new programs or projects.

At the same time, one must always bear in mind that the sophisticated quantitative techniques for decision making lack the judgment and experience of managers. Therefore, whether one is using a subjective Delphi technique or a high-powered computer program, the role of the manager in making the final forecast should never be understated.

KEY CONCEPTS

Probability Likelihood that an event will occur. The probability of future events can be estimated based on data from historical events.

Additive rule The likelihood that either one or another event will occur is the sum of the likelihood that each event will occur.

Multiplication rule The likelihood that two or more events will occur simultaneously or in sequence is the product of each event.

Subjective probability Relies not only on the scientific application of the laws of chance but also on the judgment of the manager.

Forecasting Making a prediction of some future outcome. A great number of management decisions are based on forecasts.

Trend Patterns related to the passage of time. A trend may be generally upward, constant, or downward over time.

Time series Approach to forecasting in which historical changes over time are used to help anticipate the likely result in a coming time period.

Seasonality Variations related to seasons of the year. For example, there may be more communicable diseases in the winter when people are indoors more.

Regression analysis Mathematical technique to find the unique straight line that comes closest to all the historical data points. This regression line is used to predict future events.

Curvilinear Curved line. Forecasting methods often assume that there is a straight-line relationship between changes in the variables. Sometimes the relationship is curved. A curvilinear approach to forecasting is especially useful when seasonal patterns exist.

Expected value Method used to estimate the likely value of undertaking an activity that has alternative possible outcomes. It is the weighted average of the value of each possible outcome using probabilities as weights.

Nominal group technique Method for qualitative forecasting in which a group of individuals is brought together in a structured meeting. A consensus forecast is developed.

Delphi technique Method for qualitative forecasting in which the group never meets. A consensus forecast is developed that is less biased by personalities of group members than with the nominal group technique.

Linear programming (LP) Technique to determine how best to allocate scarce resources to achieve a certain goal, which is subject to a number of constraints.

Inventory management Refers to the appropriate ordering and storage of supplies, considering the product cost, ordering costs, stockout costs, carrying costs, and quality costs.

Economic order quantity (EOQ) Approach to determine the optimal quantity for each order. It is based on creating a balance between ordering costs and carrying costs.

Gantt chart Depicts necessary activities or goals in a matrix format, with the horizontal axis indicating the time frame and the vertical axis the activities in the project.

Critical path method (CPM) Diagram or model of the sequencing of events that must be completed for successful completion of the project. Those points that must be completed prior to the next step are identified and highlighted.

PERT (program evaluation and review technique) More sophisticated version of the critical path method. All activities are noted in a network format, with events and activities identified. Estimates are made for optimistic, likely, and pessimistic actual times to complete each step.

SUGGESTED READINGS

Bauer, Jeffrey C., *Statistical Analysis for Decision Makers in Healthcare: Understanding and Evaluating Critical Information in a Competitive Market,* Richard D. Irwin, Burr Ridge, IL, October 1995.

Cleland, V.S., H.A. DeGroot, and I. Forsey, "Computer Simulations of the Differentiated Pay Structure Model," *Journal of Nursing Administration,* Vol. 23, No. 3, March 1993, pp. 53–59.

Corley, M.C., and B.E. Satterwhite, "Forecasting Ambulatory Clinic Workload to Facilitate Budgeting," *Nursing Economic$,* Vol. 11, No. 2, March-April 1993, pp. 77–81, 114.

Dennis, D.K., "Estimating Cost Behavior," In W.O. Cleverley, ed., *Handbook of Health Care Accounting and Finance,* 2nd edition, Aspen Publishers, Inc., Gaithersburg, Md., 1989, pp. 117–134.

Fass, S., "Forecasting Techniques Improve Hospital Budgeting," *Hospital Cost Management & Accounting,* Vol. 9, No. 3, June 1997, pp. 1–8.

Horngren, C.T., G. Foster, and S.M. Datar., *Cost Accounting: A Managerial Emphasis,* 9th edition, Prentice-Hall, Inc., Englewood Cliffs, NJ, 1996.

Shedlawski, J.F., "Value-added forecasting," *Hospital Materials Management Quarterly,* August 1997, pp. 50–55.

Synowiez, Barbara B., and Peter M. Synowiez, "Delphi Forecasting as a Planning Tool," *Nursing Management,* Vol. 21, No. 4, April 1990, pp. 18–19.

Wright, T., "Factors Affecting Cost of Airplanes," *Journal of Aeronautical Sciences,* Vol. 3, No. 2, 1936, pp. 122–128.

Zimmerman, S., "Forecasting and Its Importance to Health Managers in the Ever-Changing Health Care Industry," *Hospital Cost Management & Accounting,* Vol. 7, No. 12, March 1996, pp. 1–8.

CHAPTER

19

Marketing

CHAPTER GOALS

The goals of this chapter are to:

- Explain the essential elements of marketing management
- Relate the roles of nursing and marketing
- Discuss the importance of understanding the needs of customers
- Define basic marketing concepts, including the market, market segmentation, customer behavior, market measurement, market share, market research, determinant attributes, and advertising
- Define the elements of a marketing plan and discuss the role of each element
- Discuss the roles of the BCG matrix and life-cycle analysis in the development of marketing strategy
- Explain the difference between strategy and tactics and discuss the importance of tactics for carrying out strategy
- Introduce the four Ps of marketing: product, price, place, and promotion
- Discuss the implementation and control of marketing plans

※ INTRODUCTION

Virtually every organization desires to provide a high volume of services. Health care *marketing* is a management science that attempts to maintain and increase the organization's patient volume. High volume is desirable because of its financial implications, which are related to the concepts of fixed and variable costs (discussed in Chapter 7). If any costs of the organization are fixed, then increasing volume will inherently spread those costs more widely. Each unit of service will bear a smaller share of the fixed costs. The average cost per unit declines as volume increases because of the sharing of fixed costs.

For example, the costs per patient in a half-full hospital are much higher than in a full hospital because certain costs must be incurred to operate the hospital, regardless of how full it is. These include administration, heat, light, depreciation, and a wide variety of other fixed items. With fewer patients, each must cover a larger share of those costs. If the prices at which services are provided are maintained at a fairly constant level, then rising volume and declining average costs will lead to a higher profit margin per unit of service. This in turn leads to greater financial stability.

Organizations with higher volume can use their improved financial stability in a variety of ways. They can offer a wider range of services, improving health care in the community. They can offer services without an internal environment of perpetual financial crisis. This means that adequate levels of staff and improved quality of care

are more likely. Financial remuneration of employees can be determined based on factors other than what an austerity situation allows.

Many people in health care believe that the key to a successful organization is to provide high-quality care and to let potential patients know that the care is of high quality. Surprisingly, quality is not necessarily a key determining factor in the demand for an organization's health care services. To many consumers, when it comes to health care, quality goes without saying. They would not expect the government to allow any organization to offer health care services that are not of high quality. This perception may well be incorrect. However, it is a common belief.

Factors other than quality often make the difference in where a patient goes for health care services. Convenience, amenities, price, and a wide variety of other factors come into play.

Marketing is an area of management that tries to ensure that the organization achieves and maintains a high volume level. However, to the surprise of many people not familiar with marketing, the essence of marketing is not selling the organization's product. Attaining the high revenues and the profits that result from the provision of a high volume of service is more complicated than simply going out and finding customers to buy the organization's goods and services.

The concept of marketing may be counterintuitive to many nurses. Clinical education focuses on a perspective that people come for care when they are ill or want preventive services such as immunizations. Nurses are not selling patient monitoring in the same way that a department store sells shirts. However, health care organizations are selling their services, and there is nothing inherently unethical about that. If you believe that your facility provides the best care, you want potential patients to be aware of that. If your care is as good as that provided by other facilities in your area, encouraging patients to use your facility will result in higher volume, economies of scale, and ultimately lower costs and/or better services for all your organization's patients.

⁜ THE ESSENCE OF MARKETING: ASSESSING CUSTOMER NEEDS

The short-run focus of marketing efforts is on finding customers for the organization's goods and services. However, that effort is really not the main theme of marketing. Rather, the goal of marketing efforts is to enable the organization to determine what customers want or need and to develop and offer those goods or services. Selling is a minor focus of marketing, while determining what to sell is the essence of marketing.

Most nonmarketing specialists mistakenly assume that marketing consists primarily of determining what type of advertising to use and then implementing an ad campaign. The major efforts of marketing managers, however, are directed toward assessing customer needs.

Too often, organizations formed to respond to an unfilled need remain the same over time, even though they exist in a changing environment. The marketplace tends to be dynamic, in a constant state of flux. Successful organizations respond to changes in the marketplace. The sooner a health care organization can identify changing customer needs, the more promptly it can respond and the more successful it is likely to be.

Prior to the 1950s there were few if any supermarkets. Shoppers went to a variety of different stores to purchase meat, dairy products, fruits, and other groceries. The food suppliers who anticipated the notion of one-stop shopping and developed supermarkets flourished, while other food stores went out of business. The same process was true in the development of department stores.

In the 1990s, however, supermarkets and department stores were under financial pressure in the marketplace. Many affluent shoppers wanted better service than they were getting from large department stores, and they were willing to pay for it. Boutiques and other specialty stores reversed the one-stop shopping trend.

Supermarkets in wealthy neighborhoods were upscaled, particularly in the areas of service and quality. Fresh-baked breads, salad bars, and other amenities appeared in many supermarkets. The trend exhibited recognition by the companies of the changing needs and desires of their customers.

Health care organizations are similarly in a constantly changing environment. The desires of the consumers change. Most health care organizations would be quick to state that they are well aware of the constant change in the technologies and methods for providing health care. Many health care organizations are on the technological edge in providing care. However, simply deciding what a good health care product is and then setting about providing it may not be enough. Designing a better mousetrap will make you rich only if potential customers are interested in catching mice.

Focusing on customer needs often leads to the development of new products, services, and other innovations sooner than they would otherwise be adopted. This in turn makes it easier to market the organization's services. Marketing becomes more oriented to informing potential customers of what is available, rather than trying to sell what you have, whether it is what they want or not. Ultimately, such a focus on customer needs means that the organization provides service to the community rather than simply using the community to serve the needs of the organization.

UNDERSTANDING CUSTOMERS

For health care organizations, marketing represents an unusually great challenge because it is not always clear who the customer is. It is a well-known concept in health care that the physician is often viewed as the true customer, particularly by hospitals. In recent years, it has become more and more apparent that to some extent the managed care organization or insurance company is a customer of health care providers. And in some cases a relative of the patient, rather than the patient, has the decision-making power commonly associated with the ultimate customer.

If you were to buy a gift, would you consider yourself or the ultimate recipient of the gift the customer of the store selling the gift? Clearly, you are the customer. You make the decision to purchase the item. The same can be said in the case of mental health or long-term care. Often the patient lacks the capacity to make choices about the selection of a provider of health care services. For a mental health provider or nursing home, the customer often is a relative of the patient.

In marketing such services it is essential to consider the needs of the relative. Certainly, it is likely that the relative wants the patient to receive high-quality care. Beyond that, however, it may be necessary to provide additional features that make the relative feel the organization is the right one. Perhaps the organization could offer written monthly progress reports to the significant relative. Or perhaps the visiting hours could be made particularly convenient for working relatives. A simple change in visiting hours from 2 to 4 PM to 6 to 8 PM could make a difference in ultimate patient volume. The key for the organization is to know who the customer is and then to focus on the needs or desires of the customer. For most health care organizations there is more than one category of customer.

If the key customer is the insurer, that must be taken into account in the organization's decisions. Sometimes health care organizations try to respond to the needs of their potential patients, incorrectly viewing them as the decision-making customer. New buildings are built with substantial amenities that the patients want. However, patients often want more than they (or the insurers) are willing to pay for. Patients request amenities, thinking that insurance will pay for them.

Insurance companies are starting to find ways to prevent such "moral hazard" behavior. *Moral hazard* refers to the fact that people behave differently if they are insured than if they are not. For example, a homeowner is less likely to have fire extinguishers in the house if there is fire insurance on the house than if there is no insurance. A car owner is more likely to leave an expensive camera on the car seat if it is covered by theft insurance than if it is not. Similarly, patients are more likely to consume more health care services if they have health insurance. They are more likely to see a doctor for minor complaints, and they are more likely to allow the doctor to order a wide range of tests than they would if they did not have insurance.

As a result of widespread health insurance, many people have become used to receiving health care services without direct cost to themselves. Insurance companies, however, have started to encourage patients to use in-network providers or preferred providers (discussed in Chapter 2). They sometimes offer patients full reimbursement for care provided within the network and only partial reimbursement for care from other providers. In such cases the insurer may not be willing to pay for the high costs of fancy amenities. And often, given a choice of paying 30% of a hospital bill and having the amenities or going to a network provider with fewer amenities but no coinsurance, the patients choose the latter. The managed care insurance companies have so much power to steer patients to providers they prefer that it would be foolish for a marketing effort not to consider the needs and desires of the insurer as well as the patient.

The physician and more recently nurse practitioners have a dominant role in health care and cannot be ignored in any discussion of health care customers. These clinicians can steer patients to hospitals and other providers of health care services even more directly than insurers can. Some patients may have a preference for one hospital over another. On the other hand, few patients will have a preference for a particular home health agency. If the clinician refers them to a particular agency for after-hospital home care, they are likely to use that recommended agency. The marketing efforts of home health agencies must be based on the realization that a significant segment of their customers is clinicians.

Even though the services are primarily provided by nurses directly to patients, without clinician recommendations business may be lost. Marketing efforts would therefore have to focus to a great extent on clinicians. Alternatively, a home health agency might attempt to generate referrals from hospital discharge-planning nurses. In that case the nurse becomes a key customer of the agency, along with other clinicians and patients.

WHY IS MARKETING IMPORTANT FOR NURSE MANAGERS?

Keeping the Organization Current

In light of the above discussion of the main goal of marketing efforts, it should become easier to understand why marketing is important for nurse managers to comprehend. Organizations that succeed learn the lesson of marketing: that customer needs must be determined. In health care it is virtually impossible for the organization to fully understand the needs of its customers without input from the nursing staff.

The nursing staff has the pulse of the organization's customers in its hands (both literally and figuratively). Nurses constantly hear from patients and doctors what is good and bad about the organization. They have the most frequent patient contact, and the contact is of substantial duration. They are most likely to hear from the patients about what the organization should be doing better or differently. They are likely to hear from the patients about all the good things some other organization does that this one does not do.

From the marketing manager's perspective, the nursing staff can serve a significant market research role. They can listen to the patient comments and pass the information along to the marketing department. Marketing in turn can use the information to assess the changes that the organization should be making to meet the desires of the patients and physicians.

Customer needs should be a focal point of the organization. Nurses should be considering whether their activities are focused on responding to those needs. Clearly, specific activities may be required that have little direct impact on making the patient feel better. And in no case can all customer needs be satisfied regardless of cost. Nevertheless, there should be an evaluation of whether the work of a nursing unit is communicated to the patients and other clinicians so that they realize that their needs are being addressed.

A research study indicated that the single factor most often cited by patients as related to their satisfaction is staff sensitivity to inconvenience of sickness and hospitalization. As one can quickly see from the results of that study, reprinted in Table 19–1, the three most important indicators of patient satisfaction have a direct bearing on nurse treatment of patients. However, it is not strictly *clinical* treatment that is involved but rather the extent to which nurses relate to the patients' psychological needs. It would appear that the key to marketing success in health care organizations rests not so much on spending money as on having a nurturing and supportive staff attitude toward patients.

The issue of patient satisfaction is essential to every health care organization. A dissatisfied patient is not likely to return to a health care provider. That potential lost future revenue is readily apparent. However, since people talk to each other, the effects of dissatisfaction are multiplied. It has been argued that *each* dissatisfied patient might cost a hospital $400,000. The calculation is reprinted in Table 19–2.

Marketing the Importance of Nursing

Nurses do many things for patients that the patients are never aware of. One aspect of marketing should be to create a greater level of patient education concerning some of the many things nurses do for the patient behind the scenes. This can result in a more satisfied customer, which in turn can lead to additional customers later on. For example, even though in many cases patients do not pick their hospital or home health care agency, there are probably many patients who do become aware of the reputation of a hospital and then affiliate specifically with a clinician who uses that hospital. In other cases, clinicians may be affiliated with several hospitals, and patients will specify a preference when they need an elective procedure.

A vital role played by marketing is the provision of information. Customers may know what they want, but they may not understand the best way to get it. People know that when they are sick, they want to obtain the care needed to get well. The nursing profession should respond to that desire by informing the public of its role in helping them to get well.

If patients were informed of the essential role of high-quality nursing care, they would be likely to consider nursing care in their choices of health care providers. The financial remuneration of nurses is related to the demand for nurses. When demand is high and there is a shortage of nurses, salaries tend to rise. This is in line with the principles of basic economics (see Chapter 4). Therefore, it is in the interest of the nursing profession to keep the demand for nursing services high.

The demand for nursing care would be higher if people demanded that health care organizations provide high-quality nursing care. Therefore there is likely to be a direct return to all nurses from efforts made by the members of the profession to inform the public about what nurses do and why it is important to their health. One approach used to market nursing care is the American Nurses Association magnet hospitals program. In this program high-quality nursing care in hospitals is recognized via designation as a magnet hospital. This designation can be used in the hospital's marketing efforts. Marketing should not simply be something that health care organizations do as a way to compete with each other.

※ **TABLE 19–1.** *Importance of Individual Satisfaction Indicators*

Indicator	Correlation*	Indicator	Correlation*
Staff sensitivity to inconvenience of sickness and hospitalization	.94	Volunteers	.80
Staff concern for patient's privacy	.93	Information regarding diet	.79
Extent to which nurses take patient's problem seriously	.92	Likelihood of receiving food checked on the menu	.79
Time physician spends with patient	.91	Respiratory care	.79
Overall cheerfulness of hospital	.91	Speed of admissions	.79
Nurses' attention to personal and special needs	.90	Courtesy of intravenous care starter	.79
Nurses' attitude toward patient calling them	.90	Courtesy of transportation staff members	.79
Technicians' explanations of tests and treatments	.89	Length of wait for X-ray	.78
Nurses' information about tests and treatments	.88	Physical therapy	.77
Hospital's concern not to discharge patient too soon	.87	How well television worked	.75
Nurses' friendliness	.87	Skill of intravenous care starter	.75
Technical skill of nurses	.87	Social services	.73
Likelihood of recommending hospital to others	.87	Adequacy of advice for home care	.73
Courtesy of business office	.86	Nurses' attitude toward visitors	.73
Adequacy of information given to family about patient's condition and treatment	.86	Discharge waiting time	.70
		Daily cleaning of room	.69
Skill of technician taking blood	.85	Adequacy of visiting hours	.69
Courtesy of technician taking blood	.85	Noise level in and around room	.68
X-ray technicians' concern for patient's comfort	.84	Physicians' information to family	.67
Nurses' promptness in responding to call button	.84	Physicians' information to patient regarding treatments	.66
Cheerfulness of room	.82	Courtesy of information desk personnel	.64
Accommodations and comfort for visitors	.81	Quality of food	.64
Cafeteria or coffee shop rating	.81	Temperature of food	.61
Courtesy of cleaning personnel	.81	Temperature of room	.59
Courtesy of admissions personnel	.80	Physicians' concern regarding questions	.53

*The higher the correlation coefficient, the greater its importance to patients. Correlation coefficients can range from −1.0 to +1.0.

Reprinted from Rodney Ganey and Mary Malone, "Satisfied Patients Can Spell Financial Well-Being," *Healthcare Financial Management,* February 1991, p. 40, with permission of Healthcare Financial Management Association.

※ **TABLE 19–2.** *Costs of Dissatisfied Patients*

Hard Costs	
Dissatisfied patient	1
Assumed revenue associated with a typical hospitalization	× $5,000
	$5,000
Assumed average number of hospitalizations in the patient's remaining lifetime	× 5
	$25,000
Soft Costs	
Dissatisfied patient	1
Additional patients who have a significant complaint but do not register the complaint	+ 6
Significant patient complaints	7
A dissatisfied customer typically tells nine to 10 people of their dissatisfaction	× 9
People eventually receiving negative word-of-mouth information pertaining to the hospital	63
Assuming that one-fourth of the 63 people are influenced by the negative word-of-mouth to the degree that they seek hospitalization elsewhere, apply the "hard" cost assumptions from the analysis above to develop an indication of the potential opportunity cost:	
People receiving negative word-of-mouth information	63
Assumed level of influence	× .25
People choosing to be hospitalized elsewhere	16
Previously determined "hard" costs	× $25,000
Potential lost revenue	$400,000

Reprinted from Virginia Regan Rosselli, Jody Moss, and Randall Luecke, "Improved Customer Service Boosts Bottom Line," *Healthcare Financial Management*, December 1989, p. 22, with permission of Healthcare Financial Management Association.

※ MARKETING CONCEPTS

Understanding the Market

To make any assessment of the desires and needs of a group of customers, it is first necessary to understand as much as possible about the set of customers that constitutes the relevant *market*. The market is defined as the potential customers for a product or organization. Information about the market will affect not only the mix of services that should be offered but also the advertising message, price, and other critical factors.

The information about the market that is needed represents primarily demographic information. The age, race, religion, ethnic background, and mobility of the population should be assessed. The likelihood of change in the existing demographics should also be considered. The marketing efforts of the organization should also include collection of data that will help the organization assess the income and assets of the market, the educational level, and the density of the population.

Understanding the market additionally requires understanding various factors that have an impact on the types of services that can be offered and the prices that can be charged. For example, it is crucial that the organization consider available technologies as well as the wide variety of regulations that affect the organization.

In attempting to understand the market, many organizations also identify key success factors, sometimes called *determinant attributes.* Determinant attributes are factors that ultimately have an impact on a consumer's purchase decision. Generally these factors can be divided into two major types: *decision variables* and *environmental variables.* Decision variables are factors controllable by the organization that can affect volume. Environmental variables are also factors that can affect volume. They, however, are not controllable by the organization.

Data must be collected for both types of variable. Such data, for either decision or environmental variables, may require action by the organization. In the case of decision variables the organization may take steps that have a direct effect on the variable. For example, price, the amount of advertising, and the hours that a service is offered are all decision variables. Suppose that a health care organization found that patients who do not use its services would not only use them but would also be willing to pay a higher price than is currently being charged if the service were offered at more suitable hours. The organization can take a set of definite actions. It can adjust its hours of service, advertise the new hours, and raise the price to cover any higher costs associated with the new hours.

On the other hand, the general economy is not a factor within the control of the organization. However, the organization can respond to the economy. High unemployment during a recession will lead to many psychological problems. Rather than focusing as much on services for stress caused by overwork, the organization can emphasize services available for problems such as depression that result from being laid off. And it can offer to defer payment until the patient is employed. Although the organization can do little about the general economy, it can find a way to serve its community and at the same time increase its patient volume.

Market Segmentation

One essential tool of marketing is to segment the overall market. Segmentation means division of the market into several specific subsections. Some health care organizations have done this already to a great extent. Charging a low price to Blue Cross, perhaps an even lower price to an HMO, and yet a higher price to some insurers or self-pay patients represents a segmentation of the market based on the payer for the services.

By dividing the overall market a number of different objectives can be achieved. It is possible not only to charge different prices to different buyers but also to target preferred customers. For example, suppose that private insurance patients are the most profitable. The organization can target its advertising to media that primarily reach individuals who have private insurance. Advertisements can be placed in magazines read primarily by affluent individuals.

Markets can be segmented in a variety of ways. They can be divided by socioeconomic factors such as age, sex, occupation, and income, or by geography, personality traits, or buyer behavior. For example, some customers are price sensitive; others are quality sensitive; and some consider amenities important. If elderly individuals are most likely to need a service, that service can be advertised in a magazine read by the elderly. The impact of the advertisement is not dispersed over a general public, most of whom do not need the service. The result is that advertisements become more cost effective. It is not only how many people an ad reaches per dollar of cost; it also matters which people the ad reaches.

In general, segmentation is based on three factors. First, one attempts to divide the customer base into groups that have distinct and measurable needs. Second, it is vital that one can assess the specific segments. Finally, the segment must be big enough to merit a distinct effort.

Customer Behavior

Understanding how consumers behave is vital to fashioning the proper mix of services. Not only customer desires and needs but also attitudes and behavior are critical to developing a marketing plan that will create the volume of patients needed by the organization.

Consider a hospital that was losing maternity patients. The hospital was a prestigious research center, known for excellent-quality care. Yet over time its maternity volume was declining. The problem was potentially easily solvable, but the hospital was unaware of buyer behavior and therefore not tuned in to the problem. Unlike other diagnoses, for which patients are unexpectedly rushed to the hospital, maternity provides plenty of advance notice. In fact, many expectant women toured the maternity area as part of their prepared childbirth classes. However, the maternity area was not very presentable. It appeared "old." One expectant mother called it "dirty" and said she refused to deliver her baby at that hospital regardless of its reputation. A coat of paint and perhaps some minor remodeling would probably have easily paid for itself from increased patient volume. The hospital, however, failed to tune in to the effect the condition of the facilities had on preadmission visitors.

Many things affect the behavior of customers. Price, image, or an advertising message are just a few examples. Organizations need to perform market research to ascertain which factors affect consumer behavior, and how. The buying process consists of perceiving a need, getting ready to make a purchase, purchasing, consuming, and reacting after the fact. Lavidge and Steiner[1] have described the process of getting ready to make a purchase as:

Awareness → Knowledge → Liking → Preference → Conviction → and Purchase

A buyer must first perceive a need for health care services. The perceived need is not the marketer's domain. Marketing does not create needs; it satisfies them. Then there must be awareness that the provider exists and knowledge that the provider can meet the need. The buyer must like the provider enough to consider it among other possible choices. The buyer must decide that the provider is the preferred way to go. The preference must be reinforced until it becomes a conviction, and finally a purchase will take place. At any point in the process, the customer may decide to purchase a competitor's services.

Making sure that the potential buyer is aware of the health care organization as a possible source for satisfying needs is an essential role of marketing. Marketing must also put forth information that is likely to cause the buyer to like the organization's product, to prefer it, and to become convinced that the organization is the appropriate source for care. The organization must make sure that its actual production process does in fact fill the perceived need. The after-the-fact reaction of customers will influence future purchase decisions by the patient and the patient's friends and family.

Market Measurement

An important aspect of marketing is the conversion of qualitative information into quantitative estimates of demand. This is referred to as market measurement. Such measurement is made for analysis, planning, and control. Analysis is made of what services to offer. Planning is undertaken to develop the services. Control is conducted to keep performance on target.

The central aspect of market measurement is estimation of market demand. How much will be the total volume purchased by all patients in a defined market area. This measurement requires a thorough definition of the specific product or service whose demand is being estimated. It also requires a clear understanding of the period for which the estimate is being made, such as a week, month, or year into the future. The longer the period for the estimate, the less reliable the data obtained.

Environmental factors must be considered in estimating market demand. Since the demand for any service is affected by various factors outside the organization's control, the assumptions leading to a specific forecast of demand must be understood. For instance, a home health agency might plan geographical expansion into a community under the assumption that managed care organizations (MCOs) will reimburse for a certain number of home visits. If the MCOs were to change their

---

[1]Robert J. Lavidge and Gary A. Steiner, "A Model for Predictive Measurements of Advertising Effectiveness," *Journal of Marketing*, Vol. 25, October 1961, p. 59.

payment policies, the demand estimates might prove faulty. To know how much to rely on demand predictions, one must be able to assess the reasonableness of the underlying assumptions about the environment faced by the organization.

Market demand will also depend, at least to some extent, on the actions taken by the organization itself. The price charged, the advertising campaign undertaken, and other controllable factors can have an impact on market demand, and should be considered in attempting to determine it. Finding the demand for a hospital-based product may not tell the actual demand that would exist if care could be delivered to patients' homes. Estimating demand must be based on the approaches to providing the product or service that the organization is considering or intends to undertake.

Market measurement requires that demand be forecast. Forecasting demand can be done by a variety of methods ranging from crude to sophisticated. The most common of these approaches are surveys, acquisition of expert opinion, and statistical analyses.

Potential patients can be surveyed as to what they would be inclined to do under a given set of circumstances. MCOs and physicians should also be included in the survey process if they have a significant role in steering patients. It should be noted that surveying potential customers is time consuming and expensive.

Another approach would be to obtain expert opinion. For example, the organization could survey members of the nursing staff. In many instances, nurses have the closest experience with what typically happens after the introduction of new services. They may have insight into the process that occurs after the introduction of new services and the length of time before services typically reach certain levels of patient volume. They may also have insight into the attitudes of patients. For example, if one were considering how accepting patients would be of a new surgical procedure, operating room nurses who have had years of experience with surgical patients would be in a good position to provide an important perspective on what the likely acceptance of the new procedure would be. An alternative to the survey technique would be to develop focus groups to discuss the issue under consideration.

Other approaches to market forecasting include time-series analysis (discussed in Chapter 18) and regression analysis (discussed in Chapter 7). These are both sophisticated forecasting tools. However, both techniques require historical information about the items being forecast. When such data are unavailable, the time-consuming survey approach is generally used.

Market Share

Related to the concept of market measurement is *market share*. Market share represents the portion or percentage of the overall market that a specific organization controls. If half of all patients with broken legs in your area come to your ER, then you have a 50% share of the broken-leg market.

Market share is important because rather than being an absolute number, such as the number of broken legs you treat, it shows your status relative to the competition. If your total number of hospital outpatient visits is rising 4% per year, that may seem good. However, if the number of outpatient visits in your city is rising at a rate of 15% per year, then each year your hospital has a smaller share of the total market. This can be a direct warning sign that your competitors are passing you by. It can tell you about your long-term prospects if you remain as you are.

Market Research

Related to market measurement is the broader question of *market research*. This includes gathering, recording, and analyzing information to improve decisions made by the organization. Market research is needed to determine what the customer really wants and is willing to buy. The major areas for market research are advertising, business economics, products, and sales.

Advertising research focuses on issues such as the appropriate copy to use and the appropriate media for advertisements for a product or service. Business economics research considers forecasting general trends in the environment. Product research considers potential acceptance of new products, analysis of competitors' products, and other factors related to the delivery of services. Sales research focuses on issues such as market characteristics and market share.

The market research process consists of defining the problem to be investigated, constructing the model, collecting data, and interpreting data. The statement of the problem must be carefully framed, and the intended use of the research understood, to avoid wasting substantial effort. The result of the research should be to produce not just interesting information but information that is useful for making a particular decision.

A model must be constructed to ensure full understanding of all possibilities. For instance, the research might focus on the outcomes of a decision by a hospital to increase advertising to raise the hospital's profile in the community. The market research model would consider each possible ramification of the campaign. One element of the model would cover possible competitive responses. The competing hospitals might not react to the campaign, might react modestly, or might react strongly. Based on the competitive reaction, consumers might react in a variety of ways. Each possible outcome and its likelihood must be evaluated.

To evaluate the outcome of each possibility, data must be collected. They can be collected from primary sources such as observations, experiments, or surveys or from secondary sources such as existing files, service organizations that collect and sell data, or available publications. Secondary data are much easier to obtain and less costly, but they may not be relevant to the particular problem at hand. Primary data, in addition to being costly, have other inherent problems. Surveys, whether by mail, telephone, or in person, have a nonresponse rate. Are nonresponses randomly distributed? Those who feel strongly, either positively or negatively, may be more or less likely to respond. Failure to get data from that group may bias the results. Surveyors themselves may bias the results by the way they ask questions.

It is important that data collected be valid and reliable. Ensuring quality of data requires a high level of expertise. While nurse managers can help their organizations by having a basic knowledge of the field of marketing, many elements of marketing, such as market research, should be conducted by experts in the field.

It is incumbent on the organization to use market research to determine which factors are really important to the ultimate purchase decision. Therefore market research should always include analysis of the product or service's determinant attributes (discussed earlier). Depending on the product or service, this may mean considering the impact of convenience, price, special services, or any of a number of other characteristics.

Advertising

Advertising makes people aware of an organization and its products, provides knowledge about the product, and, one hopes, creates a preference for and loyalty to the organization's services. Advertising can come in the form of paid advertisements, personal selling, sales promotions, and other forms of publicity. The level of expenditures on advertising should be established so that the extra benefits from extra advertising always exceed or are at least equal to the extra cost. This is based on the concepts of marginal costs and marginal benefits (discussed in Chapter 4).

In advertising there are many critical questions to be addressed. How many people are reached by a campaign? Are they the right people? Is the message making the desired impact? It is not sufficient to have a slick presentation. The message must be designed and presented based on what is likely to work with the desired audience. The presentation and timing of the message are as important as simply reaching a large number of people.

⁂ MARKETING PLANS

Marketing is based on a strategic planning approach. Plans are made to achieve a goal. An unusual aspect of marketing plans is that they often tend to be disruptive. The plan is often aimed at making change occur. At a minimum, marketing may take patients away from competitors. Often marketing plans call for changes in the current operations of the organization. Change generally meets resistance. For the marketing plan to be effective in an environment in which reactions to the plan both internally and by competitors are likely, the plan must be carefully established.

Marketing plans should first consider the organizational mission and goals. Then internal/external analyses must be performed, a strategic marketing plan developed, and specific tactics developed. Plans must then be revised, integrated, and implemented. Finally, control and feedback are essential to an effective plan.[2]

Organizational Mission/Goals

The marketing plan should support the organizational mission. Most health care organizations have realized the importance of having a basic mission statement to guide the organization. Based on the mission statement, organizational goals can be set and strategic plans made to carry out those goals. Strategic planning is discussed in Chapter 10.

It is inappropriate to develop a marketing plan without referring to the organization's mission and strategic plan. Marketing plans often encompass major changes in product offerings, not simply the sale of existing services. Therefore the organization can easily find itself working at cross-purposes unless there is a mesh between the overall direction that the organization wants to take and the direction in which the marketing plan takes it.

Internal-External Analysis

The internal-external analysis consists of analysis of the environment, including the competition, and of the organization's internal capabilities in light of the needs and desires of the consumer. There must always be a continuing focus first and foremost on what the organization's customers need. The ability of the organization to satisfy those needs, in light of the competition, is the basis for an internal-external analysis. The opportunities and threats disclosed by this analysis must be carefully considered before any strategies can be developed. The analysis itself makes use of tools such as market measurement and market research, discussed above.

The organization's environment is a critical piece of the puzzle of trying to determine how to successfully provide services to the community. Questions about the environment that should be addressed in a marketing plan include the size of the market, the growth rate of the market, stability of prices, and the degree of competition. Factors such as social attitudes and reimbursement rules must also be considered.

The next element of the internal-external assessment is identification of the market and its needs. This assessment should include both internal and external markets. For example, if physicians are considered crucial to generating patients, they should be assessed along with patients. An example of a data collection form for identifying markets and needs is given in Exhibit 19–1.

---

[2]Hillestad, Steven G., and Eric N. Berkowitz, *Health Care Marketing Plans: From Strategy to Action*, 2nd edition, Aspen Publishers, Gaithersburg, Md., 1991, p. 54.

※ EXHIBIT 19–1. *Identification of Major Markets and Needs*

Part I—Identifying markets. A market or market segment consists of a group of people who have common demographic, specialty, or social characteristics that represent a size large enough for the organization to concentrate resources around.

Potential Markets	*Importance of Market (check one column for current and future)*						*Current Attitude Toward You (circle one number)*				
	Current			*Future*			*Very Favorable*			*Very Unfavorable*	
	High	*Med*	*Low*	*High*	*Med*	*Low*	1	2	3	4	5
Gen. medicine M.D.'s							1	2	3	4	5
Surgeons							1	2	3	4	5
OB/gyn							1	2	3	4	5
Peds							1	2	3	4	5
Other M.D.'s							1	2	3	4	5
Inpatients (by specialty)							1	2	3	4	5
Outpatients							1	2	3	4	5
Community at large							1	2	3	4	5
Donors							1	2	3	4	5
Board of directors							1	2	3	4	5
Insurance companies							1	2	3	4	5
Regulators							1	2	3	4	5
Business/ industry (specify)							1	2	3	4	5
Have no doctor market							1	2	3	4	5
HMO patients							1	2	3	4	5
Over-65 market							1	2	3	4	5
Nonuser market							1	2	3	4	5
Females							1	2	3	4	5
Males							1	2	3	4	5
Others ______							1	2	3	4	5
______							1	2	3	4	5
______							1	2	3	4	5

Part II—Based on the mix of actual and potential markets listed in Part I, indicate the size and future potential.

Key Market Segments from Part I	*Size Today*	*Future Size—Three Years*	*Your Current Market Share*
25 thru 34-year-old males - athletics	9% of metro area	14%	32% of medical care needs in sports medicine programs

Part III—Based on completion of Parts I and II, indicate the needs major market segments are likely to exhibit.

Key Market Segments	*Needs*
25 thru 34-year-old males in sports medicine program	Greater emphasis on strength, training, cardiovascular fitness

Reprinted from *Health Care Marketing Plans,* 2nd edition, by S. Hillestad and E. Berkowitz, with permission of Aspen Publishers, Inc., © 1991.

※ EXHIBIT 19–2. *Relative Competitor Assessment Form*

Competitor (specify): ______	*Much Worse*	*Somewhat Worse*		*About the Same*			*Somewhat Better*		*Much Better*
	−4	*−3*	*−2*	*−1*	*0*	*+1*	*+2*	*+3*	*+4*
1. Medical care									
A. Emergency									
B. Surgery									
C. Gen. medical									
D. Special care									
2. Nursing care									
3. Housekeeping (hospital)									
4. Food service (hospital)									
5. Staff morale									
6. Facility: Capacity/attractiveness									
7. Public relations									
8. Reputation									
9. Image (overall)									
10. Management									
11. Lab services									
12. Convenience									
13. Staff education									
14. Equipment: Capability/technology									
15 Range of services									
16. Marketing plan									
17. Ad/promo budget									

Competitive Assessment: For each competitor on which you have a Competitor Assessment form, indicate the level of competitive intensity, your share of the market, and the basis for competition.

	Competitor	*Market Share*	*Level of Competitive Intensity*					*Basis for Competition*			
			Very Intense				*Not Competitive at All*	*Product*	*Price*	*Promotion*	*Distribution*
1.	______	______	1	2	3	4	5	______	______	______	______
2.	______	______	1	2	3	4	5	______	______	______	______
3.	______	______	1	2	3	4	5	______	______	______	______
4.	______	______	1	2	3	4	5	______	______	______	______
5.	______	______	1	2	3	4	5	______	______	______	______
6.	______	______	1	2	3	4	5	______	______	______	______
7.	______	______	1	2	3	4	5	______	______	______	______
8.	______	______	1	2	3	4	5	______	______	______	______

Conclusion:

Knowing the basic markets is a critical first step. Next the markets must be fully understood. What factors result in changes in the marketplace? Are the key factors that cause the market to change related to demographics (e.g., population aging), regulatory changes (e.g., in reimbursement), or available medical services (e.g., as a result of technology)? Can the market be segmented, and if so, how attractive a market is each segment? The organization must make every effort to know not just what the markets are but why they are. What influences them and causes them to change, or to remain the same, over time?

Having gained some insight to the markets that are relevant for the organization and the needs of the market, the analysis must thoroughly examine the competition. Strengths and weaknesses of the organization vis-à-vis its competition are crucial foundations for the development of any market strategy. Exhibit 19–2 presents an example of a form that can be used to collect and record data concerning competition.

Organizations should attempt to understand any *differential advantages* they have. A differential advantage is some characteristic that provides the organization with a distinct advantage over a competitor. Such advantages might include location, cost, and services offered, among other factors. For example, a women's care center may have a distinct advantage over a general care center for treating particular problems. Organizations should constantly be attempting to develop differential advantages for themselves and trying to find ways to overcome differential advantages held by the competition. One can think of a differential advantage as creating a barrier that keeps out competition.

Just as the strengths and weaknesses of the competition must be known, so also must the organization assess its own relative merits. Being aware of the external environment is only helpful to the extent that the organization can take advantage of that information. Unless the organization conducts a thorough internal analysis of what it can and cannot do, it will be unable to take advantage of such information.

Strategic Marketing Plan

According to Hillestad and Berkowitz, many managers "call the marketing staff with the following question: 'I would like to involve you in a strategy to help our orthopedics program; could you help us put together a brochure that we can send out to doctors about the program?'"[3] The problem with this approach is that it implies that the previous two steps—evaluating the mission and goals and performing an internal-external review—probably have not been undertaken. Furthermore, the brochure represents not a strategy but a tactic.

Strategies are broader frameworks by which goals can be attained. *Tactics* represent the specific activities that must be undertaken to carry out a strategy. There are many strategic approaches that organizations can adopt. An organization can choose to charge lower prices than the competition to achieve a high market share. Or it can adopt a strategy of high prices with the expectation of a highly profitable low market share. Organizations can decide to push their product, going to the customer, or use a pull strategy, making the customer come to them.

Organizations can develop strategies to create barriers to prevent other potential providers from competing. One approach is to charge low prices to gain a large market share. Competitors are likely to be reluctant to enter a market where there is already a dominant force. Another approach to the creation of barriers is to make it costly for consumers to shift to another care provider. Yet another strategy is to offer a product that only this one organization can provide.

Sometimes strategies involve creating a high profile for quality leadership or

---

[3]Ibid., p. 107.

focusing efforts on the development of one new product. A strategy can be to become known for patient service or for convenience. A key element in setting strategies relates to the nature of the specific product or service being considered. Several techniques have been developed that can help an organization develop appropriate strategies for different products. In particular, the BCG matrix and life-cycle analysis provide excellent information for use in strategy development.

The BCG Matrix

To help organizations with strategic planning for products, the Boston Consulting Group (BCG) developed a product matrix that has become widely used in developing product strategy. The matrix considers growth potential and market share for different products or services an organization offers. The matrix is somewhat simplistic, assuming that each product or service has either a high or low market share and either a high or low potential for growth. The BCG framework is presented in Figure 19–1.

If a product has a high market share and a high potential for growth, it is considered a "star" performer in the BCG approach. It is clearly worthy of continued attention and efforts on the part of management. Just the reverse is true for a service with low current market share and low potential for growth. Management would not be using its time wisely to put substantial efforts into trying to market that product. BCG refers to such products as "dogs."

The other two cells in the matrix are less clear-cut. A product or service for which the organization has high market share but that has low growth potential is generally referred to as a "cash cow." Since there is a high market share, it is likely that the organization can charge a high price, generating substantial profits. Even if prices are not high, the high market share should mean that the organization has a cost advantage. It can spread the fixed costs over a larger number of patients, generating a lower cost per patient than is possible for competitors with smaller market share. Therefore profits should still be high for cash cows.

Cash cows not only are profitable but also throw off cash dividends. A star is profitable, but its growth may require that much of the profit be reinvested in additional capacity. Since the growth potential is low for a cash cow, it often does not require reinvestment of the cash it generates. That cash is available for providing other services.

The last cell is referred to as a "problem child." Will its high growth potential be enough to offset the disadvantage of low market share? Over time this type of service may become either a dog or a star. Careful assessment is needed before investing resources in marketing this product.

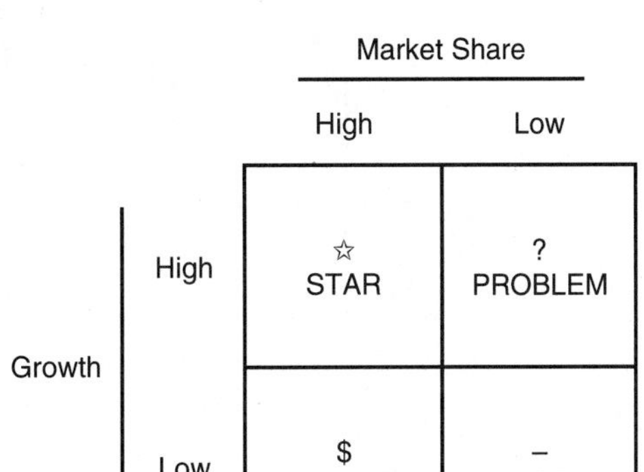

		Market Share	
		High	Low
Growth	High	☆ STAR	? PROBLEM
	Low	$ CASH COW	– DOG

FIGURE 19–1. BCG matrix.

Life-cycle Analysis

An alternative to the matrix developed by BCG is an approach called life-cycle analysis. Such analysis argues that early in the life of a new product or service the organization will have a low market share in a product that has high growth potential (BCG's problem child). This is the new-product stage of the life cycle.

If the product's introduction is successful, it will become what BCG calls a star. That will represent a period when the organization has a significant market share in a growing market. The product will be profitable and growing. This is therefore considered the growth stage of the life cycle.

At some point, the growth potential will diminish; most of the pent-up demand for the new product will have been satisfied. There will have been a spurt of growth by competitors to the point that market demand is stable and is supplied by an existing set of organizations. Each will have its own market share, but no one will be having much growth. Although BCG terms this stage a cash cow, it is not at all clear that at this mature stage in the life cycle there will be substantial profits. BCG's model simplistically assumes high or low market share. It is possible to have a number of major competitors that split the market and compete to a point at which there are few if any profits.

When the product or service starts to be replaced by a new alternative, volume drops. Since fixed costs cannot decline in the short term, profits drop sharply. It is this declining point in the life cycle of the product that BCG refers to as a dog. Figure 19–2 shows the volume potential likely at each stage in the life cycle of a product.

Strategically it is important to remain aware of the stage of each of an organization's services. When a product reaches the dog stage, or declining period, the organization should already have focused on the replacement product that consumers will need instead of the declining product and should have made substantial progress in introducing a new replacement product. Organizations that persist in simply stepping up their marketing efforts to keep selling an existing service often miss the boat. Marketing wisdom is not to sell the product you have but to provide the products and services that customers need and want. This means that marketing requires most organizations to constantly revise their thinking about what their product is and how it can best be provided to the customer.

As innovations enter the health care marketplace, they affect existing services. Figure 19–3 shows the history of diagnostic imaging. As nuclear imaging and ultrasound have become more widely used, the growth of radiography has leveled

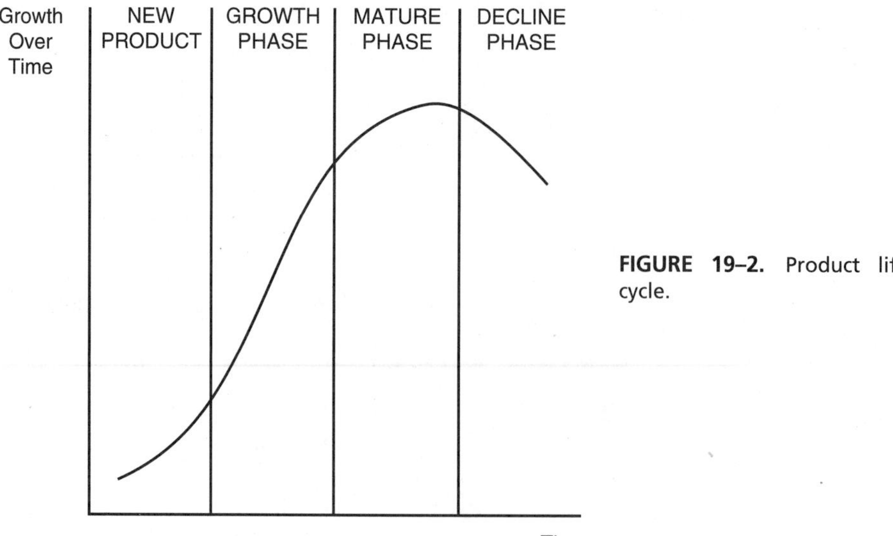

FIGURE 19–2. Product life cycle.

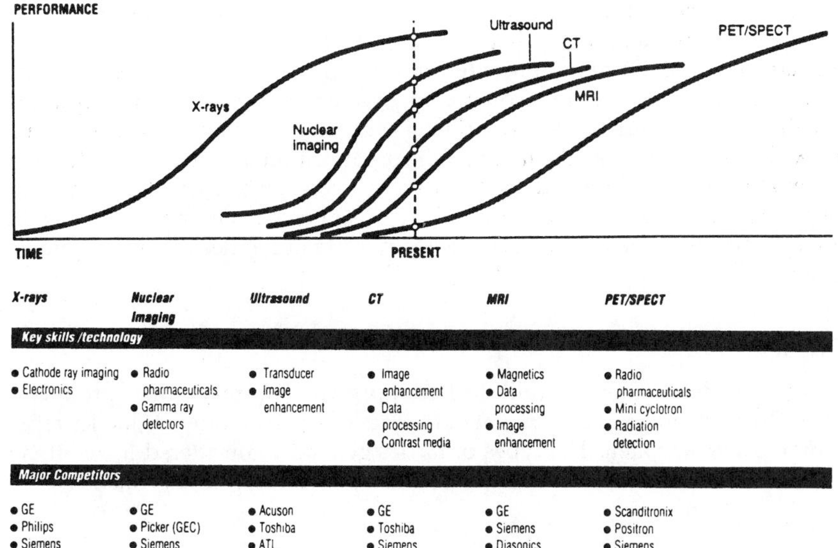

FIGURE 19–3. Development of diagnostic imaging. (Reprinted from *Health Care Forum Journal,* Vol. 32, No. 5, p. 25, with permission of the publisher, © 1989, Association of Western Hospitals.)

off. Positron emission tomography (PET) scanning, on the other hand, is still in its new-product, growth stage.

Choice of Strategy

The determination of where a product or service is in its life cycle has a direct bearing on the type of strategies that should be utilized. Early in a product's life cycle the organization's strategy should be aggressive. Introduction of the product should be rapid, in an attempt to gain dominant market share before competitors can react. However, that does not require low price. Prices can be set high if there is little competition. However, it should be realized that the higher prices are set, the more competitors are encouraged that the potential benefits make it worthwhile to enter the market for that service or product. New products require an aggressive advertising campaign to inform the public about the product.

During a product's growth stage it is important to differentiate the product or service from that of competitors. There must be some feature that will make customers prefer the product offered by the organization. Obviously, unique superiority of the product is preferable. Failing that, the organization must decide if price, convenience, or some other factor can be affected to result in customer preference.

At a mature stage in a product's life cycle, most services are well established. The focus of marketing efforts is primarily on maintaining market share. Aggressive behavior will often not be rewarded; competitors with a major stake in the same service will not likely allow significant shifts in market share. Aggressiveness may well lead to a costly battle with competitors, with little gain, if any, in volume. Marketing becomes a maintenance operation. Slight modifications are made to the product to keep it current if possible, advertising efforts are made to reinforce customer awareness, and responses are made to repel the effects of any moves by competitors.

In the declining period of a product's life cycle the organization has a difficult choice. Should the organization try to establish its own special place in the declining market; should it gradually phase out a product; or should it drop the product completely? This question can be answered only by looking at each individual case.

Sometimes, even if a product is declining on an industry-wide basis, there is room for one provider. To be that provider it must be decided whether the key characteristic of the surviving provider will be price, service, convenience, or some other factor. Before it becomes too late, the organization must build a reputation in line with that characteristic. An advertising campaign late in a product's life may be worthwhile if it can convey the fact that the organization has that special feature that the ultimate survivor in the industry must have to attract sufficient volume. Loyalty among the base of customers who are likely to still be consuming the service in five years must be developed before it becomes too late in the decline of volume for the product or service.

Tactics

Strategies define the overall desired approach to marketing products and services. To carry out the strategy a set of tactics must be employed. Tactics represent the specific actions taken. The types of tactics generally considered have often been referred to as the four Ps of marketing: *product, price, place,* and *promotion.*

Product

The product is the essential element that the marketing plan is attempting to sell. The product has been selected and developed based on prior analysis of customer needs, the organization's mission, internal-external analysis, and finally strategy. However, several tactical issues must still be addressed.

First, the organization must make a decision concerning the specific characteristics of the product, such as its quality. Will quality be the least the organization can get away with, average, or noteworthy? The actual decision relating to the level of quality is a strategic one. Carrying out the decision is tactical. How does one go about attaining a noteworthy level of quality? One approach is to attract famous surgeons to the staff and then let the public know. An alternative tactic would be to increase nursing care hours per patient day and inform the public of that fact and its positive implications. An alternative approach would be to beef up the quality assurance team. The choices of how to go about quality attainment are tactical.

Another feature is service. Again, it is a strategic question whether the organization is willing to incur the costs associated with high levels of service. But it is a matter of tactics whether service should consist of free taxi service to and from the organization. It might be worthwhile to have a host or hostess greeting patients upon arrival at the front door and taking them to admitting. Perhaps service should be provided in the form of follow-up phone calls several days after the service has been provided to ask how the patient is doing and whether any further service can be provided. In some cases a basket of fruit awaiting the patient in the room might be appropriate. The key to service is to do more than expected, to go the one extra step to make the customer take note.

Nurse managers should consider their tactics carefully, since they often come into direct contact with two different classes of customers: patients and physicians. The marketing motto "The customer is always right" can be irritating to anyone who actually must try to deal with a rude or irrational customer. Nurses, however, cope well with the irrationalities of patients, understanding how miserable it is to be sick.

One hears many anecdotes about physicians who mess up and need nurses to save the day. There is no question that nurses serve a vital role and that physicians could not get along without them. However, from a marketing perspective, that result is exactly what one would want. When physicians think they receive no direct benefit from a hospital, they start providing a greater range of patient services, including surgery, in their own offices. The reason that physicians rely on hospitals, even for outpatient surgery, is that the hospital provides some desired product or service to the physician as a customer. In many cases that desired product or service is the very nursing care that many physicians *seem* to take for granted.

As long as the physician is a key element in bringing the ultimate paying customer into a health care organization such as a hospital, the physician remains a customer, and the organization must respond by developing a set of tactics to keep the customer coming to the organization. One reason many hospitals provide unequal treatment to doctors and nurses is not a question of professionalism; it stems to a much greater extent from the fact that doctors are viewed as customers, and nurses are viewed as employees.

Viewing doctors as customers results in attempts by organizations to determine their needs. A strategy might be to increase efforts to make the organization accessible to affiliated physicians. If a particular physician wants OR time at 7 AM on Tuesdays, then a tactic to carry out the strategy is development of a specific incentive for other surgeons to use the OR on days other than Tuesday. That incentive might be a special effort to assign specific OR nurses requested by surgeons on days other than Tuesday.

Price

Price matters. Many people assume that with most of the population insured by Medicare, Medicaid, or private insurers, price does not matter. However, a growing portion of the buyers of health care services are becoming sensitive to price variations. HMOs and PPOs negotiate aggressively for the best prices they can obtain. Each organization must determine how sensitive its customers are to price and base a policy accordingly.

There are a number of different approaches to setting prices. Some organizations like to simply use a *markup.* That is, they determine the cost of providing care and raise, or mark up, the price a certain percentage over the cost. The problem with this policy is that the low-volume producer will have the highest cost (because fixed costs are not shared over a large volume of patients) and therefore the highest price. It will be difficult to increase volume and therefore reduce costs and reduce prices if you start out as a high-priced producer.

Another alternative is to charge a particularly low price, perhaps even lower than cost, to gain a substantial increase in market share. The philosophy is that even though you may lose money on each patient, as volume increases, average cost will decrease and patients will eventually become profitable at the price being charged. Further, capturing a substantial share of the market may force other providers to discontinue offering the product or service. When there are fewer providers, it may be possible to raise prices to increase the profit margin. Legal input is required to ensure that price is not set so low that it would violate antitrust laws.

Another tactic is to charge a high price, knowing that market share will be low, but planning to make a high profit on the volume achieved. This is sometimes referred to as *skimming.*

There are many other tactical approaches to price setting. The organization can charge different prices depending on the time of the day or the day of the week. For example, if an HMO wants a discounted price, a hospital that is running near capacity can offer the discount only if most patients are admitted during slower periods. For example, the HMO can agree that surgeries will be performed on weekends or other slow days or during the slower parts of the day. In this way the organization can continue to take all full-price patients at the time most convenient for the patients and their physicians. The patients with the price break will give up some convenience for the lower price.

Place

In real estate the three most important factors that establish the value of property are location, location, and location. In marketing health care services much the same is true. Traditional health care services generally expect the patient to come to the service. If the service is in an inconvenient location, it will be difficult to attract patients. While home health agencies generally visit patients, many other health care services have lagged in coming to the patient. However, more innovative approaches to health care services do attempt to bring the services closer to the patients. For example, there are now national mail-order pharmacies. Many disabled patients can avoid the high cost of a taxi to go to and from the pharmacy.

The issue of "place" is closely tied to the concept of *distribution channels*. The concept of distribution channels relates to moving the product from the producer to the consumer. How does the product get from the provider of the service to the ultimate consumer? In the case of a home care agency, the provider brings the product directly to the patient. In the case of a hospital, the patient comes to the provider. Clearly, if the distribution channel can be modified to bring the product closer to the consumer, there is a better chance of being the provider of choice.

Distribution channels are referred to as direct or indirect, depending on whether the consumer and the provider have a direct relationship or whether there is some intermediary. When a patient is admitted to a hospital on the advice of a clinician, there is an indirect channel between the patient and the hospital. The hospital is at risk if the intermediary—the clinician—decides to use a different hospital. If the hospital opens a series of clinics around the community, staffed with full-time clinician employees of the hospital, the distribution channel is direct.

Clearly, it is to the advantage of a health care provider to have a direct channel to the patient. However, this arrangement creates its own costs and risks. In the above example the hospital must take on the burden of operating a series of clinics. The clinics may be unprofitable, more than offsetting the advantage of the direct linkage. They may also alienate the other clinicians in the community who resent the hospital's competition. A hospital must adopt a strategy concerning whether it wants to establish direct channels of distribution or is willing to accept indirect channels.

One potential solution to this problem is to arrange a confederation with one or more clinician group practices. Figure 19–4 presents a possible form for such an arrangement. The group practice and the hospital each provide half the members of a management committee. The committee gives the clinician a greater amount of input in running the hospital. The hospital gains a direct distribution channel.

Once the strategic decision regarding the use of direct or indirect channels is made, tactics must be developed. If the strategy is to use direct channels, then the tactics concern the exact location of clinics and their size, staffing pattern, and hours. If the strategy is acceptance of indirect channels, then the tactics concern the actions the hospital could take to keep the referring physicians happy and ensure that they do not start referring patients elsewhere. The tactics are less certain here, and a great deal of effort must go into determining what factors influence where a clinician refers patients. If the key issue is attending to clinician needs, then someone should call the clinician periodically to ask whether the hospital is doing all it can for the clinician. If the key issue is available beds when needed, then the hospital must develop an admission process that ensures that certain clinicians always get a bed when they need it.

Which clinician should always get a bed? Should it be the one with the largest number of admissions? Or should it be a clinician with a marginal number of admissions? That is a difficult tactical issue. The clinician with the largest number of

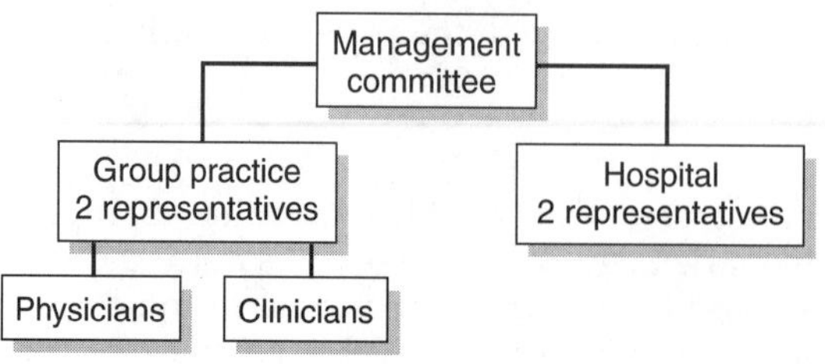

FIGURE 19–4. Direct distribution channel. (Reprinted from Deborah Arbitman and Paul King, "Affiliated Practices Can Boost Patient Referrals," *Healthcare Financial Management*, August 1990, p. 34, with permission of Healthcare Financial Management Association.)

admissions may not be in a position to move from the hospital, and a clinician with a marginal number may be quite likely to move. Health care providers must carefully consider the long-run implications of their tactics. Then they can make a reasoned decision about what approach is likely to be in the best interests of the organization.

Promotion

The last of the four tactical concerns is the one most people associate with marketing: promotion. Promotion consists of advertising, public relations, sales promotion, and personal selling. The strategy of the organization will determine which products or services will receive significant promotion in a given period. The tactical questions revolve around what combination of the four promotion approaches to use and how to go about each one.

Tactics determine whether to use print media or radio or television. Tactics focus on which newspapers or magazines, which radio or television programs, which days of the week, at which time of the day. Should nurse managers be encouraged to teach in local nursing schools as a means of public relations? Should they be paid by the health care provider while they are teaching? How much money should be spent on mass advertising and how much on a sales force?

For a home care agency, advertising creates a general public awareness. However, most patients are referred by physicians, social workers, or discharge-planning nurses. One full-time sales person will likely reach only 1,000 people per year. The advertisements that could be bought for the same money might reach hundreds of thousands. Tactically, however, one must decide which is a better buy for the money and whether the money is wisely spent on either alternative.

• • •

While the four Ps of marketing are widely discussed, it is a mistake to view marketing as a subject that can be mastered with simple tools such as a BCG matrix or by memorizing that tactics often fall under the rubric of the classic four Ps. Hillestad and Berkowitz note that every detail can have an impact on a customer, either positive or negative. Things as small as the little alligator on a sport shirt, a 30-minute pizza delivery guarantee, a call-back from a nurse, or a handwritten note to a referral physician—all examples of marketing tactics—can have an impact. The depth and breadth of marketing decisions are enormous, as are the opportunities to make mistakes. Service, design, packaging of the service, promotion, location, and pricing are all interwoven to make for hundreds of possible combinations for any given service.[4]

It should become clear that marketing does play a more substantial role than simply advertising the organization's products. Marketing is integral to deciding what products or services should be offered. When the plan is adopted, it creates change in what products and services are offered. In light of that, nursing managers should not treat informational requests from marketing as a peripheral annoyance to be handled quickly and without much thought. Six months later the decisions based on that information will come back in specific operational changes. Marketing has a significant and growing role in health care organizations, and interactions between nursing and marketing warrant careful thought and attention.

※ MARKETING FAILURES

It would be nice to believe that any organization that realizes the potential benefits of marketing will succeed in its marketing efforts. Unfortunately, that is not

---

[4]Ibid., p. 149.

always the case. History has shown that many marketing campaigns do fail. Learning from those failures should help others to avoid them.

It is true that sometimes everything will be done right and marketing efforts will still fail. However, avoiding certain common shortcomings can reduce the likelihood of that result. Specifically, common failures are often due to several specific factors.

One major problem is failure to collect data prior to making decisions. Decisions based solely on intuition may fail after substantial financial investment, when a modest amount of market research data collection could have indicated that the financial investment was unwise.

Another problem relates to errors of analysis. Data may be collected but not carefully interpreted. One key concern that managers should have is that new products and services often have strong advocates. Such people may not neutrally evaluate information, since they have a vested interest in its interpretation.

A third key element common to failure is a lack of clear objectives. Marketing should not be rushed, without careful consideration of exactly what needs to be accomplished. Focusing the marketing plan carefully on a specific set of objectives increases the likelihood of achieving them.

Finally, many organizations use incorrect tactics. It is important that carrying out the objectives of a plan be done in light of the specific clearly stated objectives. The tactics must fully and directly support the accomplishment of the goals that have been set.

※ THE ROLE OF MARKETING IN NURSE RECRUITMENT

There have been nursing shortages periodically throughout this century. When a health care provider is attempting to hire nurses, those nurses effectively become customers from a marketing perspective. In attempting to minimize the impact of a nursing shortage on an organization, a variety of marketing techniques can be used. For example, advertising is often used to attract new nurse employees, and advertising is one element of marketing.

However, marketing does not start with advertising. It starts with identification of the need or desire and the filling of that need or desire. These elements must precede advertising. Only then can a specific plan be developed regarding communication of the strengths that the organization has to offer. The role of marketing in nurse recruitment is discussed in Chapter 9.

※ IMPLICATIONS FOR NURSE MANAGERS

Marketing activities are much more highly related to nursing management than most nurses realize. The first and most vital aspect of marketing is assessing the needs and desires of the customers of the organization. Nurses are in a position to be attuned to those needs and desires, both in the case of patients and in the case of physicians.

Another major aspect of marketing is assessing the capabilities of the organization. Here again, the input of nurses is vital to gaining a clear understanding of the strengths and limitations of the organization.

The strategic and tactical issues of marketing also warrant close cooperation between nursing and marketing. Nurses are unlikely to enthusiastically work to carry out organizational strategies that they cannot support. Therefore, there should be substantive discussions between nursing and marketing as strategies are developed. Nurses should give direct input on what strategies they think are good, which ones are bad, and why. Similarly, since nursing units will be operationalizing many of the specific tactics to implement the strategies, they must have some say in the establishment of what those tactics will be.

Cost is also an important factor in marketing. The marketing department will proudly point out gains in patient volume. The nursing department will incur additional costs to implement new products, services, strategies, and tactics. There must be a clear relationship between the expectations of a marketing plan and the additional resources provided to nursing units to carry out their aspect of the plan.

Marketing plans are generally prepared by marketing experts. There will likely be times when nurses are called upon to develop a business plan for a new product or service, including aspects of the marketing plan. In such cases an understanding of the marketing concepts discussed is essential for the nurse manager. However, it would be wise for the nurse manager to employ consultants who are experts at marketing. Conducting an internal-external analysis and developing marketing strategies and marketing tactics are tasks that require a great deal of marketing experience and in-depth expertise about marketing techniques. A poor marketing plan is not necessarily better than nothing; it can mistakenly lead to the commitment of resources in a doomed venture. Working together, nurse managers and marketing managers can provide a health care organization with significant benefits from the use of marketing techniques.

Nursing departments should consider having their own marketing plan for internal marketing. The nurse's customers include other nurses, physicians, patients, and other hospital staff. Determining the needs of each customer group can improve outcomes for both the customers and nursing.

Marketing is also important as nurses become more and more entrepreneurial in their focus. There has been a growing trend of nurses starting health care businesses. These range from home care agencies to drug treatment clinics. Nurses venturing out in innovative ways will need to concern themselves with the concepts of marketing.

KEY CONCEPTS

Marketing Management science that attempts to maintain and increase the organization's patient volume. High volume is desirable because of its favorable financial implications.

Essence of marketing To enable the organization to determine what customers want or need and to develop and offer those goods or services.

Market Potential customers for a product or organization. Information about the market will affect not only the mix of services that should be offered but also the advertising message, price, and other critical factors.

Determinant attributes Factors that ultimately affect a consumer's purchase decision. There are two major types: decision variables and environmental variables. Decision variables are factors controllable by the organization that can affect volume. Environmental variables are factors that can affect volume but that are not controllable by the organization.

Market segmentation Division of the market into several specific subsections. In general, segmentation is based on three factors: each group must have distinct and measurable needs; it is vital that one can access the specific segments; and each segment must be big enough to merit a distinct effort.

Customer behavior Customers perceive a need; become aware of a provider's existence; become knowledgeable about the provider and the provider's service; develop a liking for a service and then a preference for the service, followed by a conviction to acquire that provider's service, followed by the acquisition of that provider's service; and have an after-the-fact reaction to the purchase. At any point until purchase, a customer may decide to purchase a competitor's product instead.

Market measurement Conversion of qualitative information into quantitative estimates of demand.

Market share Portion or percentage of the overall market that a specific organization controls.

Market research Gathering, recording, and analyzing information to improve decisions made by the organization. Market research is needed to determine what the customer really wants and is willing to buy. The major areas for market research are advertising, business economics, products, and sales.

Marketing plan Plan that first considers the organizational mission and goals and then, based on the results of an internal-external analysis, develops a set of strategies and tactics designed to increase the organization's volume of patients. Plans must then be revised, integrated, and implemented. Control and feedback are also essential to an effective plan.

Strategies Broad plans for the attainment of goals. Marketing strategies define the overall desired approach to marketing products and services.

Tactics Specific activities that are undertaken to carry out a strategy. The four Ps of marketing—product, price, place, and promotion—relate to tactics aimed at implementing marketing strategies.

Implementation of marketing plan Marketing plays a more substantial role than simply advertising the organization's products. When the marketing plan is adopted, it creates change in what products and services are offered. It creates changes in the way services are produced through the strategies and specific tactics it contains. It also results in changes in the allocation of resources throughout the organization.

SUGGESTED READINGS

Cooper, Philip D., "Managed Care Positives and Negatives for Health Care Marketing," *Health Marketing Quarterly,* Vol. 13, No. 2, 1995, pp. 55–61.

Gilligan, Colin, and Robin Lowe, *Marketing and Healthcare Organizations/Import London,* Scovill Patterson, New York, N.Y., September 1995.

Heater, Barbara S., "The Current Healthcare Environment: Who is the Customer?" *Nursing Forum,* July-September, Vol. 31, No. 3, 1996, pp. 16–21.

Herzlinger, Regina, *Market-Driven Health Care,* Addison-Wesley, White Plains, N.Y., 1997.

Ireson, Carol, and Diana Weaver, "Marketing Nursing Beyond the Walls," *Journal of Nursing Administration,* Vol. 22, No. 1, January 1992, pp. 57–60.

James, Genie, *Making Managed Care Work: Strategies for Local Market Dominance,* Irwin Professional Publishing, Burr Ridge, Ill., November 1996.

Kotler, Philip, and Roberta Clarke, *Marketing for Health Care Organizations,* Prentice Hall, Englewood Cliffs, N.J., January 1987.

Kotler, Philip, and Gary Armstrong, *Marketing: An Introduction,* 4th edition, Prentice Hall, Upper Saddle River, N.J., September 1996.

Kotler, Philip, *Marketing Management: Analysis, Planning, Implementation, and Control,* 9th edition, Prentice Hall, Upper Saddle River, N.J., August 1996.

Kotler, Philip, and Gary Armstrong, *Principles of Marketing,* 8th edition, Prentice Hall, Upper Saddle River, N.J., September 1998.

Morrisey, Michael A., *Managed Care and Changing Health Care Markets,* AEI Press, Washington, DC, February 1998.

Price, Courtney, *Health Care Innovation and Venture Trends,* Delmar Publishing, Belmont, Calif., May 1992.

Taylor, Tucker, "Healthcare Marketing and the Nurse Manager," *Nursing Management,* Vol. 21, No. 5, May 1990, pp. 84–85.

Vitber, Alan K., *Marketing Health Care into the Twenty-First Century: The Changing Dynamic,* Innovations in Practice and Professional Services Series, Haworth Press, Binghamton, N.Y., 1996, pp. xiv, 191.[4]

CHAPTER

20

The Nurse as Entrepreneur

CHAPTER GOALS

The goals of this chapter are to:

- Explain entrepreneur
- Describe the characteristics of nurse entrepreneurs
- Discuss opportunities for nurse entrepreneurs
- Explain legal and financial issues facing nurse entrepreneurs
- Identify the steps in developing a business plan
- Discuss pro forma financial statements
- Discuss the use of sensitivity analysis in developing a financial plan

※ INTRODUCTION

Until recently there has not been much emphasis on entrepreneurial activity in the nursing literature. An entrepreneur is "a person who organizes and manages an enterprise, especially a business, usually with considerable initiative and risk."[1] In nursing the term has come to mean a person who starts a venture that involves risk but that also offers the opportunity to make a profit or provide a new product or service or a new way to deliver a product or service. Some authors refer to entrepreneur and intrapreneur,[2] with intrapreneur referring to risk-taking and development activities within an organization and entrepreneur referring to independent activities. We use the more general term entrepreneur. Entrepreneurial activities need not be profit driven. Social entrepreneurship applies the entrepreneur's skill to develop new initiatives in not-for-profit and public organizations.

Not many years ago, nursing as a business was almost unthinkable, or at least an unpleasant thought, to nurses. Although a few nurses started for-profit home health agencies and employment agencies for temporary and other per diem staff, these nurses were unusual. It is now clear to many nurses that as health care moves in a "managed" direction and as publicly traded and other for-profit health care organizations proliferate and grow, many nurses want to be involved in entrepreneurial ventures. This chapter focuses on the characteristics of successful nurse entrepreneurs, opportunities for nurse entrepreneurs, legal and financial issues, and development of a business plan. It concludes with specific examples of nurse entrepreneurs.

---

[1] *Random House Webster's College Dictionary,* Random House, New York, N.Y., 1991, p. 447.

[2] Porter-O'Grady, Tim, "The Private Practice of Nursing: The Gift of Entrepreneurialism," *Nursing Administration Quarterly,* Vol. 22, No. 1, Fall 1997, pp. 23–29.

※ CHARACTERISTICS OF NURSE ENTREPRENEURS

Business and financial knowledge are consistently identified as skills required for the nurse entrepreneur.[3, 4] Beyond those skills, Bhide,[5] who teaches entrepreneurship at the Harvard Business School, states that there is no ideal profile for the successful entrepreneur. Others argue that nurse entrepreneurs are risk takers who are willing to assume financial as well as professional risk with the expectation that they will reap financial and professional success. Additional characteristics of entrepreneurs are imagination and creativity. Parker[6] reports that health care managers cited characteristics such as independent, accountable, champions, nontraditional, fast, gutsy, visionary, and courageous, among others, when describing entrepreneurs, as well as the less flattering terms pushy and irreverent. White and Begun[7] identify intuition as a characteristic that is important to entrepreneurship.

Having a good idea is not enough to be a successful entrepreneur. In addition to starting a business, Bhide[8] stresses the need for entrepreneurs to have management skills. Most entrepreneurial initiatives fail, not necessarily because the idea for the business was poor but because the entrepreneur did not have enough capital to keep the business going or the management skills necessary to run a new venture.

※ OPPORTUNITIES FOR NURSE ENTREPRENEURS

For nurses, entrepreneurs can be included in one of three broad categories: an individual who provides a product or service, a new organization that starts a new venture that provides a product or service, or a new venture within an existing organization. Examples include the nurse practitioner starting a patient care practice, a group of nurses developing a new incontinence product and forming a company to produce and market it, and the nurse who develops an elementary school health program within a college of nursing.

Nurses working for a for-profit company or in a business are not necessarily entrepreneurs, although they may be. A nurse can work for a for-profit pharmaceutical corporation explaining new products to physicians and nurses and not be an entrepreneur. The skills required for this position could be marketing expertise and loyalty to the corporation. The nurse manager who works to improve productivity on a nursing unit is not an entrepreneur, even though the nurse's focus may be to decrease costs. If, on the other hand, nurses work in new business or new product development and there is some financial incentive, they may be entrepreneurs, whether or not they work for a for-profit organization. Developing a community health education program for a tax-exempt, not-for-profit community hospital, especially if the program will break even financially, is an example.

Starting Your Own Business

Starting a new venture can be an exciting as well as scary prospect. The new venture can be a completely new idea, a variation on an existing idea, or an existing product or approach in a market that the nurse thinks has room for more providers or in which the nurse believes he or she can provide the product or approach more

---

[3]Ballein, Kathleen M., "Entrepreneurial Leadership Characteristics of SNEs Emerge as Their Role Develops," *Nursing Administration Quarterly*, Vol. 22, No. 2, Winter 1997, pp. 60–69.

[4]Parker, Marsha, "The New Entrepreneurial Foundation for the Nurse Executive," *Nursing Administration Quarterly*, Vol. 22, No. 2, Winter 1997, pp. 13–21.

[5]Bhide, A. "How Entrepreneurs Craft Strategies that Work," *Harvard Business Review*, March/April 1994, pp. 150–161.

[6]Parker, op cit.

[7]White, Kenneth R., and James W. Begun, "Nursing Entrepreneurship in an Era of Chaos and Complexity," *Nursing Administration Quarterly*, Vol. 22, No. 2, Winter 1997, pp. 40–47.

[8]Bhide, op cit.

efficiently. Some ventures require a huge capital investment (e.g., building a new nursing home). On the other hand, starting a consulting business out of one's home can require almost no capital and in fact may save money because of the possible tax deduction for a home office.

Deciding what to do is only one part of the process. Bhide[9] suggested three guidelines: "(1) Screen opportunities quickly to weed out unpromising ventures. (2) Analyze ideas parsimoniously. Focus on a few important issues. (3) Integrate action and analysis. Don't wait for all the answers, and be ready to change course."

The establishment of a patient care practice (private practice) by a nurse practitioner is an entrepreneurial activity. Two factors have provided the impetus for nurses to provide clinical services on their own rather than as employees. First, more nurses are educated as advanced practice nurses, and many nurses now have prescriptive privileges. Second, as of January 1998, Medicare directly reimburses advanced practice nurses for clinical care.

Another example of an entrepreneurial activity is developing a consulting practice. Porter-O'Grady,[10] in describing his career as a consultant offered practical advice about starting up. He provided two mandates: First be patient, and second the client is always right. In developing a consulting practice he suggests putting away six months of income and building a good network before starting the business. Simpson[11] described the development of a nursing informatics consulting practice. He identified job satisfaction, flexibility, and income potential as positive aspects of consulting and tough competition and business ups and downs as negative aspects.

Although developing a new product or service by a group of people is similar to developing a practice alone, the key difference of working with others is critical. Porter-O'Grady[12] advised that if one is working with a partner, it is imperative to draw up a clear contract. It is best to be clear about financial and work responsibilities and rewards before any issues arise. When we agreed to write the second edition of this book, we signed a contract with the publisher that clearly identified what we would produce, when we would produce it, and what the royalty payment would be.

Developing a product requires skills that few nurses learned in school. How to build a prototype, get a manufacturer, obtain a patent, obtain any regulatory approvals, and how to market a product or service usually require outside expertise. Nurses who develop a new continence diaper must realize that the Kimberly-Clark Corporation has been in the diaper business for a long time, has access to capital and accounting and legal expertise, and is a tough competitor.

Developing an entrepreneurial service or product within an organization in many cases is the most risk-free. At the same time the rewards may not be as great as they can be when individuals start their own companies. That does not mean it is simpler to start something new within an existing organization. In fact, this may be the most complicated of the three entrepreneurial approaches. Much depends on the arrangement that the nurse has with the organization. If part of the nurse's job is new product and service development, he or she may not assume any financial risk. A nurse can arrange for the organization to provide all of the start-up funding, but to share any profits.

An example of an entrepreneurial activity within an organization is a nurse-managed primary care center. Newland and Rich[13] described the conception,

---

[9]Ibid., page 150.

[10]Porter-O'Grady, op cit.

[11]Simpson, Roy L., "From Nurse to Nursing Informatics Consultant: A Lesson in Entrepreneurship," *Nursing Administration Quarterly*, Vol. 22, No. 2, Winter 1997, pp. 87–90.

[12]Porter-O'Grady, op cit.

[13]Newland, J.A., and E. Rich, "Nurse-Managed Primary Care Center," *Nursing Clinics of North America*, Vol. 31, No. 3, September 1996, pp. 471–486.

development, and implementation of Pace University Health Care Unit, a primary care center at Pace University. In 1977 the family nurse practitioner faculty began a nurse-managed health unit to provide a site for faculty practice and student clinical experience. Although foundations provided initial and later additional support, the expectation was that the unit would generate revenue. Pace University currently pays about two thirds of the unit's operating expenses. Other revenue comes from Medicaid, private insurance, and self-pay. The unit provides primary health care including laboratory services.

※ LEGAL AND FINANCIAL ISSUES

The entrepreneur faces many legal issues, both before starting a business and on an ongoing basis. Many of these legal issues will require consultation with an attorney. The entrepreneur is encouraged to obtain legal counsel from an attorney who specializes in business law early in the process.[14, 15] Three general legal structures are used in business: sole proprietorship, partnership, and corporation. Corporations can be for profit or not for profit. Lambert and Lambert[16] provide a detailed discussion about the advantages and disadvantages of each legal structure. A proprietorship is the least formal arrangement. An advantage of a partnership includes the availability of additional capital, but that advantage may be offset by each partner's responsibility for all of the business debts. Earnings of proprietorships and partnerships are taxed as personal income. The primary advantage of a corporation is that the owner's personal assets beyond those invested in the corporation are not at risk if the business fails. However, the corporation pays taxes on profits, and then the nurse pays taxes again on income from the corporation. Small corporations can be set up as "Sub-S" corporations, which have the legal protection of the corporate form but are taxed as if they were partnerships.

Legal issues include problems related to compliance with the numerous laws and regulations that have an impact on how a business operates. Some of these laws may not apply to businesses that have no employees aside from the principal. These laws vary from Workmen's Compensation to the Americans with Disabilities Act. Other laws relate to purchasing or leasing property, borrowing money, and consumer rights. In addition to laws that affect all businesses, there are specific laws and regulations that affect only health care organizations. Most nurses are familiar with the regulations about professional practice including malpractice; however, fewer nurses know about various state regulations such as those about care provided in ambulatory care facilities.

Although by having gotten to Chapter 20 of this book, the reader has obtained a substantial background in financial management, we still advise the nurse entrepreneur to contact an accountant early in the entrepreneurial endeavor. The accountant can provide advice on the tax and financial implications of various decisions. Should the nurse lease or buy equipment? Incorporate or start as a proprietorship? Operate locally or from a tax-advantageous location? Complete the payroll information or have the accountant do it?

Obtaining expert advice early in the business development process can save costly mistakes later on. Those nurses who develop entrepreneurial activities within an organization will most likely have the benefit of the legal and financial expertise of the organization.

---

[14]Blouin, A.S., and N.J. Brent, "The Nurse Entrepreneur: Legal Aspects of Owning a Business," *Journal of Nursing Administration,* Vol. 25, No. 6, June 1995, pp. 13–14.

[15]Lambert, V.A., and C.E. Lambert Jr., "Advanced Practice Nurses: Starting an Independent Practice," *Nursing Forum,* Vol. 31, No. 1, January-March 1996, pp. 11–21.

[16]Ibid.

⁜ BUSINESS PLAN

The creation of a business plan is essential to the development of any entrepreneurial endeavor, whether for a new health services business or a new venture with an established organization such as a hospital. Understanding the actual costs of doing business is essential to assess the likelihood of success of any new venture. Even those nurse managers who abhor the notion that providing health care is a business recognize that new services cost something. New services cannot be provided to improve the health of the community unless adequate attention has been paid to determining how those services will be paid for. A "business plan" doesn't require a "business motive."

Developing a business plan requires an understanding of the "business," the competition in the market, the projected revenue and expenses, and the time frame for achieving a break-even position. Many nurses have ventured into providing services without a firm understanding of the regulatory environment (this is especially true in home care) and without a solid base in financial management. Starting programs that fail because of inadequate financial planning does not serve the health care needs of society. It is more sensible to understand if a proposed new venture has financial flaws and work to correct them. If business planning shows that a service can only be provided at a loss, then the sources of possible subsidies should be determined before a significant amount of time, effort, and money has been invested. The depth and complexity of the business plan will vary by the venture. For ventures that will require a large capital investment, a business plan is critical. On the other hand, devoting months and months to the business plan may delay entry into the market and thus a valuable time advantage will be lost.

The plan should define the tactics that are being used to accomplish the organization's goal. It should clearly state the objectives of the proposed project and provide a link that shows how the plan's objectives will lead to accomplishment of the organization's goal.

The plan must clearly communicate the concept of the project. It must also communicate the organization's ability to carry out the project. One can think of a business plan as a document that answers the questions one should ask before investing money in a project:

- What exactly is the proposed project?
- To what extent does the organization have the capabilities to undertake the project?
- Where will the organization acquire the capabilities that it lacks?
- Will the project make or lose money?
- How much money?
- Does the organization have the financial resources to undertake the project?
- If not, where can those resources be obtained?
- How will the new product or service be marketed?
- What alternative approaches have been considered?
- Why is the proposed approach considered better than the alternatives?

The Steps in Developing a Business Plan

Project Proposal

The first step in developing a business plan is the proposal of a new product or service or expansion of an old one. Nursing is often involved in new products and services, either in a support role or as the principal proponent. For example, the addition of a new type of laser surgery would clearly have implications for nursing. Changes would likely occur in the operating room as well as the medical/surgical units. The project might be proposed by the surgeons, with the nursing department providing valuable assistance in developing the business plan. On the other hand, the decision to add an outpatient surgery unit might be suggested by the nursing director of the operating room. As such, it would be primarily a nursing business plan. Nurses can become involved in developing a variety of different programs and innovative services. Developing a new home care agency or additional home care services for an existing agency, developing a nursing agency, and developing an educational or counseling clinic are just a few examples.

Product Definition

Once a program has been proposed, the product or service must be carefully defined. What is the specific product; what are the ways it can be provided; what are the resources needed to provide it? Are the patients homogeneous or mixed in terms of diagnoses; in terms of acuity? Are the required resources limited to labor and other operating items, or are capital investments needed as well? How long will it take to get the program up and running? Are there economic or technological trends that could have an impact on patient demand in the future?

Market Analysis

Having defined the product, the next step is a market analysis. Are there people who want the product and are willing to pay for it? Can the organization create a market? How many potential buyers are there, and how many other organizations offer the product or service? What *market share* can the organization get? Market share is a percentage of the total demand or volume for the product or service. For example, if there are 10,000 patients in your community who will be treated and your organization gains a 10% market share, it will expect to treat 1,000 patients. The organization must be convinced that there will be sufficient demand to justify the investment in this project as opposed to some other project.

As part of the market study, it is necessary to consider change. Is the market likely to grow? That is, will there be a growing number of patients? Will competition grow? Will there be more and more providers competing for the patients? If so, will this organization's market share fall?

The issue of competition is critical. Is there competition? Is there the potential for competition? What will competition do when they see the new program or project? What are the strengths and weaknesses of the competition?

The market analysis must consider who the patients will be and who the payers will be. Is the population largely insured; largely indigent? Can the product be sold to a managed care organization? Having enough patients is the first step. Equally important, however, is knowing the mix of patients.

Mix of patients refers to different types of ailments and different types of payers. The types of ailments must be known so that the expected costs can be calculated. The mix of payers is also important. What percentage are Medicare patients, Medicaid, HMO, other insurance? The program's revenue can vary dramatically based on who will ultimately be responsible for paying the organization's charges. The charges represent gross revenues. Generally, however, only a portion of total charges is collected, because of government-mandated rates or special discount arrangements or because the patients are uninsured and unable to pay. The ultimate cash receipts must be known in addition to the volume of patients.

If the market analysis shows little demand or excessive competition, the planning process for this specific program may be discontinued. If it appears that there is demand for the product or service and a reasonable potential market share for the organization, the planning can continue.

Rough Financial Plan

After the market analysis is completed and indicates that demand exists for the product, a rough financial plan can be developed. The purpose of this rough plan is to determine whether the project warrants further attention. The rough financial plan revolves around an operating budget.

The operating budget includes rough estimates of both revenues and expenses. The revenues can be calculated based on the demand projections from the market analysis. The expenses can be based on rough approximations of the types and amounts of various resources needed.

The results of a rough financial plan are imprecise. The purpose of the plan is to arrive at one of three findings. The first possible finding is that the cost of the program will far exceed the revenues under any reasonable set of assumptions. In that case, managers should save their time by discontinuing the planning process if the project is being evaluated solely on financial merit. A second finding is that the program looks as if it will definitely be profitable. In that case the manager can proceed with the substantial time investment required to develop a fully detailed plan. A third finding is that it is unclear whether the project will be profitable.

The third result creates some difficulty for entrepreneurs. A major potential danger in program planning is that the manager working on the data collection will begin to push harder and harder for the project, the more time has been invested in the analysis. The more time entrepreneurs invest, the greater their psychological need to justify that investment by having the plan indicate that the project is favorable. This could result in a bias in the collection and interpretation of data concerning project feasibility.

Given the unknowns encountered in putting any new program into place, there should be a healthy degree of skepticism about the project. "If it's such a good project, why isn't someone else already doing it?" is a reasonable thought. Therefore, one should always continue with analysis cautiously. Plans should be discontinued unless factors lead the entrepreneur to believe that a more detailed analysis may in fact produce information in the project's favor.

Detailed Operations Plan

Assuming that planning for the project is still continuing after the rough financial plan, the next step is to develop a detailed operations plan.

The first element of the plan is to consider the physical location and structure required by the program or project. Next one must consider the specific human resources required. Equipment and supplies must also be taken into account. These are all direct costs of the project.

Detailed Financial Plan

Once a thorough analysis has been made concerning the various components of the proposed plan, a detailed and thorough financial plan can be developed. This financial plan incorporates all the information from the operations plan, considering the financial impact of the resources to be used. This information will ultimately be used to determine whether it is possible to go ahead with the new project.

The financial plan has three critical elements: a break-even analysis, a cash-flow analysis, and the development of a set of *pro forma* financial statements. Pro forma financial statements are predictions of what the financial statements for the project or program will look like at some point in the future.

The break-even analysis provides information on the minimum volume of patients that must be achieved for the new program not to lose money. Many new programs or projects start with low volume and gradually attract more patients. The pattern of growth in the volume of patients is predicted as part of the market analysis. Break-even analysis is valuable because combined with the volume projection it can help give the entrepreneur a sense of how long it will take before the new program stops losing money. The techniques of break-even analysis are discussed in Chapter 7.

The cash-flow analysis provides information on how much cash the program or project will spend each year, and how much cash will be received. This information is not available from the operating budget for the program. That budget will focus on revenues and expenses. However, revenues are generally received some time after the patients are treated. In many cases it takes payers (including Medicare, Medicaid, HMOs, and others) weeks or months to pay for the services provided. On the other hand, cash outlays at the beginning of the project may be substantial. In addition to paying salaries on a current basis, the organization may need to acquire supplies, equipment, and in some cases, buildings.

In the case of salaries and supplies, the time between cash payment and ultimate cash receipt may be a matter of months. In the case of buildings and equipment, substantial amounts of money may be needed to start the project, whereas the receipt of cash from the use of the buildings and equipment may stretch out over a period of years. Therefore it is important to know the amount of cash required. That information will allow one to decide if there is sufficient cash available to undertake the project. Cash budgeting is discussed further in Chapters 11 and 15.

Pro forma financial statements present a more comprehensive summary of the financial implications of the plan than is provided by the operating budget developed as part of the rough financial plan.

Pro Forma Financial Statements

Every organization has a set of financial statements that are financial summaries used to indicate the financial position of the organization at a point in time, as well as the financial results of its activities for a period of time. Often financial statements are used to indicate the organization's financial position at the end of its fiscal year, and its revenues and expenses and cash receipts and payments for an entire fiscal year. The most typically used financial statements are the balance sheet (also called the statement of financial position), the operating statement (also called the activity statement or the income statement), and the statement of cash flows (or the cash flow statement). (See Chapters 5 and 6 for a discussion of financial statements.)

When a business plan is prepared, an operating budget is developed. The operating budget provides some basic information used for developing the pro forma statements. Using the planned operating budget and the various projections and assumptions about the proposed program or project, the key financial statements are projected for each year into the future, usually for three to five years. Any predictions beyond five years are generally considered unreliable. Any predictions for fewer than three years fail to give a picture of what the financial impact of the program is likely to be once it is fully up and running.

Pro forma statements allow the user to determine some basic financial information about the proposed program or project. The pro forma balance sheets will indicate for each future year what the year-end obligations are likely to be relative to the resources. One would want to always have sufficient resources to be able to pay obligations as they become due. The pro forma statements of revenues and expenses will tell the project's expected profitability for each future year. The pro forma cash flow statements provide a summary of the information from the cash-flow analysis.

Forecasting and Capital Budgeting

The detailed financial plan, as noted above, includes a break-even analysis, a cash-flow analysis, and a set of pro forma financial statements. To get the information needed for these elements, the business plan relies heavily on several aspects of budgeting. Two critical areas of budgeting are forecasting and capital budgeting.

To prepare a cash-flow analysis and to generate pro forma financial statements, a great number of items must be forecast. These include, but are not limited to, inflation, regulation, revenues, wage rates, availability of personnel, detailed expenses, cash flows, and patient volumes. To make these forecasts, the techniques discussed in Chapter 18 are employed.

Program budgets frequently require the acquisition of capital assets. Such assets, however, require special attention because of their multiyear life and frequently high costs. The techniques of capital budgeting, which are discussed in Chapter 11, must be taken into account in preparing this part of the business plan.

Sensitivity Analysis

In developing the detailed financial plan, a helpful technique is sensitivity analysis. Sensitivity analysis is concerned with the fact that often a number of assumptions and predictions are made in calculating the financial aspects of a business plan. The number of expected patients used to develop pro forma financial statements is the result of a forecast, which may not be exactly correct. The revenues are based on a stated average charge, which is an assumption. The actual rates charged may be higher or lower. Sensitivity analysis is a process whereby the financial results are recalculated under a series of varying assumptions and predictions. This is often referred to as "what-if" analysis.

Suppose the pro forma financial statements lead one to believe that the proposed project will be a reasonable financial success. Using sensitivity analysis, one could then say, "What if managed care penetration increases by 10%? What if there are 5% fewer patients than expected? 10% fewer? What if there are 5% more patients than expected? 10% more? What if the average amount charged is raised by 10%? What if the number of staff nurses needed is three full-time equivalents (FTEs) greater than anticipated? What if the construction costs are $30,000 more than expected?"

Essentially, sensitivity analysis provides recognition of uncertainty. Uncertainty creates risk. Before a final business plan is put together and accepted, one needs to have some idea of the magnitude of risk involved. By going through the what-if analysis, one can get a sense of how unfavorable the financial results would be if some things do not occur just as hoped for or expected. If a project can show an expected favorable financial result over a range of what-if questions, it can provide an extra degree of assurance. If that is not the case, then one must carefully question whether the potential benefits are worth the risk that must be undertaken.

Examination of Alternatives

A final consideration in the development of a detailed financial plan is the examination of alternatives. There is often more than one way to implement a new service. The alternatives relate to factors such as the capacity of the service, the approach to providing the service, and the quality of the service. The business plan should be based on having selected one specific approach after having considered a wide variety of potential alternatives. Calculations regarding the costs and benefits of the various alternatives that have been considered become part of the final business plan package.

The Elements of a Business Plan Package

With business plans, as with great cooking, presentation of the finished product is an essential component of the process. Business plan development requires a significant amount of time and effort. The finished result is often a very long document. Unless carefully presented in a final package, the benefits of much of the work may be lost. When preparing a business plan for oneself, this is not critical.

The first and most critical element is a concise executive summary. The executive summary should be brief: ideally, no more than one paragraph or one page; two or three pages if absolutely necessary. The summary should convey what the project is, why it is being proposed, and what the projected most likely results are. This should be able to be done in just a few brief sentences. If the information in the summary indicates that the project is worth pursuing, the reader will read further.

The next part of a business plan should be a detailed abstract, generally about twenty or thirty pages long. The abstract should provide much greater detail than the executive summary. However, it still is a summary or abstract. It does not include all the specific documentation for the calculations that underlie the plan.

If the program is developed under the auspices of an organization, the abstract should describe the mission of the organization and the way the proposed program fits in with the mission. It should provide a description of both the product or service and its potential consumer. The abstract should explain how the new product fits in with the organization's existing services. It should explain why there is a belief that the organization has a competitive edge for this product or service that will allow it to gain and maintain a certain level of market share. The profitability of the program should be discussed in greater detail than that provided in the executive summary. The pro forma financial statements should be included.

It is essential that the abstract discuss potential risks. Regulation and other elements that would impede the project should be discussed as well. Finally, the abstract should include some estimate of the requirement for management time needed to implement the program and a statement of commitment by the manager who will bear primary responsibility for the implementation of the program.

The final part of the business plan package is the detailed analysis of each element. At this point all remaining data are included: detailed descriptions of the product and service, a detailed market research plan indicating market potential and competition, a detailed time line for implementation of the plan, a detailed marketing plan for attracting patients, and a detailed financial plan including the analyses used to develop the pro forma statements. Some of the data may be organized into appendixes to the detailed analysis.

By grouping the business plan into these three sections—executive summary, detailed abstract, and full detailed analysis—the entrepreneur allows others less familiar with the project to understand it. This will allow the project to get a fair examination, if it is within an organization, and should lead to a reasoned final decision on whether to implement the proposed program.

⋇ EXAMPLES OF ENTREPRENEURS

As discussed above, entrepreneurs take a variety of approaches to the development of their ventures and face multiple problems. Preventing potential problems is easier than solving problems once they occur. This section describes composites of nursing entrepreneurial experiences.

Example 1

Carol Aspiria expected to graduate from a master's program and become certified as a gerontological nurse practitioner. She worked as a staff nurse on a medical/surgical unit, where she earned about $50,000 per year. Her dream was to have her own practice. After she was certified, she decided to rent an office. Carol made an arrangement with a physician colleague to use a portion of her space and agreed to pay $1,000 per month for rent. Carol calculated that if she charged $30 per visit and saw 20 patients a day, her income would be $150,000 per year. This was more than enough money. What Carol failed to recognize on the revenue side was that most insurers do not pay providers for at least 90 days and that not all of them pay the full amount charged. She had also allowed herself no vacation. Carol would need income for herself during the time she waited for insurers to pay, *and* she would have to pay rent. In addition, at least for the first year it would be unlikely that she would see 20 patients per day. Although Carol knew that she would have to pay for a phone, she failed to take into account that she would need to buy a fax machine, an answering machine, paper, supplies, and many other items. Finally, Carol had planned initially to schedule her own appointments, thus saving secretarial expense. This meant she would need to complete all of the insurance forms, deal with insurance companies to get payment, and answer questions about billing from patients. All of this took time, reducing the number of patients she could see each day unless she worked extra hours. She found that she had to work 2 days a week as a staff nurse to earn additional money.

Example 2

Martha Spade, on the other hand, realized that start-up costs are extensive in any new business. She decided to work in a clinic as a nurse practitioner for a year to save money for start-up expenses and to learn how a practice works. When she started her practice, she continued to work 2 days a week in the clinic. In terms of space, she made an arrangement with a physician colleague to use her space 3 days per week and to pay the physician's secretarial staff to schedule her appointments.

Example 3

John Munchkin is a mental health advanced practice nurse. With a PhD in nursing, he works at a university and obtains a full-time salary. He sees clients in his home three evenings and one day per week. He has few additional expenses. He obtained a separate telephone line for the practice and increased his malpractice insurance and homeowners insurance. He uses an accountant to prepare his taxes. In addition, because he has a room in his house that is used only for his practice, the cost of a home office is a business expense.

Example 4

Margaret Milton is the dean of a small college of nursing. Over the past several years it has become increasingly difficult to find clinical placements for both undergraduate and graduate students. Placing nurse practitioner students was particularly difficult. At the same time she realized that the federal government had grant money to set up clinics for the underserved who had limited access to care. Dr. Milton's grant application to set up a nurse practitioner–run clinic in a housing project was funded, providing the start-up capital needed as well as 50% of the salary for a part-time nurse practitioner to get the program started. This clinic served as a training site for adult and pediatric nurse practitioners and undergraduate community health nurses. The final year of funding is next year, and Dr. Milton now realizes that the clinic's expenses continue to exceed the clinic's revenue. It is not clear that the clinic can ever break even because of the state reductions in Medicaid payments, the many uninsured people the clinic cares for, and the quality of care that the faculty insists the clinic provide. She is faced with the decision of whether to close the clinic or find other sources of funding.

• • •

The twenty-first century will be an exciting time for nursing. It is intriguing how many of the *Forbes* magazine annual list of billionaires are in businesses that were unknown twenty years ago. Thinking back only twenty years, few people had personal computers, and regular use of the Internet was unheard of. Cellular telephones and digital television were dreams. The technological and communications explosion has also had an impact on the way nurses provide care. Home health nurses carry hand-held computers, and increasing numbers of patients are treated with lasers. Creative, risk-taking nurses have the opportunity to participate in and profit from the developments of the next twenty years.

KEY CONCEPTS

Entrepreneur Person who starts a venture that involves risk but that also offers the opportunity to make a profit and/or provide a new product or service or a new way to deliver a product or service.

Business plan Detailed plan for a proposed program, project, or service, including information to be used to assess the venture's financial feasibility. The plan should clearly state the objectives of the proposed project and provide a link that shows how the plan's objectives will lead to accomplishment of the organization's goal.

Sensitivity analysis Process whereby financial results are recalculated with a series of varying assumptions and predictions

SUGGESTED READINGS

Abrams, Rhonda M., *The Successful Business Plan: Secrets & Strategies,* Oasis Press, Grants Pass, Ore., 1993.

Ballein, Kathleen M., "Entrepreneurial Leadership Characteristics of SNEs Emerge as their Role Develops," *Nursing Administration Quarterly,* Vol. 22, No. 2, Winter 1997, pp. 60–69.

Bhide, A., "How Entrepreneurs Craft Strategies that Work," *Harvard Business Review,* March/April 1994, pp. 150–161.

Blecher, Michele Bitoun, "The Nurse Will See You Now," *Hospitals and Health Networks,* Vol. 71, No. 7, April 5, 1997, pp. 96–99.

Blouin A.S., and N.J. Brent, "The Nurse Entrepreneur: Legal Aspects of Owning a Business," *Journal of Nursing Administration,* Vol. 25, No. 6, June 1995, pp. 13–14.

Brent, N.J., "Setting Up Your Own Business: Facing the Future as an Entrepreneur," *AORN Journal,* Vol. 51, No. 1, January 1990, pp. 205, 208, 210–213.

Calmelat A., "Tips for Starting Your Own Nurse Practitioner Practice," *Nurse Practitioner,* Vol. 18, No. 4, April 1993, pp. 58, 61, 64.

Campbell, K., "Intravenous Nursing Services: Strategies for Success," *Journal of Intravenous Nursing,* Vol. 19, No. 1, January-February 1996, pp. 35–37.

Campbell, Sandy, "The Newest Gatekeepers: Nurses Take on the Duties of Primary Care Physicians," *Health Care Strategic Management,* Vol. 15, No. 3, March 1997, pp. 14–15.

Chow, Gregory, "The Entrepreneurial Personality," *Nursing Administration Quarterly,* Vol. 22, No. 2, Winter 1997, pp. 30–35.

Crofts, A.J., "Entrepreneurship: The Realities of Today," *Journal of Midwifery,* Vol. 39, No. 1, January-February, 1994, pp. 39–42.

Crow, Gregory, "The Entrepreneurial Personality: Building a Sustainable Future for Self and the Profession," *Nursing Administration Quarterly,* Vol. 22, No. 2, Winter 1997, pp. 30–35.

Eaton, D.G., "Perinatal Home Care: One Entrepreneur's Experience," *Journal of Obstetrics and Gynecological Neonatal Nursing,* Vol. 23, No. 8, October 1994, pp. 726–730.

Haag A.B., "Writing A Successful Business Plan," *Journal of American Association of Occupational Health Nursing,* Vol. 45, No. 1, January 1997, pp. 25–32; 33–34.

Holman, E.J., and E. Branstetter, "An Academic Nursing Clinic's Financial Survival," *Nursing Economic$,* Vol. 15, No. 5, September-October, 1997, pp. 248–252.

Johnson J.E., "Developing an Effective Business Plan," *Nursing Economic$,* Vol. 8, No. 3, May-June 1990, pp. 152–154.

Kaplan, S.K., "The Absolutely Basic Concepts of Being a Nurse Entrepreneur," *Pediatric Nursing,* Vol. 17, No. 2, March-April 1991, pp. 179–182.

Lachman, Vicki D., "Care of the Self for the Nurse Entrepreneur," *Nursing Administration Quarterly,* Vol. 22, No. 2, Winter 1997, pp. 48–59.

Lamb, Gerri S., and Donna Zazworsky, "The Carondelet Model," *Nursing Management,* Vol. 28, No. 3, March 1997, pp. 27–28.

Lambert V.A., and C.E. Lambert Jr., "Advanced Practice Nurses: Starting an Independent Practice," *Nursing Forum,* Vol. 31, No. 1, January-March 1996, pp. 11–21.

Langton, Phyllis A., "Obstetricians' Resistance to Independent, Private Practice by Nurse-Midwives in Washington, D.C. Hospitals," *Women and Health,* Vol. 22, No. 1, 1994, pp. 27–48.

Levin, T.E., "The Solo Nurse Practitioner: A Private Practice Model," *Nurse Practitioners' Forum,* Vol. 4, No. 3, September 1993, pp. 158–164.

McNiel, N.O., and T.A. Mackey, "The Consistency of Change in the Development of Nursing Faculty Practice Plans," *Journal of Professional Nursing,* Vol. 11, No. 4, July-August 1995, pp. 220–226.

Newland, J.A., and E. Rich, "Nurse-Managed Primary Care Center," *Nursing Clinics of North America,* Vol. 31, No. 3, September 1996, pp. 471–486.

Parker, Marsha, "The New Entrepreneurial Foundation for the Nurse Executive," *Nursing Administration Quarterly,* Vol. 22, No. 2, Winter 1997, pp. 13–21.

Porter-O'Grady, Tim, "The Private Practice of Nursing: The Gift of Entrepreneurialism," *Nursing Administration Quarterly,* Vol. 22, No. 1, Fall 1997, pp. 23–29.

Shames, K., "Holistic Nurse Entrepreneur: Growing a Business," *Beginnings,* Vol. 17, No. 5, May 1997, pp. 7, 13.

Simpson, Roy L., "From Nurse to Nursing Informatics Consultant: A Lesson in Entrepreneurship," *Nursing Administration Quarterly,* Vol. 22, No. 2, Winter 1997, pp. 87–90.

Vogel, Gerry, and Nancy Doleysh, *Entrepreneuring: A Nurse's Guide to Starting a Business,* 2nd edition, NLN Press, New York, N.Y., 1994.

Vonfrolio, L.G., "Nurse Entrepreneur . . . What Are You Waiting For?" *Orthopedic Nursing,* Vol. 12, No. 2, March-April 1993, pp. 19–22.

Walker, P.H., and P. Chiverton, "The University of Rochester Experience," *Nurse Management,* Vol. 28, No. 3, March 1997, pp. 29–31.

White, Kenneth R., and James W. Begun, "Nursing Entrepreneurship in an Era of Chaos and Complexity," *Nursing Administration Quarterly,* Vol. 22, No. 2, Winter 1997, pp. 40–47.

Wilson, Cathleen Krueger, "Mentoring the Entrepreneur," *Nursing Administration Quarterly,* Vol. 22, No. 2, Winter 1997, pp. 1–12.

PART

VII

THE FUTURE

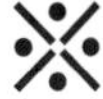

CHAPTER

21

Nursing and Financial Management: Current Issues and Future Directions

CHAPTER GOALS

The goals of this chapter are to:

- Review the current nursing literature on financial management
- Discuss the skills that will be required of nurse managers to assume an expanded role in financial management
- Discuss the pros and cons of nurses' assuming more responsibility for financial management
- Discuss the differences in responsibility for varying levels of nurse managers
- Discuss the role of the nurse as policy manager

※ INTRODUCTION

In the role of manager, nurses perform a variety of functions related to financial management. To perform these functions as efficiently as possible, nurse managers must be aware of current issues in the field of financial management in nursing. This chapter reviews current issues identified in the nursing literature. Discussion of the future of the nurse's role in financial management follows. By having a sense of the current issues and future directions in nursing as it relates to financial management, nurse managers will be in a better position to "work smarter, not harder." The most important thing for managers to avoid is complacency. The role of a manager includes innovation. Innovation, however, is only occasionally the result of inspiration; often it is the product of careful attention to the changing world and what others have done in an attempt to cope with changing realities.

There is some disagreement among nurses about whether nursing financial management is nursing or financial management. We believe nursing financial management is a blend of both fields and as such is also a subset of nursing. Many nursing leaders argue that only studies about patients (clients) and the nursing interventions associated with these clients are the purview of nursing. We believe that nursing includes the organization and delivery of nursing care. Nursing financial management is a part of that general area of nursing.

※ NURSING FINANCIAL MANAGEMENT RESEARCH

National health expenditures were more than $1.1 trillion in 1997, or almost $4,000 per person, in the United States. How to efficiently and effectively use that money is of great interest to nurses.[1] The nurse researcher can serve as a key player in both financial management of organizations and the development of public policy that impacts on financial management of organizations. If we believe that research can give us a greater understanding of the way the world works, research can be used to impact on nursing financial management. Studies about the costs of care can influence the way care is delivered and also government policy.

Review of a profession's research and literature can provide insight into the current issues in the field. Research can be described as a continuum from theoretical to applied. Most people would agree that research is the development or testing of theory. Nursing financial management research includes studies such as those that look at market behavior (how nurses respond to recruitment and retention efforts might be based on this theory), management science (how chief executive officers [CEOs] respond to first-line nurse managers having authority and responsibility for unit finances), or nursing science (how power relates to the allocation of resources in a hospital). The applied result of research in areas such as these has been included in our discussion throughout the book.

Research Taxonomies for Nursing Financial Management

There are two major taxonomies for nursing research. One was developed by Sigma Theta Tau International; the other is the Classification of Nursing-Related Dissertations (DISSER).[2] The Sigma taxonomy uses the category "systems research," and the DISSER schema uses "nurses and nursing profession." Nursing financial management falls into both these categories.

In reviewing these taxonomies, one finds that there is little research toward the theoretical end of the spectrum in the area of nursing financial management. Most financial management theoretical research takes place within the strict disciplines of accounting and finance. The research in the area of nursing financial management tends to apply theoretical developments in accounting or finance to nursing or health management in general.

There is a body of literature in applied nursing financial management research. One major element falls under the general rubric of policy and evaluation research. These studies describe how resources are allocated and explore relationships about the cost and financing of nursing care. Many of these studies look at the cost-benefit ratio of various approaches to providing nursing care, study the impact of various innovations on nursing costs, and develop instruments to measure the cost of providing care. Many of the cost studies use economic or organizational theory or both as the framework to answer questions. Others use no theoretical framework; rather, they describe the relationships among variables.

In addition to the policy and evaluation research literature, increasing numbers of articles in nursing journals are about the application of financial techniques. This is another form of applied research. Almost every issue of the major nursing management journals has at least one article on the financial aspects of nursing. Likely future trends in nursing financial management can be assessed from this applied research.

※ CURRENT ISSUES IN FINANCIAL MANAGEMENT IN NURSING

The broad categories of nursing financial management that recent literature has focused on are (1) allocation of nursing resources, (2) financial compensation and

---

[1] Levit, K., C. Cowen, B. Braden, J. Stiller, A. Sensenig, and H. Lazenby, "National Health Expenditures in 1997: More Slow Growth." *Health Affairs,* Vol. 17, No. 6, 1998, pp. 99–110.

[2] Larson, E., M. Dear, and M. Keitkemper, "Comparison of Two Schema for Classifying Nursing Research," *Image,* Vol. 23, No. 3, Fall 1991, pp. 167–170.

incentives, (3) cost-benefit ratio or cost-effectiveness, (4) approaches to decreasing the cost of care.

The allocation of nursing resources continues to be a major topic in the literature, because nursing care is perceived to be expensive and nursing shortages continue to occur cyclically. The themes include minimum staffing levels, effective and efficient levels of staffing, differentiated nursing practice, and the relationship of staffing and the organization of care to patient outcomes. There is still no agreement on what level of management should make staffing decisions or on what the minimum number of nursing hours or visits is required for groups of patients.

Financial compensation continues to be an issue. Direct Medicare reimbursement for advanced practice nurses and per visit payment to home health nurses were focuses of the late 1990s. How should nurses be compensated? What is the impact of compensation (e.g., salaries, bonuses) on productivity? Should organizations such as home health agencies provide nursing care on a capitated basis?

The cost-benefit ratio or cost-effectiveness of nursing care is an increasingly important focus. The cost-effectiveness of specific nursing interventions such as pain management as well as the cost-effectiveness of nursing care delivery models and level of practitioners will continue to be issues. What is the cost-effectiveness of unlicensed assistive personnel? Of advanced practice nurses providing care to early discharge patients? Of nurse practitioners?

Finally, decreasing the cost of nursing care is an ongoing theme, and there is still little written about increasing revenues. Nurse managers participate in decision making about how to decrease nursing costs. Approaches include using fewer nurses, variations in the configuration of nurses, and supply costs.

※ THE DEVELOPING ROLE OF THE CHIEF NURSE EXECUTIVE IN FINANCIAL MANAGEMENT

Health care organizations are dynamic; they are in a constant state of flux. To maximize opportunities in such a situation, managers must be flexible in defining their role. A decade ago nurse managers might have been astonished to be asked to participate in the development of a business plan. Yet today, chief nurse executives (CNEs) have become key players in business plan development at many hospitals and other health care organizations. The role of CNEs and other nurse managers clearly has been changing and likely will continue to change. Specifically, the CNE's role in the area of financial management is likely to continue to expand.

Although in the past the CNE might have gone to the CEO and asked for a budget of $50 million for "her" department, more often than not the CNE now attends board of trustees meeting, sits on the executive committee of the organization, and is an active voice in the decision-making process for the allocation of all the organization's resources to all departments, not just nursing. In home health agencies the management team may consist almost entirely of nurses.

In the future the responsibility and authority for financial management by nurses is likely to expand at all levels of the organization. It does not require extraordinary imagination to realize that the CNE role will expand to participating in decisions to issue bonds for financing new buildings or for merging with competitors. Topics in this book such as financial statement analysis (Chapter 6) may reflect tools needed on a frequent basis by the typical CNE within the next five years. As the role expands for top management, the role of midlevel nurse managers will also likely expand. Midlevel and first-line managers will have increasing responsibility for financial management.

Setting Organizational Policy

The CNE's role will likely expand to include a greater role in setting organizational policy about financial matters. As more CNEs participate in trustee meetings, trustees will look to the CNE for explanations about rising costs and, more important, options for restraining costs and increasing revenues. Often tactics require reorganization of the way services are provided. The CNE can play a key role in developing and proposing such strategies.

A generation of CNEs has emerged who are academically prepared to actively participate in financial management. Courses in budgeting and finance are now required in many graduate programs in nursing management. Some nurse managers are choosing joint MBA-MSN programs, and others are choosing graduate study in health management. As these educated nurses seek information on the financial operation of the organization and make informed observations, many senior financial managers will embrace their new colleagues as members of the executive team. Others will be threatened by the nurse manager's newfound knowledge and will put up subtle barriers to the nurse manager's full involvement in financial decision-making.

In the twenty-first century the cost restraints seen in the 1990s will continue. In an effort at fiscal solvency, it is likely that CEOs and boards will hold the CNE accountable for high-quality care at a cost the organization can survive with. The informed CNE must know enough about the financial condition of the organization to know with what costs it can in fact survive.

As information generation improves, the CNE has the information necessary to look at the financial management of specific units and even specific staff in the organization. The CNE will likely ask midlevel managers to assume greater accountability and responsibility for fiscal matters, although the amount of accountability at the unit level will likely continue to vary by organization. Many first-line nurse managers have expense budget responsibilities, and some, particularly in home care, have revenue responsibility as well.

Intraorganizational Responsibility for Expenses

The CNE in virtually all health care organizations is currently responsible for the direct operating expense budget of the nursing department. In many organizations the CNE is also responsible for other departments, such as the operating room or the emergency department. In almost all organizations the CNE has a high degree of control of this budget. The CNE may be told to cut 3% off the budget, but in most organizations how that is done is a department decision. In some organizations the CEO may say to cut 3% but not to cut any positions. In many organizations, salary increases are set by top management, with the CNE being intimately involved in these decisions, whether the raise is part of an organized labor settlement or not.

In most organizations the CNE has less control over indirect expenses and the allocation of those expenses to the nursing department. The CNE also has less control over the capital budget than over direct department expenses. The CEO and the chief financial officer (CFO) control the expenses of the other departments and the allocation of these expenses to nursing. Various departments and the key members of the medical staff in hospitals compete for capital. Often capital decisions are made by the CEO and the board. Since few nurses are members of the board and only slightly more are on board committees, the voice of nursing is less strong in hospital capital expenditure decision making. As more nurse executives understand capital financing, they will be in a position to lobby more forcefully for capital expenditures. As more CNEs understand supply-and-demand laws of economics, they will be able to argue regarding the likely positive organizational effects of investment in the area of nursing. As more nurses understand the allocation of indirect expenses and begin to question the allocation, the CNE's voice in these decisions may be heard.

Intraorganizational Responsibility for Revenues

Accountability for revenue is the likeliest growth area in expectations for nurse managers. The focus in the past has been to maintain costs with no reduction in quality. Many organizations focus marketing efforts on product lines. Survival has been linked to the ability to attract a sufficient volume of patients. With the wider adoption of formal structured nursing (e.g., critical paths) or interdisciplinary plans of patient care, the CNE will identify those patients the organization wants to attract and the nurse's role in that revenue generation. In home health care, CNEs almost always have this responsibility.

As patients seek more "caring" in the services provided in health facilities and as patients recognize that nursing is a key service provided, the quality of nursing care will be identified in a marketing strategy. This will enhance the power of the CNE as a key manager of highly regarded service.

Intraorganizational Role in New Ventures

As organizations seek alternatives to balancing expenses and revenues, the CNE will likely be more involved in new ventures. While in the past the CNE was told that the hospital was opening a transplant unit and that adequate staff would need to be provided, in the future the financially adept CNE will participate in the decision making about new ventures. The CNE who is familiar with business plan development and skilled at financial projections will be seen by managers as a valuable asset in the decision-making process.

Extraorganizational Changes

Along with financial responsibilities within the organization, the CNE will increasingly be involved with extraorganizational financial issues, particularly those related to reimbursement. Nurse managers will be faced with the conflict about what is of professional benefit to nursing, what is in the best interest of the nursing department, and what is in the best interest of the organization.

Cross-training of health workers and use of assistive staff are two areas where the manager faces potential conflict. Nurse managers with their roots in the profession of nursing will share the professional values associated with professional licensure. The nurse manager facing increasing salaries for professional nurses and seeing that less educated workers can be trained to perform activities formerly the purview of professional nurses will be faced with a dilemma. What does the proposed government regulation of health maintenance organizations (HMOs) mean for nursing at the hospital? Is it in the nursing department's best interest to have direct third-party reimbursement for nurses? Should the state develop an episode-based reimbursement plan for home health agencies?

Government Relations

Although professional associations such as the American Nurses Association and many nurse leaders have a long history of involvement with government, many CNEs in mid-size health organizations do not. Many reimbursement decisions are now regulated by government. The CNE of the twenty-first century must be able to interact with government officials in the executive branch as well as with legislators to influence how these reimbursement decisions are made. To do so, the CNE must understand the payment system and the financial implications of reimbursement and regulatory decisions for the health organizations with which the CNE is involved. This interaction can occur in letters, during in-person meetings with government officials, and informally at a variety of social and professional meetings.

Payer Relations

Although much of the reimbursement system is regulated by government, reimbursement decisions for individual patients are made by private insurers or by a fiscal intermediary for the government. Bills denied payment or for which payment is delayed cost health organizations a substantial amount of money.

The responsibility for collections is usually in the finance office. Clearly nurse managers do not want to become financial analysts. However, unless they understand issues of cash flow, they will not be able to assume a role in helping the organization solve cash-flow problems. The promptness and completeness with which records are generated affect the cash flow of the organization. The sophisticated nurse manager who understands cash flow will realize the benefit to the organization of working with the nursing staff to document care so as to diminish the claims that are denied or delayed. In home health care, denied claims and delayed payment are major issues threatening the fiscal viability of many agencies.

In the era of managed care, capitation for health services is a major issue. Home health agencies have capitated arrangements. Whether in home care, ambulatory care, or hospitals, capitation changes the incentives. The CNE must know the new incentives and be prepared to deal with them.

In all these areas there is a trade-off between the nurse manager's involvement in financial management and having others in the organization provide those services. We believe the days of the CNE getting a budget from the CEO are over. However, each CNE must decide the amount of information needed to effectively manage the nursing department.

※ FUTURE ROLE OF THE MIDLEVEL NURSE MANAGER IN FINANCIAL MANAGEMENT

As the CNE assumes greater responsibility for financial matters in both the nursing department and the organization, the midlevel manager can also expect to have expanded responsibilities. In most health organizations the midlevel managers and above are responsible for more than one unit. In hospitals this responsibility includes several patient care units. In a home health agency it might include responsibility for a geographic area where care is provided by ten or more nurses. Although first-line managers in most hospitals are responsible for the staffing costs on their units, the accountability of the first-line manager likely will expand also. Advanced practice nurses are setting up their own practices. In such cases a nurse may be responsible for the budget of a small business.

In decentralizing fiscal accountability the CNE must balance the cost of having a nurse manager devote time to fiscal management against the potential benefits of increased control of unit and department resources. It is likely that midlevel nurse managers and first-line managers will have more authority for staffing allocations. Units will be run more like small businesses than parts of large bureaucratic organizations. Some nurse managers may elect to hire more support staff; others may think that an all-RN staff not only provides the highest quality of care but is also most cost effective. At the same time, these managers will have greater responsibility for controlling their expenditures.

Hospitals are developing new approaches for paying nurses. For example, one approach is to pay nurses a salary rather than an hourly wage. Issues of productivity and accountability in such a payment system will challenge the nurse managers. Other hospitals are considering contracting with entrepreneurial groups of nurses to provide all the nursing care on a unit, similar to how HMOs contract with physicians to provide medical care. Many home care agencies are paying nurses on a per visit basis rather than a salary. Managers who use these approaches believe that financial incentives increase the productivity of nurses. Nurse managers from the CNE to the first-line manager will need to address the financial implications of such changes. It is not enough to know whether the staff would prefer to be salaried. Nurse managers will also have to calculate, or at least understand, the financial impact of such a change on their area.

The midlevel and first-line managers will have increased accountability for revenue as well. Historically nurse managers were held accountable for the fixed nursing personnel cost per year or, more progressively, the nursing personnel costs per patient day of care. As reimbursement moves to an episode or capitation basis, nurse managers are being held accountable for the episode of care and covered lives. The nurse managers will be held accountable for both the nursing cost associated with an episode or the group of patients and for providing an acceptable level of quality nursing care.

※ THE NURSE AS A POLICYMAKER FOR FINANCING HEALTH CARE

The focus of this book has been on financial management in a health care organization. Although this is the role most nurses will assume in financial management, there is a role for nurses in developing the external financing and regulatory systems that have an impact on organizations. Nurses can work in a variety of nonprovider settings that have a dramatic impact on people's health.

Lobbyist

Nurses serve as lobbyists to both the legislative and executive branches of all levels of government. Lobbyists often work for professional organizations such as state nurses' associations or for special interest groups such as those concerned with a particular disease or cause. Many decisions about the provision of care are directly related to the payment for that care. Many of the payment decisions are now made by government. The nurse who understands financial management can be an informed lobbyist. For example, if the state is planning to require that all Medicaid patients be part of managed care programs, what implications does this have for the nurse?

Many policy decisions affecting the financial management of health care organizations are made in industry. Pharmaceutical companies set pricing levels. Insurance companies set reimbursement policy. Major industries such as the auto industry decide which benefits will be covered. Financial consulting organizations such as the largest accounting firms employ nurses to help their clients improve operations. Nurses possessing finance skills along with their understanding of clinical care are viewed as invaluable employees in these organizations.

Policymaker

Finally, nurses can work in government and help develop the government policy for financing health care. There is a small but growing group of nurses who are knowledgeable about financial matters who work for government in financial policy development. They work in all levels of government, developing and implementing the financial policies that affect the provision of patient care. Rather than continuing to complain about the decisions government makes about financing care, the profession needs nurses who are knowledgeable about financing to make those decisions for and with us.

Many nurses say about colleagues who work in industry or government, "They've left nursing" or "They are no longer nurses." While working in industry or for government may not be providing direct patient care to an individual, we believe that nursing encompasses caring for the community as well as an individual. Nurse theorists debate what nursing is and the role of the nurse in the health of people. Is nursing caring, repatterning, and/or meeting clients' needs? However nursing is defined, it cannot be done without the provision of the resources to do so. Providing resources cannot be done without a firm understanding of financial management.

⁜ IMPLICATIONS FOR NURSE MANAGERS

As the functions of both the CNE and midlevel nurse manager expand, additional financial skills will likely be necessary. Some nurse executives obtain financial knowledge through on-the-job training. As a result, many CNEs never acquire principles and conceptual foundations of financial management and budgeting.

Some programs in nursing management prepare CNEs; others prepare first-line nurse managers. Based on a survey of nurse executives in a variety of health care settings to determine how they spend their time and on an analysis of the responses by nurse managers, nursing administration faculty, and management faculty, Scaizi and Wilson[3] discuss content that should be required in graduate programs preparing nurse administrators. Finance ranked fourth in time spent in practice setting after (1) law and health care policy, (2) organizational behavior, and (3) organizational strategy. They propose that finance should be a fundamental nursing administration content area.

The trend in the late 1970s was toward graduate programs in nursing focusing on clinical theory. As nurse managers recognized that management skills, including financial management, were necessary to be an effective manager, schools of nursing began to again include this content in their programs. Budgeting and financial management are still not required in all programs. The newly educated generation of nurse managers needs to obtain the conceptual foundations and principles to develop these skills. However, many managers currently working in health organizations do not have these skills and will be expected to obtain them either through formal academic programs or through workshops.

The late 1990s saw renewed focus on clinical expertise, and most graduate programs offered advanced practice nursing skills. These nurses also must understand financial management to meet the challenges they will face throughout their careers.

We hope this book will serve as just the beginning of your efforts to learn about financial management. We have provided the foundations. A nurse manager who has studied this book need not fear embarrassment in conversations with financial managers and other administrators. A nurse manager who has studied this book is prepared to apply the concepts of financial management to health care organizations. We hope, however, that you will continue to read, study, and learn about nursing financial management. This is a field still in its infancy. You have the opportunity to participate in the innovations still to come.

[3]Scaizi, Cynthia, and David L. Wilson, "Empirically Based Recommendations for Content of Graduate Nursing Administration Programs," *Nursing & Health Care*, Vol. 11, No. 10, December 1991, pp. 522–525.

KEY CONCEPTS

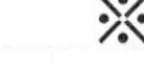

Nursing financial management research Research can be described as a continuum from theoretical to applied. Research in this area is primarily applied and focuses on nursing resource use, costing nursing care, and cost-benefit analysis.

Role of CNE in financial management This role is expanding to include participation in the major financial decisions of health organizations and setting organizational policy.

Government relations Interaction with government officials in the executive as well as the legislative branch. The CNE must understand the payment system and the financial implications for reimbursement and regulatory decisions.

Payer relations Relationship with payers is critical for the fiscal health of the organization. Nurse managers must understand payer policies about reimbursement, particularly those that affect denial of claims.

Policymaker Nurse manager can affect health care delivery as a lobbyist or financial policymaker in government.

SUGGESTED READINGS

Ballein, Kathleen M., "Entrepreneurial Leadership Characteristics of SNEs Emerge as their Role Develops," *Nursing Administration Quarterly*, Vol. 22, No. 2, Winter 1997, pp. 60–69.

Barry, Camille T., "Profiles of Nurses Professionally Involved in Public Policy," *Nursing Economic$*, Vol. 8, No. 3, May/June 1990, pp. 174–176.

Bell, Eunice A., and Barbara D. Bart, "Pay for Performance: Motivating the Chief Nurse Executive," *Nursing Economic$*, Vol. 9, No. 2, March/April 1991, pp. 92–96.

Blecher, Michele Bitoun, "The Nurse Will See You Now," *Hospitals and Health Networks*, Vol. 71, No. 7, April 5, 1997, pp. 96–99.

Bloom, J.R., J.A. Alexander, and B.A. Nuchols, "Nurse Staffing Patterns and Hospital Efficiency in the United States," *Social Science Medicine*, Vol. 44, No. 2, 1997, pp. 147–155.

Blouin A.S., and N.J. Brent, "The Nurse Entrepreneur: Legal Aspects of Owning a Business," *Journal of Nursing Administration*, Vol. 25, No. 6, June 1995, pp. 13–14.

Bodenheimer, T., and K. Sullivan, "How Large Employers are Shaping the Health Care Marketplace," *New England Journal of Medicine*, Vol. 338, No. 14, April 2, 1998, pp. 1003–1007.

Borromeo, A.R., "The Professional Salary Model: Meeting the Bottom Lines." *Nursing Economic$*, Vol. 14, No. 4, 1996, pp. 241–244.

Buerhaus, P.I., "Economics of Managed Competition and Consequences to Nurses: Part II," *Nursing Economic$*, Vol. 12, No. 2, 1994, pp. 292–298.

Campbell, Sandy, "The Newest Gatekeepers: Nurses Take on the Duties of Primary Care Physicians," *Health Care Strategic Management*, Vol. 15, No. 3, March 1997, pp. 14–15.

Caroselli, C. "Economic awareness of nurses: Relationship to Budgetary Control," *Nursing Economic$*, Vol. 14, No. 5, 1996, pp. 292–298.

Crowell, Daina M., "Organizations *Are* Relationships: A New View of Management," *Nursing Management*, Vol. 29, No. 5, May 1998, pp. 28–29.

DeGroot, H.A., "Patient Classification Systems and Staffing: Part I, Practice and Promise," *Journal of Nursing Administration*, Vol. 24, No. 9, 1994, pp. 43–51.

DeGroot, H.A., "Patient Classification Systems and Staffing: Part II, Practice and Promise," *Journal of Nursing Administration*, Vol. 24, No. 10, 1994, pp. 17–23.

Eaton, D.G., "Perinatal Home Care: One Entrepreneur's Experience," *Journal of Obstetrics and Gynecological Neonatal Nursing*, Vol. 23, No. 8, October 1994, pp. 726–730.

Ervin, N., W. Chang, and J. White, "A Cost Analysis of a Nursing Center's Services," *Nursing Economic$*, Vol. 16, No. 6, 1998, pp. 307–312.

Ethridge, Phyllis, "A Nursing HMO: Carondelet St. Mary's Experience," *Nursing Management*, Vol. 22, No. 7, July 1991, pp. 22–27.

Finkler, S., C. Kovner, J. Knickman, and G. Hendrickson, "Innovation in Nursing: A Benefit/Cost Analysis," *Nursing Economic$*, Vol. 12, No. 1, 1994, pp. 25–29.

Gebulski-Alexander, Catherine, "The Nurse Executive in the 21st Century: How Do We Prepare?," *Nursing Administration Quarterly*, Vol. 22, No. 1, Fall 1997, pp. 76–82.

Grandinetti, Deborah A., "Will Patients Choose NPs Over Doctors?" *Medical Economics*, Vol. 74, No. 14, July 14, 1997, pp. 134–151.

Holman, E.J., and E. Branstetter, "An Academic Nursing Clinic's Financial Survival," *Nursing Economic$*, Vol. 15, No. 5, September-October 1997, pp. 248–252.

Huston, C.L., "Unlicensed Assistive Personnel: A Solution to Dwindling Health Care Resources or the Precursor to the Apocalypse of Registered Nursing," *Nursing Outlook*, Vol. 44, No. 2, 1996, pp. 67–73.

Kirk, R., *Managing Outcomes, Process, and Cost in a Managed Care Environment*, Aspen, Gaithersburg, Md., 1997.

Kovner, C.T., and J. Schore, "Differentiated Levels of Nursing Workforce Demand," *Journal of Professional Nursing,* Vol. 14, 1998, pp. 242–253.

Lambert, V.A., and C.E. Lambert, Jr., "Advanced Practice Nurses: Starting an Independent Practice," *Nursing Forum,* Vol. 31, No. 1, January-March 1996, pp. 11–21.

Levit, K., C. Cowen, B. Braden, J. Stiller, A. Sensenig, and H. Lazenby, "National Health Expenditures in 1997: More Slow Growth," *Health Affairs,* Vol. 17, No. 6, 1998, pp. 99–110.

Newland, J.A. and E. Rich, "Nurse-Managed Primary Care Center," *Nursing Clinics of North America,* Vol. 31, No. 3, September 1996, pp. 471–486.

Prescott, P.A., K.L. Soeken, and M. Griggs, "Identification and Referral of Hospitalized Patients in Need of Home Care," *Research in Nursing and Health,* Vol. 18, No. 2, 1995, pp. 85–95.

Shames, K., "Holistic Nurse Entrepreneur: Growing a Business," *Beginnings,* Vol. 17, No. 5, May 1997, pp. 7, 13.

Simpson, R.L., "Outsourcing: Should Nursing Care?" *Nursing Management,* Vol. 26, No. 4, 1995, pp. 22–24.

Walker, P.H., and P. Chiverton, "The University of Rochester Experience," *Nursing Management,* Vol. 28, No. 3, March 1997, pp. 29–31.

OTHER RESOURCE

Health Care Financing Administration, at http:\\www.hcfa.gov.

Glossary

A

ABC *See* activity-based costing.

accounting System for keeping track of the financial status of an organization and the financial results of its activities.

accounting controls Methods and procedures for the authorization of transactions, safeguarding of assets, and accuracy of accounting records.

accounting cost Measurement of cost based on a number of simplifications, such as an assumed useful life for a piece of equipment.

accounting cycle Period of time from when cash is spent to acquire resources to provide care until cash is received in payment for the services provided.

accounting rate of return (ARR) Profitability of an investment calculated by considering the profits it generates, as compared with the amount of money invested.

accounts payable Amounts owed to suppliers (such as a per diem agency or a medical supply company).

accounts receivable Money owed to an organization or individual in exchange for goods and services provided.

accrual accounting Accounting system that matches revenues and related expenses in the same fiscal year by recording revenues in the year in which they are earned (whether received or not) and the expenses related to generating those revenues in the same year.

accrue Increase or accumulate in advance.

accumulated depreciation Total amount of depreciation related to a fixed asset that has been taken over the years the organization has owned that asset.

activity accounting Method of tracking costs and other information by focusing on the activities undertaken to produce the good or service.

activity-based costing (ABC) Approach to determining the cost of products or product lines using multiple overhead allocation bases that relate to the activities that generate overhead costs.

acuity Measurement of patient severity of illness related to the amount of nursing care resources required to care for the patient.

acuity subcategory Amount that would have been budgeted for the actual output level if the actual acuity level had been correctly forecast.

acuity variance Variance resulting from the difference between the actual acuity level and the budgeted level; the difference between the flexible budget and the value of the acuity subcategory.

ADC *See* average daily census.

additive rule Likelihood of either one event or another event's occurring is the sum of the likelihood of each event occurring.

administration Management.

administrative control Plan of organization (e.g., formal organization chart concerning who reports to whom) and all methods and procedures that enable management planning and control of operations.

adverse selection "A tendency for utilization of health services in a population group to be higher than average. From an insurance perspective, adverse selection occurs when persons with poorer-than-average life expectancy or health status apply for, or continue, insurance coverage to a greater extent than do persons with average or better health expectations."[1]

---

[1]This term has been quoted from Lawrence Bartlett, Patricia Hitz, and Renee Simon, Appendix A—Glossary of Common Managed Care Terms, in *Assessing Roles, Responsibilities, and Activities in a Managed Care Environment: A Workbook for Local Health Officials,* Agency for Health Care Policy and Research, Department of Health and Human Services, AHCPR Publ. No. 96-0057, July 1996.

age-of-plant ratio *See* plant-age ratio.

aging schedule Management report that shows how long receivables have been outstanding since a bill was issued.

algebraic distribution Cost-allocation approach that uses simultaneous equations to allocate nonrevenue cost center costs to both nonrevenue and revenue cost centers in a manner that does not create distortions.

allowance for bad debts *See* allowance for uncollectible accounts.

allowance for uncollectible accounts Estimated portion of total accounts receivable that is expected to not be collected because of bad debts; sometimes called allowance for bad debts.

allowances Discounts from the amount normally charged for patient care services. These discounts are sometimes negotiated (e.g., with HMOs or Blue Cross), and other times are mandated by law (e.g., Medicare, Medicaid).

all-payer system System of payment where all payers use the same payment method for paying for health care services.

ALOS *See* average length of stay.

alternative workers Use of workers not traditionally used to provide care. Includes workers who are less skilled than professional nurses but who may be able to assume some activities traditionally performed by RNs.

ambulatory care "All types of health services which are provided on an outpatient basis, in contrast to services provided in the home or to persons who are inpatients. While many inpatients may be ambulatory, the term ambulatory care usually implies that the patient must travel to a location to receive services which do not require an overnight stay."[2]

amortization Allocation of cost of an intangible asset over its lifetime.

annuity Series of payments or receipts, each in the same amount and spaced evenly over time (e.g., $127.48 paid monthly for 3 years).

annuity payments *See* annuity.

any willing provider law "Laws that require managed care plans to contract with all health care providers that meet their terms and conditions."[3]

ARR *See* accounting rate of return.

assets Valuable resources; they may be either physical, having substance and form such as a table or building, or intangible, such as the reputation the organization has gained for providing high-quality health care services.

audit Examination of the financial records of an organization to discover material errors, evaluate the internal control system, and determine if financial statements have been prepared in accordance with generally accepted accounting principles.

auditor Person who performs an audit.

audit trail Set of references that allows an individual to trace back through accounting documents to the source of each number used.

average cost Full cost divided by volume of service units.

average daily census Average number of inpatients on any given day; patient days in a given time period divided by number of days in the time period.

average length of stay Average number of patient days for each patient discharged; number of patient days in a given time period divided by number of discharges in that time period.

axiom Unproved but accepted assertion that is either self-evident or a mutually accepted principle.

B

bad debts Operating expenses related to care provided to patients who ultimately do not pay the provider, although they were expected to pay. Amounts included in revenues but never paid are balanced by the charge to bad debts.

---

[2]Ibid.
[3]Ibid.

balance sheet Financial report that indicates the financial position of the organization at a specific point in time; officially referred to as the statement of financial position.

benefit-cost philosophy Viewpoint that one should never spend more to collect cost information than the value of the information.

Blue Cross Major provider of hospitalization insurance to both individuals and groups. For most hospitals, one of the largest sources of revenue.

board-designated Portion of the fund balance that the board has identified and a corresponding amount of assets that the board has restricted for a specific purpose; sometimes called board-restricted.

board of directors *See* board of trustees.

board of trustees Governing body that has the ultimate responsibility for decisions made by the organization.

board-restricted *See* board-designated.

bondholder Creditor of the organization who owns one of the organization's outstanding bonds payable.

bonding of employees Insurance policy that protects the organization against embezzlement and fraud by employees.

bond payable Formal borrowing arrangement in which a transferable certificate represents the debt. The holder of the bond may sell it, in which case the liability is owed to the new owner.

bonus systems Method to provide incentive for employees to improve performance. Employees receive financial payment, shares of stock, or other remuneration if certain targets are achieved or exceeded.

breakeven analysis Technique for determining the minimum volume of output (e.g., patient days of care) necessary for a program or service to be financially self-sufficient.

breakeven point *See* breakeven volume.

breakeven time (BT) Amount of time before the present value of cash inflows is at least equal to the present value of cash outflows.

breakeven volume Volume needed to just break even. Losses are incurred at lower volumes, and profits at higher volumes.

budget Plan that provides formal, quantitative expression of management's plans and intentions or expectations.

budgeting Process whereby plans are made and then an effort is made to meet or exceed the goals of the plans.

building fund Restricted fund containing assets that can be used only to acquire buildings and equipment.

business plan Detailed plan for a proposed program, project, or service, including information to be used to assess the venture's financial feasibility.

C

cafeteria plan Method of providing fringe benefits in which the employee chooses from a variety of options those fringe benefits that the employee wants.

capital acquisitions *See* capital assets.

capital assets Buildings or equipment with useful lives extending beyond the year in which they are purchased or put into service; also referred to as long-term investments, capital items, capital investments, or capital acquisitions.

capital budget Plan for the acquisition of buildings and equipment that will be used by the organization for one or more years beyond the year of acquisition. Often a minimum dollar cutoff must be exceeded for an item to be included in the capital budget.

capital budgeting Process of proposing the purchase of capital assets, analyzing the proposed purchases for economic or other justification, and encompassing the financial implications of accepted capital items into the master budget.

capital equipment Equipment with an expected life beyond the year of purchase. Such equipment must generally be included in the capital budget.

capital investments *See* capital assets.

capitalism *See* market economy.

capital items *See* capital assets.

capitation "A method of payment for health services in which an individual or institutional provider is paid a fixed amount for each person served, without regard to the actual number or nature of services provided to each person in a set period of time. Capitation is the characteristic payment method in certain health maintenance organizations. It also refers to a method of Federal support of health professional schools. Under these authorizations, each eligible school receives a fixed payment, called a 'capitation grant,' from the Federal government for each student enrolled."[4]

career ladder Approach to promotion and compensation that allows a worker to progress in an organization or a field.

carrying costs of inventory Capital costs and out-of-pocket costs related to holding inventory. Capital cost represents the lost interest because money is tied up in inventory. Out-of-pocket costs include such expenses as insurance on the value of inventory, annual inspections, and obsolescence of inventory.

carve out "Regarding health insurance, an arrangement whereby an employer eliminates coverage for a specific category of services (e.g., vision care, mental health/psychological services, or prescription drugs) and contracts with a separate set of providers for those services according to a predetermined fee schedule or capitation arrangement. 'Carve out' may also refer to a method of coordinating dual coverage for an individual."[5]

case management "The monitoring and coordination of treatment rendered to patients with a specific diagnosis or requiring high-cost or extensive services."[6]

case mix "A measure of the mix of cases being treated by a particular health care provider that is intended to reflect the patients' different needs for resources. Case-mix is generally established by estimating the relative frequency of various types of patients seen by the provider in question during a given time period and may be measured by factors such as diagnosis, severity of illness, utilization of services,"[7] and patient characteristics.

case-mix index Measurement of average complexity or severity of illness of patients treated by a health care organization.

cash Money on hand, plus cash equivalents, such as savings and checking accounts and short-term certificates of deposit.

cash basis Accounting system under which revenues are recorded when cash is received and expenses are recorded when cash is paid. This system is not generally allowed because it does not adequately match revenues and related expenses in the same year.

cash budget Plan for the cash receipts and cash disbursements of the organization.

cash budgeting Process of planning the cash budget.

cash disbursement Outflow of cash from the organization.

cash equivalents Savings and checking accounts and short-term certificates of deposit; items that are quickly and easily convertible into cash.

cash flow Measure of the amount of cash received or disbursed at a given point in time, as opposed to revenues or income, which frequently are recorded at a time other than when the actual cash receipt or payment occurs.

cash management Active process of planning for borrowing and repayment of cash or investing excess cash on hand.

cash payment *See* cash disbursement.

cash receipt Inflow of cash into the organization.

census Number of patients occupying beds at a specific time of day (usually midnight).

CFO *See* chief financial officer.

charge master List of an organization's prices for each of its services.

charity care Care provided to patients who are not expected to pay because of limited personal financial resources.

---

[4]Ibid.
[5]Ibid.
[6]Ibid.
[7]Ibid.

chart of accounts Accounting document that assigns an identifying number to each cost center and each type of revenue or expense. These code numbers are assigned to all financial transactions. By looking at any code number and referring to the chart of accounts, one would know exactly which cost center was involved and the specific type of revenue or expense.

chief financial officer (CFO) Manager responsible for all financial functions of an organization.

chief nurse executive (CNE) Top-level nurse manager responsible for all nursing functions in the organization. This includes all nursing care provided to clients.

CNE *See* chief nurse executive.

coefficient of determination Measure of the goodness of fit of a regression; generally referred to as the "R-squared."

coinsurance Percentage of a patient's health services charge that must be paid by the patient.

collateral Specific asset pledged to a lender as security for a loan.

collection period Time from when a patient bill is issued until cash is collected.

commercial paper Form of short-term borrowing in which the borrower issues a financial security that can be traded by the lender to someone else.

committed costs Costs that cannot be changed in the short run.

common size ratio Class of ratios that allows one to evaluate each number on a financial statement relative to the size of the organization. This is accomplished by dividing each financial statement number by a key number from that statement, such as total assets or total revenues.

competitive strategy Organization's plan for achieving its goals, specifically, what will be sold and to whom.

compound interest Method of calculating interest that accrues not only on the amount of the original investment but also on the interest earned in interim periods.

congruent goals *See* goal congruence.

conservatism principle Financial statements must give adequate consideration to the risks faced by the organization.

constant dollars Dollar amounts that have been adjusted for the effects of inflation.

consumer Person who receives services from a health care provider; this includes not only patients but also health workers.

contingency Event that may or may not occur.

continuous budgeting System in which a budget is prepared each month for a month one year in the future. For example, once the actual results for this January are known, a budget for January of next year is prepared.

continuous quality improvement (CQI) A philosophy concerning the production of an organization's goods and services that proposes that there should be a constant focus on improvement in the quality of the product or service.

contractual allowances Discounts from full charges, available to governments and some other third-party payers.

contribution margin Amount by which the price exceeds the variable cost. If the contribution margin is positive, each extra unit of activity makes the organization better off by that amount.

contribution from operations Contribution margin from the routine annual operations of the organization.

control Attempt to ensure that actual results come as close to planned results as possible.

control chart Graph of variances that indicates upper and lower limits. A variance should be investigated if either of the limits is exceeded.

controllable Items over which a manager can exercise a degree of control.

control limit Amount beyond which a variance should be investigated.

co-payment Dollar amount that must be paid each time a health service is used.

corporation Business owned by a group of persons (shareholders or stockholders) who have limited liability; owners are not liable for more than the amount invested in the firm.

cost Amount spent on something. Costs have two stages: acquisition cost and expired cost. When some asset or service is purchased, it has an *acquisition cost.* If the item is an asset, it will appear on the balance sheet at its cost until it is used up. Once the asset is used up, it becomes an *expired cost,* or an expense.

cost accounting A subset of accounting related to measuring costs to generate cost information for reporting and making management decisions.

cost accounting system Any coherent system designed to gather and report cost information to the management of an organization.

cost allocation Process of taking costs from one area or cost objective and allocating them to others.

cost base Statistic used as a basis for allocation of overhead (e.g., patient days, labor hours).

cost behavior Way that costs change in reaction to events within the organization.

cost-benefit analysis Measurement of the relative costs and benefits associated with a particular project or task.

cost of capital Cost to the organization of the money used for capital acquisitions; often represented by the interest rate that the organization pays on borrowed money.

cost center Unit or department in an organization for which a manager is assigned responsibility for costs.

cost driver Activity that causes costs to be incurred.

cost-effective Approach that provides care as good as any other approach but at a lower cost, or an approach that provides the best possible care for a given level of cost.

cost-effectiveness Measure of whether costs are minimized for the desired outcome.

cost-effectiveness analysis Technique that measures the cost of alternatives that generate the same outcome. *See also* cost-effective.

cost estimation Process of using historical cost information to segregate mixed costs into their fixed and variable components and then using that information to estimate future costs.

cost finding Process that finds the costs of units of service (e.g., lab tests, x-rays, routine patient days) based on allocation of nonrevenue cost center costs to revenue centers.

cost measurement Process of assessing resources consumed and assigning a value to those resources.

cost objective Any particular item, program, or organizational unit for which we wish to know the cost.

cost pass-through Payment by a third party, which reimburses the health care organization for the amount of costs it incurred in providing care to patients.

cost-per-hire ratio Costs related to advertising vacancies, using placement firms, interviewing and processing potential candidates, traveling, and moving, all divided by the number of individuals hired.

cost pool Any grouping of costs.

cost of product What the organization must pay for the product; can be affected by quantity discounts.

cost reimbursement Revenue based on paying the organization for the costs incurred in providing care to patients.

cost reporting Process of conveying information about the cost of resources consumed relative to a specific cost objective.

cost-volume-profit relationship Relationship of how costs, volume, and profits are interrelated.

CPM *See* critical path method.

CQI *See* continuous quality improvement.

cr. Credit.

credit Bookkeeping term for an increase in an item on the right side of the fundamental equation of accounting, or a decrease in an item on the left side.

creditors People or organizations to whom the organization owes money.

critical path An indication in the critical path method of essential steps, a delay in which will cause a delay in the entire project.

critical path method (CPM) Program technique that indicates the cost and time for each element of a complex project and indicates cost/time tradeoffs where applicable.
cross-subsidization of costs Situation in which some patients are assigned more costs than they cause the organization to incur, and others are assigned less.
current assets Resources the organization has that either are cash or can be converted to cash within one year or that will be used up within one year. Current assets are often referred to as short-term or near-term assets.
current liabilities Obligations that are expected to be paid within one year.
current ratio Current assets divided by current liabilities.
curvilinear Curved line. Most statistical methods described assume that there is a straight-line relationship between changes in variables; sometimes the relationship is curved.
curvilinear forecasting Forecasting using curved lines to make estimates of future values.

D

data base Compilation of related information systematically organized.
days-receivable ratio Accounts receivable divided by patient revenue per day; a measure of how long it takes on average until revenues are collected.
debit Bookkeeping term for an increase in an item on the left side of the fundamental equation of accounting or a decrease in an item on the right side.
debt Liability.
debt-to-equity ratio *See* total debt-to-equity ratio.
debt service Required interest and principal payments on money owed.
debt service coverage ratio Cash available to pay interest and principal payments divided by required interest and principal payments; a measure of the ability of the organization to meet required debt service.
decentralization Delegation of decision-making autonomy downward within the organization.
decision package Zero-based budgeting term referring to a package of all the information to be used in ranking alternatives and making a final decision.
decision variables Factors controllable by the organization that can affect volume.
decreasing returns to scale Extremely large volume may lead to increasing cost per unit produced due to capacity constraints or shortages of labor or supplies.
deductible Amount that must first be paid by an insured individual before insurance covers any costs; usually the first $100 or $200 or $500 per year for health insurance.
deferred revenues Items that will become revenue in the future when the organization provides goods or services. These are liabilities until the goods or services are provided.
deficit Excess of expenses over revenues. This term sometimes is used to refer to the current year or budgeted year and sometimes to the deficit accumulated over a period of years.
Delphi technique Technique sometimes employed for forecasting that uses an expert group, which never meets, to generate written information as the basis for making a decision. When used in forecasting, each member's written forecast is distributed to all members of the group, along with the reasoning behind it. This process is repeated several times, and eventually a group decision is made.
demand Amount of the good or service that consumers are willing to acquire at any given price.
demand curve Quantity (horizontal axis) desired by consumers for any given price (vertical axis).
demographics Characteristics of the human population, including age, sex, growth, density, distribution, and other vital statistics.
dependent variable Item whose value is being predicted.
depreciate Decline in value or productive capability.
depreciation Allocation of a portion of the cost of a capital asset into each of the years of the item's expected useful life.

depreciation expense Amount of the original cost of a fixed asset allocated as an expense each year.

determinant attributes Factors that ultimately affect a consumer's purchase decision. There are two major types: decision variables and environmental variables.

diagnosis-related groups (DRGs) System that categorizes patients into specific groups based on their medical diagnosis and other characteristics, such as age and type of surgery, if any. Currently used by Medicare and some other hospital payers as a basis for payment.

differential advantage Characteristic that provides the organization with a distinct advantage over a competitor; advantages might include location, cost, services offered, and other factors.

differential costs *See* incremental costs.

direct costs (1) Costs incurred within the organizational unit for which the manager has responsibility are referred to as direct costs of the unit; (2) costs of resources used for direct care of patients are referred to as the direct costs of patient care.

direct distribution Allocation of nonrevenue center costs directly and only to revenue centers.

direct expenses Expenses that can be specifically and exclusively related to the activity within the cost center; *see also* direct costs.

direct labor Labor that is a direct cost element.

direct labor cost Cost of direct labor.

direct labor dollars *See* direct labor cost.

direct labor hours Number of hours of direct labor consumed in making a product or providing a service.

disbursement Cash payment.

discount rate Interest rate used in discounting.

discounted cash flow Method that allows comparisons of amounts of money paid at different times by discounting all amounts to the present.

discounting Reverse of compound interest; process in which interest that could be earned over time is deducted from a future payment to determine how much the future payment is worth at the present time.

discretionary costs Costs for which there is no clear-cut relationship between inputs and outputs. The treatment of more patients does not necessarily require more of this input; use of more of this input does not necessarily allow for treatment of more patients.

disequilibrium Situation in which the quantity demanded at the current price is not the same as the quantity suppliers want to provide at that price. In such a situation there is pressure to either raise or lower the price until an equilibrium is achieved.

distribution channels Way a product moves from producer to consumer.

distributional efficiency Ability of the market to allocate resources to different individuals in an efficient manner.

divergent goals *See* goal divergence.

dividend Distribution of profits to owners of the organization.

double distribution Allocation approach in which all nonrevenue centers allocate their costs to all other cost centers once, and then a second allocation takes place using either step-down or direct distribution.

double-entry accounting Whenever a change is made to the accounting equation, at least one other change must be made as well to keep the equation in balance.

dr. Debit.

DRGs *See* diagnosis-related groups.

E

economic goods Goods or services acquired by consumers to provide physical or psychic benefit.

economic order quantity (EOQ) Approach to determine the balance between ordering costs and carrying costs.

economics Study of how scarce resources are allocated among possible uses.

economies of scale Cost of providing a good or service falls as quantity increases because fixed costs are shared by the larger volume.

effectiveness A measure of the degree to which the organization accomplishes its desired goals.

efficiency A measure of how close an organization comes to minimizing the amount of resources used to accomplish a result.

efficiency ratios Class of ratios that examines the efficiency with which the organization uses its resources in providing care and generating revenues.

efficiency variance *See* quantity variance.

elasticity of demand Degree to which demand increases in response to a price decrease or decreases in response to a price increase.

electronic data Data that are computerized.

employee benefits Compensation provided to employees in addition to their base salary (e.g., health insurance, life insurance, vacation and holiday pay).

employees per occupied bed (EPOB) Total number of paid full-time equivalents (FTEs) divided by the average daily census.

endowment fund Restricted fund that contains the endowment assets that belong to the organization; only earnings may be removed from this fund under normal conditions.

engineered costs Costs for which there is a specific input-output relationship.

entity Specific individual, organization, or part of an organization that is the focus of attention; accounting must be done from the perspective of the relevant entity.

environmental variables Factors that can affect an organization but that are not controllable by the organization.

EOQ *See* economic order quantity.

EPOB *See* employees per occupied bed.

equilibrium Situation in which the quantity of a good or service offered at the stated price is the same as the quantity that buyers want to purchase at that price.

equity (1) Fairness. (2) Ownership; e.g., the share of a house that is owned by the homeowner free and clear of any mortgage obligations is the homeowner's equity in the house.

evaluative budgeting Approach to allocating resources based on the idea that each element of expenditure for each unit or department is explained and justified.

event Occurrence that is beyond the control of managers; often referred to as a state of nature.

exception report List of only those individual items, such as variances, that exceed a specified limit.

expected value Weighted average of possible outcomes, using known or subjective probabilities as weights.

expenditure Payment, often used interchangeably with expense.

expense centers *See* cost centers.

expenses Costs of services provided; expired cost.

expired cost *See* cost.

external accountant Accountant hired by an organization to perform an audit of the organization's financial records.

external costs Costs imposed on individuals and organizations resulting from the actions of an unrelated individual or organization. *See also* externality.

externality Secondary effect of an action by an individual or organization that presents additional costs or benefits to those affected.

F

factoring Selling the organization's accounts receivable, usually for less than their face value.

favorable variance Variance in which less was spent than the budgeted amount.

feedback Information about actual results given to avoid past mistakes and improve future plans.

fee-for-service System in which there is an additional charge for each additional service provided (as opposed to a prepaid system, in which all services are included in exchange for one flat payment).

fiduciary Relating to holding something in trust; a fiduciary is a trustee who maintains assets in trust.

FIFO *See* first-in, first-out.

financial accounting System that records historical financial information, summarizes it, and provides reports of what financial events have occurred and the financial impact of those events.

financial ratios Ratios developed using data from the organization's financial statements prepared for external users.

financial statements Reports that convey information about the organization's financial position and the results of its activities.

financing accounts receivable Borrowing money and using the organization's accounts receivable as security or collateral for a loan.

first-dollar coverage Insurance coverage that has no deductible or co-payment; the insurance company pays the "first dollar."

first-in, first-out (FIFO) Method of accounting for inventory that assumes we always use up the oldest inventory first.

first-line manager Person responsible for one patient care unit, area, or group of nursing staff.

fiscal Financial.

fiscal year One-year period defined for financial purposes. A fiscal year may start at any point during the calendar year and ends one year later; for example, fiscal year 2001 with a June 30 year end refers to the period from July 1, 2000, through June 30, 2001.

fixed assets Assets that will not be used up or converted to cash within one year; sometimes referred to as long-term assets.

fixed costs Costs that do not change in total as volume changes within the relevant range.

flexible budget Budget that is adjusted for volume of output.

flexible budget variance Difference between actual results and the flexible budget.

flexible budgeting Process of developing a budget based on different workload levels. Often used after the fact to calculate the amount that would have been budgeted for the actual workload levels attained. Depends heavily on the existence of variable costs.

float (1) Interim period from when a check is written until the check is cashed and clears the bank. (2) Movement of staff from one unit or department to another.

forecast Prediction of some future value such as patient days, chest tubes used, or nursing care hours per patient day.

forecasting Process of making forecasts.

forecast interval Range of values surrounding a forecast for which there is a specified probability that the actual result will fall within the range.

for-profit Organization whose mission includes earning a profit that may be distributed to its owners.

free enterprise *See* market economy.

fringe benefits *See* employee benefits.

FTE *See* full-time equivalent.

full cost Total of all costs associated with an organizational unit or activity; includes direct and indirect costs.

full-time equivalent (FTE) Equivalent of one full-time employee working for one year. This is generally calculated as forty hours per week for fifty-two weeks, or a total of 2,080 paid hours. This includes both productive and nonproductive (e.g., vacation, sick, holiday, education) time. Two employees each working half-time for one year are the same as one FTE.

fully integrated Hospital information system in which all the components are able to communicate with each other; health care provider offering full range of health care services.

fund accounting System of separate financial records and controls; assets of the organization are divided into distinct funds with separate bank accounts and a complete separate set of financial records.

fundamental equation of accounting Assets equal liabilities plus fund balance.

fund balance Owner's equity in a not-for-profit organization.

future value (FV) Amount a sum of money will grow to be worth at some point in the future.

G

GAAP *See* generally accepted accounting principles.

Gantt chart Depicts necessary activities or goals in a matrix format, with the horizontal axis indicating the time frame and the vertical axis the activities in the project.

general journal First place that financial transactions are entered into the accounting records; chronological listing of all financial transactions.

general operating fund Unrestricted fund used for the day-in and day-out operations of the organization.

generally accepted accounting principles (GAAP) Set of rules that must be followed for the organization's financial statements to be deemed a fair presentation of the organization's financial position and results of operations.

goal congruence Bringing together the goals, desires, and needs of the organization with those of its employees.

goal divergence Natural differences between the goals, desires, and needs of the organization and those of its employees.

going-concern principle Assumption that the numbers reported on a financial statement are those of an organization that will continue in business for the foreseeable future. If the organization is not a going concern, that must be noted on the financial statements or the accompanying notes.

goodwill Intangible asset that represents a measure of the value of the organization that goes beyond its specific physical assets.

gross patient revenues Charges for health care services provided. Note that most providers do not collect this gross amount because of discounts, bad debts, charity care, and other allowances to customers and third-party payers.

group-rated Price charged for insurance based on the experience of the group.

H

health insurance Insurance that pays part or all of the costs of specified health care services.

Health Care Financing Administration (HCFA) Federal agency that administers the Medicare program.

health maintenance organization (HMO) "An entity with four essential attributes: (1) an organized system providing health care in a geographic area, which accepts the responsibility to provide or otherwise assure the delivery of (2) an agreed-upon set of basic and supplemental health maintenance and treatment services to (3) a voluntarily enrolled group of persons, (4) for which services the entity is reimbursed through a predetermined fixed, periodic prepayment made by, or on behalf of, each person or family unit enrolled. The payment is fixed without regard to the amounts of actual services provided to an individual enrollee. Individual practice associations involving groups or independent physicians can be included under the definition."[8]

Health Plan Employer Data and Information Set (HEDIS) "A core set of comparable performance measures of managed care plans on quality, access, patient satisfaction, membership, utilization, finance, and descriptive information on health plan management and activities. HEDIS was developed by the National Committee for Quality Assurance (NCQA) to enable employers to compare the value of their health care dollar across a variety of health care plans."[9]

---

[8]Ibid.

[9]Ibid.

HEDIS *See* Health Plan Employer Data and Information Set.
hierarchy Structure that establishes the authority and responsibility of different individuals within an organization.
HMO *See* health maintenance organization.
hourly rate Allocation method that assigns costs to units of service based on the amount of time required to provide a treatment or procedure.
hours per patient day Paid hours divided by patient days.
HPPD *See* hours per patient day.
hurdle rate *See* required rate of return.

I

incentives Activities, rewards, or punishments that make it in the individual's interest to act in a desired manner.
income Excess of revenues over expenses for a specific period.
increasing returns to scale *See* economies of scale.
incremental budgeting Approach to resource allocation that simply adds an additional percentage or amount onto the prior year's budget allocation, without investigation of whether the continuation of the amounts authorized in the prior year's budget are warranted.
incremental costs Additional costs that will be incurred if a decision is made that would not otherwise be incurred by the organization.
indemnity Compensation for losses incurred, usually a dollar amount.
independent variable Variable used to predict the dependent variable.
indexing for inflation Adjustment of historical information for the impact of changes in price levels.
indirect costs (1) costs assigned to an organizational unit from elsewhere in the organization are indirect costs for the unit; (2) costs within a unit that are not incurred for direct patient care are indirect costs of patient care.
indirect expenses *See* indirect costs.
indirect method Method for measuring cash flows that starts with the operating revenues and expenses and reconciles to actual cash flows.
inputs Resources used for treating patients or otherwise producing output; examples include paid nursing hours, chest tubes, and IV solutions.
institutional cost report Document prepared by many health care organizations for submission, as required, to third-party payers such as Medicare, Medicaid, and Blue Cross.
intangible asset Asset without physical substance or form.
integrated services network (ISN) "A network of organizations, usually including hospitals and physician groups, that provides or arranges to provide a coordinated continuum of services to a defined population and is held both clinically and fiscally accountable for the outcomes of the populations served."[10]
interest coverage ratio Cash available to pay interest divided by interest; a measure of the organization's ability to meet its required interest payments.
internal accountant Accountant who works for an organization, recording financial information throughout the year.
internal control System of accounting checks and balances designed to minimize both clerical errors and the possibility of fraud or embezzlement; the process and systems that ensure that decisions made in the organization are appropriate and receive appropriate authorization. Requires a system of accounting and administrative controls.
internal rate of return (IRR) Discounted cash-flow technique that calculates the rate of return earned on a specific project or program.
inventory Materials and supplies held for use in providing services or making a product.
inventory carrying costs *See* carrying costs of inventory.

---

[10] Ibid.

inventory costing Process of determining the cost to be assigned to each unit of inventory, generally for financial statement purposes.
inventory management The appropriate ordering and storage of supplies.
inventory ordering costs *See* ordering costs.
inventory valuation Process of determining the cost of inventory used and the value of inventory assets.
investment centers A responsibility center that not only controls its revenues and expenses but the level of capital investment as well.
investments Stocks and bonds that the organization does not intend to sell within one year.
IRR *See* internal rate of return.

J

job-cost sheet Management document used to accumulate all of the materials and labor used for a specific job.
job-order costing Approach to product costing that directly associates the specific resources used for each job with that job.
joint costs Fixed costs required for the treatment of several types of patients; elimination of any one of those types of patients would have no effect on these costs.
journal entry Entry into the general journal or a subsidiary journal.
justification Explanation used in defending a proposed budget or in explaining variances that have occurred.
just-in-time (JIT) inventory Approach to inventory management that calls for the arrival of inventory just as it is needed, resulting in zero inventory levels.

L

last-in, first-out (LIFO) Inventory valuation method that accounts for inventory as if the most recent acquisitions are always used prior to inventory acquired at an earlier date and still on hand.
learning curve *See* learning curve effect.
learning curve effect Hypothesis that with each doubling of output, the cost per unit falls systematically.
lease Agreement providing for the use of an asset in exchange for rental payments.
ledger Accounting book for keeping track of increases, decreases, and the balance in each asset, liability, revenue, expense, and fund balance account.
length of stay (LOS) Number of days a patient is an inpatient; generally measured by the number of times the patient is an inpatient at midnight; *see also* average length of stay.
liabilities Legal financial obligations an organization has to outsiders; essentially, money the organization owes to someone.
LIFO *See* last-in, first-out.
line item Any resource that is listed as a separate line on a budget.
linearity Straight line relationship.
linear programming (LP) Technique to determine how best to allocate scarce resources, subject to constraints, to optimize a certain goal.
line function Element of running an organization that implies direct authority, in contrast with the staff function, which is consultative and without direct authority. Nursing is a line department.
line item Any resource listed separately on a budget; for example, all nursing labor for a unit may appear in aggregate (one line item), or head nurse costs may appear separately from RN costs and from LPN costs (resulting in three line items). Further subdivisions of nursing cost create additional line items.
line manager Manager of a line department or unit of the organization; *see also* line function.
lines of authority Formal lines of authority may be either direct (full authority), such as the associate director of nursing reporting to the chief nurse executive, or indirect (limited authority), such as the director of dietary reporting to the chief of the medical staff.

liquid assets Cash or other assets that can quickly be converted to cash to meet the short-term liabilities of the organization.
liquidate Convert into cash.
liquidity ratios Class of ratio that examines the ability of the organization to meet its obligations in the coming year.
lock box Post office box that is emptied directly by the bank. The bank removes the receipts and credits them directly to the organization's account.
long-range budget Plan that covers a period of time longer than one year, typically three, five, or ten years.
long-range planning Planning process that focuses on general objectives to be achieved by the organization over a period of typically three to five years; often referred to as strategic planning.
long run *See* long term.
long term Period longer than one year.
long-term assets *See* capital assets.
long-term investment *See* capital assets.
long-term liabilities Obligations that are not expected to be paid for more than one year.
LOS *See* length of stay.
lower of cost or market Marketable securities and investments are recorded on financial statements at their cost or the market value, whichever is lower. This treatment results from the principle of conservatism.

M

managed care "Systems that integrate the financing and delivery of health care services to covered individuals by means of arrangements with selected providers to furnish comprehensive services to members; explicit criteria for the selection of health-care providers; significant financial incentives for members to use providers and procedures associated with the planned and formal programs for quality assurance and utilization review."[11]
managed care organization (MCO) Insurance and provider organization that adheres to principles of managed care. *See also* managed care.
management by objectives (MBO) Technique in which a supervising manager and the subordinate manager agree upon a common set of objectives upon which performance will be measured.
management control system Complete set of policies and procedures designed to keep operations going according to plan.
management information system System designed to generate information for managers. This term is commonly used for computerized systems for generating information.
management letter Letter from the certified public accountant (CPA) to the management of the organization discussing weaknesses in the internal control system that were revealed as part of an audit.
management role Three of the most essential elements are planning, control, and decision making.
managerial accounting Generation of any financial information that can help managers to manage better.
managerial hierarchy Structure that establishes the authority and responsibility of various persons within the organization.
managerial reports Reports that provide information to help managers run the organization more efficiently.
margin At the edge; usually refers to the effects of adding one more patient.
marginal benefit *See* marginal utility.
marginal cost Additional amount that must be spent to acquire or produce one more unit.

---

[11]Ibid.

marginal cost analysis Process for making decisions about changes should be based on the marginal costs of the change rather than on the full or average costs.
marginal costs Change in cost related to a change in activity; includes variable costs and any additional fixed costs incurred because the volume change exceeds the relevant range for existing fixed costs.
marginal utility Additional benefit or utility gained from purchase of one more unit of a particular item.
market Potential customers for a product or organization.
marketable investments Investments that are bought and sold in financial markets, making them readily convertible to cash.
marketable securities Investments in stocks and bonds that the organization intends to sell within one year.
marketing Management science that attempts to maintain and increase the organization's sales volume.
market economy System in which individuals can choose whether to invest their wealth or capital in a business venture, workers can choose whether to work for that venture at the wages offered, and consumers can choose whether to buy the products of the venture at the seller's price.
market failure Situations in which the free market does not operate efficiently.
market management Approach to product-line management that focuses mainly on creating an increased external market.
market measurement Conversion of qualitative information into quantitative estimates of demand.
market segmentation Division of the market into specific subsections.
market share Portion or percentage of the overall market that a specific organization controls. If half of all patients with broken legs come to your ER, you have a 50% share of the broken leg market.
market size variance Variance caused by the existence of a greater or smaller number of patients in the community than was expected.
markup Certain percentage added to the cost of a product or service to establish its selling price.
master budget Set of all of the major budgets of an organization; generally includes the operating budget, long-range budget, program budgets, capital budget, and cash budget.
material Amount of money substantial enough that an error of that magnitude in the financial statements would cause a user of the statements to make a different decision than would be made if the user had known the correct information.
matrix distribution *See* algebraic distribution.
matrix management System in which a manager has responsibility that cuts across department lines.
MBO *See* management by objectives.
MCO *See* managed care organization.
Medicaid (Title XIX) "A Federally aided, State-operated and administered program which provides medical benefits for certain indigent or low-income persons in need of health and medical care. The program, authorized by Title XIX of the Social Security Act, is basically for the poor. It does not cover all of the poor, however, but only persons who meet specified eligibility criteria. Subject to broad Federal guidelines, States determine the benefits covered, program eligibility, rates of payment for providers, and methods of administering the program."[12]
Medicare Federal program under the Social Security Administration that pays for medical care for the aged and permanently disabled.
Medicare cost report Institutional cost report prepared for Medicare.

[12]Ibid.

Medicare loss ratio Amount of the health care premium that is spent on medical care, as opposed to health plan administration and profits.

Medicare risk contract Contract between the Medicare program and an HMO to provide all medically necessary benefits to any Medicare beneficiary who is enrolled in the plan in exchange for a monthly capitated payment.

microcosting Process of closely examining the actual resources consumed by a particular patient or service. Microcosting tends to be extremely costly and is generally done only for special studies.

midlevel nurse manager Person responsible for nursing functions on more than one nursing unit or area.

mission Set of primary goals that justify an organization's existence, such as providing high-quality hospital care to the surrounding community or providing research and education.

mission statement Statement of the purpose or reason for existence of an organization, department, or unit. Provides direction regarding the types of activities that the organization should undertake.

mixed costs Costs that contain an element of fixed costs and an element of variable costs, such as electricity. A unit or department budget as a whole represents a mixed cost.

monitoring and control ratios Cost accounting ratios that can be used to generate information to aid managers in monitoring and controlling various aspects of the organization's operations.

monopoly Sole seller, who therefore has the power to set prices at a higher-than-equilibrium level.

monopsony Market in which there is only one buyer.

moral hazard Fact that people behave differently if they are insured than if they are not. Patients are more likely to consume more health care services if they have health insurance.

mortgage payable Loan that is secured by a specific asset.

moving average Method of averaging out the roughness caused by random variation in a historical series of data points.

multiple distribution The double distribution and the algebraic or matrix distribution approaches to cost allocation.

multiple regression analysis Form of regression analysis that uses more than one independent, or causal, variable. This can result in a better result than using only one variable.

multiplication rule Likelihood of two or more events' occurring simultaneously or in sequence is the product of probability of each event.

N

near term *See* current assets.

negotiative budgeting Approach to resource allocation in which the amount allocated to a unit or department is based on a process of negotiation.

net cash flow Net difference between cash receipts and cash payments.

net income Revenue less expense; profit.

net patient revenues Gross revenues less contractual allowances, bad debts, and charity care.

net present cost Aggregate present value of a series of payments to be made in the future.

net present value (NPV) Present value of a series of receipts less the present value of a series of payments.

network cost budgeting Combines the techniques of network analysis with cost accounting to generate the most cost-effective approach to carrying out a project.

net working capital Current assets less current liabilities.

nominal group technique Forecasting technique in which a group of individuals is brought together in a structured meeting and arrives at a group consensus forecast.

noncontrollable Item a manager does not have the authority or ability to control.

nonoperating revenue Categorization that no longer appears on the statement of revenues and expenses. All revenues are operating, unless they are incidental and peripheral to the organization, in which case they are shown as gains.

nonproductive time Sick, vacation, holiday, and other paid nonworked time.

nonrevenue cost center Cost center that does not charge directly for its services; its costs must be allocated to a revenue center to be included in the organization's rates.

nonroutine decisions Management decisions that are not made on a routine, regularly scheduled basis.

normality Element of specification analysis that requires that there be a normal distribution of historical points around the regression line.

not-for-profit Organization whose mission does not include earning a profit for distribution to owners. A not-for-profit organization may earn a profit, but such profit must be reinvested for replacement of facilities and equipment or for expansion of services offered.

note payable Written document representing a loan.

NPV *See* net present value.

NRG *See* nursing resource grouping.

nurse executive Senior nurse responsible for managing the nursing services of an entire organization; *see also* chief nurse executive.

nurse manager Person responsible for organizational unit, program, or department.

nursing resource grouping (NRG) Classification of patients into homogeneous groups based on nursing care consumed. Any patient in an NRG consumes a set of nursing resources similar to those of any other patient in that NRG.

O

objective function Equation that states the relationship between the objective in a linear programming problem and the other variables in the process. The objective is the item, the value of which we wish to optimize.

objectives Specific targets to be achieved to attain goals.

one-shot Budget that is prepared only once rather than on a regular basis (e.g., monthly or annually).

operating Related to the normal routine activities of the organization in providing its goods or services.

operating budget Plan for the day-in and day-out operating revenues and expenses of the organization. It is generally prepared for one year.

operating expenses Costs of the organization related to its general operations.

operating margin Operating income (revenues less expenses, before other gains or losses) divided by revenue; a profitability measure.

operating revenues Revenues earned in the normal course of providing the organization's goods or services.

operations Routine activities of the organization related to its mission and the provision of goods or services.

opinion letter Letter from the CPA to users of the organization's audited financial statements providing expert opinion as to whether the financial statements are a fair presentation of the financial position and results of operations of the organization, in accordance with generally accepted accounting principles.

opportunity cost A measure of cost based on the value of the alternatives that are given up in order to use the resource as the organization has chosen.

opportunity costs of inventory Carrying costs or costs of having money tied up in inventory rather than in a revenue-producing endeavor such as an interest-bearing bank account.

ordering costs Costs associated with an order of inventory (e.g., clerk time for preparation of a purchase order).

OTPS Other than personnel services.

outcome Result; can be affected by management actions, in contrast to events, which are defined as occurrences beyond the control of managers.

outputs Product or service being produced (e.g., patients, patient days, visits, operations).

overapplied or underapplied overhead Amount that the actual overhead costs differ from the amount of overhead applied to units of service.

overhead Indirect costs. Often cannot be easily associated with individual patients, even by a job-order type of detailed observation and measurement. Overhead costs therefore require some form of aggregation and then allocation to units, departments, and ultimately patients or other units of service.

overhead application Process of charging overhead costs to units of service based on a standard overhead application rate.

overhead application rate Amount charged per unit of service for overhead; calculated using a cost base.

overhead costs *See* overhead.

owner's equity Residual value after the liabilities of an organization are subtracted from the assets. Represents the portion of the assets owned by the organization itself or its owners.

P

partial productivity A portion of the total productivity; total outputs divided by some subpart of total inputs.

partnership Business owned by a group of persons (partners) who have unlimited liability; partners may be sued for all liabilities of the firm. *See also* corporation.

pass-through costs *See* cost pass-through.

patient care variance Extent to which paid, worked, productive time is actually consumed in the process of direct patient care as opposed to other activities.

patient classification System for distinguishing among different patients based on their acuity, functional ability, or resource needs.

patient day One patient occupying one bed for one day.

patient mix *See* case mix.

patient mix variance Variance from the organization's expected patient case mix.

patient revenue per day Total patient revenue divided by the number of days in the year.

patient revenues *See* gross patient revenues and net patient revenues.

payback Capital budgeting approach that calculates how many years it takes for a project's cash inflows to equal or exceed its cash outflows.

payer Individual or organization that provides money to pay for health care.

per diem Daily charge. Refers to (1) the charge per day for routine care and (2) agency nurses who work day to day.

per diem method Approach used to allocate department costs to units of service if the surcharge, hourly rate, and relative value unit methods do not reasonably apply.

performance budget Plan that relates the various objectives of a cost center with the planned costs of accomplishing those activities.

period costs Costs that are treated as expense in the accounting period that they are incurred, regardless of when the organization's goods or services are sold.

periodic inventory *See* perpetual *vs* periodic inventory.

perpetual *vs* periodic inventory Under the perpetual inventory method, the organization keeps a record of each inventory acquisition and sale, so it always knows how much has been sold and how much is supposed to be in inventory; under the periodic method, the organization records only purchases and uses a count of inventory to determine how much has been sold and how much is on hand.

personnel Persons employed by an organization.

PERT *See* program evaluation and review technique.

PHO *See* physician-hospital organization.

physician-hospital organization (PHO) "A legal entity formed by a hospital and a group of physicians to further mutual interests and to achieve market objectives. A PHO generally combines physicians and a hospital into a single organization for the purpose of obtaining payer contracts. Doctors maintain ownership of their practices and agree to accept managed care patients according to the terms of a professional services agreement with the PHO. The PHO serves as a collective negotiating and contracting unit. It is typically owned and governed jointly by a hospital and shareholder physicians."[13]

---

[13]Ibid.

planning Deciding upon goals and objectives, considering alternative options for achieving those goals and objectives, and selecting a course of action from the range of possible alternatives.

plant Building.

plant-age ratio Accumulated depreciation of buildings and equipment divided by annual depreciation expense; an approximation for the average age of physical facilities.

posting Process of transferring all parts of a journal entry to the specific ledger accounts that are affected by the entry.

PPO *See* preferred provider organization.

PPS *See* prospective payment system.

preferred provider organization (PPO) "Formally organized entity generally consisting of hospital and physician providers. The PPO provides health care services to purchasers usually at discounted rates in return for expedited claims payment and a somewhat predictable market share. In this model, consumers have a choice of using PPO or non-PPO providers; however, financial incentives are built in to benefit structures to encourage utilization of PPO providers."[14]

premium Payment to an insurance company for coverage for a set period.

prepaid assets Assets that have been paid for and not yet used but that will be used within one year. This includes items such as fire insurance premiums or rent paid in advance.

prepaid group plan *See* health maintenance organization.

present cost *See* net present cost.

present value Value of future receipts or payments discounted to the present.

preventive controls *See* accounting controls.

price variance Portion of the total variance for any line item that is caused by spending a different amount per unit of resource than had been anticipated (e.g., higher or lower salary rates, higher or lower supply prices).

principal The amount of money borrowed.

private insurers Insurance companies that are not part of the government.

probabilistic estimate Estimate based on a manager's subjective estimate of what is most likely to occur.

probability Likelihood of an event's occurring. The probability of future events can be estimated based on data from historical events.

process costing Approach to product costing based on broad averages of costs over a large volume of units of service.

product costing Determination of the cost per unit of service. Job-order costing measures separately the cost of producing each job, whereas process costing is based on costs averaged across a large number of units of service. An individual patient or group of patients of a similar type may be considered a job.

product costs Costs that are treated as part of the product and that do not become expenses until the product is sold.

production function Financial implications of making and distributing a product.

product line Group of patients who have some commonality (e.g., a common diagnosis) that allows them to be grouped together.

product-line costing "Determination of the cost of providing care to specific types of patients. This approach is sometimes aided by the use of standard cost techniques, such as Cleverley's model of standard treatment protocols."[15]

productive time Straight time and overtime worked.

productive *vs* nonproductive variance Variance caused by an unexpected amount of nonproductive hours.

productivity Ratio of any given measure of output to any given measure of input over a specified period.

---

[14]Ibid.

[15]Cleverley, William O., "Product Costing for Health Care Firms," *Health Care Management Review*, Vol. 12, No. 4, fall 1987.

productivity measurement Measurement of productivity.

profit Amount by which an organization's revenues exceed its expenses.

profitability analysis Analysis of the profits related to a specific program, project, or service under existing conditions or under a specific set of assumptions.

profitability ratio Class of ratios that evaluates the profitability of the organization.

profit center Responsibility unit that is responsible for both revenues and expenses. Health care organizations have referred to profit centers as revenue centers, emphasizing that a specific charge for such centers will appear on patient bills.

profit margin Excess of revenue over expense divided by total revenue; an indication of the amount of profits generated by each dollar of revenue.

profit sharing plan Incentive arrangement under which executives receive a portion of an organization's profits that exceed a certain threshold.

pro forma financial statements Financial statements that predict what the financial statements for a project, program, or organization will look like at some point in the future.

program (1) Sequence of instructions for a computer to do a task; (2) project or service that cuts across departments.

program budget Plan that looks at all aspects of a program across departments and over the long term.

program evaluation and review technique (PERT) Multibranch programming technique designed to predict total project completion time for large-scale projects and to identify paths that have available slack.

programming (1) Process of deciding what major programs the organization will commence in the future; (2) development of computer software instructions.

property, plant, and equipment Land, buildings, and pieces of equipment owned by an organization.

proprietary *See* for-profit.

proprietorship Business owned by one individual.

prospective payment Payment based on a predetermined price for any particular category of patient (e.g., a particular DRG) as opposed to reimbursement based on the costs of care provided to the patient.

prospective payment system (PPS) Approach to paying for health care services based on predetermined prices.

provider Health care worker or health care organization that dispenses health care to people.

Q

quality costs Costs incurred to ensure that a product is of the required quality. May include costs such as inspection or replacement or harm to the patient created by using a product of inferior quality.

quality driver Factor that is critical to the level of quality of a product or service.

quantity variance Portion of the total variance for any line item that is caused by using more input per unit of output (e.g., patient day) than had been budgeted.

quick ratio Cash plus marketable securities plus accounts receivable, all divided by current liabilities.

R

r^2 (R squared) Regression analysis statistic that can range from a low of zero to a high of 1.0. The closer it is to 1.0, the more of the variability in the dependent variable has been explained by the independent variable(s).

rate setting Process of assigning prices to the units of service of the revenue centers. Prices must be set high enough to recover the organization's total financial requirements.

rate variance Price variance that relates to labor resources. In such cases it is typically the hourly rate that has varied from expectations. *See also* price variance.

ratio One number divided by another.

ratio analysis Widely used managerial tool that compares one number with another to gain insights that would not arise from looking at either of the numbers separately.

ratio of cost to charges (RCC) Method used to convert a patient's bill to the patient's costs by applying the ratio of the organization's costs to its charges.

RCC *See* ratio of cost to charges.

reciprocal distribution *See* algebraic distribution.

recruitment Effort directed at getting potential employees to become employees.

regression analysis Statistical model that measures the average change in a dependent variable associated with a one-unit change in one or more independent variables.

regulation Government rule that has the force of law.

relative value unit (RVU) scale Arbitrary unit scale in which each patient is assigned a number of relative value units based on the relative costs of different types of patients. For example, if nursing care costs twice as much for type A patients as for type B patients, then type A patients will be assigned a number of relative value units twice as high as that assigned to type B patients.

relevant costs Only those costs that are subject to change as a result of a decision.

relevant range Range of activity that might reasonably be expected to occur in the budget period; range of activity within which fixed costs do not vary.

repurchase agreement Flexible bank-related financial investment instrument. Can be for periods as short as one day.

required rate of return Interest rate that must be achieved for a capital project to be considered financially worthwhile; also called hurdle rate.

residual Portion left over; when liabilities are subtracted from assets, the leftover or residual value is the fund balance or owner's equity.

residual income (RI) Profits from a project in excess of the amount necessary to provide a desired minimum rate of return.

responsibility accounting Attempt to measure financial outcomes and assign those outcomes to the individual or department responsible for them.

responsibility center Part of the organization, such as a department or a unit, for which a manager is assigned responsibility. Health care organizations generally have cost centers and revenue centers.

restricted funds Funds whose assets are limited as to their use. If the restriction is placed by the donor, it can be removed only by the donor; however, if the assets are restricted by the board, the restriction may be removed by the board.

retention Continued employment; often measured as the converse of turnover or staff leaving an organization.

retrospective patient classification Categorization of patients into a patient classification based on the nursing care needs that were met.

return on assets (ROA) Profit divided by total assets; a measure of the amount of profit earned for each dollar invested in the organization's assets.

return on investment (ROI) Ratio that divides the amount of profit by the amount of investment. Just as an individual would measure the success of a personal investment, so an organization would use ROI to measure the yield received relative to an amount of money invested.

revenue Amounts of money an organization has received or is entitled to receive in exchange for goods or services provided.

revenue center Unit or department that is responsible and accountable not only for costs of providing services but also for the revenues generated by those services.

revenue variances Assessment of how much of the variance between expected and actual revenues results from changes in the total health care organization demand in a given geographic region, a health care organization's share of that total demand, its mix of patients, and the prices for each class of patient.

RI *See* residual income.

risk sharing "The distribution of financial risk among parties furnishing a service. For example, if a hospital and a group of physicians from a corporation provide health care at a fixed price, a risk-sharing arrangement would entail both the hospital and the physician group being held liable if expenses exceed revenues."[16]

---

[16]Ibid.

ROA *See* return on assets.
ROI *See* return on investment.
rolling budget System in which a budget is prepared each month for a month one year in the future. For example, once the actual results for this January are known, a budget for January of next year is prepared.
RVU *See* relative value unit scale.

S

safety stock Minimum inventory that an organization attempts always to maintain on hand; would be dipped into only when an event arises that would, in the absence of a safety stock, have resulted in a stockout.
seasonality Predictable pattern of monthly, quarterly, or other periodic variation in historical data within each year.
seasonalization Adjustment of the annual budget for month-to-month seasonality.
segment *See* market segmentation.
segmentation *See* market segmentation.
self-pay patients Patients who are responsible for payment of their own health care bills because they do not have private insurance and are not covered by either Medicare or Medicaid.
semi-fixed cost *See* step-fixed.
semi-variable cost *See* mixed cost.
sensitivity analysis Process whereby financial results are recalculated under a series of varying assumptions and predictions. This is often referred to as "what if" analysis.
service unit (SU) Basic measure of an item being produced by an organization (e.g., patient days, home care visits, hours of operations).
short run *See* short term.
short term Period of time shorter than the long term; *see also* long-term.
short-term assets *See* current assets.
simple linear regression Regression analysis that uses one dependent and one independent variable and produces predictions along a straight line.
simulation Mathematical approach that processes a number of different estimates a large number of times and projects the likelihood of various aggregate outcomes.
sinking fund Segregated assets to be used for replacement of plant and equipment.
skimming Charging a high price knowing that market share will be low but planning to make a high profit on the volume achieved.
slack time Waiting time between activities in a network analysis.
social costs *See* external costs.
solvency Ability to meet current and future obligations.
solvency ratios Class of ratios that evaluate the organization's ability to meet its obligations as they come due over a time frame longer than one year.
special purpose budget Any plan that does not fall into one of the other specific categories of budgets.
special purpose funds Assets restricted to a particular purpose (e.g., government grant research projects, student loans, establishment of a new burn care unit).
specific identification Inventory valuation method that identifies each unit of inventory and tracks which specific units are on hand and which have been sold.
spending variance Equivalent of the price or rate variance for fixed and variable overhead costs.
spreadsheet Large ledger sheet often used by accountants for financial calculations. Spreadsheets are often computerized now and are prepared using programs such as Excel or LOTUS 1-2-3.
staff function Provision of auxiliary assistance or service to the line managers and their departments. Finance is a staff function. Units designated to provide staff functions do not provide direct patient care.

staff manager Manager with no direct line responsibility for running the organization. Most nurse managers are line managers; the director of nursing education and the director of nursing recruitment are examples of staff positions.

standard cost Expectation of what it should cost to produce a good or service, usually on a per unit basis. They are targets, often established based on industrial engineering studies.

standard cost profile Costs, fixed and variable, direct and indirect, of producing each service unit (SU); *see also* standard treatment protocol.

standard treatment protocol Set of intermediate products or service units (SUs) consumed by a patient in each product line.

statement of financial position Financial report that indicates the financial position of an organization at a specific point in time; often referred to as the balance sheet.

state of nature *See* event.

step-down Method of cost allocation in which nonrevenue centers allocate their costs to all cost centers, both revenue and nonrevenue, that have not yet been allocated. Once a nonrevenue center allocates its costs, no costs can be allocated to it.

step-fixed Cost that is fixed over short ranges of volume but varies within the relevant range; sometimes referred to as step-variable.

step-variable *See* step-fixed.

stock option plan *See* stock plan.

stockout costs Costs incurred when supply is needed but not available. If the supply is needed for patient care, it often must be purchased at a higher price from a local vendor.

stock plan Bonus arrangement that provides shares of stock as part of an executive incentive system.

stop-loss coverage "Insurance coverage purchased by a health plan from an insurance company to reimburse the plan for the cost of benefits paid out to an individual or account that has exceeded what the plan expected to pay out. It stops the insurance company's loss. It is also known as reinsurance or risk-control insurance."[17]

strategic budget *See* long-range budget.

strategic business unit Approach to product-line management in which managers look not only at marketing but also at allocation of resources and profitability.

strategic management Process of setting the goals and objectives of an organization, determining the resources to be allocated to achieving those goals and objectives, and establishing policies concerning getting and using those resources.

strategic planning Process of setting long-term goals and designing a plan to achieve those goals; often referred to as long-term planning.

strategies Broad plans for the attainment of goals. Marketing strategies define the overall desired approach to marketing products and services.

SU *See* service unit.

subcategory Device to allow separation of the flexible budget variance into the price variance and the quantity variance. The actual quantity of input per unit of output, multiplied by the budgeted price of the input, times the actual output level.

subjective probability Relies not only on the scientific application of the laws of chance but also on the judgment of the manager.

subsidiary journal Detailed journals in which original entries are first made, with only a summary total entry being made to the general journal. For example, a sales journal would list each patient bill, with only a summary of total of revenue recorded in the general journal.

subsidiary ledger Ledgers in which detailed information is recorded, with only a summary being posted to the general ledger. For example, a subsidiary accounts receivable ledger would keep track of each patient's receivable separately, and the general ledger would show only the total increase or decrease in receivables.

---

[17]Ibid.

substitute Economic good that can be used as an alternative to another economic good.
sunk costs Costs that already have been incurred and will not be affected by future actions.
supply Amount of a good or service that all suppliers in aggregate would like to provide for any given price.
supply curve Quantity that would be offered by suppliers at any given price.
support cost center Cost center that is not a revenue center.
surcharge method Approach to cost allocation in which a revenue center compares its costs excluding inventory with the inventory cost and determines a proportional surcharge.
surplus *See* profit.

T

tactics Specific activities undertaken to carry out a strategy.
taxes payable Taxes owed to local, state, or federal government.
template Customized computer program application that gives a framework to which managers can add variables to perform computerized analysis.
third-party payer "Any organization, public or private, that pays or insures health or medical expenses on behalf of beneficiaries or recipients. An individual pays a premium for such coverage in all private and in some public programs; the payer organization then pays bills on the individual's behalf. Such payments are called third-party payments and are distinguished by the separation among the individual receiving the service (the first party), the individual or institution providing it (the second party), and the organization paying for it (third party)."[18]
time and motion studies Industrial engineering observations of the specific time and resources consumed for some activity.
time-series analysis Use of historical values of a variable to predict future values for that variable without the use of any other variable other than the passage of time.
time value of money Recognition that money can earn compound interest, and therefore a given amount of money paid at different points in time has a different value; the further into the future an amount is paid, the less valuable it is.
Title XIX (Medicaid) "The title of the Social Security Act which contains the principal legislative authority for the Medicaid program and therefore a common name for the program."[19]
total costs Sum of all costs related to a cost objective.
total debt-equity ratio Total liabilities divided by fund balance. The higher this ratio, the less borrowing capacity the organization has left.
total financial requirements (TFR) Financial resources needed to provide for the present and future health care needs of the population served by the organization.
total productivity Ratio of total outputs to total inputs; amount of output per unit of input.
total quality management (TQM) A philosophy that prevention of defects is cheaper than cure; TQM focuses on doing things right initially and avoiding having to do them a second time.
total variance Sum of the price, quantity, and volume variances; the difference between the actual results and the original budgeted amount.
TQM *See* total quality management.
trade credit Accounts payable; generally no interest is charged for a period of time, such as one month.
transfer prices Amounts charged to one responsibility center for goods or services acquired from another responsibility center in the same organization.
trend Patterns related to the passage of time. For example, although there are daily fluctuations in the census, the pattern of the census is relatively stable.
true costs Actual resources consumed. Measurement of unique true costs is rarely possible:

---

[18] Ibid.
[19] Ibid.

no matter how accurate accounting information is, there always will be different assessments of cost in different situations. Even beyond this, however, true costs do not exist because accounting can never do more than approximate economic cost.

turnover Employees who leave employment in an organization.

U

uncontrollable *See* noncontrollable.

unfavorable variance Variance in which more is spent than the budgeted amount.

uniform reporting Approach to have health care organizations improve comparability of financial information from organization to organization by completing uniform accounting reports.

unit of service *See* service unit.

unrestricted funds Funds whose assets may be used for any normal purpose; usually only the general operating fund is unrestricted.

unsecured note Loan secured without collateral.

use variance Another name for quantity variance; so called because the quantity variance focuses on how much of a resource has been used; see also quantity variance.

utility Physical or psychic benefit one receives from goods or services.

V

value-added Costs that directly affect the quality of patient care. Many TQM initiatives focus on identifying value-added costs as opposed to non-value-added costs.

variable billing System in which the amount billed to each patient for nursing care per patient day varies based on the differing resource consumption of different patients.

variable costs Costs that vary in direct proportion with volume.

variance Difference between budget and actual results.

variance analysis Comparison of actual results as compared with the budget, followed by investigation to determine why variances occurred.

vendor Supplier, such as a pharmaceutical company or hospital supply company.

volume variance Amount of variance in any line item that is caused simply because the workload level changed.

W

wages payable Amounts owed to employees.

wealth Value of all resources a consumer currently owns.

weighted average method Inventory valuation method that accounts for inventory as if the inventory gets mixed together and each unit is unidentifiable.

weighted procedure method Approach to allocating a cost center's costs to units of service based upon a special study that establishes the relative costliness of each type of service the center performs.

Winters' forecasting method Statistical forecasting method that predicts seasonal patterns particularly well.

working capital Current assets and current liabilities of an organization.

working capital management Management of current assets and current liabilities of an organization.

working capital method Method for measuring cash flows that focuses on working capital.

workload Volume of work for a unit or department. There should be a direct relationship between the workload and the amount of resources needed; therefore a workload measure such as patient days is inferior to one such as patient days adjusted for average patient acuity.

work measurement Technique that evaluates what a group of workers is doing and attempts to assess the number of workers needed to accomplish the tasks efficiently.

work sampling Approach to determining time and resources used for an activity based on observations at intervals of time rather than continuous observation.

Y

year-to-date Sum of the budget or of actual values for all months from the beginning of the year through the most recent period for which data are available, or of both.

Z

ZBB *See* zero-base budgeting.

zero balance accounts System in which separate accounts are maintained at a bank for each major source of cash receipt and for major types of payments; at the close of each day, the bank, using computer technology, automatically transfers all balances, positive or negative, into one master concentration account. Any borrowing or investing of cash can then be done against that one account.

zero-base budgeting (ZBB) Program budgeting approach that requires an examination and justification of all costs rather than just the incremental costs and that requires examination of alternatives rather than just one approach.

Index

Note: Page numbers in *italics* refer to illustrations; page numbers followed by a t refer to tables.

C

D

E

P

Q

R

S

ISBN 0-7216-7714-2